Evaluation of Herbal Medicinal Products

Evaluation of Herbal Medicinal Products

Perspectives on quality, safety and efficacy

Edited by
Pulok K Mukherjee
Director, School of Natural Product Studies, Jadavpur University, Kolkata, India

Peter J Houghton
Emeritus Professor in Pharmacognosy, Pharmaceutical Sciences Division, King's College London, London, UK

ondon • Chicago

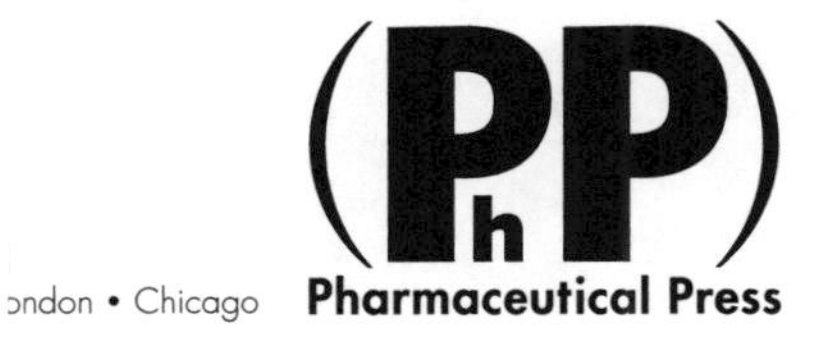

Published by the Pharmaceutical Press
An imprint of RPS Publishing

1 Lambeth High Street, London SE1 7JN, UK
100 South Atkinson Road, Suite 200, Grayslake, IL 60030-7820, USA

(PP) is a trade mark of RPS Publishing
RPS Publishing is the publishing organisation of the Royal Pharmaceutical Society of Great Britain

First published 2009

Typeset by J&L Composition, Scarborough, North Yorkshire
Printed in Great Britain by Cromwell Press Group, Trowbridge

ISBN 978 0 85369 751 0

A catalogue record for this book is available from the British Library

Contents

Preface

It would be impossible in one book to cover every possible aspect of the evaluation of herbal medicinal products. Apart from the large number of plant species used throughout the world for medicinal purposes, there are many disease states, geographical regions and cultural considerations.

Consequently, some will be disappointed that a topic has not been included, which they think important, while others will think that a particular geographical area, disease state or analytical method has been overemphasised or neglected!

We make no pretence of claiming that this volume is comprehensive, and recognise that there are many interesting and exciting developments in analytical approaches and biological studies which are barely mentioned.

However, we hope that this collection of articles gives a sufficient overview of approaches to the evaluation of herbal medicinal products to enable others to produce similar articles to make the picture more complete.

Our aim is to improve the level of understanding of the various avenues that are needed to provide a fully rounded evaluation of these materials, so that they can be used with greater confidence, because of improved quality and an increasing scientifically sound evidence base.

Pulok K Mukherjee
Peter J Houghton

Contributors

Bolanle A Adeniyi

Departments of Pharmacy Practice, and Medicinal Chemistry and Pharmacognosy, UIC PAHO/WHO Collaborating Center for Traditional Medicine, University of Illinois at Chicago, College of Pharmacy, 833 South Wood Street, Chicago, IL 60612, USA

O P Agarwal

Indian Council of Medical Research, Ansari Nagar, New Delhi 110 029, India

K F H Nazeer Ahmed

School of Natural Product Studies, Department of Pharmaceutical Technology, Jadavpur University, Kolkata 700 032, India

Stanley O Aniagu

Molecular Pathobiology Group, School of Biosciences, University of Birmingham, Birmingham, UK

Rudolf Bauer

Institute of Pharmaceutical Sciences, Department of Pharmacognosy, Universitätsplatz 4/1, 8010 Graz, Austria

Ezra Bejar

Herbalife International, Century City, CA 90067, USA

Albert J J van den Berg

Section Medicinal Chemistry and Chemical Biology, Department of Pharmaceutical Sciences, Faculty of Sciences, Utrecht University, Utrecht, The Netherlands and b PhytoGeniX BV, Utrecht, The Netherlands

Cees J Beukelman

Section Medicinal Chemistry and Chemical Biology, Department of Pharmaceutical Sciences, Faculty of Sciences, Utrecht University, Utrecht, The Netherlands and b PhytoGeniX BV, Utrecht, The Netherlands

Sujit K Bhattacharya

ICMR Virus Unit, I D & B G Hospital Campus, Beliaghata, Kolkata 700 010, India

Tuhin Kanti Biswas

J B Roy State Ayurvedic Medical College and Hospital, 170–172, Raja Dinendra Street, Kolkata 700 004, India

Shrabana Chakrabarti

S N Pradhan Centre for Neurosciences, University of Calcutta, 244B Acharya J C Bose Road, Kolkata 700 020, India

Sekhar Chakraborty

ICMR Virus Unit, I D & B G Hospital Campus, Beliaghata, Kolkata 700 010, India

Debprasad Chattopadhyay

ICMR Virus Unit, I D & B G Hospital Campus, Beliaghata, Kolkata 700 010, India

Raymond Cooper

PhytoScience Inc, PO Box 1935, Los Altos CA 94023, USA

Larry H Danziger

Departments of Pharmacy Practice, and Medicinal Chemistry and Pharmacognosy, UIC PAHO/WHO Collaborating Center for Traditional Medicine, University of Illinois at Chicago, College of Pharmacy, 833 South Wood Street, Chicago, IL 60612, USA

Cynthia L Darlington

Department of Pharmacology and Toxicology, School of Medical Sciences, University of Otago Medical School, Dunedin, New Zealand

Sonali Das

ICMR Virus Unit, I D & B G Hospital Campus, Beliaghata, Kolkata 700 010, India

Rajendra M Dobriyal

Herbal Research Labs, Hindustan Unilever Research Center, 64 Main Road, Whitefield, Bangalore 560 066, India

Brian J Doyle

Departments of Pharmacy Practice, and Medicinal Chemistry and Pharmacognosy, UIC PAHO/WHO Collaborating Center for Traditional Medicine, University of Illinois at Chicago, College of Pharmacy, 833 South Wood Street, Chicago, IL 60612, USA

Cristobal Fraga

Department of Physiology, University of Santiago de Compostela, Spain

A Gantait

School of Natural Product Studies, Department of Pharmaceutical Technology, Jadavpur University, Kolkata 700 032, India

Anwarul Hassan Gilani

Natural Product Research Division, Department of Biological and Biomedical Sciences, Aga Khan University, Karachi 74800, Pakistan

R Govindarajan

National Botanical Research Institute, Rana Pratap Marg, Lucknow 226 001, India

Wandee Gritsanapan

Department of Pharmacognosy, Faculty of Pharmacy, Mahidol University, 447 Sri-Ayuthaya Road, Ratchatevi, Bangkok 10400, Thailand

S Bart A Halkes

Section Medicinal Chemistry and Chemical Biology, Department of Pharmaceutical Sciences, Faculty of Sciences, Utrecht University, Utrecht, The Netherlands and b PhytoGeniX BV, Utrecht, The Netherlands

K B Harikumar

Amala Cancer Research Centre, Thrissur 680 555, Kerala, India

P J Houghton

Department of Pharmacy, King's College London, Franklin Wilkins Building, 150 Stamford Street, London SE1 9NH, UK

Tianan Jiang

Life Extension Inc, 1100 West Commercial Boulevard, Fort Lauderdale, FL 33309, USA

Ki Sung Kang

Institute of Natural Medicine, University of Toyama, 2630 Sugitani, Toyama, 930-0194, Japan

David O Kennedy

Brain, Performance and Nutrition Research Centre, Northumbria University, Newcastle upon Tyne NE1 8ST, UK

Arif-ullah Khan

Natural Product Research Division, Department of Biological and Biomedical Sciences, Aga Khan University, Karachi 74800, Pakistan

Burt H Kroes

Medicinal Chemistry and Chemical Biology Section, Department of Pharmaceutical Sciences, Faculty of Sciences, Utrecht University, Utrecht, The Netherlands

N Satheesh Kumar

School of Natural Product Studies, Department of Pharmaceutical Technology, Jadavpur University, Kolkata 700 032, India

V Kumar

School of Natural Product Studies, Department of Pharmaceutical Technology, Jadavpur University, Kolkata 700 032, India

Ramadasan Kuttan

Amala Cancer Research Centre, Thrissur 680 555, Kerala, India

Talash Anne Likimani

Herbalife International, Century City, CA 90067, USA

Chang-Xiao Liu

Tianjin Institute of Pharmaceutical Research, Tianjin 300193, China

Tracie Locklear

Departments of Pharmacy Practice, and Medicinal Chemistry and Pharmacognosy, UIC PAHO/WHO Collaborating Center for Traditional Medicine, University of Illinois at Chicago, College of Pharmacy, 833 South Wood Street, Chicago, IL 60612, USA

Gail B Mahady

Departments of Pharmacy Practice, and Medicinal Chemistry and Pharmacognosy, UIC PAHO/WHO Collaborating Center for Traditional Medicine, University of Illinois at Chicago, College of Pharmacy, 833 South Wood Street, Chicago, IL 60612, USA

Mohua Maulik

Indian Council of Medical Research, New Delhi, India

Subir Kumar Maulik

Department of Pharmacology, All India Institute of Medical Sciences, New Delhi, India

Royce Mohan

Departments of Ophthalmology & Visual Science and Pharmaceutical Sciences, Angiogenesis Discovery Research, Lexington, KY 40536-0305, USA

Kakali Mukherjee

School of Natural Product Studies, Department of Pharmaceutical Technology, Jadavpur University, Kolkata 700 032, India

Pulok K Mukherjee

School of Natural Product Studies, Department of Pharmaceutical Technology, Jadavpur University, Kolkata 700 032, India

DB Anantha Narayana

Herbal Research Labs, Hindustan Unilever Research Center, 64, Main Road, Whitefield, Bangalore 560 066, India

Lara O Orafidiya

Department of Pharmaceutics, Obafemi Awolowo University, Ile-Ife, Nigeria

Srikanta Pandit

J B Roy State Ayurvedic Medical College and Hospital, Kolkata 700 004, India

Alexander G Panossian

Swedish Herbal Institute Research and Development, Gothenburg, Sweden

Bhushan Patwardhan

Interdisciplinary School of Health Sciences, University of Pune, Pune, India

Roman Perez-Fernández

Department of Physiology, University of Santiago de Compostela, Spain

Werayut Pothitirat

Department of Pharmacognosy, Faculty of Pharmacy, Mahidol University, 447 Sri-Ayuthaya Road, Ratchatevi, Bangkok 10400, Thailand

K C Preethi

Amala Cancer Research Centre, Thissur 680 555, Kerala, India

P Pushpangadan

Amity Institute for Herbal and Biotech Products Development, Mannamoola, Peroorkada, Trivandrum-5, Kerala, India

Gulam Nabi Qazi

Hamdard University, Hamdard Nagar, New Delhi, India

Sujay Rai

School of Natural Product Studies, Department of Pharmaceutical Technology, Jadavpur University, Kolkata 700 032, India

Vietla S Rao

Department of Physiology and Pharmacology, Faculty of Medicine, Federal University of Ceara, Rua Cel Nunes de Melo-1127, Porangabussu; Fortaleza, CE, Brazil

José-Luis Ríos

Departament de Farmacologia, Facultat de Farmàcia, Universitat de Valància, Spain

B P Saha

School of Natural Product Studies, Department of Pharmaceutical Technology, Jadavpur University, Kolkata 700 032, India

Kumar N Satheesh

School of Natural Product Studies, Department of Pharmaceutical Technology, Jadavpur University, Kolkata 700 032, India

Samuel Seoane

Department of Physiology, University of Santiago de Compostela, Spain

Christine M Slover

Departments of Pharmacy Practice, and Medicinal Chemistry and Pharmacognosy, UIC PAHO/WHO Collaborating Center for Traditional Medicine, University of Illinois at Chicago, College of Pharmacy, 833 South Wood Street, Chicago, IL 60612, USA

Paul F Smith

Dept. of Pharmacology and Toxicology, School of Medical Sciences, University of Otago Medical School, Dunedin, New Zealand

Nai-Ning Song

Tianjin Institute of Pharmaceutical Research, Tianjin 300193, China

Roy Upton

Registered Herbalist, Executive Director, American Herbal Pharmacopoeia, Scotts Valley, CA, USA

Ashok Vaidya

ICMR Advanced Centre of Reverse Pharmacology, MRC-KHS, Vile Parle, Mumbai, India

M Venkatesh

School of Natural Product Studies, Department of Pharmaceutical Technology, Jadavpur University, Kolkata 700 032, India

Eva M Vigo

Department of Physiology, University of Santiago de Compostela, Spain

A Wahile

School of Natural Product Studies, Department of Pharmaceutical Technology, Jadavpur University, Kolkata 700 032, India

Eva M Wenzig

Institute of Pharmaceutical Sciences, Department of Pharmacognosy, Universitätsplatz 4/1, 8010 Graz, Austria

Jenneke A Wijbenga

Scientific Institute Dutch Pharmacists, The Hague, The Netherlands

Georg C Wikman

Swedish Herbal Institute Research and Development, Gothenburg, Sweden

Edwin van den Worm

Section Medicinal Chemistry and Chemical Biology, Department of Pharmaceutical Sciences, Faculty of Sciences, Utrecht University, Utrecht, The Netherlands

Pei-Gen Xiao

Institute of Medicinal Plants, Chinese Academy of Medical Science, Beijing, 100094, China

Noriko Yamabe

Institute of Natural Medicine, University of Toyama, 2630 Sugitani, Toyama, 930-0194, Japan

Erdem Yesilada

Yeditepe University, Faculty of Pharmacy, Kayisdagi, 34755 Istanbul, Turkey

Takako Yokozawa

Institute of Natural Medicine, University of Toyama, 2630 Sugitani, Toyama, 930-0194, Japan

Yiwen Zheng

Department of Pharmacology and Toxicology, School of Medical Sciences, University of Otago Medical School, Dunedin, New Zealand

Glossary

Adverse drug reaction (ADR) In the pre-approval clinical experience with a new medicinal product or its new usages, particularly as the therapeutic dose(s) may not be established, all noxious and unintended responses to a medicinal product related to any dose should be considered adverse drug reactions. The phrase 'responses to a medicinal product' means that a causal relationship between a medicinal product and an adverse event is at least a reasonable possibility, i.e., the relationship cannot be ruled out.

Adverse event (AE) An AE is any untoward medical occurrence in a patient or clinical investigation subject who has been administered a pharmaceutical product but which does not necessarily have a causal relationship with this treatment. An AE can therefore be any unfavourable and unintended sign (including an abnormal laboratory finding), symptom, or disease temporally associated with the use of a medicinal (investigational) product, whether or not related to the medicinal (investigational) product (see the ICH guidance for *Clinical Safety Data Management: definitions and standards for expedited reporting*, E2A, 1994).

Botanicals Plant-based or -derived ingredients. Any product that is made from plants or herbs. Botanicals are obtained from plant material and may include leaves, roots, bark and/or seeds. The plant material is typically processed by milling and/or extraction to produce the botanical dietary ingredient, aroma, herbal medicinal product or traditional herbal medicine.

Clinical trial/study Any investigation in human subjects intended to discover or verify the clinical pharmacological, and/or other pharmacodynamic effects of an investigational product(s), and/or to identify any adverse reactions to an investigational product(s), and/or to study absorption, distribution, metabolism, and excretion of an investigational product(s) with the object of ascertaining its safety and/or efficacy. The terms 'clinical trial' and 'clinical study' are synonymous.

Dietary supplement A product taken by mouth that contains a 'dietary ingredient' intended to supplement the diet. The 'dietary ingredients' in these products may include: vitamins, minerals, herbs or other botanicals, amino acids, and substances such as enzymes, organ tissues, glandulars, and metabolites. Dietary supplements can also be extracts or concentrates, and may be found in many forms such as tablets, capsules, soft gels, gel caps, liquids, or powders. They can also be in other forms (such as a bar) but if they are, information on their label must not represent the product as a conventional food or as a sole item of a meal or diet.

Directive 99/83/EEC on 'well-established use' The Directive permitted the use of bibliographic references in place of pharmacological and toxicological testing of HMPs and the results of clinical trials for products that have already been on sale in the European Union as a medicinal product, for not less than 10 years. Volume 2A of the Notice to Applicants clarifies the legal background of bibliographic applications as follows: 'Where the constituent or constituents of the medicinal product have a well-established medicinal use, with recognised efficacy and an acceptable level of safety, demonstrated by detailed references to published literature'.

Good clinical practice (GCP) A standard for the design, conduct, performance, monitoring, auditing, recording, analyses, and reporting of clinical trials, which provides assurance that the data and reported results are credible and accurate, and that the rights, integrity, and confidentiality of trial subjects are protected.

Herbal medicinal product (HMP) Any medicinal product (q.v.) exclusively containing as active ingredients one or more herbal substances or one or more herbal preparations, or one or more such herbal substances in combination with one or more such herbal preparations.

Herbal preparations Preparations obtained by subjecting herbal substances to treatments such as extraction, distillation, expression, fractionation, purification, concentration or fermentation. These include comminuted or powdered herbal substances, tinctures, extracts, essential oils, expressed juices and processed exudates.

Herbal substances All mainly whole, fragmented or cut plants, plant parts, algae, fungi, lichen in an unprocessed, usually dried form, but sometimes fresh. Certain exudates that have not been subjected to a specific treatment are also considered to be herbal substances. Herbal substances are precisely defined by the plant part used and the botanical name according to the binomial system (genus, species, variety and author).

Independent Ethics Committee (IEC) An independent body (a review board or a committee, institutional, regional, national, or supranational), constituted of medical/scientific professionals and nonmedical/nonscientific members, whose responsibility it is to ensure the protection of the rights, safety, and well-being of human subjects involved in a trial and to provide public assurance of that protection, by, among other things, reviewing and approving/providing favourable opinion on the trial protocol, the suitability of the investigator(s), facilities, and the methods and material to be used in obtaining and documenting informed consent of the trial subjects.

Medicinal product '[Any substance] . . . presented for treating or preventing disease . . . [and which may be] administered . . . with a view to . . . restoring, correcting or modifying physiological functions.'

Multicentre trial A clinical trial conducted according to a single protocol but at more than one site and, therefore, carried out by more than one investigator.

Protocol A document that describes the objective(s), design, methodology, statistical considerations, and organisation of a trial. The protocol usually also gives the background and rationale for the trial, but these could be provided in other protocol referenced documents. Throughout the ICH *Good Clinical Practice: consolidated guideline* E6(R1) (1996) GCP guidance, the term 'protocol' refers to protocol and protocol amendments.

Quality assurance (QA) All those planned and systematic actions that are established to ensure that the trial or experiment is performed and the data are generated, documented (recorded), and reported in compliance with good clinical practice (GCP) or good laboratory practice (GLP) and the applicable regulatory requirement(s).

Quality control (QC) The operational techniques and activities undertaken within the quality-assurance system to verify that the requirements for the quality of the trial-related activities have been fulfilled.

Randomisation The process of assigning trial subjects to treatment or control groups, using an element of chance to determine the assignments in order to reduce bias.

Regulatory Authorities Bodies having the power to regulate. In the ICH GCP guidance the expression 'Regulatory Authorities' includes the authorities that review submitted clinical data and those that conduct inspections. These bodies are sometimes referred to as Competent Authorities.

Serious adverse event (SAE) or serious adverse drug reaction (serious ADR) Any untoward medical occurrence that at any dose:

- results in death
- is life-threatening
- requires inpatient hospitalisation or prolongation of existing hospitalisation

- results in persistent or significant disability/incapacity or
- is a congenital anomaly/birth defect.

Source documents Original documents, data, and records (e.g., hospital records, clinical and office charts, laboratory notes, memoranda, subjects' diaries or evaluation checklists, pharmacy dispensing records, recorded data from automated instruments, copies or transcriptions certified after verification as being accurate and complete, microfiches, photographic negatives, microfilm or magnetic media, radiographs, subject files, and records kept at the pharmacy, at the laboratories, and at medico-technical departments involved in the clinical trial).

Traditional herbal medicinal products HMPs fulfilling certain criteria:

- used exclusively for traditional indications
- for use without the supervision of a medical practitioner
- not subject to prescription control
- for oral or external use or inhalation
- a qualifying period of time has elapsed – the 30-year requirement
- traditional use data show safety and efficacy to be plausible in the proposed conditions of use
- combinations with vitamins and minerals where their presence is ancillary to the herb.

Well-being (of the trial subjects) The physical and mental integrity of the subjects participating in a clinical trial.

Part I

Overview of various types of traditional medicine

1

The worldwide phenomenon of increased use of herbal products: opportunities and threats

Pulok K Mukherjee and Peter J Houghton

Introduction

One of the phenomena of the last three decades has been the huge increase in use of 'herbal products'. These can be defined as plants, parts of plants or extracts from plants that are used in healthcare or in combating disease. To avoid confusion with culinary herbs, herbs and plant extracts that have some association with medical uses are referred to as 'herbal medicinal products' (HMPs). Many of the plant species used have been used for centuries in a limited part of the world but the increase in global travel and communications has resulted in many of these now being used worldwide. HMPs form the largest part of what is sometimes called complementary and alternative medicine (CAM), and are at one end of a continuum from 'healthy foods' through 'nutraceuticals' to 'herbal medicinal products', i.e. products that have mainly a use in treating or preventing disease. A similar strand of continuity exists between purely cosmetic agents, products that address an aesthetically unpleasant skin condition with medical dimensions, e.g. sun-protection agents and topical preparations for treating skin diseases and other conditions.

It is somewhat ironic that this 'return to nature', as far as medicinal substances are concerned, has occurred at a time when medicine has become increasingly technologically sophisticated, both in the equipment and products used for diagnosis and treatment, and also in the design and research into the mechanisms underlying disease. Such research has led to the introduction of 'designer drugs' with selective actions and high potency and, for many disease states, the fruit of this is evident in the majority of patients who survive longer or lead more pleasant lives than would have been the case two generations ago.

However, it should not be forgotten that these advances in medicine and therapy are easily available to only a minority in the world as a whole. In many places, mainly in developing countries, but also in pockets in every affluent society, herbal products are the major, if not the only, source of medication, for economic or geographical reasons. This is in contrast to the more affluent areas of the globe where they are used as a matter of choice rather than necessity. Several different reasons have been put forward for the resurgence of interest in and use of HMPs. These include a reaction against the serious side-effects sometimes observed when orthodox drugs are used, especially the more potent ones; the inability of Western medicine to treat some diseases satisfactorily, especially chronic conditions such as eczema and arthritis, and the generally mistaken idea that 'natural' must be better or safe.

The sales figures for HMPs indicate their widespread and increasing use, e.g. US$ 257 million in the USA in 2004 (Blumenthal, 2005), record sales in 2006 from Boots, a UK chain of pharmacies (Newswire, 2006). Medicinal plants and herbs are increasingly seen as high-value crops and a growing number of species are under cultivation (Cavaliere, 2007). However, many HMPs are still obtained from wild, as opposed to cultivated, plants, and this is causing much concern in conservation circles, both from the narrow perspective of species becoming rare or extinct, but also from the wider perspective of habitat and environmental damage.

The increase in interest in and use of HMPs is not only reflected in rising sales figures for these products but in other areas as well. Some good-quality, thoroughly researched reference books have appeared in recent years and editions subsequent to the first have appeared quite rapidly. A selection is shown in Table 1.1. It should be noted that, although they share some common features with 'classic' pharmacognosy texts, they are distinct in concentrating more on reports of pharmacological and clinical studies, including toxicity studies, than botanical or chemical descriptions.

The need for new editions is due to the rapid increase in scientific research, and consequent publication of research papers in refereed journals dealing with medicinal plants. In recent years several new titles, e.g. *Journal of Ethnopharmacology*, *Phytotherapy Research, Phytomedicine* have joined long-running publications such as *Planta Medica, Phytochemistry* and *Journal of Natural Products*. For practically all such titles, the impact factor, a controversial indicator of citation and scientific importance of a journal, has risen steadily in recent

Table 1.1 A selection of reference books dealing with herbal products

Title	Authors/Editors	Publishers	Year
British Herbal Compendium Vol. 2	Bradley P	British Herbal Medicine Association, Bournemouth, UK	2006
ESCOP Monographs 2nd edn.		Thieme, Stuttgart, Germany	2003
Principles and Practice of Phytotherapy	Mills S and Bone K	Churchill Livingstone, London, UK	2000
Herbal Medicines 3rd edn.	Barnes J. Anderson LA and Phillipson JD	Pharmaceutical Press, London, UK	2007
Potter's Herbal Cyclopedia	Williamson EM	Daniel, Saffron Walden, UK	2003
Herbal Drugs and Phytopharmaceuticals 3rd edn.	Wichtl M	Medpharm Press, Stuttgart	2004
PDR for Herbal Medicines 2nd edn.		Medical Economics Company, New Jersey, USA	2000
Pharmacology and Applications of the Chinese Materia Medica Vols 1 and 2	Chang H-M and But P P-H	World Scientific , Singapore	1987
Herbal Medicine – a concise overview for professionals	Williamson EM	Butterworth-Heinemann, London, UK	2000

years. A good example of this is the *Journal of Ethnopharmacology*, for which the impact factor has doubled in the past ten years.

There is also increasing interest from legislators, funding bodies for research and organisations concerned with health policy and regulatory affairs. Government funding has been made available in the USA for the NIH (National Institutes of Health) to carry out clinical trials on some widely used herbs, e.g. *Ginkgo* and *Echinacea*. In the European Union a new category of licensed medicines, based on traditional use, was introduced in 2005 under the Traditional Medicines Directive and, under the Framework 7 programme funding, has been included for collaborative research into traditional Chinese medicine. In the UK, the House of Lords (the Upper Chamber of Parliament) conducted a wide-ranging consultation under its Commission on Complementary and Alternative Medicine, which was published in 2000 and this was followed by some funding from UK government for CAM research, although not in the areas recommended as priority by the report (Anon., 2003). Many national governments in developing countries are showing interest in the inclusion of formulations based on traditional herbal medicines into their healthcare programmes, but probably the greatest commercial thrust is coming from the Far East, especially from the Peoples' Republic of China, where US$3.6 million has been allocated for the modernisation of TCM as a focal point in the current Five Year Plan (Normile, 2003).

India has produced a well-regarded healthcare system and traditional medicines play a vital role in primary healthcare. Ayurveda is one of the oldest systems of the world and Ayurvedic physicians prefer to dispense drugs prepared by their own hands; they do not rely upon the products manufactured by pharmaceutical industries. Owing to commercial orientation and increasing demand for natural products, a few pharmacies are preparing unethical products, which results in an embarrassing position for physicians and patients. To overcome this, there is a need to fix certain standards for these natural products. Provisions relating to the manufacture and control of Ayurvedic, Siddha and Unani (ASU) drugs have been prescribed in the Drugs and Cosmetics Act 1940. In addition to these specifications, the Government of India has recently introduced regulations for Good Manufacturing Practice (GMP) on ASU products in Gazette Notification of Government of India, Extraordinary (dated 23 June, 2000 vide GSR No 560E). This is an important step in improving the quality and standards of ASU drugs being manufactured in about 9000 licensed ASU pharmacies in the country and in reassuring the public that these medicaments are effective and safe (Mukherjee, 2002; Mukherjee and Wahile, 2006).

It is against this background that this book has been conceived and the timeliness of producing such a volume is emphasised when the opportunities and threats that the current situation presents are considered.

Establishing standards for herbal products: the place of pharmacopoeial monographs

It has often been stated that any assessment of safety or efficacy of any pharmaceutical must also take into account the quality of the material used. Standards for minimum acceptable quality are conventionally laid down in pharmacopoeial monographs, which provide a summary of the acceptable substance and give details of relevant tests to determine its identity, the presence and acceptable levels of impurities and to check that the levels of 'actives' are sufficient to achieve the desired effect (and, in some instances, are low enough to prevent toxic effects). Any sample should be checked against all the tests specified, and should comply with them, before it can be labelled as being of pharmacopoeial quality.

It is important to note that the term 'monograph' is used for two somewhat different types of specifications. A pharmacopoeial monograph, e.g. as found in the British or European pharmacopoeias, gives only details of the tests to be used to establish quality, with perhaps very brief notes about its use. The other type of monograph is more concerned with comprehensive information about a plant and will include information about its chemical constituents, pharmacology, toxicology and clinical studies and usage.

Pharmacopoeial monographs deal with all types of pharmaceuticals and those dealing with medicinal plant material have been included since the earliest editions of official monographs, i.e. those recognised legally at a national or international level. It is fascinating to trace the evolution of a monograph for one particular medicinal plant since it reflects developments in analytical techniques, the increasing knowledge of the chemical compounds present and the growing body of knowledge that links the compounds present to the desired biological or clinical effect.

However, the monographs of earlier pharmacopoeias dealt with 'classic' plant drugs but did not cover many of the herbal products that are now used and with which this book is concerned. Many new monographs have had to be written, and many are also awaiting construction, because of this. The problem is accentuated because of international trade and the speed with which a new product may become established without adequate standards being available. Although pharmacopoeias may have been compiled for such drugs, they have often not covered all the possible aspects seen in a good-quality monograph. Examples included the early editions of the British herbal pharmacopoeia and the Chinese pharmacopeia, which were concerned almost exclusively with macroscopical and microscopical tests to determine the correct botanical identity, with sometimes some thin-layer chromatography for identity based on chemical profile, but not always of those compounds considered to be responsible for the activity, and therefore the efficacy. Tests for impurities were limited to such crude assessments as ash values and assay procedures were almost entirely absent.

More recent editions of the *British Pharmacopoeia* and *European Pharmacopoeia* have included monographs for many more herbal drugs and more sophisticated chromatographic methods, especially liquid chromatography, have been introduced for both identity tests, tests for impurities and for assay procedures. These approaches are dealt with to some extent in this book, but it should be noted that tests involving biological activity are very unusual in pharmacopoeial monographs, so greater attention is paid to tests for biological activity relevant to the reputation and claims for treating particular diseases associated with the herbal drug in question, since collation of these aspects in a book is not common.

The proper use of traditional medicine

In addition to so many benefits, there are also risks associated with the different types of traditional and complementary medicines. A number of reports have revealed examples of incorrect use of traditional medicines by consumers, including incidents of overdose, unknowing use of suspect or counterfeit herbal medicines, and unintentional injuries caused by unqualified practitioners. Although consumers today have widespread access to various traditional and complementary treatments and therapies, they often do not have enough information on what to check when using them, to avoid unnecessary harm. In this context, the World Health Organization has developed guidelines, which provide governments and other stakeholders with the general principles and activities necessary for the development of reliable consumer information. The document will also be a useful reference to consumers in guiding them on the information they need to have, to choose a traditional or complementary therapy that is safe and effective. Although consumer information cannot compensate for poor products or inadequate practices, it can help consumers gain increased knowledge about the benefits and potential risks of therapies and where to find reliable sources of information.

Types of consumer information required may vary from country to country, depending on a number of factors such as cultural and traditional influences, health system structure and the pattern of traditional and complementary medicine use. It also outlines the general principles and activities for ensuring reliable information, such as how to develop reliable knowledge, how to disseminate the information and regulatory measures to be followed for information and advertisement. It also suggests the topics to be considered when developing consumer information promoting proper use of traditional and complementary medicines, i.e. where and how to find good information, therapeutic claims and corresponding levels of evidence (quality, precautions, adverse events, toxic therapies, interaction and contraindication and dosages), procedure-based therapies, practitioners, pricing and health insurance coverage.

Opportunities

As mentioned above, there has probably not been a time in the past hundred years or more when the potential of herbal medicine as a source of novel chemical entities for drug lead molecules and novel types of medicines has aroused so much interest and therefore presented opportunities for their introduction as part of mainstream medicine.

Increasing acceptance medically of 'polypharmacy' in treatment

The introduction of combination therapies for many major diseases in Western medicine has removed something of the stigma of 'polypharmacy' from herbal medication. This was highlighted by a serious proposal in the *British Medical Journal* to introduce the 'polypill', containing a mixture of six different pharmaceuticals, to reduce the risk of cardiovascular disease by 80% in patients over 55 (Wald and Law, 2003). This article received much publicity and was hailed by the editor as possibly the most important paper for 50 years. Extra interest was added in the fact that three of the drugs incorporated in the 'polypill' were at doses of only a half those recommended therapeutically, thus raising the possibility of synergism occurring.

Synergy and polyvalency

Synergy occurs when two compounds are given together to give a greater pharmacological effect than would be expected from their activities at the same dose when given alone. More details are given in Chapter 6. Recent developments in quantifying and demonstrating synergism mathematically (Berenbaum, 1989) are likely to stimulate more research and for synergism in herbal extracts to be taken more seriously. Polyvalency, also discussed more fully in Chapter 6, occurs when the overall effect observed can be ascribed to a mixture of activities caused by different components in the extract. Such a multitargeted approach, inherent in polyvalency, increases the likelihood of some sort of positive response for patients with a presenting symptom which might be due to any one of a variety of factors. In addition, polyvalency is less likely to result in resistance developing in target infectious or parasitic organisms. It has been noted that the defence mechanisms of plants usually rely on a mixture of weakly active compounds rather than a single, very potent product and this has been suggested as a paradigm for treatment of human disease (Schmidt *et al.*, 2007).

Increased awareness of prevention strategies

Another paradigm shift in orthodox medicine has been the attention paid to drugs that activate or protect the defence, protective and repair mechanisms of the body rather than destroy the damaging agents (Wagner, 2003). An example of this is the great amount of interest in antioxidants. These are hypothesised to prevent the attack and damage caused by reactive oxygen species to cell membranes, enzymes and DNA, which is currently considered to be an important aspect of the aetiology of many diseases, including cancer, neurodegenerative disease and inflammatory conditions. This approach of aiding the natural means of defence and stimulating repair has long been a salient feature of Western herbalism, so the attitude of mainstream clinicians and researchers to HMPs, which might display less rapid and less spectacular results characteristic of such effects, is likely to be more sympathetic than would have been the case a generation ago.

Increasing clinical evidence for efficacy

Another opportunity for herbal products is the clinical efficacy that has been demonstrated for some preparations in disease states where conventional therapy is less than ideal, either because it is not very effective or because associated side-effects and toxicity occur. Several such disease states are chronic and the effects of long-term use of xenobiotics are unknown. Although many studies in recent years have demonstrated this for HMPs unfamiliar to Western orthodox medicine (see Table 1.2), it should not be forgotten that some have held pride of place as the preferred medication for a long time, Senna as a laxative probably being the best example. The success of a Chinese formula in treating severe atopic eczema in children (Sheehan, Atherton *et al.*, 1992) was probably the trigger for the huge increase in use of TCM in the UK over the past 15 years. Continued high sales of HMPs such as St John's wort, Saw Palmetto and Ginkgo suggest that many people derive real benefit from using them. It has been pointed out that there is an increasing body of evidence for the efficacy of some HMPs (Ernst, 2000) and this is bound to stimulate more clinical trials by groups previously not interested in this type of medication. Trials on HMPs have been collated in several recent publications and the major ones of these are listed in Table 1.2.

As evidence for the efficacy of extracts increases, the debate has intensified between viewing extracts of plants in their own right as medicines or of using them as sources for active compounds for development into more conventional single chemical entity (SCE) pharmaceuticals (Mills and Canter, 2007). Probably both views are correct, depending on the particular case in point. The pharmaceutical industry appears to go through cycles of interest and uninterest in natural products as a source of lead molecules, the rises in interest usually being stimulated by the success of SCE compounds such as paclitaxel or artemisinin. At present there is much concern about the decreasing portfolio of promising molecules as far as most major pharmaceutical companies are concerned and the natural world is once again receiving interest (Rouhi, 2003; Schmidt *et al.*, 2007). The anti-inflammatory diterpenes from *Tripterygium wilfordii* have been highlighted as interesting leads, as have the antidiabetic flavonoids from *Artemisia dracunculus* (Schmidt *et al.*, 2007) but attention is also being paid to sources of novel compounds from organisms other than the flowering plants, such as microorganisms, insects and marine organisms (Rouhi, 2003).

On the other hand, despite much research, the search for one active compound in an extract that clearly shows activity has often been fruitless. In this latter situation, the regulatory and analytical systems discriminate against the adoption of such extracts as bona fide medicinal substances on a par with SCEs. Robust and meaningful analytical approaches, as well as results from good clinical studies, of many such HMP extracts are needed to strengthen the case for closely defined mixtures to be accepted as well as SCE drugs. Progress is being made, as noted in an interesting paper (Tyler, 1999) which addressed many of the points to be considered before HMPs would be taken seriously by mainstream medicine.

Consumer choice

An important consideration in the market economies that dominate most of the Western world is consumer choice. The attraction of 'natural' medicines, chiefly plant extracts, for consumers has several irrational

Table 1.2 A selection of monographs and papers dealing with clinical trials on herbal products (see also books mentioned in Table 1.1)

Title	Authors/Editors	Journal or Publisher	Year
Handbook of Clinically Tested Herbal Remedies Vols 1 & 2	Barrett M	Haworth Herbal Press, New York, USA	2004
Cochrane Reviews		http://www.cochrane.org/reviews/	Various
The clinical efficacy of herbal treatments — an overview of recent systematic reviews	Ernst E	*Pharmaceutical Journal* 262: 85–87	1999
Systematic reviews of herbal medicines — an annotated bibliography	Linde K et al.	*Forschende Komplementärmedizin und Klassische Naturheilkunde* 10 (suppl. 1): 17–27	2003
The efficacy of herbal medicine — an overview	Ernst E	*Fundamental and Clinical Pharmacology* 19: 405–409	2005
Quality control of herbal drugs	Pulok K Mukherjee	Business Horizons Ltd, New Delhi	2002

aspects (e.g. that 'chemical' means 'bad') but it is not surprising, in view of the cost and safety concerns of many drugs produced by the pharmaceutical industry, that HMPs are generally viewed as much safer, even if not so potent, alternatives. There is therefore scope and opportunity for commercial promotion of HMPs and this has been very noticeable over the past twenty years, not only in the pharmaceutical arena but also in cosmetics and foods.

Threats

Extravagant claims

The mistaken idea that 'natural is completely safe', as well as 'natural' being a more 'comfortable' word than 'synthetic', has been exploited to the full by advertisers and commerce in many parts of the world. Medicinal claims are allowed in many developed countries for products licensed as medicines only but, in less-controlled environments, extravagant claims are made. Even in developed countries, clever wording and innuendoes can raise expectations of what using a product will achieve. Such 'hype' is particularly noticeable in advertisements for cosmetic and personal care products but is often encountered in areas of commerce notoriously difficult to control, such as mail order sales over the internet. All these instances raise the spectre of 'snake oil' and associated practices, where often worthless materials were sold with quasi-miraculous claims, which were such a feature of 19th century frontier life in the USA. It is probably true to say that legislation in many countries still has this type of unsubstantiated claim very much in mind in its general attitudes to herbal medicines. The scientific establishment usually reacts in scepticism and cynicism against extravagant claims with the result that 'the baby is thrown out with the bathwater' and potentially useful herbs are dismissed by those in positions of authority without much thought or serious scientific investigation.

Lack of sufficient evidence base

Medical, pharmaceutical and other scientific organisations may not have such a prejudiced view as that expressed above, but are frequently frustrated by the lack of good evidence for claims made. Scientific, 'evidence-based' grounds are often not substantial enough to the use of a herb for a condition in which it is purported to bring about relief. Placebo-controlled, randomised, double-blind crossover clinical trials are still reckoned as the gold standard for proving efficacy and, although, as noted above, an increasing number are being reported for herbal materials (see Table 1.2), good-quality studies exist for a comparatively small number and meta-analyses for even fewer. In many reported trials reported numbers are quite small, no placebo or equivalent drug is used to compare and endpoints are not clearly defined. For several widely used HMPs, e.g. Echinacea, the clinical evidence for efficacy is equivocal and the failure of some well-publicised trials to demonstrate any significant effect, e.g. on St John's wort carried out by the National Institutes of Health in the USA (Hypericum Depression Trial Study Group, 2002), has been seen as one of the causes of the downturn in sales in recent years of some HMPs.

Poor-quality materials

The lack of standards for HMPs in many countries means that wide variability exists in the quality of plant material used to make commercial products. In extreme cases, the incorrect species or part of the plant is used, but more often the material consists of the correct plant material with low amounts of the compounds considered to be responsible for the biological activity. In these situations, it is unlikely that the recommended dose of plant material will have sufficient amounts present for any clinical effect and, in some cases, it might be possible that resistance or immunity builds up. Poor quality might also occur if the HMP is contaminated with mould, insects or other infestations that produce toxic effects.

Such contamination of herbal material has been documented throughout history but, in recent years another type has occurred. The so-called 'herbal' material is mixed with, or replaced by, synthetic pharmaceuticals that show the activity claimed for the herbal. The most common cases are the addition of steroids such as betamethasone to anti-inflammatory 'herbal' topical preparations for skin complaints, such as eczema, and incorporation of large amounts of sildenafil in 'herbal' tablets for male impotence.

It is not surprising that such blatant cases of adulteration make many medical practitioners wary of using or recommending herbal products. The situation is compounded in many developed countries by the general lack of personnel with skills in knowing how to analyse such products or having expertise in performing and interpreting the analyses. With such ignorance, it is not difficult for poor-quality material to enter the market without being detected.

A common criticism of many clinical studies carried out on HMPs is that those running the trials do not appreciate the need to define the material being tested in terms of its botanical identity, freedom from possible contaminants and in the profile and amounts of the major constituents present. If these trials are reported in the literature, they mean very little if the material is not defined, because it would be impossible to obtain consistent replicate results without knowing if the plant materials used were of similar profile. Ideally, they should be 'standardised', i.e. the concentrations of 'active' compounds are defined within fairly strict limits and the relative amounts of the different ingredients is the same for every batch.

Concerns over safety

Safety is closely linked with good quality. HMPs are generally regarded as 'safe' by the public because they are 'natural', and consequently instances of adverse effects arising from their use attract attention. In recent years there have been some serious cases of harm occurring to those taking HMPs, probably the most notorious being the irreparable kidney damage induced in women in Belgium who were taking a Chinese herbal mixture as a slimming aid (Vanherweghem *et al.*, 1993). Such events have often led to HMPs being restricted in their sale or being taken off the market completely. In many cases the observed toxicity is not actually due to the true herb itself, but has occurred because the wrong plant was used, or some other toxic substance was added to a HMP formulation. The severe renal damage that occurred in the case noted above is an example of use of the wrong plant and is thought to be due to a confusion over the Chinese names of the herbs. The roots of *Stephania tetranda*, known as 'fang ji' should have been used in the formula, but appear to have been substituted with *Aristolochia fangchi* roots, known as 'fang chi', which contain the cytotoxic and nephrotoxic aristolochic acids. Numerous cases of toxicity have been reported because of the presence of heavy metals, such as lead, mercury and arsenic, often added because these materials are used therapeutically in some Asian systems of medicine. Another serious problem, referred to above, is the undeclared addition of synthetic, 'orthodox' pharmaceuticals to allegedly herbal products with the resulting risks of adverse effects, build-up of resistance or interaction with other medication.

However, it is important to accept that even if the correct herbal material is used, with no added substances, safety may be compromised. There is a variety of reasons for this, including the herb containing a level of actives higher than usual, the presence of bioactive compounds other than those having the desired activity and interaction with other medication. This last aspect has attracted quite a lot of attention in recent years with the huge increase in the use of HMPs by those also on orthodox medication. Interaction may be additive, where an exaggeration of the activity caused by the conventional medicine is noted, leading to overdose, or there may be a negative interaction, where the herb has an opposite effect to the orthodox drug, and so decreases its activity to a level where its efficacy is severely compromised.

The presence of other ingredients in the formula of a HMP may affect the plasma levels of the actives. If absorption from the gut into the bloodstream is reduced by compounds such as tannins, the levels may be too low for a therapeutic effect, while the presence of some other substances, e.g. black pepper (*Piper nigrum* fruits) may accelerate absorption and cause the bioactive substances in the blood to reach dangerously high levels. Similar negative and positive effects occur when metabolising enzymes in the liver are up-regulated or inhibited respectively or when excretion through the kidneys is increased or decreased.

Legislative and commercial pressures

The regulatory status of HMPs varies quite widely across the world and it is impossible to summarise briefly. In the developed world, the procedures for medicines to be 'officially' recognised have generally been designed with SCE drugs in mind and required studies in adsorption, metabolism and excretion are difficult to apply to HMPs. The problem also exists of allowing for variation in content between batches, while also defining the extract in terms of minimum levels of 'active' ingredients, often complicated by the fact that the actives may comprise a variety of compounds and are often not completely known. New developments in defining extracts by metabolomics are providing a fresh approach to this but, as yet, these advances have not been adopted by regulatory authorities. (*Metabolomics* – are the study and portrayal of all the secondary metabolites present in a plant extract by methods linking analysis with chemometrics and principal-component analysis.)

If HMPs are to be awarded a status on a par with SCE medicines, then considerable costs have to be incurred in doing the necessary work to construct the portfolio of data required by regulators. With SCE medicines, this is carried out by the large pharmaceutical companies, who are able to recoup the sums extended by sales of the medicine for its first few years, and protection from competitors marketing a similar product by patents and intellectual property rights (IPR).

This is much more difficult for products consisting of plant parts or crude extracts, and the situation is complicated by the fact that any IPR for traditional medicines should take the original owners of the information and use into consideration. Much has been written in the past two decades on 'biopiracy' in the context of traditional medicines and is discussed comprehensively in three special issues of *Journal of Ethnopharmacology* (volume 51, issues 1–3, 1996) and updated more recently (Soejarto *et al.*, 2005). Protection against this was a major part of the Convention on Biological Diversity signed in Rio de Janeiro in 1992, but it has proved to be somewhat controversial, since claims have been made that it has prevented, rather than stimulated, research and development of traditional medicines on a scientific basis. The uncertainty of gaining IPR on a product is one reason why many pharmaceutical companies avoid introducing extracts and herbal formulas into their portfolio of products. The consequence of this is that many products sold in developed countries are not marketed as 'medicines' but terms such as 'food supplements' are used. This not only reduces the perceived risks in the eyes of the public but also means that the product is subject to less stringent quality-control measures. Definition of a product as other than a medicine also broadens the range of outlets from where they can be obtained. In the UK, for example, as well as in many other countries, many 'conventional' medicines can only be obtained from a pharmacy, but products classed as 'food supplements' can be obtained from supermarkets and grocery stores.

In less-regulated and less-developed economies, the problems are different, since much supply at a local level is done as a family business, and consumerism is not a major factor, as most purchasers and users are in close contact socially with the suppliers. However, urbanisation breaks this immediate link and its dramatic increase in most developing countries has been matched by a rise in trade based on 'processed' herbs and HMPs very similar to that seen in developed countries. The huge problem posed by 'fake drugs' in many developing countries includes HMPs, and cheap substitutes and adulterated material are often encountered, as noted above. The concern that arises from this is being expressed in legislation, but often it is the enforcement of this legislation that is a problem, rather than its enactment (Harding, 2006).

Threats to conservation

The rise in use of HMPs has meant that increased amounts of plant material are required to satisfy consumer demand. Although many herbs and medicinal plants are cultivated, particularly now in countries such as India and China, the majority are gathered from the wild in developing countries, and are a valuable source of extra income for the local population, many of whom are subsistence farmers. Sustainable harvesting may be practised for plants used within a particular cultural group, and often is reflected in religious and other restrictions and rituals. However, when an outside market opens up, with the prospect of financial gain, and perhaps for plants not used by the group, these traditional controls may be discarded. What is also serious is the fact that collectors who may invade the area are unsympathetic to the local sustainable practices and consequently overcollect, possibly leading to extinction of the species in that area and destruction of the habitat. Such overcollection has made several medicinal plant species very rare in the wild in many parts of the world and efforts to reverse the situation, or prevent it happening, have been the focus of conservation organisations such as Worldwide Fund for Nature.

Shortages arising from overcollection, or from natural disasters in major growing areas, will inevitably lead to uncertainty over supply, with consequent higher prices and general volatility in the market. Shortages of genuine material also increase the risk of poor-quality, worthless or even dangerous material being supplied instead of the authentic products.

Cultivation is one obvious answer to some of these problems but it is not always possible to activate immediately on agronomic grounds. Not all medicinal species are easily adapted to plantation agriculture, since they may flourish best in association with a variety of other species.

Conclusions

Herbal medicinal products occupy a significant place in consumer consciousness in the developed world and are important in healthcare in most developing countries. There is increasing interest from the medical and scientific communities in giving them a place in evidence-based medicine, and this is consolidated by a more sympathetic attitude on the part of regulatory authorities than has previously been the case.

However, major obstacles exist in both the developed and developing world, to the acceptance by scientists, the medical establishment, legislators and regulators, of HMPs as substances equivalent to 'orthodox' medicines. Many of the concerns which need to be addressed come under the categories of quality, safety and efficacy. This book has been conceived as a way of bringing contemporary attitudes, discoveries and knowledge in these fields to the attention of health professionals and other scientists, as well as the informed general public. It is hoped that the recognition of what is already known will not only stimulate interest in use and acceptance of more HMPs but also encourage greater research to give a firmer scientific foundation to the use of many others.

Acknowledgement

The authors wish to express their gratitude to the Commonwealth Scholarship Commission, Association of Commonwealth Universities, UK, for the Commonwealth Academic Staff Fellowship Award to Dr. Pulok K. Mukherjee.

References

Anon. (2003). UK government funds CAM research. *Focus Alternative Compl Ther* 8: 397–401.

Sheehan MP, Atherton DJ *et al.* (1992). *Br J Dermatol* 126: 179–184.

Berenbaum MC (1989). What is synergy? *Pharmacol Rev* 41: 93–141.

Blumenthal M (2005). Market report. *Herbalgram* 66: 63.

Cavaliere C (2007). AHPA publishes 2004–2005 wild plant tonnage survey. *Herbalgram* 75: 12–13.

Ernst E (2000). Herbal medicines: where is the evidence? *BMJ* 321: 395–396.

Harding A (2006). Dora Akunyili: scourge of Nigerian drug counterfeiters. *Lancet* 367: 1479.

Hypericum Depression Trial Study Group (2002). Effect of *Hypericum perforatum* (St John's wort) in major depressive disorder. A randomised controlled trial. *JAMA* 287: 1807–1814.

Mills S, Canter PH (2007). Does the future of phytomedicine lie in using plants to isolate bioactive components? *Focus Altern Complement Ther* 12: 88–90.

Newswire (2006). Brits on a herbal high. http://www.prnewswire.co.uk/cgi/news/release?id=184420 (accessed 15 Aug 2007).

Normile D (2003). The new face of Traditional Chinese Medicine. *Science* 299: 188–190.

Rouhi AM (2003). Betting on natural products for cures. *Chem Eng News* 81: 93–94.

Schmidt BM, Ribnicky DM, Lipsky PE *et al.* (2007). Revisiting the ancient concept of botanical therapeutics. *Nature Chem Biol* 3: 360–366.

Soejarto DD, Fong HSS, Tan GT *et al.* (2005). Ethnobotany/ethnopharmacology and mass bioprospecting: Issues on intellectual property and benefit-sharing. *J Ethnopharmacol* 100: 15–22.

Tyler VE (1999). Phytomedicines: Back to the future. *J Nat Prod* 62: 1589–1592.

Vanherweghem JL, Depierreux M, Tielemans C *et al.* (1993). Rapid progressive interstitial renal fibrosis in young women: association with slimming regimen including Chinese herbs. *Lancet* 341: 135–139.

Wagner H (2003). Phytomedicine in the twenty-first century: new developments and challenges. *Focus Altern Complement Ther* 8: 392–396.

Wald NJ, Law MR (2003). A strategy to reduce cardiovascular disease by more than 80%. *BMJ* 326: 1419–1423.

2

Developing herbal medicinal products with quality, safety and efficacy: from field to bedside, with particular reference to the situation in India

Pulok K Mukherjee, A Wahile, M Venkatesh, A Gantait, BP Saha and OP Agarwal

Introduction

History records the fact that almost every culture around the world has noted the contribution of herbs and their use as foods and medicines. The oldest prescriptions, found on Babylonian clay tablets and the hieratic writing of ancient Egypt on papyrus, display numerous ancient pharmaceutical and medicinal uses of botanicals and foods. It should be noted that, until the 19th century, almost nothing was known about the composition of food, and the nutritional requirements of humans and food were accepted mainly on the basis of the history of use. While some herbal medicinal products (HMPs) have long been used both as foods and medicine, others have no significant history of use as food ingredients. The present insights into the nutrient composition of food and the nutritional requirements of humans are significant and are having a considerable impact on feeding habits. HMPs may be parts of plants, simple extracts or isolated active constituents, although usually the last group is not included in the definition of HMP. HMPs are regulated either as food or as medicinal products according to the regulations of a particular country and in the latter case often with simplified registration procedures. These differences in regulatory status are caused by differences in traditional use, in cultural and historical background, in scientific substantiation and in enforcement of current legislation (Bast *et al.*, 2002).

Studies on chemical ecology can identify materials of potential benefit to humanity, either in terms of agriculture or pharmaceutical development. The current view of many ecologists is that, although secondary metabolites may not have been produced mainly for the defence of the organism, a large subset of them are maintained because they do improve the fitness of the produce to survive. Acceptance of this idea makes it clear that secondary metabolites are characterised by a high degree of biological activity. This worldwide botanical cornucopia includes many reliable medicines. The World Health Organization (WHO) records the fact that 80% of the world population still relies on botanical medicines (Mukherjee *et al.*, 1998a; Mukherjee, 2002a).

Because of commercial orientation and the increasing demand for natural products, a paucity of well-qualified and trained personnel in herbal industries and the lack of harmonised regulations in various countries, the quality of the herbal products available in the market is unreliable and sometimes misleading. Therefore, it is essential that the information provided to healthcare professionals and consumers be unbiased, accurate, trusted and guarantees optimum quality, safety and efficacy.

Development of biologically active plant products

Although traditional medicines have been used for centuries by many civilisations in the world, scientific research and development in phytotherapy have suffered through lack of patent protection and diversity and the relatively small scale of the industries involved, compared with the conventional pharmaceutical industries. Moreover, traditional medicines are extensively used in the treatment of various ailments, but evidence-based recommendations are lacking. Established guidelines for assessing the efficacy and safety of phytomedicine, although scientifically consistent, are claimed by some to impose impracticable financial demands on licence holders. To prove the efficacy of the herbal drugs, good clinical research is needed but to produce the results carrying sufficient statistical weight is expensive and laborious and the cost of undertaking research studies may not be justified commercially. It is difficult to patent herbs and the size of the market is not comparable with most patentable conventional drugs. Being a mixture of complex chemicals, the herbs as a whole will have different properties from that of any single constituent acting alone. The action of the latter will not predict the effect of the former, particularly if the experimental evidence is based on work done on laboratory animals.

The strategy for deriving a single molecule as a therapeutic product is fairly well known. There are some steps such as synthesis or isolation from a natural source, identifying hits through in-vitro and in-vivo screening, converting hits into leads and then lead optimisation, pharmacokinetic study of the optimised lead, toxicological evaluation and eventual subjection to the various phases of clinical trials. However, in the case of HMPs, the strategy for developing them as licensed medicines is not well understood, largely because hardly any HMPs have successfully been introduced as such, especially in Western countries. Each country has its own strategy for product development, since the window of opportunity in herbal medicine is very large, but difficulties abound, not least that herbal products are generally kept as a trade secret, and knowledge of useful herbs is not always shared, something that has to happen if HMPs are to be viewed seriously as important in healthcare globally. A well-accepted product development strategy should be introduced, so that new HMPs can be developed and evaluated. This is essential, because the European Union, to use as an example, now requires much from the herbal product manufacturers, as described in their recent guidelines, but has not come up with a road map that will help the producers of HMPs in developing countries to meet their expectations (Mukherjee and Wahile, 2006a).

Herbal extracts are complex mixtures, so high sensitivity and miniaturised assays are required, together with innovative technologies, e.g. immunochemical and enzymatic methods coupled with online chemoanalytical systems, high-performance liquid chromatography (HPLC)-based assays used directly for a wide range of mechanism-based and cellular assays. Many pharmaceutical companies now prefer prefractionated extracts or pure compounds libraries in lead discovery, because of the low 'hit' rate in high-throughput screening technology (HTS, see p. 53) with crude extracts (Bindseil *et al.*, 2001). The most fruitful approach has been suggested to be a combination of pure compounds, fractions and extracts and a differential use thereof, depending on the target and the screening format (Potterat and Hamburger, 2008).

Limitations of traditional experience in developing HMPs

Although many conventional drugs or their precursors are derived from plants, there is a basic difference between administering a pure chemical substance and the same chemical in a plant matrix. Herbal products represent a number of unique problems in quality control because of the nature of herbal ingredients present therein. The constituents responsible for the claimed therapeutic effects are often unknown and the complex composition of drugs that are used in the form of whole plant, plant parts or the extracts obtained therefrom raises unique standardisation problems.

Another limitation concerns safety. Herbal prescribers and their consumers are less likely to detect some types of adverse reactions to herbal medicines than other types of medicine. Recognition will be particularly difficult, when the signs and symptoms are not unusual in the population and could thus be ascribed to alternative causes. Although long-standing experience may tell much about striking and predictable acute toxicity, it is a less reliable tool for the detection of reactions that occur uncommonly, develop very gradually or need a prolonged latency period, or that are inconspicuous (De Smet, 1995). An appealing example of inconspicuous toxicity is the fact that traditional eye medicines may damage the eye by a direct action of toxic substances introduced into the conjunctival sac, by the introduction of microorganisms leading to infection, by physical trauma resulting from the application, or indirectly by delaying the patient's presentation to a clinic for therapy. Epidemiological research has shown that a quarter of the corneal ulcers and childhood blindness in rural Africa is associated with the instillation of traditional eye medicines (Yorston and Foster, 1994; Courtright *et al.*, 1994; Lewallen and Courtright, 1995).

Safety claims on herbal medicines cannot be based on traditional empiricism. Not all HMPs have firm roots in traditional practices, and this may well be an underestimated issue. When traditional source plants are extracted in a non-traditional way (e.g. by resorting to a non-polar solvent such as hexane), the question arises whether this non-traditional extract is just as safe as the traditional one. Until recently, the ostrich fern *(Matteuccia struthiopteris)* was generally considered to be a non-toxic, edible plant with a history of use as a spring vegetable that went back to the 1700s. However, recent observations of serious gastrointestinal toxicity following the consumption of lightly sautéed or blanched ostrich fern shoots suggest that this vegetable is only safe when it is thoroughly cooked before use (Srinivasan, 2006). Sometimes a compound found as a herbal ingredient may have no medicinal tradition at all, and its route of administration or dose level may be quite different from that used in a traditional setting. A troubling example is that high-dose supplements of beta-carotene, taken alone or with vitamin A or vitamin E, increase rather than decrease the incidence of lung cancer in people at high risk of this disease although there was some epidemiological evidence that a diet rich in plants containing carotenoids was associated with a decreased occurrence of cancer (Marwick, 1996). Moreover, the administration form also differs based on the application pattern, e.g. most of the Ayurvedic and Siddha preparations of the Indian systems of medicine are used in traditional medicine by mixing the same with different solvents or adjuvants called 'Anupan' such as milk, honey, etc. While exploring those, the same drug may be used with other anupan which does not comply with the traditional concepts, and so the chances of adverse reaction, or less activity than the original HMP cannot be overlooked (Mukherjee, 2001, 2002b).

Establishing the quality of herbal products

Definition and characterisation of the material is necessary prior to the assessment of the relevance of available efficacy and safety data. It is also important that the material used and available commercially should be consistent with the evaluated material, because any significant change in quality would trigger the need for a re-evaluation of the relevance of the safety and efficacy data. There is a general, worldwide consensus on how to control the quality of herbal medicinal products, although considerable effort is necessary to guarantee a constant and adequate quality. Specifications and analysis of the preparations of multi-component drugs involve complicated factors and use of herbal materials of good quality, along with proper control of the manufacturing processes, are prerequisites for quality control. Several parameters for quality control of herbal medicine are given in Figure 2.1. In the Indian situation, where preparations of the herbal drugs are based on the selected prescriptions, manufacturers are requested to obtain the approval of statutory authorities by submitting a form containing the name, components and their specifications, the method of preparation, dosage and applications, efficacy, method and period of storage, specification and testing methods for the preparation. In the case of preparations not based on the selected prescriptions, and those combining herbal drugs or their extracts with synthetic drugs, the basis of the composition and literature or records to clarify the efficacy and safety are also requested redundant (Bast *et al.*, 2002; Srikumaran, 2006).

Evidence to support the safety of a botanical product may come from a wide variety of data, including documented traditional use, experimental studies, clinical trials and other human data such as case reports and epidemiological data.

Scientific monographs from the European Scientific Cooperative On Phytotherapy and the World Health Organization, for example, offer a valuable and updated overview on published scientific literature, which may be used in support of the demonstration of the safety and efficacy of a botanical product in a bibliographical application. These monographs may help to avoid duplication of work and bring about gradual harmonisation in the evaluation of medicinal products. In principle, human clinical data provide the most reliable source of information to assess the benefit and safety of a product, but old reports and studies that do not agree with the current state of the art, where studies are placebo-controlled, should be viewed sceptically and it should be established by expert judgement whether

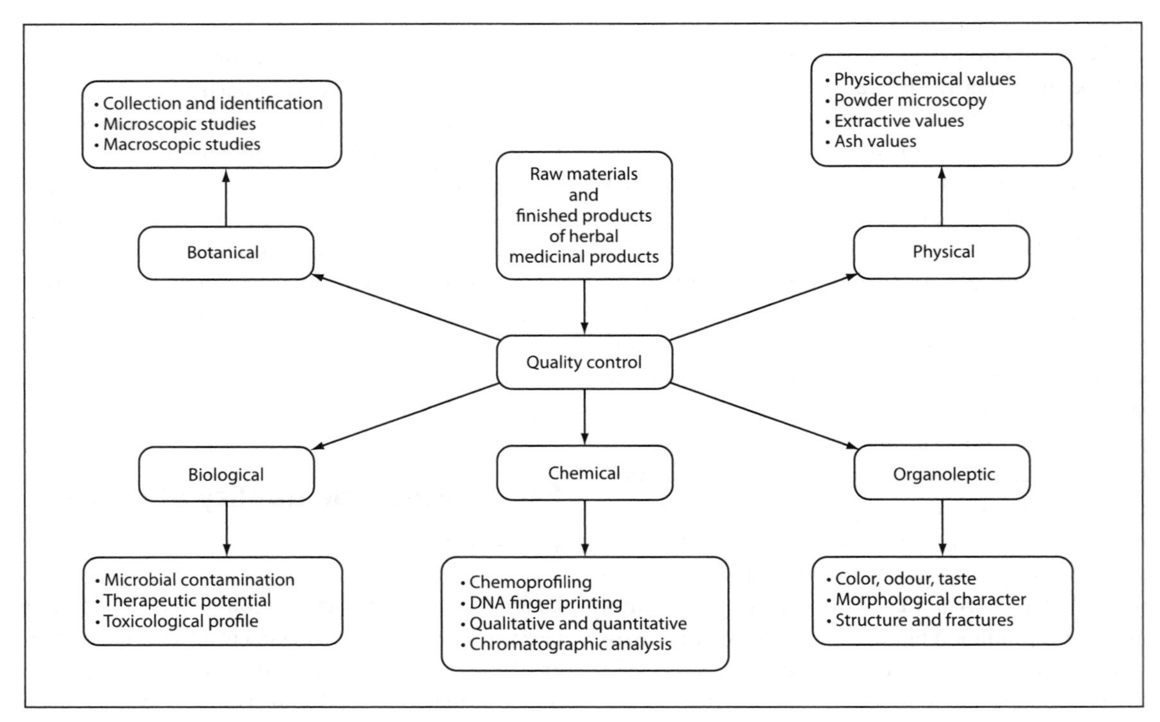

Figure 2.1 Quality control methods in evaluating herbal medicinal products.

the bibliographic data can demonstrate a sufficient level of safety and efficacy (Barnes, 2003a).

Documentation on traditional use may include:

- proper identification of the botanical used
- determination of parts used
- preparation process of the botanical ingredients
- formulation of the traditional product
- mode (route, schedule, and dose) of administration of the preparation
- indications of use of the botanical/preparation
- traditional geographical areas and populations in which such use occurred
- time span and extent of use of the botanical product
- contraindications and adverse effects that have been associated with use in humans and animals.

Quality control of herbal medicines is a critical and essential issue to be considered in assuring the therapeutic efficacy, safety and to rationalise the use of HMPs in healthcare. The challenges faced in the quality control of herbal drug preparations are described further in Figure 2.2 and also discussed in Chapters 27 and 28.

In traditional herbal medicines in the Indian subcontinent, the quality control aspect has been considered from inception by the religious experts or the medicine men using the herb for diseases, and later by the physicians known as *vaidyas* and *hakims*. However, modern concepts require necessary changes in their approach. For example, the quality control of traditional herbal medicines, the traditional methods of preparations are studied and documented and then this information is interpreted properly in terms of modern assessment (Mukherjee, 2002b). Adulterants, and more often, the incorrect identification of the herbs, are the causes of low quality in herbals.

Although a consumer of an officially approved herbal medicine should not have to be concerned about the correct identity of the ingredients, this is a primary concern when an individual goes out into the field to collect his own herbs. Austrian physicians recently described a case of a very young boy who developed veno-occlusive disease of the liver after long-term consumption of a tea prepared from *Adenostyles alliariae*. This herb had been erroneously gathered by the boy's parents instead of coltsfoot (*Tussilago farfara*) and it contains a greater amount of hepatotoxic pyrrolizidine alkaloids than coltsfoot (De Smet, 1989; Sperl *et al.*, 1995). Botanical misidentification can be problematic not only with self-collected plants, but also with commercially

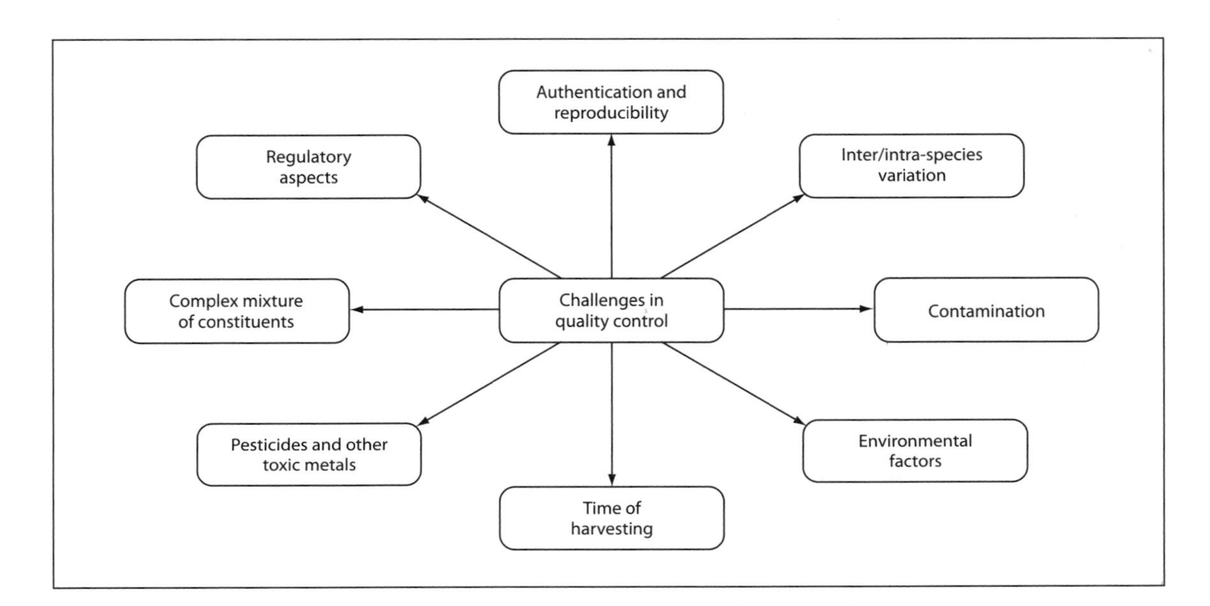

Figure 2.2 Challenges in quality control of herbal medicines.

available materials. German researchers recently exposed, for instance, that *Sarothamni scoparii* flos does not always originate from *Sarothamnus scoparius* ('Besenginster') but may also come from *Spartium junceum* ('Spanischer Ginster') (Schier *et al.*, 1994). Because the flowers of *Spartium junceum* are rich in toxic quinolizidine alkaloids of the cytisine type (Greinwald *et al.*, 1990), this adulteration could cause poisoning and thus be clinically relevant. Problems with the botanical quality of crude plant drugs may be even more pertinent in the case of traditional Chinese and Indian systems of medicine. The quality of prepackaged herbal products may also be a problem, in particular in countries where those products are not generally categorised as medicines. As a result, they remain exempt from governmental approval processes so that their quality is essentially uncontrolled and this is the prevailing situation in so many developed and developing countries (Tyler, 1995; Mukherjee *et al.*, 2006c).

Herbal medicines should be free not only from botanical contaminants, but also from residual pesticides or fumigating agents and from pathogenic microorganisms or microbial toxins. There are evidences, for instance, that medicinal plant materials from India and Sri Lanka can be contaminated with toxigenic fungi *(Aspergillus*, *Fusarium*). Since aflatoxin B has sometimes been recovered from such materials in potentially unsafe amounts, it would certainly be prudent to improve their storage conditions (Abeywickrama and Bean, 1991). Of great practical concern is the presence, intentionally or by accident, of toxic metals (such as lead and arsenic) or conventional pharmaceuticals (e.g. corticosteroids and non-steroidal anti-inflammatory drugs) in certain herbal medicines of Asian origin (De Smet, 1996). Although these hazards have been denounced for more than two decades now, they continue to pose an occasional threat to public health (Gertmner *et al.*, 1995; Shaw *et al.*, 1995). The contamination of herbal medicines with pharmaceuticals is not necessarily limited to products of Oriental origin but it is higher because, in these cases, of the lower stringencies of rules and regulation governing the quality of the herbals in different countries (Natori *et al.*, 1980; Espinoza *et al.*, 1995).

There are various aspects which have to be considered for optimising the quality of HMPs.

Good agricultural practices

Good agricultural practice (GAP) aims to meet consumer needs for products that are of high quality, safe and produced in an environmentally and socially responsible way.

WHO has developed a series of technical guidelines relating to the quality control of herbal medicinal plants grown in commercial plantations. These facilitate technical support for development of methodology to monitor or to ensure product safety, efficiency and quality, preparation of guidelines, and promotion of exchange of information (WHO, 2003). The guidelines cover techniques and measures required for the appropriate cultivation and collection of medicinal plants, documentation of necessary data and information during their processing. Good agricultural and collection practices for medicinal plants are only the first steps in quality assurance but play an important role in the protection of natural resources of medicinal plants for sustainable use.

GAP includes identification and authentication of cultivated medicinal plants, certification of seeds and other propagation materials, intensive care and management of cultivation, harvesting during the optimal season to ensure best quality of herbals and adequate knowledge of growers and producers on these aspects. The quality of the herbal medicines may be affected based on the methods adopted in the cultivation and harvesting methods of herbs. Auditing notebooks for the interpretation of the technical requirements of GAP to the specific situation of each farm are very important and these do not involve much investment and financial constraints as organisational burdens for farmers, especially those regarding the management of information. Various steps are to be followed for the achievement of GAP, combining scientific expertise and a comprehensive knowledge of herbal plant cultivation for translation into operational guidelines relevant to the regional context (WHO, 2003).

Good collection practices

Between 70% and 90% of the plant species used medicinally are commercially obtained by collecting the drugs in the natural habitat. The practice of collecting plant materials is not uniform throughout the world and good collection practice (GCP) is an important criterion in this respect and should be carried out as part of GAP. Collection practices should ensure the long-term survival of wild populations and their associated habitats and management plans should provide a framework for setting sustainable harvest levels and describing appropriate practices that are suitable for each medicinal plant species and plant part used. GCP should also include collection of permits from government authorities and land owners, technical planning with knowledge of geographical distribution, population density of the target medicinal plant species and essential information on the target species.

Macroscopical and microscopical evaluation

Organoleptic evaluation of herbal drugs is a primary means that includes evaluation parameters such as colour, size, odour and taste, and surface characteristics (texture and fracture).

Macromorphological evaluation is different for different parts of crude drugs – e.g. for crude drugs from barks, they are nature of curvature, surface characteristics, fracture characteristics and characteristics of transverse surfaces. Similarly microscopical evaluation is still of great importance in evaluation of crude drugs and nowadays a range of techniques are applied. More details on botanical techniques are given in Chapters 27 and 28.

Good manufacturing practices

Requirements and methods for quality control of finished herbal products, particularly for combining/mixing herbal products, are far more complex than for chemical drugs. Unlike conventional drugs, which are usually produced from synthetic materials by means of reproducible manufacturing techniques and procedures, herbal drugs are prepared from materials of natural origin obtained from various regions, varying climatic conditions and times of collection. However, alterations to quality might also arise during the processing stage by which the HMP is produced, so good manufacturing practice (GMP) is one of the most important tools to ensure the quality of the manufactured herbal drugs. To promote and improve the quality of herbal medicines, WHO has developed GMP guidelines for the manufacture of herbal medicines (WHO, 1996; 2002), which direct that materials should be handled in a fashion that is not detrimental to the product. After the arrival of the product for processing, the herbal material should not come directly into contact with humans and it should not be exposed to sun. Because of the high degree of initial microbial contamination of herbal materials, specific and detailed requirements have been developed to cover microbial contamination of equipment, air, surfaces, personnel and also for utilities, ancillary and supporting systems (Mukherjee *et al.*, 2005). The guidelines emphasise minimising the use of water for cleaning the herbal material and recommend an air duster or air shower. The presence of other plant materials of different species or different plant parts should be avoided during the process to avoid contamination, and the time limit mentioned in the master record should not be exceeded, to ensure the quality. The methods followed for standardisation should be documented and the blending process should be adequately controlled and documented and should be tested for conformity to the established specification. Any one specification batch should not be blended with other batches for the purpose of meeting specifications, except for standardisation of the content of the constituents with known pharmaceutical therapeutic effect. Where particular physical attributes are critical, blending should be validated to show uniformity of the combined batch and the validation should include testing of these critical attributes.

The WHO 2002 guidelines emphasise that operations on different products should not be carried out simultaneously or consecutively in the same room unless there is no risk of cross-contamination and when dry materials are used in production, special precaution should be taken to prevent the generation and dissemination of dust.

Standardisation of chemical aspects using marker analysis

For standardisation and quality assurance purposes, three attributes, i.e. authentication, purity and assay are desirable. Authentication, as the name suggests, relates to proving that the material is true, that is, it corresponds to the claimed identity. Purity pertains to evaluating that there are no adulterants present in the plant material and it can be evaluated by classic pharmacognostic procedures such as microscopy, ash values and other tests, for example, extractive values. The assay part of standardisation is chemical and biological profiling by which the chemical and biological effects could be assessed and effective doses are established. Safety for use could also be assessed through this parameter. In biological assays, the drug activity is evaluated through a pharmacological model but this is seldom used because biological testing is highly subjective in nature, subject to much variation in response and there are strict regulatory controls on animal testing. Therefore, the development of standardisation procedures for quality control through biological assays is significant but difficult (Bauer, 1998; Mukherjee, 2003b).

Chemical studies, on the other hand, are versatile and can be put to good use in standardisation, and are still the major technical approach used. Fingerprints can be generated for qualitative assessment. As far as quantitative assessment is concerned, the concentrations of the secondary metabolites, which are considered to be the active constituents of herbal drugs, are studied and used to provide standardisation procedures. The compounds in question are called 'marker' compounds. Of these marker compounds, some are therapeutically active, and others may not be active, but when used should be present in abundant quantity (Shu, 1998; Mukherjee, 2002a). Marker analysis may help in different ways, e.g. to assess potency, anticipate the active constituents, and ensure the quality and consistency of botanical raw materials and finished products. They may also help in detecting the adulterants and monitoring decomposition, essential in the stability study of herbals and deciding the shelf-life of a product (Tamizhmani, 2003). Several aspects on this context are illustrated in Figure 2.3.

Chromatographic testing of herbal medicines can be carried out for two purposes: identification and potency determination. Among the chromatographic methods for analysis of marker components, thin-layer chromatography is significant because it is simple, cost-effective, reproducible and visualisable. Further, fingerprinting of the chromatographic patterns and quantitative analysis of markers is possible using a densitometric scanner. The use of chromatographic fingerprinting for herbal drugs serves not only in identification but also assessment

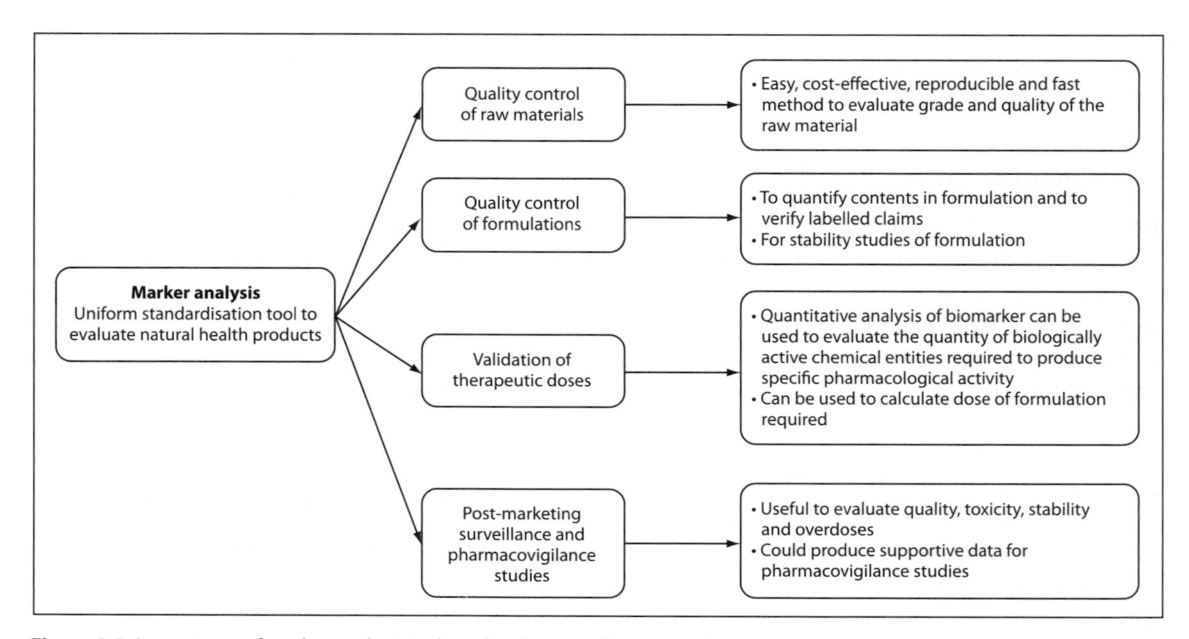

Figure 2.3 Importance of marker analysis in drug development from natural resources.

of the stability of the chemical constituents observed by chromatography (Mukherjee *et al.*, 2006b). Marker compounds and chromatographic profiles may be used to evaluate the quality of products from herbal growers and suppliers, to standardise raw materials, and control formulation and tablet content uniformity.

Unfortunately, the development of a biomarker for this paradigm is not an easy task because of the complex interplay of many variables in this approach. The biomarkers may act in combination with other chemical entities, via poorly understood mechanisms of synergy or antagonism, to be responsible for the efficacy of the standardised extracts for any particular therapeutic area or disease (Mills and Kerry, 2000). To define any molecule as a biomarker entails thorough research, and theoretically several biomarkers are desirabed to be relevant for the rational use of any given standardised extract (Keug *et al.*, 1996; Lazarowych, 1998).

Minimising risk

This consideration introduces the second step that should be taken towards safer herbal medicines. Herbal producers and sellers should ban unsafe remedies and discourage unsafe practices, but, unfortunately, the introduction of herbal medicine-like products into the market in many developing countries is not adequately monitored. This unsatisfactory situation could be greatly improved by the creation of a special licensing system for herbal medicines, such as is being developed in Europe. Such a system would not only help to exclude preparations from herbs with known toxicity, but would also provide a valuable tool to improve HMP quality, particularly since health problems arising from use of HMPs are often due to contaminants rather than the declared ingredients (WHO, 2000; Mukherjee, 2002b).

Not only the quality of a finished herbal product is important, but also the quality of the consumer information about that product. Understandable warnings in the package insert can certainly help to reduce the risk of inappropriate uses and adverse reactions (De Smet, 1994, 1996). The German health authorities have limited the indication of herbal anthranoid laxatives to constipation that has not responded to bulk-forming therapy. In addition, they have imposed restrictions to the laxative use of most anthranoid-containing herbs, that is, not to be used for more than 1–2 weeks without medical advice, not to be used in children under 12 years of age, and not to be used during pregnancy or lactation. This example illustrates that herbal health risks do not always require a full ban of specific herbal ingredients but can sometimes be reduced by appropriate warnings in the product information.

A striking feature of certain restrictive measures is that they are limited to one particular herb, without taking into account that the toxic constituents of that herb also occur in other medicinal plants. For instance, when the German health authorities announced their ban of herbal medicines prepared from the madder root, *Rubia tinctorum* (Pressedienst, 1993) because of its mutagenic anthranoids, they paid no attention to the occurrence of these compounds in other rubiaceous plants that serve as medicines in the Far East, e.g. *Morinda umbellata*, *Rubia cordifolia*, *Hymenodictyon excelsum* and *Damnacanthus indicus* (Kawasaki *et al.*, 1992).

Safety of herbal products

How safe are HMPs?

Very few herbal drugs have been subjected to systematic toxicological and nutritional assessment, yet, because of their long history, customary preparation and use and absence of evidence of harm, they are generally regarded as safe to consume. This long 'history of safe use' of herbal drugs forms the benchmark for the comparative safety assessment of newer herbal products. Apart from these observations, the other important factors in establishing a history of safe use are the results of animal studies and observations from human exposure (Walker, 2004). With the availability of herbal drugs from the fieldside to the bedside, via the internet site, care must be taken to ensure the safety of herbal drugs, since the regulations for herbal drugs are increasing day by day. Chapter 30 also deals with toxicological aspects of HMPs.

While the safety of some herbal medicines can be compromised by deficient product quality, other herbal products are dangerous, even if they have excellent quality. Yohimbe products rich in yohimbine will be less safe for over-the-counter use than products containing no or negligible amounts of this alkaloid (De Smet, 1994b). Likewise, the Chinese *Tripterygium* preparations that occasionally surface in the Netherlands, will particularly entail the risk of serious health problems (e.g. gastrointestinal disturbances, skin rashes, immunosuppression, blood disturbances, amenorrhoea, and oligospermia), when their quality is immaculate because of high levels of compounds with a narrow therapeutic index (De Smet, 1995).

The problems of the safety of herbals should not be ignored (De Smet, 1993). The information collected during the pre-marketing phase of any drug is inevitably incomplete with regard to possible adverse reactions; tests in animals are insufficiently predictive of human safety; in clinical trials patients are selected and limited in number; the conditions of use differ from those in clinical practice and the duration of trials is limited; and information about rare but serious adverse reactions, chronic toxicity, use in special groups (such as children, the elderly or pregnant women) or drug interactions is often incomplete or not available. Because the general public think that herbal remedies are 100% safe, they often take them without any medical advice and treat them like food. Consequently, the occurrences of side-effects, toxicity and drug interaction are not documented (Mukherjee *et al.*, 2006a). Phyto-pharmacovigilance is needed in every country, because there are differences between countries (and even regions within countries) in the occurrence of adverse drug reactions, and other drug-related problems and methods of data acquisition, handling and evaluation have to be developed, including the collection of consumer comments regarding non-prescription products.

Toxicity of herbals

All xenobiotics are toxic if they accumulate beyond the normal level in to the physiological system, as in the incident in the 1990s in Singapore, Hong Kong and also in Belgium, when women treated with a Chinese herbal preparation suffered from renal failure caused by the presence of the toxic material aristolochic acid, in a plant drug marketed and indicated for slimming (Meyer *et al.*, 2000). Therefore the importance of controlling the correct identification of herbal preparation should be taken into account from the very beginning (Schiltera, 2003; Khan, 2006). In addition to the problem of incorrect plant identification, some mixtures may be toxic, particularly if they are misused.

Risk assessment

Generally, for herbs or complex extracts, it is not possible to make a risk assessment on the basis of a single active component, because more than one may be of toxicological significance and matrix effects may affect bioavailability. The risk assessment/safety evaluation relates to the material as consumed; thus data applicable to the finished products are of major importance. Detailed analytical and other data are required to give assurance that the material tested provides relevant information, bearing in mind the possibility of matrix effects, e.g. on bioavailability, absorption and pharmacokinetic behaviour (Kroes, 2004).

Continual review and assessment of the safety of botanicals is needed, with an emphasis on surveillance of the use of these products to identify unknown hazards or risks and address them expeditiously.

Herbal toxicity and the consumer

The chance that a herbal medicine produces an adverse reaction depends not only on the herbal medicine and its dosage but also on consumer-bound parameters, such as age, genetics and concomitant diseases. For instance, the risk that the alkaloid berberine in Chinese *Coptis* species elicits jaundice seems to be most substantial in infants who are deficient in glucose-6-phosphate dehydrogenase (Yung *et al.*, 1990; Chan, 1993).

Herb–drug interactions

Herb–drug interactions may have little or no effect in patients and some are harmless. For those drug–drug interactions that are potentially harmful, the effects may only occur in a small proportion of patients. However, serious interactions can occur and these may be life-threatening.

An overview of the adverse drug interactions between herbal preparations and conventional medicines has been described by De Smet *et al.* (1996) and many other possibilities are listed in Barnes *et al.* (2006). Although it is sometimes the conventional medicine that increases the toxicity of a herbal compound, it is more likely that a herbal preparation interferes with the effects of a conventional drug. For instance, the root of *Salvia miltiorrhiza* (Danshen), which has been used traditionally in China for the treatment of coronary diseases, can enhance the anti-coagulant activity of warfarin when both drugs are taken together (Lo *et al.*, 1994). Herbal laxative preparations reportedly caused abdominal pain and diarrhoea in some patients. Any laxative or bulk-forming agents will speed intestinal transit, and thus may interfere with the absorption of almost any intestinally absorbed drug, thus eliminating drugs too quickly and diminishing their therapeutic effect because of reduced plasma concentrations. Patients with impaired renal or liver functions or who are elderly are at most risk from drug interactions and may be more prone to adverse effects (Chavez, 2006). Healthcare professionals providing pharmaceutical medicines for the treatment of diseases should be aware that concomitant use of herbal remedies can cause problems. Similarly herbalists treating patients should be aware of potential herb–drug interactions. There is limited information available in the literature concerning the interaction of herbal medicines and conventional medicines and much of it is speculative rather than arising from reports.

Establishing the efficacy of herbal products

Many complementary medicines, particularly herbal medicines, have a long history of traditional use. However, the efficacies of most of these are unproven. The lack of evidence does not necessarily mean that complementary medicines lack efficacy or are unsafe, but that rigorous clinical investigation has not yet been undertaken and that extensive surveillance of the use of these drugs has not yet been carried out.

Even though some standardised herbal extracts have undergone extensive clinical investigation, evidence of efficacy should be considered to be extract-specific. At most, evidence should be extrapolated only to preparations of the same herb with a very similar profile of constituents (Busse, 2000; Barnes, 2003a).

Clinical research and efficacy studies

One of the fundamental dogmas of clinical pharmacology is the rigorous assessment of the mechanism of action of drugs, their efficacy, kinetics and safety using evidence from well-designed studies. The safety and efficacy of the herbal products may also be determined by the pattern and concentration of the chemical components that they contain. Any evidence of efficacy, safety and quality for herbal medicines has until recently been anecdotal, or empirical at best, and rarely based on rigorous prospective randomised controlled trials. The situation is now changing but most clinical trials of herbal medicine have focused on either standardised extracts of single herbs or standardised formulas, reflecting increased sponsorship of such studies by manufacturers in the increasingly important over-the-counter market. Evidence from clinical studies of single herb extracts or standardised formulas cannot be generalised to individualised herbal medicine, and claims by practitioners that the latter has an evidence base requires confirmation (Scholten, 2001). In addition, no references to pharmacological and clinical data obtained with 'concentrated extracts of different composition' should be made for traditional preparations. This would generate the wrong impression that safety and efficacy are comparable.

Phytoequivalence

Herbal medicinal products (HMPs), after meeting the standards of quality and safety, have to face the pharmacological basis for efficacy. Pharmacological study can be pharmacodynamic and pharmacokinetic. In recent years numerous studies investigating the pharmacodynamic effects of HMPs have been performed but not much information is available on pharmacokinetics.

Considering phytoequivalence, one of the problems that the herbal industry faces is that of ensuring consistency in raw material availability and quality. Because of a lack of sufficient amounts of raw material, pharmaceutical companies may use an equivalent substitute herb, where the same marker is present in sufficient concentration. There is much debate on whether such a replacement is justified. One school of thought argues that, as the marker compound is considered responsible for biological activity, the original herb can be substituted by one containing the same amount of marker compound. The other school of thought contends that, as well as the marker compound, other constituents which are naturally present affect the activity, and these may not be present in the substitute herb. It is our view that an indiscriminate use of substituted material where the marker compound is present in sufficient quantity must be prevented unless bioequivalence studies are undertaken, as is done for generic single chemical entity drugs.

The pharmacokinetic study of HMPs is extraordinarily complex, owing to the presence of many components in a mixture. Concentrations of single compounds are low and plasma concentration of those constituents is often in the range of micro- to picograms per litre, so the analytical techniques to be employed should be sensitive enough to detect the presence of the compounds at that level. Modern instruments such as gas chromatography-mass spectrometry (GC-MS)/MS or HPLC-MS/MS are used to accomplish this target (Bhattaram *et al.*, 2002). However, different compounds have different bioavailabilities and so will complicate the design of pharmacokinetic studies. Different approaches are possible for the study of phytoequivalence depending on the types of preparations. If the constituent responsible for an activity is known, then equivalence studies could be performed in the same way as with allopathic drugs. However, if the constituents responsible for activity are not known, then only data acquired with defined chemical constituents can be used, but this is insufficient – data obtained with bioassays or pharmacological studies are more reliable.

Comparison of a phytogeneric and an innovator formulation can only be extrapolated if the following are performed (Loew and Kaszkin, 2002):

- pharmaceutical equivalence
- biopharmaceutical equivalence
- bioequivalence with different end points
- clinical studies.

The constituents of an extract can be divided into active and accompanying substances or coeffectors. Coeffectors may have an influence on the physicochemical properties such as stability, solubility, or the half-life of the active compounds. There are several examples in the literature showing improvement of solubility and bioavailability of single compounds because of the presence of coeffectors. Saponins increase the absorption of corticosteroids, some antibiotics, flavones, phytosterols, and silicic acid. The concentration of kavain and yangonin in mouse brain samples is higher after administration of a *Piper methysticum* extract than after administration of the purified single compounds in the same amount.

The improved bioavailability of ascorbic acid from a citrus extract compared with pure ascorbic acid is explained by an increased absorption and an improved stability of vitamin C in the presence of several flavonoids contained in the citrus extract. However, the mechanism of interaction and the coeffectors were not identified. One approach to identify the chemical structure of a coeffector was recently performed by Butterweck *et al.* (1998; 2003) in studies on *Hypericum perforatum* and its constituent hypericin. A better understanding of the pharmacokinetics and bioavailability of natural compounds can help in designing a rational dosage regimen, and potential botanical product–drug interactions can be predicted (Butterweck and Derendorf, 2006).

Once activity is established by clinical trials, it is necessary to standardise that activity to make certain that a uniform amount of it is present in each dosage unit. This can be a very complex matter with herbal products, the activity of which is not due to a single chemical entity but to a mixture of constituents, some of which have not yet been identified. At the present time, most herbal products are standardised on the basis of the concentration of a single active or marker compound in a concentrated extract. If the active or the marker compound is present in appropriate quantity, it is assumed that all the other necessary components are also represented and uniform activity is assured (Mukherjee *et al.*, 2006a). However, the use of pharmacological and clinical methods, linked to a qualitative and quantitative chemical profile of all the significant constituents by some method such as HPLC-MS or GC-MS, is the better approach to achieve phytoequivalence.

Without rigorous phytoequivalence studies, the results of a clinical trial performed with a particular brand of herbal medicine product cannot be easily or reliably extrapolated to other brands of herbal medicine products.

The need for herbal pharmacovigilance

Herbal pharmacovigilance should be explored in every way for safer herbal medicinal products for the community. There is no standard procedure evidence for recording and monitoring of adverse drug reactions in most countries. In this context, instead of mistaking the absence of reliable evidence as the green signal for commercial exploitation, herbal pharmacovigilance lends a note of caution. By analogy with conventional pharmacovigilance, herbal pharmacovigilance aims at the detection of serious adverse reactions, at the quantification of their incidence, and at the identification of contributive and modifying factors. A classic and inexpensive tool of pharmacovigilance is spontaneous reporting, on a voluntary basis, by health professionals, consumers or other parties who observe or experience a suspected or possible adverse reaction during daily practice (Barnes, 2003b; Kayne, 2006). Such reporting should come not only from healthcare providers, but also from herbal prescribers and herbal manufacturers. Herbal companies should be legally bound to report suspected adverse reactions to their products to the competent authorities, just as is now required from synthetic drug manufacturers. All should recognise that the reporting of suspected adverse reactions to their herbal medicines is an act of courage, which will eventually increase rather than decrease the respectability of professional herbalists and HMP manufacturers.

This problem can be exemplified by the situation regarding the hepatotoxic potential of the wall germander *(Teucrium chamaedrys*). There was animal evidence to suggest that the hepatotoxicity of the wall germander resided in its terpenoids and other medicinally used *Teucrium* species contain similar terpenoids (Kouzi *et al.*, 1994), but no one used this to question the safety of this herb in humans. Eventually a report on hepatitis associated with the use of *Teucrium polium* was published (Mattei *et al.*, 1995), but it required further clarification by the European Commission before the hepatotoxicity of this herb was established.

Traditional experience can bring such dose-dependencies to light and it may help to identify means of processing that reduce the likelihood of acute problems. However, not all adverse reactions occur immediately after they are administered and the importance of delayed reactions has recently been underlined by a retrospective study, covering clinical safety trials, which linked the occurrence of muscular weakness caused by hypokalaemia with long-term use of herbal anthranoid laxatives.

Herbal pharmacovigilance, however, is not a negative tool but a neutral one, especially when it identifies a new serious herbal health risk. Pharmacovigilance can also be reassuring, however, by providing evidence that certain herbal health risks are absent or negligibly small. Thus, it can help to boost one of the major claimed features of phytotherapeuticals, namely their relative safety when compared with conventional pharmaceuticals.

Acknowledgement

The authors are thankful to the All India Council for Technical Education, New Delhi, Government of India for financial support through a research grant.

References

Abeywickrama K, Bean GA (1991). Toxigenic *Aspergillus flavus* and aflatoxins in Sri Lankan medicinal plant material. *Mycopathologia* 113: 187–90.

Anonymous (1992). *Quality Control Methods for Medicinal Plant Materials*. World Health Organization document, WHO/PHARMA/92.559/rev.1, World Health Organization, Geneva.

Anonymous (2003). *WHO guidelines on good agricultural and collection practices (GACP) for medicinal plants.* World Health Organization, Geneva.

Barnes J (2003a). Quality, efficacy and safety of complementary medicines: fashions, facts and the future. Part I: Regulation and quality. *Br J Clin Pharmacol* 55: 226–233.

Barnes J, Anderson LA, Phillipson JD (2006). *Herbal Medicines*, 3rd edn. Pharmaceutical Press, London.

Barnes J (2003b). Quality, Efficacy and Safety of Complementary Medicines: fashions, facts and the future. Part II. Regulation and quality. *Br J Clin Pharmacol* 55: 331–340.

Bast A, Frank Chandler R, Choy PC *et al.* (2002). Botanical health products, positioning and requirements for effective and safe use. *Environmental Toxicology and Pharmacology* 12: 195–211.

Bauer R (1998). Quality criteria and standardization of phytopharmaceuticals: can acceptable drug standards be achieved? *Drug Inform J* 32: 101–110.

Bhattaram VA, Graefe U, Kohlert C *et al.* (2002). Pharmacokinetics and bioavailability of herbal medicinal products. *Phytomedicine* 9 Suppl 3: 1–33.

Bindseil KU, Jakupovic J, Wolf D *et al.* (2001). Pure compound libraries; a new perspective for natural product based drug discovery. *Drug Discov Today* 6: 840–847.

Busse W (2000). The significance of quality for efficacy and safety of herbal medicinal products. *Drug Inform J* 34: 15–23.

Butterweck V, Petereit F, Winterhoff H, Nahrstedt A (1998). Solubilized hypericin and pseudohypericin from *Hypericum perforatum* exert antidepressant activity in the forced swimming test. *Planta Med* 40: 291–294.

Butterweck V, Lieflander-Wulf U, Winterhoff H, Nahrstedt A (2003). Plasma levels of hypericin in presence of procyanidin B2 and hyperoside: a pharmacokinetic study in rats. *Planta Med* 69: 189–192.

Butterweck V, Derendorf H (2006). Pharmacokinetics of Botanical Products. In: *Herbal Supplements – Drug Interactions*, eds Y.W.F. Lam, S.M. Huang and S.D. Hall. Taylor & Francis Group, New York, pp. 205.

Chan E, (1993). Displacement of bilirubin from albumin by berberine. *Biol Neonate* 63: 201–208.

Chavez ML, Jordan MA, Chavez PI (2006). Evidence-based drug–herbal interactions. *Life Sci* 78: 2146–2157.

Courtright P, Lewallen S, Kanjaloti S, Divala DJ (1994). Traditional eye medicine use among patients with corneal disease in rural Malawi. *Br J Ophthalmol* 74: 810.

De Smet PAGM (1989). Drugs used in non-orthodox medicine. In: *Side Effects of Drugs – Annual 13*. Dukes MNG, Beeley L (eds.) Elsevier, Amsterdam, pp. 442–473.

De Smet PAGM (1993). Scutellaria species. In: *Adverse Effects of Herbal Drugs*. De Smet PAGM, Keller K, Hänsel R, Chandler RF (eds.). Volume 2. Springer-Verlag, Heidelberg, pp. 289–296, 317.

De Smet PAGM (1994a). Mangaanintoxicatie door het gebruik van Chien Pu Wan tabletten. *Ned T Geneeskd* 138: 2516–2517.

De Smet PAGM (1995). Health risks of herbal remedies. *Drug Safety* 13: 81–93.

De Smet PAGM, D'Arcy PF (1996). Drug interactions with herbal and other non-orthodox drugs. In: *Drug interactions*. Wellington PJ, D'Arcy PF (eds.) Springer Verlag, Heidelberg, pp. 327–352.

De Smet PAGM, Smeets OSNM (1994b). Potential risks of health food products containing yohimbe extracts. *BMJ* 309: 958.

Espinoza EO, Mann MJ, Bleasdell B (1995). Arsenic and mercury in traditional Chinese herbal balls. *N Engl J Med* 333: 803–804.

Gertmner E, Marshall PS, Filandrinos D, Potek AS, Smith TM (1995). Complications resulting from the use of Chinese herbal medications containing undeclared prescription drugs. *Arthritis Rheum* 38: 614–617.

Greinwald R, Lurz G, Witte L, Czygan FC (1990). A survey of alkaloids in *Spartium junceum* L. (Genisteae-Fabaceae). *Z Naturforsch Sect C Biosci* 45: 1085–1089.

Kawasaki Y, Goda Y, Yoshihira K (1992). The mutagenic constituents of *Rubia tinctorum*. *Chem Pharm Bull* 40: 1504–1509.

Kayne S (2006). Problems in the pharmacovigilance of herbal medicines in the UK highlighted. *Pharmaceut J* 276: 543–545.

Keug W, Lazo O, Kunze L (1996). Potentiation of the bioavailability of daidzin by an extract of *Radix puerariae*. *Proc Natl Acad Sci USA* 93: 4284–4288.

Khan IA (2006). Issues related to botanicals. *Life Sci* 78: 2033–2038.

Kouzi SA, McMurtry RJ, Nelson SD (1994). Hepatotoxicity of germander (*Teucrium chamaedrys* L.) and one of its constituent neoclerodane diterpenes teucrin A in the mouse. *Chem Res Toxicol* 7: 850–856.

Kroes R, Walker R (2004). Safety issues of botanicals and botanical preparations in functional foods. *Toxicology* 198: 213–220.

Lazarowych NJ, Pekos P (1998). Use of fingerprinting and marker compounds for identification and standardization of botanical drugs: strategies for applying pharmaceutical HPLC analysis to herbal products. *Drug Inform J* 32: 497–512.

Lewallen S, Courtright P (1995). Peripheral corneal ulcers associated with use of African traditional eye medicines. *Br J Ophthalmol* 79: 343–346.

Lo ACT, Chan K, Yeung JHK, Woo KS (1994). The effects of Danshen (*Salvia miltiorrhiza*) on pharmacokinetics and pharmacodynamics of warfarin in rats. *Eur J Drug Metab* 37: 1197–1200.

Loew D, Kaszkin M (2002). Approaching the problem of bioequivalence of herbal medicinal products. *Phytother Res* 16: 705–711.

Marwick C (1996). Trials reveal no benefit, possible harm of beta carotene and vitamin A for lung cancer prevention. *JAMA* 275: 422–423.

Mattei A, Rucay P, Samuel D, Feray C, Reynes M, Bismuth H (1995). Liver transplantation for severe acute liver failure after herbal medicine (*Teucrium polium*) administration. *J Hepatol* 22: 597.

Meyer MM, Chen TP, Bennett WM (2000). Chinese herb nephropathy. *BUMC Proc* 13: 334–337.

Mills S, Kerry B (2000). *Principles and Practice of Phytotherapy*. Churchill Livingstone, NY, pp. 22–25.

Mukherjee PK, Sahu M, Suresh B (1998a). Indian herbal medicines – a global approach. *Eastern Pharmacist* 21– 23.

Mukherjee PK (2001). Evaluation of Indian traditional medicine. *J Drug Inform USA*, 35: 631–640.

Mukherjee PK (2002a). Problems and prospects for the GMP in herbal drugs in Indian Systems of Medicine. *J Drug Inform USA*, 63: 635–644.

Mukherjee PK (2002b). *Quality Control of Herbal Drugs – an approach to evaluation of botanicals.* Business Horizons. New Delhi: India, pp. 230–250.

Mukherjee PK, Verpoorte R (eds) (2003a). *GMP in Herbal Drugs.* Business Horizons, New Delhi, pp. 45–60.

Mukherjee PK (2003b). Exploring botanicals in Indian system of medicine – regulatory perspectives. *Clin Res Regul Affairs J* 20: 249–263.

Mukherjee PK, Mukherjee K (2005). Evaluation of botanicals – perspectives of quality, safety and efficacy. In: *Advances in Medicinal Plants*, Vol 1, Prajapati ND, Prajapati T, Jaypura S (eds). Asian Medicinal Plants, pp. 87–110.

Mukherjee PK, Wahile A (2006a). Perspectives of Safety for Natural Health Products. In: *Herbal Drugs – A Twenty first Century Perspective.* Sharma RK, Arora R (eds). Jaypee Brothers Medicinal Publishers Ltd., New Delhi, pp. 50–59.

Mukherjee PK, Wahile A, Kumar V, Rai S, Mukherjee K (2006b). Marker profiling for a few botanicals used for hepatoprotection in Indian system of medicine. *Drug Inform J* 40: 131–139.

Mukherjee PK, Wahile A (2006c). Integrated approaches towards drug development from Ayurveda and other Indian systems of medicines. *J Ethanopharmacol* 103: 25–35.

Mukherjee PK, Rai S, Kumar V, *et al.* (2007). Plants of Indian origin in drug discovery. *Expert Opin Drug Deliv Discov* 2(5): 633–657.

Natori S (1980). Application of herbal drugs to health care in Japan. *J Ethanopharmacol* 2: 65–70.

Potterat O, Hamburger M (2008). Drug discovery and development with plant-derived compounds. In: *Progress in Drug Research, Natural Compounds as Drugs,* Volume 1, Eds. F. Petersen and R. Amstutz. Birkhäuser Verlag AG, Basel, pp. 53.

Pressedienst BGA (1993). *Widerruf der Zulassung für Krappwurzelhaltige Arzneitmittel angeordnet.* Bundesgesundheitsamt, Berlin, 15.

Schier W, Sachsa B, Schultze W (1994). Aktuelle Verfälschungen von Arzneidrogen. 5. Mitteilung – Birkenblätter, Orthosiphonblätter, Besenginsterblüten, Wohlriechendes Gänsefusskraut und Isländisches Moos. *Dtsch Apoth Ztg* 134: 4569–4576.

Schiltera B, Andersson BC, Anton CR *et al.* (2003). Guidance for the safety assessment of botanicals and botanical preparations for use in food and food supplements. *Food Chem Toxicol* 41: 1625–1649.

Shaw D, House I, Kolev S, Murray V (1995). Should herbal medicines be licenced? *BMJ* 311: 451–452.

Shu YZ (1998). Recent natural products based drug development: A pharmaceutical industry perspective. *J Nat Prod* 61: 1053–1071.

Sperl W, Stuppner H, Gassner I *et al.* (1995). Reversible hepatic veno-occlusive disease in an infant after consumption of pyrrolizidine-containing herbal tea. *Eur J Pediatr* 154: 112–116.

Srikumaran M (2006). Proposed rule: Current good manufacturing practice in manufacturing, packing, or holding dietary ingredients and dietary supplements. *Life Sci* 78: 2049–2053.

Srinivasan V (2006). Challenges and scientific issues in the standardization of botanicals and their preparations. United States Pharmacopeia's dietary supplement verification program – A public health program. *Life Sci* 78: 2039–2043.

Tamizhmani T, Mukherjee PK, Manimaran S, Suresh B (2003). Indian Herbal Drug Development – Problems and Prospects. *Pharma Times* 34: 13–15.

Tyler VE (1995). Herbal remedies. *J Pharm Technol* 11: 214–220.

Walker R (2004). Criteria for risk assessment of botanical food supplements. *Toxicol Lett* 149: 187–195.

WHO (2003). *Guidelines on Good Agricultural and Collection Practices (GACP) for Medicinal Plants,* World Health Organization, Geneva, pp. 1–69.

WHO (2002). *Traditional Medicine Strategy 2002–2005.* Geneva, WHO (document reference WHO/EDM/TRM/2002.1).

WHO (2000). *General Guidelines for Methodologies on Research and Evaluation of Traditional Medicine.* Geneva, WHO (document reference WHO/EDM/TRM/2000.1).

WHO (1998). *Quality Control Methods for Medicinal Plant Materials.* World Health Organization, Geneva.

WHO (1996). *Good Manufacturing Practices: Supplementary Guidelines for the Manufacture of Herbal Medicinal Products.* Annex 8 of WHO Expert Committee on Specifications for Pharmaceutical Preparations. Thirty-fourth Report. Geneva, World Health Organization (WHO Technical Report Series, No. 863) (F/S).

WHO (1991). *Guidelines for the Assessment of Herbal Medicines.* Geneva, WHO (document reference WHO/TRM/91.4).

Yeung CY, Lee FT, Wong HN (1990). Effect of a popular Chinese herb on neonatal bilirubin protein binding. *Biol Neonate* 58: 98–103.

Yorston D, Foster A (1994). Traditional eye medicines and corneal ulceration in Tanzania. *J Trop Med Hyg* 97: 211–214.

3

Natural remedies from Turkey: perspectives of safety and efficacy

Erdem Yesilada

Introduction

Although recently developed tools, such as computer-aided molecular drug design or high-throughput screening techniques, have increased the success rate in the discovery of novel bioactive molecules, traditional remedies are still among the most reliable sources in the discovery and development of new medicines.

During the history of humankind, the Middle East has played a key role in the development of contemporary medicine. From Hippocrates to Dioscorides, Avicenna to Rhazes, many pioneers of medicine lived and practised in the area. The historical development of traditional Islamic medicine that prevailed in the middle and southern parts of the region is well-summarised in the reports of Abu-Rabia (2005), Brewer (2004) and Saad *et al.* (2005).

The rich traditional and cultural diversities, which originated from the widespread nomadic lifestyle once common in the region, have generated a vast wealth of traditional knowledge. The wide range of climatic zones from subtropical to continental or maritime to desert in the region has produced a large flora, e.g. the Anatolian peninsula records about 11 000 higher plant taxa and more than 1100 are noted for their uses as medicinal remedies (Yesilada and Sezik, 2003), whereas the number of plant species reported in the region from Syria and Iraq down to the Arabian peninsula is only about 2600, of which 700 are noted as medicinal plants (Saad *et al.*, 2005). The number of plant-originated substances that are sold in *akhtar* (*attarah*) shops in Jordan was reported to be around 286 (Lev and Amar, 2002).

Ethnobotanical information shows diversity, depending upon the locality where the survey was carried out. In cities or towns, the main addresses for supplying the plant remedies are akhtar shops, spice shops or bazaars, where mainly unani medicine is practised. Along with the local or nationwide remedies, some imported plant materials, such as ginseng, may even be purchased from these places. For example, *ud-ül kahir* (*Anacyclus pyrethrum*, Asteraceae) or *misvaq* (*Salvadora persica*, Salvadoraceae) do not grow in Anatolia (the Asian part of Turkey), but those plants are imported and sold in akhtar shops in Turkey. In villages or in small towns, the villagers prefer to collect wild plants growing in the vicinity, instead of purchasing from akhtars. Knowledge of the utilisation of these plant remedies in these small settlement units is generally acquired from ancestors, and has been practised over a long period, remaining mostly undocumented. Consequently, the list of herbal materials and usages suggested by the herbalists in Turkey (Baser *et al.*, 1986) were found to be remarkably different compared with those reported as folk medicine (Yesilada and Sezik, 2003).

Although a number of attempts have been made to document the regional wealth of ethnobotanical knowledge in the Middle East, most were carried out using the traditional healers or materials sold in akhtars as a source of information (Azaizeh *et al.*, 2003). As an exception, particularly in the past two decades, the ethnobotanical characteristics of Turkish folk medicine have been investigated and documented by several research groups in Turkey through scientific field surveys (Yesilada and Sezik, 2003). With regards to the general status of folk medicine in the middle and southern parts of the Middle-East, Yesilada (2005) and Saad *et al.* (2005) brought attention to the insufficient amount of scientific research for documents and evaluation of the folkloric information in their reports. Moreover, they also pointed out that, owing to various factors, such as over-harvesting of wild species, detrimental climatic and environmental changes, migration from urban to larger centres, and the modernisation of the society, there is rapid disappearance of this wealth of heritage and they urged scientists to document the real folklore information as soon as possible.

Apart from these factors, the central parts of the region have faced drastic changes in recent decades, e.g. wars, political and military events, and extensive immigrations, so the sociocultural mapping in the region has been affected severely. In Israel, Jewish immigrants from all over the world, as well as minorities, mainly Arabs in origin, have at least partially maintained their culture and tradition, including traditional medicine. Because of the mutual interactions between these diverse cultures, the present traditional knowledge of healing in Israel might possibly be a reflection of cross-cultural influences (Lev, 2006).

Azaizeh *et al.* (2003) pointed out the practitioners' lack of knowledge of plant identification and of good treatments, which indicates that the material prescribed and practised by these practitioners might be false and might have unwanted toxic effects. However, peasants or nomadic people have acquired knowledge from their ancestors, and are more experienced in the application of herbal remedies, but make less use of written material; so documentation to preserve this folkloric herbal information is extremely important.

To demonstrate the regional richness of the traditional health heritage, some particular examples of the appraisal of Turkish traditional medicine are summarised below.

Evaluation of the herbal remedies used in diabetes mellitus

Diabetes mellitus is of growing public concern worldwide because it causes severe complications, including blindness, and cardiac and kidney diseases. Owing to the requirement for lifelong, continuous medication, traditional remedies have found widespread application in combating complications of diabetes in particular, especially in rural areas or in the patients who do not have medical insurance to cover the high costs of conventional drugs. According to a rough estimate, over 1200 plant species have been recorded in use worldwide for their alleged hypoglycaemic activity (Marles and Farnsworth, 1995).

In a recent study, Otoom *et al.* (2006) reported the results of a cross-sectional study in the management of diabetes in Jordan. The study was conducted by interviewing 310 patients living in cities. It was found that 31% of those interviewed had used herbal products (96 patients) and the most commonly used herbs by patients in Jordan were listed. Furthermore, it was found that 47.9% used herbs on a daily basis, following advice from friends, and that 86.5% were satisfied with the results in diabetes control. Some of the crude herbal drugs cited were also included in the list of herbal materials sold by herb dealers (akhtars) in Turkey (Baser *et al.*, 1986), even in other remote

Islamic countries such as Morocco (Tahraoui *et al.*, 2007). The hypoglycaemic activity of several of the herbs mentioned has some scientific basis (Mukherjee *et al.*, 2006). An unusual amino acid, 4-hydroxyisoleucine, with significant antidiabetic and antidyslipidaemic activities, was isolated from the seeds of fenugreek (Fowden *et al.*, 1973; Narender *et al.*, 2006). Broca *et al.* (2000) reported that the major isomer of this amino acid, that is *2S, 3R, 4S*, induces insulin secretion through a direct effect on pancreatic beta cells in rats and humans. Recently, the soluble dietary fibre fraction of fenugreek has been reported for its hypoglycaemic, insulinaemic, hypolipidaemic and antiplatelet effects in a type II diabetes model (Hannan *et al.*, 2003).

Thymoquinone was isolated as the active antidiabetic component of black cumin oil (El-Mahmoudy *et al.*, 2005). The hyperglycaemic and hypoinsulinaemic responses to streptozotocin were significantly abrogated in rats co-treated with thymoquinone, and this abrogating effect has persisted for one month after stopping treatment. It was emphasised that the protective value of thymoquinone against the development of type I diabetes mellitus is achieved via nitric oxide inhibitory pathway.

The effect of stinging nettle, *Urtica dioica* on lowering blood glucose has been noted in old writings such as those of Avicenna. Bnouhamm *et al.* (2003) demonstrated that aqueous extract of the leaves had a significant antihyperglycaemic effect, which might be caused in part by the reduction of intestinal glucose absorption. Farzami *et al.* (2003) isolated an active fraction F1 from the aqueous extract with a significant effect on insulin secretion from the Langerhans islets. This extract was also shown to improve the blood lipid profile in rats fed with a high-fat diet, since significant decreases in total cholesterol, low-density lipoprotein cholesterol, low-density/high-density lipoprotein cholesterol ratio and plasma total apo B were observed. Although the active ingredients of *U. dioica* are still unknown, Kavalali *et al.* (2003) reported that the lectin fraction from *Urtica pilulifera* L., which acts through increasing the insulin secretion from the islets, is the active component in streptozotocin-induced diabetic rats.

However, the active ingredients in the other remedies against diabetes listed above for Jordan have not been defined so far. Some examples of ethnopharmacological studies from Turkish traditional remedies, which have been used to alleviate diabetes symptoms, are given below.

Gentiana olivieri (Oliver's gentian)

In east and south-east Anatolia, a macerate called *afat,* prepared from the flowering aerial parts of *Gentiana olivieri* Afan (Gentianaceae), is locally popular for lowering the blood glucose in type II diabetes, and dried herbs are sold in akhtar shops and bazaars (Baser *et al.*, 1986). A scientific investigation was conducted on the material to evaluate this information (Sezik *et al.,* 2005). Although tea prepared from the plant is used in folk medicine, the activity of the aqueous extract was not noteworthy, but the methanol extract showed potent hypoglycaemic activity in the oral glucose tolerance test. The methanol extract was then submitted to bioassay-guided fractionation procedures by using successive chromatographical techniques to give a C-glycosylflavone, isoorientin, as the active ingredient. The antidiabetic activity of the compound was potent, providing 77% inhibition in blood glucose concentration, when administered for 15 days to streptozotocin-diabetic rats at a dose of 15 mg/kg body weight. Isoorientin also showed potent anti-hypertriglyceridaemic (50% inhibition) and anti-hypercholesterolaemic (35% inhibition) activities. The authors suggested that the effect of isoorientin on type II diabetes might be due to its potent antioxidant activity, which was previously reported by Orhan *et al.* (2003). The presence of the chemically stable sugar moiety in the molecule may facilitate the transport and accumulation in beta cells of the Langerhans islets and restore the oxidative damage. As another possible mechanism, isoorientin may sensitise the insulin receptor to insulin or stimulate the stem cells of islets of Langerhans in the pancreas of streptozotocin-diabetic rats, so restoring plasma levels of insulin or it may result in the improvement of carbohydrate metabolic enzymes towards the re-establishment of normal blood glucose levels.

Myrtus communis (myrtle)

A tea prepared from *Myrtus communis* L. (Myrtaceae) leaves or the volatile oil, obtained from the leaves by steam distillation, is used to lower blood glucose level (Baytop, 1999). Elfellah *et al.*

(1984) reported a potent hypoglycaemic activity for ethanol/water extract of the leaves in streptozotocin-induced diabetic mice but this was inactive in normoglycaemic mice. Önal *et al.* (2005) reported that the aqueous extract of the leaves had α-glucosidase inhibitory activity *in vitro* as potent as acarbose, a well-known α-glucosidase inhibitory agent.

The hypoglycaemic activity of the volatile oil (myrtle oil) in normal and alloxan-diabetic rabbits was investigated by Sepici *et al.* (2004; 2007). Myrtle oil was inactive in normoglycaemic rabbits as expected, but a good hypoglycaemic activity was observed 4 h after the administration to diabetic animals in 50 mg/kg dose. A more pronounced effect was observed on subacute administration for a week. In addition to hypoglycaemic activity, myrtle oil also showed a mild hypotriglyceridemic activity, but did not affect serum insulin concentration in normal and alloxan diabetic rabbits. The authors claimed that the reduction in blood glucose level may be due to the reversible inhibition of α-glycosidases present in the brush-border of the small intestinal mucosa, a higher rate of glycolysis as envisaged by the higher activity of glycokinase, as one of the key enzymes of glycolysis, and an enhanced rate of glycogenesis, as evidenced by the higher amount of liver glycogen present after myrtle oil administration.

Evaluation of the anti-inflammatory and antinociceptive potential of Turkish medicinal plants

Inflammatory conditions are the most common disorders frequently treated with traditional remedies. In particular rural people are exposed to several forms of inflammatory diseases during daily life: abscesses and inflammatory wounds, as well as rheumatic or back pain. Consequently, home-made remedies of either plant or animal origin are frequently employed to alleviate these symptoms. To emphasise the importance and effectiveness of the traditional remedies, several examples of ethnopharmacological studies are given below.

Ecballium elaterium (squirting cucumber)

Ecballium elaterium A. Rich., squirting cucumber (Cucurbitaceae), is a widespread plant particular to Eastern Mediterranean territories and a well-known remedy since the time of Hippocrates. The fruit juice, elaterium, was used as a powerful hydragogue cathartic agent as well as a diuretic in kidney inflammations. However, frequent uses or larger doses should be avoided since they lead to severe effects on the gastrointestinal system. Dioscorides described other applications for the powdered elaterium (precipitated part of the fruit juice) which, when mixed with milk and dropped into nostrils, 'cleared away icterus' and a 'headache of long continuance' (Guenther, 1934). In Middle-Eastern societies, including Turkey, the use against jaundice and liver cirrhosis has been widely practised since antiquity, through intranasal aspiration of the fruit juice, and a potent antihepatotoxic activity was reported due to its cucurbitacin B, a triterpenoid constituent (Agil *et al.*, 1999). Pre- and post-treatment with elaterium (dried fruit juice) and cucurbitacin B reduced carbon tetrachloride-induced hepatotoxicity, as evidenced by the reduction in the abnormally increased alanine aminotransferase enzyme level.

Post-treatment administration of cucurbitacin B caused a significant reduction in the degree of steatosis observed in a control group of animals, which were treated only with carbon tetrachloride. It is concluded that elaterium and cucurbitacin B had preventive and curative effects against carbon tetrachloride-induced hepatotoxicity.

In Turkey, a similar application for the fresh fruit juice into nostrils has been suggested for the treatment of sinusitis, as a popular folk remedy throughout the Anatolian peninsula. This application of fruit juice is uncommon in any other country except Turkey and the east Aegean islands. However, the medical case described by Dioscorides as 'headache of long continuance' is known to be the main symptom of sinusitis. Since Dioscorides was born and lived in southern Anatolia (Anazarba), it has been speculated that this application has been practised for at least 2000 years in Anatolia.

Despite widespread application, this practice often causes life-threatening uvular oedema (Eray *et al.*, 1999; Satar *et al.*, 2001) because of the high cytotoxicity of cucurbitacins contained in the fruit juice. Raikhlin-Eisenkraft and Bentur (2000) described the symptoms of 13 patients who were exposed to the undiluted fruit juice: Within minutes of exposure, the patients exhibited irritation of mucous membranes of various degrees of severity, manifested as oedema of pharynx, dyspnoea, drooling, dysphagia, vomiting, conjunctivitis, corneal oedema and erosion, depending on the route of the exposure. Recovery began within several to 24 hours after administration of oxygen, steroids, antihistamines and β-2-agonists.

To solve this problem, Sezik *et al.* (1984) carried out clinical studies on volunteers to determine a proper and non-toxic dose of the drug for the treatment of sinusitis, and through the application of properly diluted juice into voluntary patients, they observed a good recovery in 87% of the treated patients with acute maxillary sinusitis. To disclose its efficacy several successive studies have been carried out. The fruit juice showed a potent inhibitory activity against acetic acid-induced vascular permeability in mice and through bioassay-guided fractionation and isolation procedures, cucurbitacin B was isolated and defined as the main anti-inflammatory principle (Yesilada *et al.*, 1988). The anti-inflammatory profile of the fruit juice and cucurbitacin B were further evaluated using several in-vivo models on bradykinin-, serotonin-, and carrageenin-induced hind-paw oedema models in mice (Yesilada *et al.*, 1989). Results of the study suggested that some constituents other than cucurbitacin B could contribute to the anti-inflammatory activity of the fruit juice. However, the other cucurbitacins, i.e. E, I and D, were found to be completely inactive for anti-inflammatory activity (Yesilada *et al.*, 1988). Further studies still need to be conducted on cucurbitacin B to evaluate its potential histopathological toxicity on nasal aspiration and effects on cytokine profile, to disclose efficiency in sinusitis treatment.

Cistus laurifolius (rockrose)

Rockrose, *Cistus laurifolius* L. (Cistaceae), is a widespread plant in Mediterranean countries and is used as a remedy for a great many ailments. An aqueous extract from the flowers of the plant is suggested to treat ulcers, while a warm decoction of the leaves is used as a bath to relieve rheumatic pain or wilted fresh leaves are applied on joints (Yesilada *et al.*, 1995). To prove its efficiency in rheumatic disorders, methanolic and aqueous extracts and fractions obtained from the leaves were tested against interleukin (IL)-1α, IL-1β and tumour necrosis factor (TNF)-α. Methanolic extract and lipophilic solvent fractions (i.e. hexane and chloroform) showed a significant inhibitory activity against IL-1α and 1β, but proved to be ineffective on TNF-α (Yesilada *et al.*, 1997c). The aqueous extract of the plant was also found to possess significant in-vivo antinociceptive activity (Ark *et al.*, 2004).

Sambucus nigra and *S. ebulus* (elderberry)

Flowers or aerial parts of *Sambucus* species (Caprifoliaceae) are used in traditional medicines for various ailments and act as diuretics, laxatives, diaphoretics and expectorants. In Turkey, there are two species: *S. nigra* and *S. ebulus*. Leaves of both species are known as *karahekim* or Black Physician by the inhabitants in some districts, referring to their diverse biological activities and the blackish appearance of stems during drying, caused by their rich coumarin content and black fruits. In particular, black fruits are used for the treatment of haemorrhoids, the leaves of both species against snake bite, or a bath prepared from the fresh herbs or leaves is used to palliate rheumatic and catarrhal symptoms (Sezik *et al.*, 1991). It has also been reported that *S. ebulus* herb is used in the treatment of gastric ulcers (Sezik *et al.*, 1992). A potent anti-inflammatory activity was determined against carrageenin-induced inflammations for the ethanolic extract of *S. nigra* leaves (Yesilada and Sezik, 1990). Methanol extract as well as chloroform and *n*-butanol fractions showed remarkable inhibitory activity on TNF-α, but remained ineffective on IL-1α and 1β (Yesilada and Sezik, 1990).

Anti-inflammatory activity of *S. ebulus* aerial parts was evaluated by Yesilada (1997a) by using in-vitro (phospholipase A_2-inhibitory activity) and in-vivo test models (carrageenin- and serotonin-induced hindpaw oedema, adjuvant-induced arthritis). The methanol extract and its *n*-butanol fraction were found to possess significant anti-inflammatory activity. Through bioassay-guided fractionation and isolation procedures on butanol fraction, chlorogenic acid was isolated as the anti-inflammatory principle. However, this was not the sole active ingredient, since the chloroform and remaining aqueous fractions were also found to possess significant activity. It was noteworthy that methanol extract and butanol fraction showed remarkable activity in the carrageenin-induced paw oedema model when applied topically, which supported the traditional application mode: a poultice prepared from the leaves is applied externally to the affected joint. The methanol extract showed a more pronounced inhibitory activity than aqueous extract against IL-1α and 1β. This extract was further fractionated through successive solvent extractions. The hexane fraction and, to a lesser degree, the chloroform fraction showed inhibitory effects on IL-1α, 1β and TNF-α (Yesilada *et al.*, 1997c). These data also supported the folkloric application that non-polar ingredient(s) might be active. However, in a recent study, Ebrahimzadeh *et al.* (2006) reported that the hexane extract from the leaves did not show any anti-inflammatory activity against the carrageenin-induced oedema model. This is probably due to the inconvenience of the carrageenin model in revealing the activity. In a previous study, the hexane fraction was also found ineffective against paw oedema models (Yesilada, 1997a). In Iran, rhizomes of the plant have also been used for similar purposes and Ahmadiani *et al.* (1998) evaluated possible analgesic and anti-inflammatory effects of *S. ebulus* rhizome on chronic (formalin test) and acute (tail flick) pain models in rats. Accordingly, a significant analgesic activity was reported for methanol extract at 100 and 200 mg/kg intraperitoneal doses, which act through a central mechanism.

Daphne oleoides

In Turkish folk medicine, *Daphne oleoides* Schreber ssp. *oleoides* (Thymelaeaceae) leaves are used externally in rheumatism and oedema, and abdominal pain, while the roots have uses against high fever in malaria. Roots of the plant were shown to possess potent inhibitory activity on macrophage-derived cytokines, IL-1α and TNF-α biosynthesis (Yesilada *et al.*, 1997c). In particular, the methanol extract and its hexane and chloroform fractions were very active on these cytokines. This result is in good agreement with the recommended folkloric utilisation route of the material. The poultice obtained by boiling the whole plant is applied to the body, while the patient also takes a bath using the warm aqueous extract for the treatment of rheumatism. Since lipophilic compounds could pass the skin barrier easily, such an application seems reasonable. In a subsequent study, through activity-guided isolation procedures and chemical isolation techniques, 17 compounds were isolated and their structures were elucidated (Yesilada *et al.*, 2001): diterpenoids-genkwadaphnin and 1,2-dehydrodaphnetoxin and a coumarin derivative, daphnetin showed potent inhibitory activity and were found to be the main active ingredients. Other compounds present were shown to possess moderate inhibitory activity and may have a contributory role in the effect of the remedy.

Veronica anagallis-aquatica (water speedwell)

The high humidity and low temperatures in winter in northwest Anatolia in Turkey are associated with a high incidence of rheumatic disorders, and herbal remedies are frequently used to alleviate such symptoms. *Veronica anagallis-aquatica* L. (Scrophulariaceae) is one of these remedies; aerial parts are boiled in milk and the poultice thus obtained is applied to the abdomen for abdominal pain or its warm decoction (without removing the boiled herbs) is used as a bath remedy to alleviate rheumatic pain (Fujita *et al.*, 1995). To evaluate this information, antinociceptive and anti-inflammatory activities of the aerial parts were studied using *p*-benzoquinone-induced writhing reflexes and carrageenin-induced paw oedema tests, respectively. Through bioassay-guided fractionation and isolation procedures, iridoid glucosides were isolated as the active antinociceptive and anti-inflammatory principles, which supported the folkloric utilisation (Küpeli *et al.*, 2005). The activity of these molecules was found to be independent of their hydroxyl substitution in benzyl group, but dose-dependent. These compounds were also found to be safe and did not induce any apparent toxicity or gastric damage.

Nerium oleander (oleander)

Despite the widespread distribution of oleander, *Nerium oleander* L., (Apocynaceae) in the Mediterranean region, it has seldom been reported as a folk remedy because of its poisonous constituents. During our expeditions in northwest Anatolia, a local woman described how fresh oleander flowers are put in alcohol in the summer and kept as a home-made remedy to alleviate the severe pain and paralysis that intermittently occurred in her legs. We did not rate this application at first, but while referring to the database of Turkish folk medicine (TUHIB), we found a similar use described by another informer in Antalya (South Anatolia), in which flowers kept for 40 days in olive oil are applied to joints to treat rheumatic pain (Yesilada, 2002). Moreover, leaves or flowers are used to stop pain or eczema, and the sap obtained from fresh leaves for abscess or rheumatism was also recorded. To evaluate this information, both aqueous and ethanol extracts of oleander leaves were tested and both were shown to possess significant antinociceptive activity against *p*-benzoquinone-induced writhings, that of the ethanol extract being more pronounced (Erdemoglu *et al.*, 2003). However, both extracts of leaves were shown to induce gastric ulcerogenicity in mice and they were ineffective against carrageenin-induced paw oedema. Nonetheless, either fresh or dried flowers of oleander exhibited a potent antinociceptive activity and the activity of ethanol extract was more remarkable even than that of aspirin, the reference drug, without inducing any visual gastric toxicity. The ethanol extracts of fresh or dried flowers also showed a potent anti-inflammatory activity, but the aqueous extract was found to be ineffective. Experimental results have clearly confirmed that liposoluble fractions of flowers, similar to ethanol or olive oil extracts used in folk medicine, possess remarkable antinociceptive and anti-inflammatory activities (Erdemoglu *et al.*, 2003).

Berberis crataegina (barberry)

In Urgut bazaar (Uzbekistan), on a herb dealer's counter, we found some small, packed, black, tough material that was recommended for lumbago. This was the concentrated aqueous root extract of zirk (*Berberis asiatica*). Various *Berberis* species (Berberidaceae) have been used for the treatment of various inflammatory diseases in Eastern traditional medicines (from the Middle East to central Asia). In Azerbaijan, *Berberis vulgaris* L. barks are used for fever and rheumatism (Damirov *et al.*, 1988), whereas in Uzbekistan, *B. oblonga* roots find uses for low back pain (Sezik *et al.*, 2005) and in Pakistan, *B. lycium* Royle is used to treat rheumatism and muscular pain (Ikram *et al.*, 1966). However, the active constituents have not been defined thus far.

To evaluate this information, a study was conducted on the roots of *B. crataegina*, a common plant in Anatolia. Extracts and fractions from the roots were shown to possess a potent inhibitory effect against carrageenin- and serotonin-induced hind-paw oedema, acetic-acid-induced increased vascular permeability, castor-oil-induced diarrhoea and Freund's complete adjuvant (FCA)-induced arthritis models (Yesilada and Küpeli, 2002). Through bioassay-guided fractionation procedures berberine was isolated as the main active ingredient. This compound also showed antinociceptive activity, which was assessed by the inhibitory activity on acetic-acid-induced writhing reflexes and antipyretic activity on FCA-induced increased fever. In a follow-up study, anti-inflammatory, antinociceptive and antipyretic effects of six isoquinoline alkaloids, namely berberine, berbamine, palmatine, oxyacanthine, magnoflorine and columbamine were compared (Küpeli *et al.*, 2002). All alkaloids inhibited inflammation in varying degrees, and berberine, berbamine and palmatine were shown to possess significant and dose-dependent inhibitory activity against serotonin-induced hind-paw oedema on oral and topical applications and acetic-acid-induced increase in vascular permeability on oral administration. Moreover, these three alkaloids were also shown to possess dose-dependent antinociceptive and antipyretic activity. However, all alkaloids induced gastric lesions in varying degrees.

Studies on the gastro-protective and antiulcer activity of Turkish folk remedies

Field expeditions in Turkey have revealed that a high number of plant remedies have been used as folk remedies against gastrointestinal complaints, i.e. gastric pain, abdominal pain, indigestion, haemorrhoids, constipation, diarrhoea, etc. Among these, we interpreted the complaints of 'gastric pain' as a possible sign of peptic ulcer in contemporary pathological terms, and so have studied extracts of some of these plants for the assessment of antiulcer activity using several in-vivo models.

Experimental material was selected according to the results of preliminary bioassay tests (Yesilada *et al.*, 1993; Gürbüz *et al.*, 2002; 2003; 2005). Those possessing significant antiulcer activity have been processed further for the evaluation of the activity.

Cistus laurifolius (rockrose)

Flowers and flower buds of *Cistus laurifolius* L. (Cistaceae) are used in the treatment of peptic ulcers in South Anatolia (Honda *et al.*, 1996). Interestingly, the same use for this plant was also described in *Materia Medica* by Dioscorides (Guenther, 1934). Dioscorides (AD 20–79) was born and lived in Anazarba, a town near Adana province, indicating that this application had been practised for at least 2000 years in the same region.

The suggested application was as follows: the aqueous extract, prepared by boiling, is kept in a cool place (nowadays preferably in a refrigerator). The patient drinks this remedy whenever she or he feels thirsty, without limitation, instead of water. In a preliminary testing against water immersion and restraint-induced stress ulcer model in rats, the methanolic extract showed toxicity because of the extraction of resinous constituents. Although the inner surface of the mucous membrane of the stomach was free from ulcers, there were some haemorrhagic lesions on the outer muscular layer (Yesilada *et al.*, 1993). These animals also suffered from severe diarrhoea. In a lower dosage, however, the methanol extract was found to be totally ineffective. On the other hand, the aqueous extract showed a potent and dose-dependent antiulcer activity. At a high dose (1020 mg/kg) 100% inhibition was observed in ulcer score, while activity decreased to 65% at a half-dose (520 mg/kg). These results strongly supported the traditional means of application.

In a follow-up study, the aqueous extract was further fractionated through solvent extraction with *n*-butanol (saturated with water) and water. The latter was also precipitated with ethanol to give H_2O-precipitate and a H_2O-upper layer. The H_2O-precipitate fraction showed a potent antiulcer activity against water immersion and restraint-induced stress ulcer model in rats (98.6% inhibition at 183 mg/kg dose), while the other two fractions were found to be toxic in equal dose levels. In a half-dose administration, however, fractions were not toxic but the activity was poor (Yesilada *et al.*, 1997b). The active fraction also showed similar activity on subcutaneous administration revealing that the activity was not due to any local effect, i.e. by protection of gastric mucosa from the irritating factors, etc.

To evaluate the activity profile of the H_2O-precipitate, a wide range of in-vivo experimental models have been tested. Models and inhibitory percentages were found as follows: pyloric ligation-induced ulcerogenesis (94.6%), indometacin-induced ulerogenesis (84.6%), cysteamine-induced duodenal lesions (82.8%) and ethanol-induced ulcerogenesis (59.1%). Test material was found ineffective against serotonin-induced ulcerogenesis. In-vivo results were also confirmed by histopathological examination. As for biochemical parameters no effect on gastric secretion volume was observed but there was a significant change in the gastric acidity.

Results have clearly supported the traditional means of preparation of the remedy and its application. The polysaccharide fraction and probably the major constituents present showed its activity partially through modulating the gastric prostaglandin level and neutralising the gastric acid.

Spartium junceum (Spanish broom)

Interesting information also recorded in southern Anatolia was that an infusion of flowers of Spanish broom, *Spartium junceum* L. (Fabaceae), is used for the treatment of gastric ulcers (Yesilada *et al.*, 1993). Since the plant is known to contain cytisine-type alkaloids, which are reportedly toxic at a higher dose (Baytop, 1999), we considered that this might be a false interpretation. However, a preliminary testing of methanol and aqueous extracts showed remarkable and dose-dependent inhibitory rates against water immersion and restraint-induced stress ulcer models (Yesilada *et al.*, 1993).

To evaluate the antiulcerogenic activity, flowers were first extracted with methanol and then the plant residue was re-extracted with water (E-H_2O). The methanol extract was further submitted to successive solvent extractions to obtain hexane, ethylacetate and remaining H_2O fractions. Hexane and ethylacetate fractions possessed weak activity, while the remaining H_2O fraction was found to be toxic to rats, all experimental animals had died within 15 min after administration. E-H_2O extract exerted very high inhibitory activity (100%) on stress-ulcer. This later extract was subjected to further processing through Amberlite ion-exchange and then Sephadex LH-20 column chromatograpy to yield an active fraction (Yesilada *et al.*, 2000a).

This active fraction showed remarkable activity against stress-induced (94.6%), ethanol-induced (100%) and pyloric ligation-induced (83.9%) ulcers. Also the gastric juice volume, gastric pH, gastric acidity and peptic activity were inhibited significantly. This active fraction yielded a new triterpene saponin, named spartitrioside, showing 98.3% inhibition against the stress ulcer model (Yesilada and Takaishi, 1999).

Recently the role of active oxygen species in the pathogenesis of various gastric mucosal injuries activity has been widely discussed. Some antioxidants were reported to show an in-vivo protective effect against acute mucosal injuries induced by active oxygen species. To evaluate the role of antioxidant principles on the antiulcerogenic activity of *Spartium junceum* flowers, free-radical scavenging activity was studied. Through activity-guided fractionation and isolation procedures, several flavonoid glycosides with antioxidant activity were isolated (Yesilada *et al.*, 2000b). This study also revealed that flavonoid components in the extract may make a contribution to the antiulcerogenic activity of the flowers because of their potent antioxidant activity.

Centaurea solstitialis ssp. *solstitialis* (yellow starthistle)

In Turkey, fresh spiny flowers of *Centaurea solstitialis* L. spp. *solstitialis* (CSS) (Asteraceae) are recommended by the local people to be swallowed while soft, after rolling up into pills in the hand, for the treatment of peptic ulcers as a folk remedy (Yesilada *et al.*, 1995). A potent antiulcerogenic activity of the aqueous and methanolic extracts from spiny flowers was found against a water immersion and immobilisation-induced stress ulcer model in rats (Yesilada *et al.*, 1993). The chloroform fraction of the methanol extract from the aerial parts of CSS was also shown to possess potent inhibitory activity against *Helicobacter pylori* (Yesilada *et al.*, 1999). The ethanolic (80%) extract from flowering herb was subjected to successive fractionation procedures. Among the successive solvent extractions with organic solvents, the chloroform extract showed the highest inhibition (99.5%) against ethanol-induced ulcerogenesis (Yesilada *et al.*, 2004). Two sesquiterpene lactones were found as active components but other solvent extracts and fractions were also found to possess antiulcerogenic activity, so more work needs to be done in this context.

Momordica charanthia (bitter melon)

Momordica charantia L. (Cucurbitaceae) fruits are purported to possess a wide range of biological activities, in particular detailed investigations have been carried out on antidiabetic activities and the fruits have been proven to possess remarkable hypoglycaemic properties, both *in vivo* and in clinical studies (Dans *et al.*, 2007). Although the plant is not native to Turkey, the fruits are frequently used in folk medicine in the western parts of Anatolia. However, most of the medicinal features of the fruits known worldwide are not recognised in the Turkish folk medicine. The matured fruits are used externally for the rapid healing of wounds and internally for the treatment of peptic ulcers (Baytop, 1999). Whole matured fruits are sliced and put inside a jar of virgin olive oil or almond oil and left in sunshine until the seeds melted after about 2 or 3 weeks, when they are homogenised by pressing with a spoon. The ointment is kept at home to use when necessary for the rapid healing of wounds, abscesses and eczematous skin by applying twice a day, externally, or administered orally on an empty stomach every morning before breakfast against peptic ulcers. Because of its popularity, the plant is cultivated in the fields in the Marmara region.

However, in a previous study, the antiulcerogenic activity of the oily extract of the fruit, as well as solvent extracts with hexane, chloroform, ethanol and water, were found to be ineffective against immobilisation plus cold-induced stress and indometacin-induced ulcer models in rats (Yildirim, 1994). The author suggested that the healing effect of the fruit might be due to its oily vehicle or even to a placebo effect.

Considering the possibility that the model employed by these researchers may not be the correct activity assessment of the material, we carried out further experiments using another experimental model based on cytoprotective activity, i.e. the ethanol-induced ulcerogenesis model, in rats (Gürbüz *et al.*, 2000). The olive oil extract of fruits showed a dose-dependent and significant antiulcerogenic activity. The dried fruits were also found to be remarkably active when mixed with filtered honey; 100% inhibition was observed compared with honey as vehicle control. In both experiments the vehicles themselves, i.e. olive oil and honey, also exhibited some inhibitory activity against this model of ulcer, 58.1% and 94.3%, respectively, when compared with ulcer index obtained through the administration of 0.5% carboxymethyl cellulose suspension.

A high concentration of carotenoids was detected in the active ethanol extract of *M. charantia* fruits. Carotenoids are known to possess potent antioxidant activity and have been reported to prevent the gastric mucosa from the development of injury induced by various noxious agents (Kiraly *et al.*, 1992). For the evaluation of the role of antioxidant components, the active ethanol extract was also tested in the diethyldithiocarbamate-induced (DDC) ulcerogenesis model, and found to give 78.4% inhibition of gastric lesions. On the other hand, the activities of active ethanol extract and olive oil extract were tested in a more severe gastric ulcer model, hydrochloric acid plus ethanol-induced ulcerogenesis in indometacin-pretreated rats. The olive oil extract was ineffective against this model but the ethanol extract showed 45.8% inhibition. Moreover, chloroform fraction of the fruits showed some inhibitory activity against standard and clinical strains of *Helicobacter pylori* (Yesilada *et al.*, 1999b).

Hypericum perforatum (St John's wort)

St John's wort, *Hypericum perforatum* L. (Guttiferae), has recently gained much attention because of its proven effects in psychiatric problems, particularly as an antidepressant. Oily preparations of the material are also claimed to be effective internally in dyspeptic complaints, and externally for the treatment and post-therapy of acute and contused injuries, myalgia and first-degree burns (Blumenthal, 1998). In the akhtar shops in Turkey, the plant is recommended as an antidepressant, against bed-wetting in children and as a treatment for diarrhoea (Baser *et al.*, 1986). However, in Turkish folk medicine, people use the plant for a different purpose: the oily extract or tea prepared from these species are popularly used for the treatment of gastric ailments, i.e. internally for peptic ulcers and externally for wound healing (Yesilada *et al.*, 1993).

To evaluate this information, the antiulcerogenic effect of the ethanol extract from the flowering herbs of *H. perforatum* was studied and a dose-dependent and significant (82.8–97.8% inhibition) activity was observed against ethanol-induced ulcerogenesis in rats (Yesilada and Gürbüz, 1998). The extract was then fractionated by successive solvent extractions and ether fraction showed the highest inhibitory rate (86% inhibition), but more polar fractions were also found to possess some activity (between 49 and 71% inhibition), suggesting that different components of the plant may have a role in the antiulcerogenic activity. Moreover, chloroform and butanol fractions showed a considerable anti-*Helicobacter* activity.

Antihepatotoxic activity of Turkish folk remedies

The liver is the vital organ in the body for the metabolic, secretory and excretory functions. Because of the negative effects of chemotherapeutics, pesticides or environmental toxins, etc. on its functioning, supportive therapies are frequently required. Although conventional medicine does not provide many remedies against liver disorders, folk remedies have long been used for such purposes. Since lay people generally could not distinguish and define an activity related to this organ, a wide variety of parameters should be evaluated for the selection of such remedies, i.e. folk remedies used to treat anaemia, liver insufficiency, allergies and as a blood-purifier or panacea.

To select remedies with a hepatoprotective effect, a preliminary screening study was carried out on seven plant materials selected using the above criteria (Aktay *et al.*, 2000). Four out of seven were found to possess remarkable antihepatotoxic activity against carbon tetrachloride-induced hepatotoxicity, which was also confirmed by histopathological examination. Activity was assessed by monitoring the changes in plasma and hepatic tissue malondialdehyde (evidence of lipid peroxidation) as well as plasma enzyme levels; alanine transferase (ALT) and aspartate transferase (AST). Among these plants, the ethanol extract from the flowering herbs of *Gentiana olivieri*

Griseb. (Gentianaceae) and *Fumaria vailantii* Lois. (Fumariaceae) were found to possess pronounced activity.

Gentiana olivieri extract was then submitted to bioassay-guided fractionation procedures using the above-mentioned methods for antihepatotoxic activity assessment (Orhan *et al.*, 2003). A C-glycosylflavone, isoorientin, was isolated as an active component of the plant. This compound significantly reduced the hepatotoxicity induced by carbon tetrachloride in rats on subacute administration for 5 days. Isoorientin showed 75.0% and 80.8% inhibition, respectively, on increased plasma ALT and AST levels, and significantly reduced the tissue glutathione level after hepatotoxin challenge.

Conclusions

A list of natural remedies found in the akhtar shops (herbalists) in Turkey was reported by Baser *et al.* (1986). In addition, detailed field surveys were conducted on Turkish folk medicine for compilation of plant remedies used by rural people in villages or towns, either by our research team or by several other researchers, and the results have been published in international or national journals (Yesilada and Sezik, 2003). If the lists of remedies are compared, striking discrepancies can be distinguished between the uses suggested by herbalists and those in folk medicines (Table 3.1). (The sample plants are selected from those examined in this chapter.) Therefore, in our published studies on Turkish ethnobotany, the knowledge obtained from herbalists or traditional healers and those from rural people has always been treated separately.

Lists of plant- and animal-originated or inorganic drugs in the shops of herbalists in some Middle Eastern countries, i.e. Syria and Yemen (Honda *et al.*, 1990), Iran and Egypt (Ahmed *et al.*, 1979) and Jordan (Lev and Amar, 2002), have been published by several authors. Furthermore, there are several studies reporting the results of interviews with traditional healers (Ali-Shtayeh *et al.*, 2000). However, there seems to be a great deficiency in the documentation of herbal folklore from rural inhabitants. Therefore, it is important to conduct field studies in nomadic or rural societies, to document this knowledge before it vanishes because of the pressures of modernisation.

Plants offer a wide range of active constituents for exploring new leading drug molecules. Traditional medicines, either supplied from traditional healers, herbalists or rural people, are accepted as the most reliable and logical route to realise this goal. The Middle East, as the origin of the oldest civilisations in history, as well as in cultural diversity, has harboured a vast heritage of traditional remedies. Documentation and, in particular, appraisal of this knowledge through advanced ethnopharmacological

Table 3.1 Comparative uses of several plant remedies in Turkish folk medicine and in akhtar shops

Plant name	Use in akhtars	Use in Turkish folk medicine
Cistus sp.	Headache or earache	To treat peptic ulcer or against rheumatic pain
Spartium junceum	To pass kidney stones	Gastric pain
Centaurea sp.	Bloating	Against fever, headache, peptic ulcer
Berberis sp.	Liver and gall disorders	Rheumatic pain, low-back pain
Nerium oleander	Pain	Paralysis
Daphne sp.	Not found	Rheumatism
Veronica sp.	Not found	Rheumatism
Hypericum sp.	Depressions, diarrhoea	Peptic ulcer, wound healing
Sambucus nigra	Rheumatism	Rheumatism, haemorrhoids, gastric pain

surveys may lead to the discovery of new drug candidates to improve the quality of human life as well as effective armaments to combat diseases.

References

Abu-Rabia A (2005). Urinary diseases and ethnobotany among pastoral nomads in the Middle East. *J Ethnobiol Ethnomed* 1: 1–3.

Agil A, Miró M, Jimenez J, *et al.* (1999). Isolation of an anti-hepatotoxic principle from the juice of *Ecballium elaterium*. *Planta Med* 65: 673–675.

Ahmadiani A, Fereidoni M, Semnanian S, *et al.* (1998). Antinociceptive and anti-inflammatory effects of *Sambucus ebulus* rhizome extract in rats. *J Ethnopharmacol* 61: 229–235.

Ahmed MS, Honda H, Miki W (1979). *Herb Drugs and Herbalists in the Middle-East*. Tokyo: Institute for the Study of Languages and Cultures of Asia and Africa. Studia Culturae Islamicae No. 8.

Aktay G, Deliorman D, Ergun E, *et al.* (2000). Hepatoprotective effects of Turkish folk remedies on experimental liver injury. *J Ethnopharmacol* 73: 121–129.

Ali-Shtayeh MS, Yaniv Z, Mahajna J (2000). Ethnobotanical surbey in the Palestinian area: a classification of the healing potential of medicinal plants. *J Ethnopharmacol* 73: 221–232.

Ark M, Ustün O, Yesilada E (2004). Analgesic activity of *Cistus laurifolius* in mice. *Pharm Biol* 42: 176–178.

Azaizeh H, Fulder S, Khalil K, *et al.* (2003). Ethnobotanical knowledge of local practitioners in the Middle-Eastern region. *Fitoterapia* 74: 98–108.

Baser KHC, Honda G, Miki W (1986). *Herb Drugs and Herbalists in Turkey*. Tokyo: Institute for the Study of Languages and Cultures of Asia and Africa. Studia Culturae Islamicae No. 27.

Baytop T (1999). *Phytotherapy in Turkey, Past and Present*. Istanbul: Istanbul Universitesi Yayinlari.

Blumentahl M (1998). *The Complete German Commission E Monographs*. Boston: American Botanical Council Integrative Medicine Communications.

Bnouham M, Merhfour FZ, Ziyyat A, *et al.* (2003). Antihyperglycaemic activity of the aqueous extract of *Urtica dioica*. *Fitoterapia* 74: 677–681.

Brewer H (2004). Historical perspectives on health: Early Arabic medicine. *J Roy Soc Promot Health* 124: 184–187.

Broca C, Manteghetti M, Gross R, *et al.* (2000). 4-Hydroxyisoleucine: effects of synthetic and natural analogues on insulin secretion. *Eur J Pharmacol* 390: 339–345.

Dans AM, Villarruz MV, Jimeno CA, *et al.* (2007). The effect of *Momordica charantia* capsule preparation on glycemic control in type 2 diabetes mellitus needs further studies. *J Clin Epidemiol* 60: 554–559.

Damirov IA, Prilipko II, Shukurov DZ, *et al.* (1988). *Lekarstvenniye rasteniya Azerbaybjana*. Baku: Maarif Publ., 319.

Ebrahimzadeh MA, Mahmoudi M, Salimi E (2006). Anti-inflammatory activity of *Sambucus ebulus* hexane extracts. *Fitoterapia* 77: 146–148.

Elfellah MS, Akhtar MH, Khan MT (1984). The antidiabetic effect of the ethanol-water extracts of *Myrtus communis* using streptozotocin-induced hyperglycaemia in mice. *J Ethnopharmacol* 11: 275–281.

El-Mahmoudy A, Shimizu Y, Shiina T, *et al.* (2005). Successful abrogation by thymoquinone against induction of diabetes mellitus with streptozotocin via nitric oxide inhibitory mechanism. *Immunopharmacology* 5: 195–207.

Eray O, Tunçok Y, Günerli A, *et al.* (1999). Severe uvular angioedema caused by intranasal administration of *Ecbalium elaterium*. *Vet Hum Toxicol* 41: 376–378.

Erdemoglu N, Küpeli E, Yesilada E (2003). Anti-inflammatory and antinociceptive activity assessment of plants used as remedy in Turkish folk medicine. *J Ethnopharmacol* 89: 123–129.

Farzami B, Ahmadvand D, Vardasbi S, *et al.* (2003). Induction of insulin secretion by a component of *Urtica dioica* leaves extract in perifused islets of Langerhans and its in vivo effects in normal and streptozotocin diabetic rats. *J Ethnopharmacol* 89: 47–53.

Fowden L, Pratt HM, Smith A (1973). 4-hydroxyisoleucin from seed of *Trigonella foenum-graecum*. *Phytochemistry* 12: 1707–1711.

Fujita T, Sezik E, Tabata M, *et al.* (1995). Traditional medicine in Turkey VII. Folk medicine in middle and west Black Sea regions. *Econ Bot* 49: 406–422.

Guenther R (1934). *The Greek Herbal of Dioscorides*. Oxford: University Press.

Gürbüz I, Akyüz Ç, Yesilada E, *et al.* (2000). Anti-ulcerogenic effect of *Momordica charantia* L. fruits on various ulcer models in rats. *J Ethnopharmacol* 71: 77–82.

Gürbüz I, Ustun O, Yesilada E, *et al.* (2002). In vivo gastroprotective effects of five Turkish folk remedies against ethanol-induced lesions. *J Ethnopharmacol* 83: 241–244.

Gürbüz I, Ustun O, Yesilada E, *et al.* (2003). Anti-ulcerogenic activity of some plants used as folk remedy in Turkey. *J Ethnopharmacol* 88: 93–97.

Gürbüz I, Özkan AM, Yesilada E, *et al.* (2005). Anti-ulcerogenic activity of some plants used in folk medicine of Pinarbasi (Kayseri, Turkey). *J Ethnopharmacol* 101: 313–318.

Hannan JMA, Rokeya B, Faruque O, *et al.* (2003). Effect of soluble dietary fibre fraction of *Trigonella foenum graecum* on glycemic, insulinemic, lipidemic and platelet aggregation status of type 2 diabetic model rats. *J Ethnopharmacol* 88: 73–77.

Honda G, Miki W, Saito M (1990). *Herb Drugs and Herbalists in Syria and North Yemen*. Institute for the Study of Languages and Cultures of Asia and Africa. Studia Culturae Islamicae 39, Tokyo.

Honda G, Yesilada E, Tabata M, *et al.* (1996). Traditional medicine in Turkey. VI. Folk medicine in West Anatolia, Afyon, Kütahya, Denizli, Mugla, Aydin provinces. *J Ethnopharmacol* 53: 75–87.

Ikram M, Ehsanul M, Warsi SA (1966). Alkaloids of *Berberis lyceum* Royle-1. *Pakistan J Sci Indian Res* 9: 343–346.

Kavalali G, Tuncel H, Göksel S, *et al.* (2003). Hypoglycaemic activity of *Urtica pilulifera* in streptozotocin-diabetic rats. *J Ethnopharmacol* 84: 241–245.

Kiraly A, Suto G, Vincze A, *et al.* (1992). Correlation between the cytoprotective effect of β-carotene and its gastric mucosal level in indomethacin-treated rats with or without acute surgical vagotomy. *Acta Physiol Hung* 80: 213–218.

Küpeli E, Kosar M, Yesilada E, *et al.* (2002). A comparative study on the anti-inflammatory, antinociceptive and antipyretic effects of isoquinoline alkaloids from the roots of Turkish *Berberis* species. *Life Sci* 72: 645–657.

Küpeli E, Harput US, Varel M, *et al.* (2005). Bioassay-guided isolation of iridoid glucosides with antinociceptive and anti-inflammatory activities from *Veronica anagallis-aquatica* L. *J Ethnopharmacol* 102: 170–176.

Lev E, Amar Z (2002). Ethnopharmacological survey of traditional drugs sold in the Kingdom of Jordan. *J Ethnopharmacol* 82: 131–145.

Lev E (2006). Ethno-diversity within current ethnopharmacology as part of Israeli traditional medicine. A review. *J Ethnobio Ethnomed* 2: 1–31.

Marles RJ, Farnsworth NR (1995). Antidiabetic plants and their active constituents. *Phytomedicine* 2: 137–189.

Mukherjee PK, Maiti K, Mukherjee K, *et al.* (2006). Leads from Indian medicinal plants with hypoglycemic potentials. *J Ethnopharmacol* 106: 1–28.

Narender T, Puri A, Shweta KT *et al.* (2006). 4-hydroxyisoleucine an unusual amino acid as antidyslipidemic and antihyperglycemic agent. *Bioorg Med Chem Let* 16: 293–296.

Orhan Deliorman D, Aslan M, Aktay G, *et al.* (2003). Evaluation of hepatoprotective effect of *Gentiana olivieri* herbs on subacute administration and isolation of active principle. *Life Sci* 72: 2273–2283.

Otoom SA, Al-Safi SA, Kerem ZK, *et al.* (2006). The use of medicinal herbs by diabetic Jordanian patients. *J Herbal Pharmacother* 6: 31–41.

Önal S, Timur S, Okutucu B, *et al.* (2005). Inhibition of α-glucosidase by aqueous extracts of some potent antidiabetic medicinal herbs. *Prep Biochem Biotechnol* 35: 29–36.

Raikhlin-Eisenkraft B, Bentur Y (2000). *Ecbalium elaterium* (squirting cucumber) – remedy or poison? *J Toxicol Clin Toxicol* 38: 305–308.

Saad B, Azaizeh H, Said O (2005). Tradition and perspectives of Arab Herbal Medicine: A review. *eCAM* 2: 475–479.

Satar S, Gökel Y, Toprak N, Sebe A (2001). Life-threatening uvular angiodema caused by *Ecbalium elaterium*. *Eur J Emerg Med* 8: 337–339.

Sepici A, Gürbüz I, Cevik C, *et al.* (2004). Hypoglycaemic effects of myrtle oil in normal and alloxan-diabetic rabbits. *J Ethnopharmacol* 93: 311–318.

Sepici-Dincel A, Acikgöz S, Cevik C, Sengelen M, Yesilada E (2007). Effects of in vivo antioxidant enzyme activities of myrtle oil in normoglycaemic and alloxan diabetic rabbits. *J Ethnopharmacol* 110: 498–503.

Sezik E, Kaya S, Aydan N (1984). The effect of *Ecbalium elaterium* fruits in the treatment of sinusitis. In: Baser K H C, Kırımer N, eds. *Proceedings of IVth Meeting of Plant Originated Drug Raw Materials.* Eskisehir: Anadolu University, p. 65.

Sezik E, Tabata M, Yesilada E, *et al.* (1991). Traditional medicine in Turkey I. Folk medicine in Northeast Anatolia. *J Ethnopharmacol* 35: 191–196.

Sezik E, Zor M, Yesilada E (1992). Traditional medicine in Turkey II. Folk medicine in Kastamonu province. *Int J Pharmacognosy* 30: 233–239.

Sezik E, Aslan M, Yesilada M, *et al.* (2005). Hypoglycaemic activity of *Gentiana olivieri* and isolation of the active constituent through bioassay-directed fractionation techniques. *Life Sci* 76: 1223–1238.

Tahraoui A, El-Hilaly J, Israili ZH, *et al.* (2007). Ethnopharmacological survey of plants used in the traditional treatment of hypertension and diabetes in south-eastern Morocco (Errachidia province). *J Ethnopharmacol* 11: 105–117.

Yesilada E, Tanaka S, Sezik E, *et al.* (1988). Isolation of an anti-inflammatory principle from the fruit juice of *Ecbalium elaterium*. *J Nat Prod* 51: 504–508.

Yesilada E, Tanaka S, Tabata M, *et al.* (1989). Anti-inflammatory effects of the fruit juce of *Ecbalium elaterium* on edemas in mice. *Phytother Res* 3: 75–76.

Yesilada E, Sezik E (1990). Screening of some Turkish medicinal plants which are used in the treatment of some inflammatory diseases for their anti-inflammatory activities. *Planta Med* 56: 659.

Yesilada E, Sezik E, Fujita T, *et al.* (1993). Screening of some Turkish medicinal plants for their anti-ulcerogenic activities. *Phytother Res* 7: 263–265.

Yesilada E, Honda G, Sezik E, *et al.* (1995). Traditional medicine in Turkey V. Folk medicine in inner Taurus Mountains. *J Ethnopharmacol* 46: 133–152.

Yesilada E (1997a). Evaluation of anti-inflammatory activity of a Turkish medicinal plant: *Sambucus ebulus*. *Chem Nat Prod* 13: 696–697.

Yesilada E, Gürbüz I, Ergun E (1997b). Effects of *Cistus laurifolius* L flowers on gastric and duodenal lesions. *J Ethnopharmacol* 55: 201–211.

Yesilada E, Ustün O, Sezik E, *et al.* (1997c). Inhibitory effects of Turkish folk remedies on inflammatory cytokines: interleukin-1α, interleukin-1β and tumor necrosis factor α. *J Ethnopharmacol* 58: 59–73.

Yesilada E, Gürbüz I (1998). Evaluation of the anti-ulcerogenic effect of the flowering herbs of *Hypericum perforatum*. *J Fac Pharm Gazi Univ* 15: 25–31.

Yesilada E, Takaishi Y (1999a). A saponin with anti-ulcerogenic effect from the flowers of *Spartium junceum*. *Phytochemistry* 51: 903–908.

Yesilada E, Gürbüz I, Shibata H (1999b). Screening of Turkish anti-ulcerogenic folk remedies for anti-*Helicobacter pylori* activity. *J Ethnopharmacol* 66: 289–293.

Yesilada E, Takaishi Y, Fujita T, *et al.* (2000a). Antiulcerogenic effects of *Spartium junceum* flowers on in vivo test models in rats. *J Ethnopharmacol* 70: 219–226.

Yesilada E, Tsuchiya K, Takaishi Y, *et al.* (2000b). Isolation and characterization of free radical scavenging flavonoid glycosides from the flowers of *Spartium junceum* by activity-guided fractionation. *J Ethnopharmacol* 73: 471–478.

Yesilada E, Taninaka H, Takaishi Y, *et al.* (2001). In vitro inhibitory effects of *Daphne oleoides* ssp. *oleoides* on inflammatory cytokines and activity-guided isolation of active constituents. *Cytokine* 13: 359–364.

Yesilada E (2002). Biodiversity in Turkish folk medicine. In: Sener B, ed. *Biodiversity: Biomolecular aspects of biodiversity and innovative utilization*. London: Kluwer Academic/Plenum Publishers, 119–135.

Yesilada E, Küpeli E (2002). *Berberis crataegina* DC. root exhibits potent anti-inflammatory, analgesic and febrifuge effects in mice and rats. *J Ethnopharmacol* 79: 237–248.

Yesilada E, Sezik E (2003). A Survey on the traditional medicine in Turkey: semi-quantitative evaluation of the results. In: Singh V K, Govil J N, Hashmi S, Singh G, eds. *Ethnomedicine and Pharmacognosy: Recent Progress in Medicinal Plants. Vol.VII*. Houston, Texas: Studium Press, LLC, 389–412.

Yesilada E, Gürbüz I, Bedir E, *et al.* (2004). Isolation of anti-ulcerogenic sesquiterpene lactones from *Centaurea solstitalis* L. ssp. *solstitialis* through bioassay-guided fractionation procedures in rats. *J Ethnopharmacol* 95: 213–219.

Yesilada E (2005). Past and future contributions to traditional medicine in the health care system of the Middle-East. *J Ethnopharmacol* 100: 135–137.

Yildirim OF (1994). *Studies on the Effect of Momordica Charantia L. on the Experimentally Induced Peptic Ulcer in Rats*. Masters thesis, Gazi University, Institute of Medical Sciences.

4

Traditional Chinese medicines: the challenge of acceptance by Western medicine

Chang-Xiao Liu, Pei-Gen Xiao and Nai-Ning Song

Introduction

Chinese materia medica is an important part of Chinese traditional and herbal medicine and Chinese civilisation. The first book on Chinese materia medica, *Herbal Classics of the Divine Plowman* (*Shen-nong Bencao Jing*), known as 'the canon of materia medica' was composed in the second century BC under the pseudonym of Shennong, 'the Holy Farmer'. China remains one of the leading nations in the use of medicinal plants and recently developments have occurred so that medicinal plants still play an outstanding role in official health services in China. More than five thousand species have been identified as medicinal plants in China and the last edition of the Chinese pharmacopoeia (PRC Pharmacopoeia Committee, 2005) recorded more than 1146 Chinese drugs originating from medicinal plants, although it should be noted that the division between foods and medicine is less than in many other cultures (Liu and Xiao, 1992; Liu *et al.*, 2000).

The discovery of drugs is accredited to the emperor Shennong, who tried hundreds of herbs and tested seventy poisons in a day. The first book on Chinese materia medica, believed to have been written about 2000 years ago, is named *Shennong Bencao Jing (Shennong Herbs)*. It represents a systematic account of all knowledge related to the application of drugs in that period in Chinese history. Unfortunately, the original text was lost long ago and what is available today is a script re-edited during the Ming and Qing dynasties from quotations contained in many other classics.

The Chinese pharmacopoeia has made big changes to its format in recent editions (PRC Pharmacopoeia Committee, 1953, 1963, 1977, 1985, 1990, 1995, 2000, 2005). The 1977 edition of the Chinese pharmacopoeia was issued in two volumes, the first being devoted to Chinese materia medica and described 744 drugs and 270 compound formulations. These numbers increased with subsequent editions. A recent survey of editions of pharmacopoeias of the People's Republic of China (PRC), showed that at least 80% of Chinese traditional and herb drugs are from plant origin (PRC Pharmacopoeia Committee, 1953, 1963, 1977, 1985, 1990, 1995, 2000, 2005; Liu *et al.*, 2000a).

Commonly used Chinese materia medica comprise about 500 species (Liu and Xiao, 1986, 1992, 2000). The plants' phyla contain over 11,000 medicinal plant species (Table 4.1).

The 2000 edition of the PRC's pharmacopoeia listed 531 kinds of drugs from a variety of plant families. Those containing over 100 medicinal plant species are listed in Table 4.2; genera with over 15 medicinal plant species, and so a higher proportion of therapeutic members, are listed in Table 4.3.

The large numbers of species mentioned is due to the wide range of habitats in China and the fact that China has a long history in the effective use of traditional Chinese medicine. The Chinese government has emphasised the systematisation of traditional Chinese medicines (TCM) and raising it to higher levels, so TCMs and their preparations are now widely accepted throughout the PRC.

Table 4.1 An overview of Chinese medicinal plants

Origin	Number of medicinal plant species
Thallophytes	467
Bryophytes	48
Pteridophytes	455
Gymnosperms	126
Angiosperms	
Dicotyledons	8598
Monocotyledons	1429
Total	11 118

Table 4.2 Families containing over 100 medicinal plant species mentioned in the Chinese pharmacopoeia

Family	Medicinal species/genera	Example of important medicinally used genera
Compositae	778/155	*Artemisia, Senecio, Aster, Saussurea, Atractylodes*
Euphorbiaceae	160/39	*Euphorbia, Glochidion, Croton, Mallotus*
Labiatae	436/75	*Fritillaria, Polygonatum, Smilax, Ophiopogon, Veratrum, Allium*
Leguminosae	490/107	*Cassia, Sophora, Crotalaria, Glycyrrhiza, Indigofera, Astragalus, Aconitum, Delphinium, Thalictrum*
Liliaceae	358/46	*Crataegus, Prunus, Rosa, Chuenomeles, Rubus, Potentilla*
Orchidaceae	287/76	*Dendrobium, Gastrodia, Habenaria, Liparis, Bletilla*
Papaveraceae	135/15	*Corydalis, Meconopsis, Papaver*
Polygonaceae	123/8	*Rheum, Polygonum, Fagopyrum*
Ranunculaceae	420/34	*Clematis, Anemone, Coptis, Salvia, Rabdosia, Nepeta, Clinopodium, Scutellaria, Thymus*
Rosaceae	360/39	*Dendrobium, Gastrodia, Habenaria, Liparis, Bletilla*
Rubiaceae	219/59	*Uncaria, Hedyotis (Oldenlandia), Morinda, Rubia, Gardenia*
Saxifragaceae	155/24	*Astilbe, Bergenia, Hydrangea, Saxifrage*
Umbelliferae	234/55	*Angelica, Heracleum, Bupleurum, Feruls, Ligusticum, Peucedanum*

Table 4.3 Genera containing over 15 medicinal species and with a higher proportion of therapeutic members

Genus	Species/total species	Main ethnopharmacological data
Aconitum	46/167	Anodyne; antirheumatic
Aralia	19/30	Dispelling; internal cold; arrow poison; asthmolytic; cardiotonic
Aristolochia	31/39	General tonic; antirheumatic; promote circulation for various infections; snakebite; abdominal treatment
Berberis	67/200	Antidysentery; various infections; antipyretic; antidote
Codonopsis	26/50	Tonic; invigorates the functions of the digestive system; for weakness
Corydalis	73/150	Anodyne; treatment of coronary heart diseases; febrile and detoxicant
Delphinium	35/113	Anodyne; antirheumatic
Dendrobium	35/60	Tonic; for febrile diseases with thirst and dry mouth; dry cough and chronic tidal fever
Hypericum	16/50	Antimicrobial; emenogogue; treatment of hepatitis
Lysimachia	28/50	Invigorating blood circulation and eliminating blood stasis; asthmolytic; for menstrual disorders
Rabdosia	30/90	Antimicrobial; anticancer; febrifugal; detoxicant
Salvia	41/78	Antimicrobial; treatment of coronary heart disease
Swertia	22/70	Treatment of hepatitis; bitter-tonic; febrifugal and detoxicant
Thalictrum	39/67	Antipyretic; antimicrobial; for various infections; anticancer
Gentiana	53/247	Antipyretic; antidote; stomachic; anti-inflammatory
Scutellaria	33/102	Antipyretic; antidote; promote circulation

Sustainability of resources of medicinal materials

The pathways of development of resources

Medicinal resources are the basis of development and application of TCM. The resources included in Chinese crude drugs are geo-authentic (*Di Dao*) crude drugs; conservation and implementation; introduction; acclimatisation and cultivation; and good agricultural practice (GAP). Geo-authentic crude drugs comprise part of Chinese crude drugs, but should be differentiated from 'ordinary' Chinese crude drugs in that they have specific germ plasma, production sites, and/or specific production techniques and processing methods.

Owing to the destruction of forests, overgrazing of meadows, expansion of industry and urbanisation, as well as excessive collection in the wild of rare and endangered plants or animals, the natural resources of medicinal plants or animals are being reduced day by day. There has therefore been an urgent need to draw up necessary plans for medicinal resource utilisation and conservation.

Conservation and implementation

Although abundant and rich, resources of medicinal plants are not unlimited and must be protected by law as well as by people. Collection of any medicinal plant should be guided by precise knowledge of the species, including its locality, time of maturation, the parts to be collected, and its conservation needs. Steps should be taken to avoid over-exploitation and excessive collection. The gathering of rare and endangered species, such as *Panax ginseng* C.A. Mey., *Coptis chinensis* Franch., *Gastrodia elata* Bl. and *Paris polyphylla* Sm., should be prohibited and gene banks of medicinal plants have already been set up in some instances to preserve the gene pool.

Introduction and acclimatisation

Several plants listed in the ancient Chinese materia medica were actually of foreign origin and even today are imported to some extent, e.g. American ginseng from North America. To meet the market demand, several botanical gardens in China have introduced these plants for acclimatisation, aimed at eventual plantations, e.g. *Panax quinquefolium* L., *Amomum kravanh* L. and *Strychnos nux-vomica* L. This policy also includes non-official crude drugs of wild origin, which have been used by people for practical medication, e.g. *Schisandra chinensis* Baill., *Gentiana scabra* L., *Cistanche desreticola* Murr., *Asarum sieboldii* Miq., *Scutellaria baicalensis* Georgi.

Cultivation

The increasing use of medicinal plants in China necessitates cultivation of the most commonly used ones to guarantee supplies. About 100 species of medicinal plants are under cultivation, covering some 460 000 hectares (Liu and Xiao, 1995). The most important cultivated medicinal plants are *Panax ginseng* C.A. Mey., *Panax notoginseng* (Burt.) F.H. Chen, *Astragalus mongholicus* Koidz., *Angelica sinensis* (Oliv.) Diels, *Coptis chinensis* Franch., *Codonopsis pilosula* (Franch.) Nannf., *Rehmannia glutinosa* Libosch. *f. hueichingensis* (Chao et Schih) Hsiao, *Paeonia suffruticosa* Andr., *Cinnamomum cassia* Bl., *Amomum villosum* Lour. and *Atractylodes macrocephala* Koidz.

Several wild-growing medicinal plants, which are needed in vast quantities, are not cultivated, e.g. *Glycyrrhiza uralensis* Fisch., *Rheum palmatum* L., *Poria cocos* (Schw.) Wolf, *Dioscorea nipponica* Makino. As an approach to GAP, modern biological technology has been used for tissue culture in propagating *Lithospermum erythrorhizon* Sieb. et Zucc., *Panax quinquefolium* L., *Corydalis yanhusuo* and *Scopolia tangutica* Maxim.

Sustainability for resources

Sustainability of medicinal plant materials will become an important future criterion for success in the application of TCMs as a major marketed entity, since taking a plant from only wild sources, such as the forests or the meadows, can almost eliminate that plant, if cultural techniques for crop development are not introduced.

In the nationwide general investigation for medicinal plant materials in 1983, 12 809 kinds of plant resources in China were counted. However, the number decreased by half in less than 20 years so that, in an investigation done in 2001, there only remained about 6000 kinds of medicinal plant materials according to ingredients for prescription. Since medicinal plant materials are basic items in the modernisation of TCM, it is necessary to achieve the continuous use of the resources. To ensure the quality and quantity of TCMs, the need for standardised culturing of medicinal plants has emerged. In 2002, the Chinese State Food and Drug Administration (SFDA), formulated a guideline for good agricultural practice for Chinese crude drugs (SFDA, 2002). In 2004 the World Health Organization (WHO) issued a set of guidelines for good agricultural and collection practices for medicinal plants (GACP) (World Health Organization, 2004). These guidelines are specially aimed at the protection of medicinal plants or animals and the promotion of their cultivation, collection, and use in a sustainable manner which conserves the medicinal resource and the enviroment. There now are 448 bases for growing medicinal plants under GAP distributed in the 24 provinces. In 18 selected provinces, the area under fully controlled cultivation reaches nearly a million square kilometres.

The GAP policy was passed by the SFDA in 2002 and is designed to regulate the production of Chinese crude drugs, ensure their quality and facilitate the standardisation and modernisation of TCMs. GAP is applicable to producers of Chinese crude drugs for the entire production process of Chinese crude drugs.

Producers should adopt standardised management and quality control measures to ensure continuing resources of natural crude drugs and protect the ecological environment, as well as to achieve sustainable utilisation based on the principle of 'maximum sustainable yield'.

The environmental conditions of production sites for Chinese crude drugs should meet the requirements of the related national standards for atmospheric conditions, air quality, soil quality and irrigation. According to the growing needs for medicinal plants, appropriate areas for cultivation should be determined and standard operating procedures for cultivation should be formulated. Types, period and amount of fertilisation should be determined subject to the nutritional requirements of medicinal plants and soil fertility. Organic manure should be the main fertilising agent, and fertilisers should be applied sparingly in accordance with the growing needs of plants. Field management should be strengthened in accordance with the characteristic changing of medicinal plants and their parts for use, furthermore topping, deflowering, pruning, shading and other measures should be carried out appropriately to adjust the growth of plants, so as to increase the yield of the crude drugs and maintain the consistency of quality.

Integrated pest management should be adopted for the control of diseases and pests. If necessary, minimum effective input of certain high-efficacy, hypotoxic and low-residue pesticides can be used according to the Regulations for Pesticides Management of the PRC, so as to reduce residues of pesticides, avoid heavy metal contamination and protect the ecological environment.

Collection of wild and semi-wild medicinal plants or animals should conform to the principle of 'maximum sustainable yield'. Fostering, rotation and conservation should be planned and carried out to benefit propagation and renewal of resources. Appropriate collection periods (season and years) and methods should be determined in accordance with the quality and yield of the plants with reference to traditional experience, etc. After being collected, the medicinal parts should be selected, washed, cut or trimmed. Those that need drying should use appropriate methods and techniques, with controlled temperature and humidity. Contamination should be prevented and degradation of active constituents should be avoided.

Producers should establish a quality management department that is responsible for supervision and quality control for the entire production process, and should have adequate staff, premises, instruments and equipment to meet the requirements of the scale of production and species identification. This department is responsible for monitoring the environment, hygiene, testing production and packaging materials, as well as the crude drugs. All of these must be adequately documented.

Traditional processing of Chinese crude drugs and pharmacological effects

The processing of Chinese crude drugs means preparing Chinese materia medica with techniques according to the theories of traditional Chinese medicine, to meet clinical requirements of dispensing prescriptions and making ready-made medicines.

The processing of Chinese crude drugs is a complicated job, which may consist of cleansing, cutting into smaller pieces with a guillotine, reducing toxicity, changing their property, enhancing therapeutic activities, improving unpleasant taste or smell, and separating different parts of a drug for different uses. Cleansing and trimming includes selecting, sieving, winnowing, shaking, brushing, wiping or scraping, digging, squeezing, rubbing, picking, tearing and peeling, striking, embracing, rolling and tying, washing, floating, soaking, rinsing, filtering, moistening and retting. Refining of prescribed powder medicines may be achieved by burning over flames, drying over a small fire, sunning, airing, staining, etc. Cooking includes stir-frying, scalding, simmering or baking in hot ashes, roasting, broiling with fluid substances in a pan, calcining, quenching, steaming, boiling, reproducing, reducing into powder after removal of oil or reparation of frost-like powder fermentation, germination, efflorescence and squeezing juice.

Safety aspects

Recent trends in the scope of pharmacovigilance

Pharmacovigilance is a science and activity relating to the detection, assessment, understanding and prevention of adverse effects or any other possible drug-related problems. Signal-reported information is a possible causal relationship between an adverse event and a drug, which was unknown or incompletely documented previously. Usually more than a single report is required to generate a signal, depending upon the seriousness of the event and the quality of the information.

The Erice Declaration sets out the principles of good communication practices in pharmacovigilance. It states that industrialists, doctors, and patients had different — but not contradictory — points of view when questions of drug safety are at issue. Trust and partnerships between the groups were considered important, and a wider public debate was deemed desirable, to help the public better understand risk. Crisis management is also an important matter where communication plays a major role. Several aspects of the communication of benefit–risk information were outlined in the Declaration. During drug therapy, adverse events are frequent. Frequently, several drugs are given at the same time as combined therapy, and concurrent medicines are provided simultaneously for opportunistic infections. All of these factors make the evaluation of the safety of the compound complicated. The numbers of patients in clinical trials and the duration of treatment should be maximised, while exclusions should be minimised. Safety data should be collected and analysed, and the relevance of surrogate markers be questioned. Post-authorisation safety surveillance is important and has to be planned in advance.

Adverse event/adverse experiences

These are defined as any untoward medical occurrence that may present during treatment with a pharmaceutical product but that does not necessarily have a causal relationship with this treatment.

Side-effects

These may be the many unintended effects of a pharmaceutical product occurring at doses normally used in humans, which are related to the pharmacological proprieties of the drug. Essential elements of this definition are the pharmacological nature of the effect, which means that the phenomenon is unintended, and there is no overt overdose.

Adverse reactions

These are responses to a drug which are noxious and unintended, occurring at doses normally used in humans for the prophylaxis, diagnosis, therapy of disease, or for modification of physiological function.

Pharmacovigilance concerns cover herbal medicines and any significant enhancement of health system performance can be achieved by preventing adverse events in particular, and improving patients' safety and healthcare quality in general.

To develop global norms, the following aspects should be emphasised:

- the development of standards and guidelines for definition, measurement and reporting of adverse events
- the provision of support to countries in developing reporting systems taking preventive action
- the promotion of framing of evidence-based policies, including global standards that will improve patient care, with particular emphasis on such aspects as product safety, safe clinical practice and safe use of medicinal products and medical devices
- the creation of a culture of safety within healthcare organisations.

In recent years, extensive attention has been paid to the safety of traditional Chinese medicine in China and throughout the world. Despite the large numbers of plants used in TCM, less than 1% are classified as toxic. Traditionally, there existed '18 incompatible medicinal herbs' and '19 mutual restraining medicinal herbs', which were the sum of clinical experience for drug inter-reaction and coadministration of herbs. Severe side-effects may occur when two incompatible or mutual restraining drugs are used in coadministration.

The TCM materials that have attracted attention because of its toxicity are species of *Aristolochia*. Clinically, the renal toxicity induced by *Caulis aristolochiae manshuriensis* was first reported over 40 years ago (Wu, 1964) and later by Zhou *et al.* in 1979 and 1988. The renal toxicity induced by medicinal plants was called Chinese herb nephropathy by foreign researchers and it was concluded that the nephropathy was mainly induced by the aristolochic acid contained in *Akebia quinata* Decne. and *Cocculus laurifolius* DC. Therefore, in some investigations, it was suggested that 'Chinese herb nephropathy' be renamed aristolochic acid nephropathy. Recent studies showed that aristolochic acid present in *Aristolochia debilis* Sibe. et Zucc. and *Aristolochia fungchi* YC Wuex LD Chow et SM Hwang induces renal toxicity. The report produced enormous effects in the TCM market all over the world.

Safety issues may arise from the following conditions:

- overdose administration
- administration for a long time
- unsuitable combinations with other drugs
- use of different drugs from related species, e.g. *Bupleurum longnirudium* is used instead of *Bupleurum chinensis* or *Bupleurum scorzomerifolium*, *Aristolochia fungchi* YC Wuex LD Chow et SM Hwang used instead of *Stephania tetrandra* S. Moore
- preparation of the herbs
- the patient's individual differences in drug reaction, pharmacogenes, metabolism, and allergic functions.

Facing these issues, Chinese researchers have applied modern scientific methods to understand the safety of TCM, such as fingerprint techniques to control quality and production practice. In clinical studies, doctors must implement GCP ethically and in clinical therapy, carry out individual therapeutic principles according to the theory of TCM. In basic research on the safety of TCM, toxicology, toxicokinetics and pharmacokinetics, metabolomics and metabonomics methods are used to test the toxicity, effectivity and mechanism of action, enzyme inhibition and induction methods to investigate drug–drug reactions. The induction and inhibition of TCM on cytochrome P450 activities is of particular importance. The information from these studies suggests that TCM with conventional therapeutic products may increase the plasma levels of some therapeutic agents, which would increase the risk for serious drug adverse events in patients. Conversely, the interaction between TCM and conventional therapies may also affect the safety profile of the TCM, highlighting a need for healthcare professionals to recognise and understand the potential risk of TCM herb–drug interactions (Ge *et al.*, 2005; Liu, 2005; Lu *et al.*, 2005).

Conventional recognition of the safety of Chinese herbal medicines

In *Shennong's Canon of Chinese Materia Medica* (AD 1000), the 365 sorts of Chinese drugs recorded were divided according to their toxicity and property into three groups:

- Group 1 (120 drugs) comprises those that are least toxic, are non-toxic, of high safety, beneficial to the human body, suitable to be taken frequently, and functioning as nourishing and tonic agents. Examples include *Radix Ginseng*, *Radix Salviae Miltiorrhiza*, *Radix Achyranthis Bidentatae*, *Colla Corli Asini* and *Radix Glycyrrhizae*.
- Group 2 (120 drugs) could or could not be toxic, meaning that if the drugs are correctly used, they are non-toxic. Examples are *Radix Lithospermi* and *Radix Trichosanthis*.
- Group 3 (another 120 drugs) are usually toxic and not suitable for long-term intake, and include *Radix Dichroae* and *Radix Pulsatillae*.

This recognition of the toxicity and safety of Chinese drugs has been successful in clinical practice, and handed down from generation to generation. Among the 534 kinds of Chinese herbal drugs in the present pharmacopoeia of the PRC, there are 49 with high toxicity, e.g. *Semen Strychni*, *Rhizoma Pinellae*, *Caulis Aristolochiae Manshuriensis*, *Radix Aconiti*, *Radix Sophorae Tonkinensis* and *Rhizoma Anemones Raddeanae*, and 22 with slight toxicity, e.g. *Radix Zanthoxyli*, *Rhizoma Dryopteris Crassi rhizomatis* and *Cortex Meliae*, the other 463 being non-toxic. However, this conventional recognition of the toxicity and safety of Chinese drugs is based on traditional experience and can no longer meet the demands of modern society (Xiao and Liu, 2004), so a re-evaluation is necessary.

Understanding of the safety matters of Chinese medicines

As the case stands, TCMs do have adverse effects. A total of 6061 cases of intoxication and adverse effects from Chinese drugs were reported between 1915 and 1994, among which 2217 cases were reported in the 1980s, and 3272 in the four years from 1991 to 1994 (Yuan, 2000). Therefore, wide attention has been paid to this problem and many papers have been published (Wang and Lu, 1999; Wang and Ren, 2002; Yu *et al.*, 2003).

Because the quality of TCM is very variable, quality and standardisation of Chinese drugs are stressed as of major importance in the National Program for Modernisation of Traditional Chinese Medicine (2002–2010). Application of various codes of good practice has established a good basis for safe usage of Chinese herbal medicines. In 2001, the Chinese government released its Drug Administration Act and Drug Registration Regulation to standardise the research, development and marketing of new drugs of chemical products and traditional Chinese medicines, which specified documents with scientific test data (SFDA, 2002).

Measures for strengthening the safety of Chinese medicines

Unfortunately publicity for TCM preparations is sometimes one-sided and promotes them as 'pure natural drugs without any toxic adverse effect'. To repudiate this, the potential toxic side-effects and adverse reactions should be stressed, and commonly used herbs should comply with acceptable processes of purification and production of dosage forms.

A five-grade evaluation system for safety, which may act as a reference for further study, correction and supplementation is put forward below.

Grade I

- Herbs that have been regarded as foods for a long time, but have some medical function, where LD_{50} was not detected in animal studies, or the maximum tolerant dosage is more than 10 g/kg.
- Long-term toxicity (30 days feeding) was not detected, with no evident adverse effect and toxicity when 100 times the human adult dosage was administered.
- The 'three-genesis' test (carcinogenesis, teratogenesis and mutagenesis) was negative.

Inclusion of herbs in this grade is based on *Ingredients of Foods in China* (Yang *et al.*, 2002).

Grade II

- Herbs that have served both as foods or medications historically, with LD_{50} more than 10 g/kg.
- Long-term toxicity could not be detected (30 days feeding), with no evident adverse effect and toxicity when 100 times the human adult dosage was administered.
- The three-genesis test was negative.

Inclusion of herbs in this grade is based on Document file No. 51 (Ministry of Health, 2002).

Grade III

- This grade includes herbs taken as health-giving food for a long time, such as drug diet or drug tea, which have some therapeutic functions and effects. No toxic-adverse effects were found when more than 2 g/kg of the extract or more than 5 g/kg of crude drug was administered.
- Long-term toxicity could be detected (30 days feeding): mild, nonfatal, reversible adverse effect, and toxicity could be detected when 100 times the human adult dosage was administrated.
- The three-genesis test was negative.

Inclusion of herbs in this grade is based on Document file No. 51 (Ministry of Health, 2002).

Grade IV

- Herbs that have evident medical function or effect, possess active ingredients of intensive pharmaceutical effect, are liable to lead to toxic adverse effects when improperly used; LD_{50} could be detected.

- Long-term toxicity could be detected (30 days feeding) in its extract when the dosage is less than 2–5 g/kg; nonfatal, non-incapacitant adverse reaction could be caused by 50 times the dosage for human adults, but no evident toxic adverse effect is found in administration of 30 times the dosage for human adults.
- Some types could induce a positive reaction in the three-genesis test.

Grade V

- Drugs with evident toxic adverse effects, being mildly, moderately or potently toxic when given by different routes, containing ingredients (such as digitoxin) with potent toxicity, easy to induce toxic-adverse effect; LD_{50} of the extract less than 1 g/kg, and that of the crude drug less than 2 g/kg.
- Long-term toxicity (30 days feeding) could be detected; 30 times the dosage for human adults could induce toxic adverse, or even fatal, incapacitant and irreversible reaction.
- Positive reaction to the three-genesis test; maternal perinatal toxicity tests show mother–child inter-generational toxicity.

According to the principles of evidence-based medicine, the causes and characteristics of adverse reactions to Chinese herbs should be determined by literature review and meta-analyses, to work out methods and programmes for prevention. Ideally large sample sizes and multifactor statistical management of the results should be used.

China established a nationwide adverse drug reaction surveillance system in 2003 and up to 2007, case reports concerning adverse reactions to Chinese drugs accounted for 10–14% of the total, which is significantly lower than those about chemical agents, reflecting that, as to safety, Chinese drugs are still better than chemical agents. The system of circulating information about adverse reaction of drugs was created at that time, with six issues released so far, and reported eight Chinese drugs with adverse reaction and one kind containing aristolochic acids. Renal damage by Longdan Xiegan pill has been notified, for which active measures were taken by the State Bureau of Foods and Drugs Supervision and Administration.

On an international level, China is involved with the WHO Forum on Harmonization of Herbal Medicine (FHM) and also with a technical cooperation programme with WHO, the *Guidance for Safety of Commonly Used Chinese Herbal Medicines (Chinese Diagram)*.

Research and development of new drugs

Many pharmacologically active compounds from plants have the potential to become single chemical entity drugs. About 140 new drugs have originated directly or indirectly from Chinese medicinal plants by means of modern scientific methods, demonstrating that these herbs are an important source of new drugs.

Alkaloids are an important group and include the benzylisoquinoline type, potentially serving as the basis of new drugs for analgesic, sedative, antimicrobial and cardiovascular ailments. The tropane-type alkaloids such as anisodamine and anisodine isolated from *Scopolia* are attractive for their effect on microcirculatory systems. The diterpene-type alkaloids isolated from *Aconitum* and *Delphinium* provide a starting point in the quest for more effective anodyne, antiarrhythmia and cardiotonic drugs, while the alkaloids related to harringtonine have potential antileukaemic action. Among phenolic compounds, several flavonoids such as scutellarin, icariin, isorhanetin and puerarin, and the coumarins such as daphnetin and daphnoretin, need to be considered for their cardiovascular activity. Within the terpenoids, many monoterpenes display effects against respiratory problems and can perhaps be used in the development of more favourable remedial medicines. Several peroxide substances, such as quinhuosu (artenisin-in) and yingzhaosu A, hold promise as antimalarial agents.

Since 1949 there have been many scientific reports on Chinese medicinal plants, and this forms a solid platform for further work (Xiao, 1983; 1986; 1988; Xiao and Fu, 1986; Liu and Xiao, 1992; 1993; 2000; Xiao and Liu, 1999; Liu, 1987; Liu *et al.*, 2000).

Pathways for research and development from TCMs

The numerous prescriptions, folk drugs and herbal drugs play an important role in maintaining people's health. They are also the resources for research and development of new drugs; pathways for discovery and development of new drugs from Chinese traditional and herbal drugs are discussed below.

Research conducted under the guidance of experiences of TCMs

There is no record of the term 'chronic mylocytic leuk[a]emia' in the classics of TCM. However, based on the theories and methods of TCM diagnosis, this condition can be diagnosed and treated according to the symptoms involved. A complex prescription, 'Dnggui-Luhui' pills, has been used for this purpose and was confirmed with a clinical trial on 22 patients. The prescription consists of:

- *Angelica sinensis* (root)
- *Aloe vera* (dried juice)
- *Gentiana acabra* (fructus)
- *Gardenia jasminoides* (root)
- *Scutellaria baicalensis* (root)
- *Phellodendron amurense* (stem bark)
- *Coptis chinensis* (rhizome)
- *Rheum palmatum* (root and rhizome)
- Indigo Naturalis, a product derived from the leaves of *Saphicacanthus cusia*
- *Aucklandis lappa* (root).

Subsequent experimentation conducted with the animal model of leukaemia 7212 (L7212) in mice revealed that only Indigo Naturalis among the ingredients of the prescription was effective, but that it was accompanied with some side-effects.

In an effort to increase the therapeutic effect and reduce the side-effects, further study of Indigo Naturalis has been done. Indirubin was identified as the active anticancer principle. The compound showed various inhibitory activities against leukaemia in animal studies and toxicological studies showed that, when it was given daily for a month at an oral dose of 100–500 mg/kg, no toxicological reactions were observed. A clinical trial was carried out in 314 cases of chronic myelocytic leukaemia and 82 patients achieved complete remission with a further 87 having partial remission and other beneficial effects, although side-effects such as abdominal pain and diarrhoea sometimes occurred. Indirubin has been shown to have similar therapeutic effect as myleran in the treatment of chronic myelocytic leukaemia. It possesses neither serious side-effects nor inhibition of bone marrow.

It is not necessary to repeat here the story of the development of artemisinin from the Chinese traditional antimalarial drug, *Artemisia annua*, to a globally accepted antimalarial.

Exploration of ancient literature of TCM in modern clinical studies

In the ancient classic *Shanghanlun* (*Treatise on Febrile Diseases*, edited by Zhang Zhong-Jing), it was recorded that Gegen Decoction, a decoction of the root of *Pueraria lobata*, was recommended for the treatment of stiffness and soreness in the neck. A series of clinical trials of preparation of *Pueraria lobata* gave satisfactory results and the active isoflavone components of this plant were isolated, e.g. daidzin and puerarin. Pharmacological studies revealed that either the total isoflavone or the single compound puerarin was capable of increasing the cerebral and coronary blood flow, decreasing the oxygen consumption of the myocardium, increasing the blood oxygen supply and depressing the production of lactic acid by the blood oxygen-deficient heart muscle, all of which could help explain its effects.

'Wuweizi' (Fructus *Schizandra Chinensis*), a Chinese traditional drug commonly used as an astringent, was found in clinical use to exhibit therapeutic effects on certain types of hepatitis, particularly in lowering the elevated serum glutamic pyruvic transaminase (SGPT) levels. This effect immediately aroused the interest of doctors as well as pharmacologists. It was found that the active principles responsible for lowering elevated SGPT levels were a series of lignans, of which schizandren B, schizandrol B and schizandrin C showed the best protective activity against liver damage induced by chemical substances.

'Lingzhicao' (Ganoderma), a fungus, has been regarded as a panacea in TCM and widely used in folklore for neurasthenia, chronic hepatitis, cardiovascular disease and chronic ulcers of the digestive system. Clinical studies of the water-soluble preparation of *Ganoderma capense* showed that it had a satisfactory effect on progressive muscular dystrophy and atrophic myotonia.

Drugs used by smaller ethnic groups in the PRC

Scopolia tangutica Maxim. ('Tangchom Nagbo') is a drug used by the doctors of traditional Tibetan medicine in Qinghai. Overdosage of this medicine causes the symptoms characteristic of atropine-like toxicity. Phytochemical investigation revealed that besides hyoscyamine and scopolamine, the plant contained the tropane alkaloids anisodamine and anisodine. Both are weaker in action than atropine and scopolamine in the central and peripheral nervous systems. Clinically anisodamine has been used for the treatment of septic shock from toxic bacillary dysentery, fulminant epidemic meningitis and haemorrhagic enteritis. Anisodine is used for the treatment of migraine and diseases of the fundus occuli caused by vascular spasm, organophosphorus poisoning, and acute paralysis caused by cerebral vascular accident, it is also being used as the chief component in Chinese traditional anaesthesia.

Active compounds isolated from TCMs

Of about 250 pharmacologically active compounds that have been reported from Chinese materia medica, 100 or so have been subjected to systematic chemical, pharmacological and clinical studies.

Table 4.4 shows the chemical nature of these pharmacologically active principles from Chinese medicinal plants (Liu *et al.*, 2000).

Classification of pharmacological activities

About 140 single chemical entity drugs have been discovered directly or indirectly from Chinese materia medica plants by means of modern scientific methods. By pharmacological classification, 36 affect the cardiovascular system, 23 are anticancer drugs, 21 affect the nervous system, 15 the respiratory system, 18 are antimicrobials, 14 are used for the digestive system, 9 for eliminating parasites, 5 for contraception, and 1 as an eye medicine (Liu and Yaniv, 2005).

Recent trends in research and development

Quality assurance of TCM products

Developing a new preparation from a medicinal product used for a long time in traditional Chinese medicine to meet present-day international standards of quality, safety and efficacy, and quality standardisation is a very important guarantee.

Table 4.5 shows the most important methods used in quality and standardisation. Great progress in quality studies has been achieved through the application of specific and selective methods, using a combination of high-performance liquid chromatography (HPLC) with ultraviolet, mass spectrometry (MS), or nuclear magnetic resonance (NMR). The standardisation methods are used to establish stan-

Table 4.4 The pharmacologically active principles in traditional Chinese medicines

Chemical type		Number of compounds
Alkaloids		202
Terpenes	Monoterpenes	27
	Sesquiterpenes	32
	Diterpenes	33
	Triterpenes	43
Cardiac glucosides		23
Phenolic compounds	Quinones	25
	Flavonoids	34
	Coumarins	27
	Lignans	21
	Phenyl propanoids	17
	Other	48
Acids and miscellaneous		34
Total		571

Table 4.5 Application of modern analytical methods in the quality assesssment and standardisation of traditional Chinese medicines

Method classification	Analytical method
Chromatography	Thin-layer chromatography (TLC) Thin-layer electrophoresis (TLE) High-performance liquid chromatography (HPLC) Gas chromatography (GC) Capillary electrophoresis (CE) Capillary electrochromatography (CEC) Isotachophoresis (ITP)
Mass spectrometry	Mass spectrometry (MS)
Nuclear magnetic resonance	Nuclear magnetic resonance (NMR)
Combination	HPLC coupled with MS, with MS/MS, with NMR, with UV/MS/NMR/FT-ICR

dards or fingerprints of the extract of crude drugs and preparations of TCMs. In the 2005 edition of the Chinese pharmacopoeia, HPLC was used for quality control in 77% of crude drugs of TCMs, and 94% of patent drugs and preparations.

Molecular–biological technical application in pharmacological profiles

The development and introduction of molecular biological methods with highly selective and sensitive bioassays into the screening of plant extracts or compounds from TCMs has revolutionised research. New methods on aspects such as gene, receptor and signal transduction levels provide a much better understanding of the mechanisms of action of an active compound. The new methods have revealed that the pharmacological potential of plant extracts and their preparations is greater than previously supposed.

High-throughput screening technology (HTS) is a relatively new approach, developed in the 1990s. The technology is based on the theoretical principles of drug discovery through application of multidisciplinary knowledge and integration of various advanced technologies, thereby forming a rapid, effective, and large-scale drug screening system. With the application of technology platforms based on molecular and cell biology, many new therapeutic targets, such as genes, receptors, and enzymes, have been identified and validated for drug discovery. The HTS system applied in natural product research can decrease the amount of testing samples that are difficult to isolate and purify, by using microgram quantities. Therefore, the technology is an effective tool in the early stage of drug discovery and development form TCMs.

In modern research into TCM, more screening and isolation efforts are necessary to evaluate the pharmacological and pharmacokinetic profile of extracts, preparations or active compounds. An example is the recent studies on a fixed herbal complex that has a reputation in TCM for the prevention and therapy of stroke. The herbal complex consists of eight herbs (root of *Salvia miltiorrhiza*, Rhizoma Ligustic ('Cum Chuanxiong'), root of *Paeonia rubra*, root of *Angelica pubescens*, root of *Stephania tetrandra*, ramulus of *Uncaria rhynchophylla*, rhizome of *Gastrodia elata*, and root of *Panax ginseng*).

As a result of the detailed chemical and pharmacological studies, the researchers were able to assign defined pharmacological effects to the individual herbs and their major active compounds, which in turn had a direct relevance for stroke prevention and therapy (Gong and Sucher, 1999). The clinical efficacy of this herb complex was explained by a pharmacokinetic or pharmacodynamic synergism.

Achievements in single chemical entity drug discovery and development

Salvicine

Salvicine, a diterpenoid compound, is a new topoisomerase II inhibitor and induces topo II-mediated DNA breaks (Meng *et al.*, 2001) (Figure 4.1). It is a stucturally modified derivative of a natural product from the Chinese traditional medicine *Salvia prionitis* Hance (Labiatae) (Huang *et al.*, 1990). Its pharmacological activity was evaluated against a panel of human tumour cells (Meng *et al.*, 2001) and xenografts (Qing *et al.*, 1999). Salvicine is equipotent to etoposide against three leukaemia cell lines (Zhang *et al.*, 1999). Additionally, salvicine has a prominent cytotoxic effect on multidrug-resistant cell lines. Salvicine, like most chemotherapeutic drugs, exerts

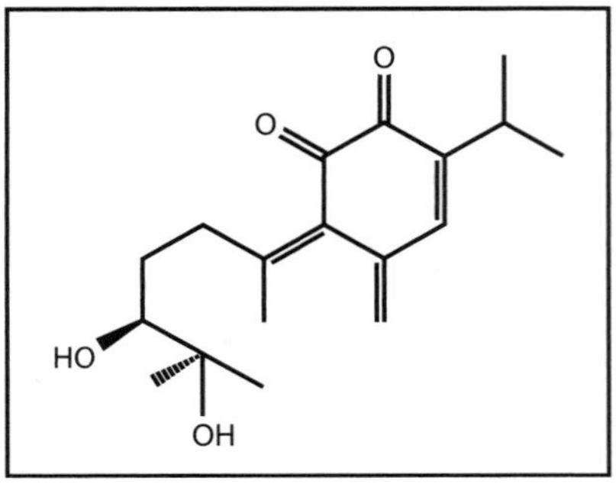

Figure 4.1 Salvicine.

its antitumour effect by inducing cancer cell apoptosis, and salvicine is equally effective at inducing apoptosis in K562 and K562/A02 cells (Qing *et al.*, 2001) and in HL60 cells (Meng *et al.*, 2001; Liu *et al.*, 2002). This compound has now entered clinical trials in patients with cancer.

Schiprizine

Schiprizine, or ZT-1 a derivative of huperzine A (Hup A), is a novel potent cholinesterase (ChE) inhibitor, which is rapidly transformed into the active metabolite Hup A, from a Chinese club moss (Figure 4.2). ZT-1 was selected from over 100 Hup A derivatives initially identified at our institute and in-vitro pharmacological tests have shown that it produces a marked concentration-dependent inhibition of acetylcholinesterase. In-vivo investigations have shown that ZT-1 is equipotent to Hup A and more potent than donepezil and tacrine (Zhu *et al.*, 1999, 2000; Anon., 2004). The preclinical studies have been finished in China and Phase I clinical trials have also been completed in Switzeland and China (Wei *et al.*, 2006; Xu *et al.*, 2005). A clinical Phase II trial, for the treatment of Alzheimer's disease, is being conducted in patients with mild-to-moderate symptoms (Anon., 2004).

Bromotetrandrine

Stephania tetrandra, containing bisbenzylisoquinoline alkaloids, has been used as an anti-inflammatory and analgesic medicine in the PRC (Figure 4.3). Recent studies have shown that the alkaloids enhanced the cytotoxicity of anticancer drugs in P-glycoprotein-dependent tumour cells. The multidrug resistance of the constituent tetrandrine and its derivatives showed that bromotetrandrine BrTet showed significant reversal of multidrug resistance *in vitro* and *in vivo* (Wang *et al.*, 2005), and clinical trials are in progress (Xiao *et al.*, 2004, 2005; Jin *et al.*, 2005).

Kanglaite injection prepared from Coix seeds

Coix seeds come from *Coix Lacryma-jobi* L. subsp. *Ma-yuen* (Romanet) T. Koyama (family *Gramineae*). In traditional Chinese medicine, coix seeds serve several functions, e.g. they stimulate function of the spleen and lung, remove heat (which helps in the drainage of pus) and induce diuresis but latterly an extract (Kanglaite) has been developed as an

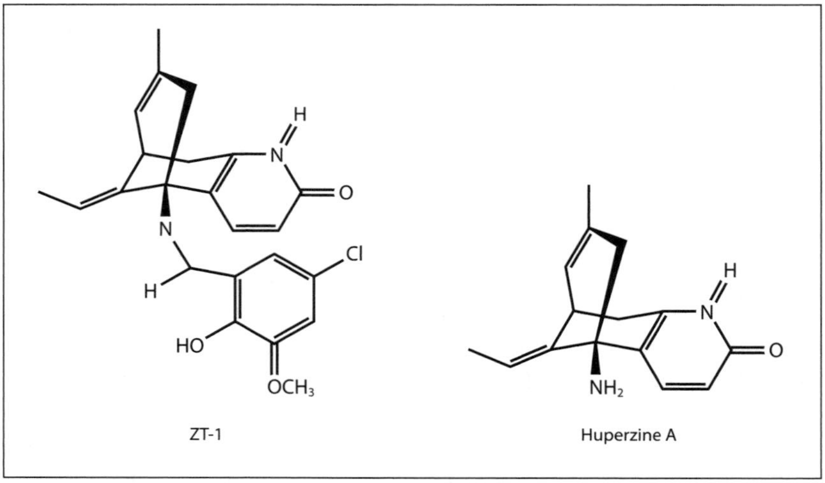

ZT-1

Huperzine A

Figure 4.2 The chemical structures of schiprzine (ZT-1) and huperzine A.

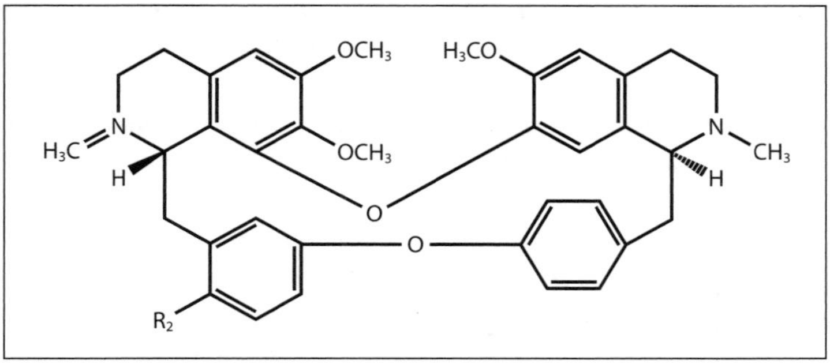

Figure 4.3 Chemical structure of bromotetrandrine. (R_1 = Br, R_2 = H).

anticancer drug. The mechanism of action of kanglaite injection is as follows. The drug:

- inhibits the mitosis of tumour cells during G_2/M phases
- induces apoptosis of tumour cells
- affects the genetic expression of tumour cells by up-regulating FAS/Apo-1 gene expression and down-regulating Bc1–2 gene expression
- inhibits tumour angiogenesis
- counteracts the cachexia of cancers
- reverses the multiresistance of tumour cells to anticancer drugs and the resistance modification in some chemotherapeutics.

Kanglaite injection has been successfully applied in the treatment of a variety of malignant tumours. The prospective, randomised and large-scale clinical studies have been carried out in 1408 cases. Clinical studies have shown that kanglaite could not only inhibit cancer cells but also enhance immunity. Moreover, kanglaite has synergistic and toxicity-reducing effects when combined with chemo- or radiotherapy. It could also relieve pain, improve the patient's quality of life and extend survival time (Li, 1998; Qian, 1998; Shen, 1998; Jin, 1999; Li, 2006).

Berbamine

Berbamine is a bisbenzylisoquinoline alkaloid (Figure 4.4) from *Berberis* spp. (Liu *et al*., 1991). From an economical viewpoint it was valuable that *Berberis* resources were comprehensively utilised to develop new drugs and new pharmacological activities (Liu, 2000b). Pharmacological studies showed that berbamine possesses a significant leukogenic effect in rats and dogs injured by anticancer agents and radioactivity and in clinical trials, a transleukogenic effect was demonstrated in 405 patients with leucopenia. It is also used as an adjuvant to chemotherapy or radiotherapy to protect the haematogenic function of bone marrow.

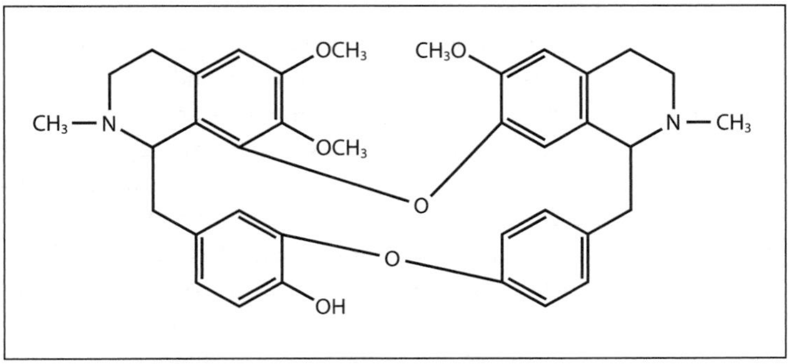

Figure 4.4 Chemical structure of berbamine.

Challenges in modern research and development

As well as its exploitation within China as a source of novel, single chemical entity drugs, TCM has also attracted interest internationally.

The first challenge: discovery and development of new drugs from TCMs

TCM development has entered a new stage of research with development from tradition to science. A major difference between the old and present-day drug development is probably that in the past, people tested the medicines directly on humans, whereas nowadays the starting point is screening at the molecular or cellular level.

The effectiveness of TCM products in the treatment of a variety of ailments and diseases has been established empirically over thousands of years. Novel standardisation methods will significantly raise the medical potential and quality of TCM. Utilising DNA fingerprinting techniques and developing cutting-edge genechip-based applications will assure standardisation for the quality of botanicals and products of TCM. Using modern molecular biology techniques, different species of commonly used TCM are being studied to identify species-specific markers. Application of this information will mean that different genera of these drugs, as well as different families and species, can be distinguished.

For example, using distinct complementary DNA sequence information derived from *Fritillaria cirrhosae* D. Don and *Fritillaria thunbergii* Miq., a silicon-based genechip was manufactured, which contained different oligonucleotide probes corresponding to the different species of *Fritillaria* plants. Thus, the genechip was used to demonstrate its capability to detect the sequence-specific probes correctly. This is useful in the development of genechip technology as a standardisation tool for other phytopharmaceutical materials. This standardisation tool can also be applied to drug discovery research. Genechip technology will be an important part of research for biologically active fractions and compounds. We envisage that the successful development of TCM will gain its own niche in today's fast-changing pharmaceutical industry.

A process system of discovery and development of new drugs from TCM has been established in many institutions in China. Figure 4.5 presents a basic process for the study of new drugs from medicinal plants used in TCM (Liu *et al.*, 2007).

In drug discovery, the active compounds obtained by in-vitro or in-vivo bioassay are isolated and then pharmacology, toxicity and safety, as well as clinical trials of the selected active compounds are performed. Where possible, an active compound and its analogues are subjected to structure–activity relationship studies to obtain more effective and safe compounds. In a traditional medicine system, pharmacological evaluation of extracts or active compounds may lead to the establishment of standardised extracts or pure compounds. In this case, these substances and their formulations can be used in pharmacology, toxicity and clinical trials.

Using the above methods in combination with clinical trials and in-vitro and in-vivo pharmacological studies, related data can be obtained about the activity of medicinal plants and their extracts. Moreover, using the systems biology approach for the organism and combining this with metabolomics data for different extracts of the medicinal plant or fractions, compound–activity relationships can be discerned. Metabolomics/metabonomics of medicinal plants is rapidly developing and it will be a key technology in the system biology in studies of activity, action mechanism, drug interaction, drug safety and relationships of medicinal plants with the environment.

The second challenge: safety of TCM products

In many parts of the world, phytotherapeutical products are only over-the-counter products. The clinical safety and interactions of these products have become an issue, one which requires careful monitoring and reporting, followed by substantial scientific study and communication to effect public awareness and enhance safety. In the PRC, the government has also issued a set of guidelines for studies of the safety and efficacy of TCM products (SFDA, 2005) and a basic process for evaluation of TCMs for facilitating the regulation and registration of TCM products has been introduced (Liu *et al.*,

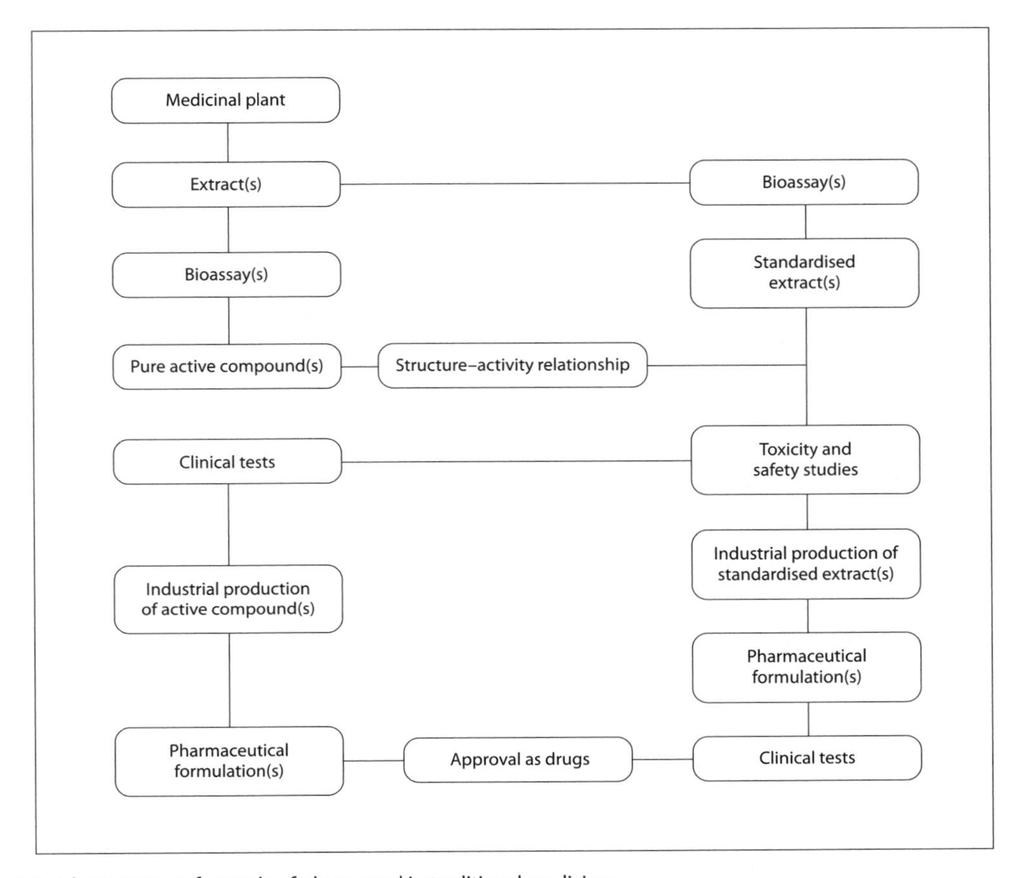

Figure 4.5 A basic process for study of plants used in traditional medicines.

2007). These aims are an important start, but are not adequate for the continuous improvement of TCM products in healthcare.

A comprehensive programme for safety evaluation of products based on traditional medicines is needed for consumers in the PRC and worldwide. The first key factor is to obtain standardised and controlled products or preparations of TCM of good quality for safety evaluation studies. They must be free of contaminants such as insects, herbicides and pesticides, solvent residues, heavy metals, aflatoxins and other toxic microbial metabolites and radioactivity (Liu *et al.*, 2007).

The third challenge: application of modern techniques and methods

Studies in TCM must face the challenge of the application of modern technological advances.

Modern techniques and methods are rapidly developing and now it is possible to measure gene expression, the proteome and metabolomics/metabonomics. These methods open a complete new world of possibilities to study the activity, mechanism of action, safety and efficacy of TCM. It will give researchers opportunities to better understand the mode of action by comparing the changes in the transcriptome, proteome and metabolomic/metabonomic patterns in comparison with those observed with known drugs. In system biological studies, the application of metabonomic methods to analyse urine samples makes it possible to identify biomarkers by nuclear magnetic resonance or liquid chromatography-MS/MS analyses, thus allowing the diagnosis of a variety of diseases, the measurement of possible liver or kidney toxicity, and the mechanism of action.

Metabolomics will be a key technology in the systems biology approach to studies of medicinal plants. Chromatography, mass spectrometry and nuclear magnetic resonance spectrometry methods are currently being used in metabolomics by measuring a selected group of metabolites in an organism qualitatively and quantitatively, and measuring fingerprints of metabolites and identifying all compounds in cells, organism, or parts of medicinal plants. This systems biology approach is a major challenge for the coming years in studying TCM and the development of such '-omics' can influence several areas of drug discovery and development.

Metabonomics can be applied at any stage in drug discovery and development processes, for example:

- predictive biomarkers for drug-related effects in animal models
- understanding the biochemical mechanisms of action to target-organ or to target-organ pathologies in animals to humans
- developing biomarkers for toxicities in non-clinical development
- predictive biomarkers for drug-related effects in humans during Phase II and Phase III clinical trails (Liu, 2004a, 2004b, 2005c, 2005d; Liu *et al.*, 2004).

Metabonomics technology has been applied in studies of the mechanism of action of complex Gensing ('Shen-Mai') injection for the treatment of cardiac disease and Complex Uncaria stem mixture for the treatment of hyperactivity syndrome in children (Liu, 2004a; Huang *et al.*, 2005; Wu, 2005).

Chinese medicine and pharmacology are a great treasure house, and efforts should be made to explore them and to raise them to a higher level. Recalling the research and development of new drugs from Chinese traditional and herbal drugs, it can be seen that exploration and research with natural drugs is an important pathway for new drug research.

References

Anon. (2004). ZT-1, a new treatment for Alzheimer's disease. http://www.debiopharm.com.

Chen CH (1984). Biological activities and medicinal potentialities of diterpene alkaloids. *Chin Trad Herb Drugs* 1: 180–184.

Cheng PY, Lin YL, Xu GY (1984). New diterpenoids of *Rabdosia macrocalyx*, the structure of macrocalin A and B. *Acta Pharm Sin* 19: 593–598.

Cheng ZL, Huang BS, Zhu DY *et al.* (1981). Studies on the active principles of *Aristolochia debilis.* II. 7-hydroxy aristolochic acid A and 7-methyloxy aristolochia acid A. *Acta Chim Sin* 39: 237–242.

Deng SX, Mo YJ (1979). Pharmacological studies on *Gastrodia eleta* Bleme. I. The sedative and anticonvulsant effect of synthetic gastrodin and its genin. *Acta Botan Yunnan* 1: 66–73.

Dong ZT, Jiang WD (1982). Effects of danshensu on isolated swine coronary artery perfusion preparation. *Acta Pharm Sin* 17: 226–228.

Duan YC, L, i CH, Chen SY (1957). A preliminary study of anthelmintic action of potassium quisquqalate. *Acta Pharm Sin* 5: 87–91.

Ge ZQ, Yuan YJ, Liu CX (2005). Effects of traditional and herbal medicines on cytochrome P450 activities. *Asian J Drug Metabol Pharmacokinet* 5: 3–16.

Geng JY, Huang WQ, Ren TC *et al.* (1990). *Medicinal Herbs.* New World Press, Beijing, pp. 12–262.

Gong X, Sucher NJ (1999). Stroke therapy in traditional Chinese medicine (TCM): prospects of drug discovery and developments. *Trends Pharmacol Sci* 20: 191–196.

Group of Pharmacology Beijing Medical College (1982). Anticonvulsive and sedative actions of piperine. *J Beijing Med Colleg* (4): 217–220.

Hu BZ, Xu RS, Chen GJ *et al.* (1979). The structure, identification and pharmacological actions of l-dicentrine. *Chin Pharm Bull* 14: 110–111.

Hunan Institute of Pharmaceutical Industry (1978). Pharmacological investigation of the pressure action of *Citrus aurantium. Science Bull Sin* 23: 58–62.

Huang BH, Chen WS, Hu Y *et al.* (1981). A study on the chemical constituents of *Ardisia japonica. Acta Pharm Sin* 16: 27–30.

Huang XL, Wang XM, Huang Y *et al.* (1990). Structural elucidation of salproplactone. *Acta Bot Sin* 32: 490–491.

Huang YR, Wei GL, Xiao SH *et al.* (2005). Studies on pharmacodynamics and its biochemical mechanism of Ucncaria-stem mixture for treating children's hyperactivity syndrome by metabonomic method. *Chin Trad Herb Drugs* 36 (3): 301–305.

Jiang Y, Zhao XR, Wu QX *et al.* (1982). Pharmacological actions of dehydrocorydaline on the cardiovascular system. *Acta Pharm Sin* 17: 61–65.

Jin J, Wang FP, Wei H, Liu GT (2005). Reversal of multidrug resistance of cancer through inhibition of P-glycoprotein by 5-bromotetrandrine. *Cancer Chemther Pharmacol* 55: 179–188.

Jin HC (1999). Study on biological sensitivity enhancing effect of Kanglaite injection in human colon carcinoma cells. *J Pract Oncol* 14: 308–310.

Kin KC, Wang YE, Hsu B (1964). Some neuropharmacological actions of rotundine. *Acta Pharm Sin* 11: 754–761.

Li C, Du FF, Chen Y, Xu *et al.* (2004). A sensitive method for the determination of the novel cholinesterase inhibitor ZT-1 and its active metabolite huperzine A in rat blood using liquid chromatography/tandem mass spectrometry. *Rapid Commun Mass Spectr* 18: 651–656.

Li DH, Hao XG, Zhang SK *et al.* (1981). Antitumor action and toxicity of iriquinone. *Acta Pharmacol Sin* 2: 131–134.

Li DP (2006). Research advance on ethnopharmacology, pharmacodynamics, pharmacokinetics and clinical therapeutics of Coix seed and its preparation, Kanglaite injection. *Asian J Drug Metab Pharmacokinet* 6: 5–22.

Li JC, Liu CJ, An XZ *et al.* (1982). Studies on the antitumor constituent of *Rabdosia japonica* (Burm. F.) Hara. I. The structure of rabdosin A and B. *Acta Pharm Sin* 17: 682–687.

Li TD (1998). *Collection of the studies of Kanglaite injection against tumors.* Zhejiang University Press, Hangzhou, pp. 184–191.

Liu CX (1987). Development of Chinese medicine based on pharmacology and therapeutics. *J Ethnopharmacol* 19: 119–123.

Liu CX (1988). *On Chinese Traditional Medicines.* Tianjin Institute of Pharmaceutical Research, Tianjin, pp. 1–180.

Liu CX (2000a). Ethnopharmacology, pharmacology and clinical application of medicinal plants in China. *Studies on Pharmacology and Pharmacokinetics.* Hong Kong Medical Publisher, Hong Kong, pp. 56–134.

Liu CX (2000b). Studies on plant resources, pharmacology and clinical treatment with berbamine. *Studies on Pharmacology and Pharmacokinetics* Hong Kong Medical Publisher, Hong Kong, pp. 154–160.

Liu CX (2004a). Application of metabonomics in drug discovery and development. In: He, F.C. ed. *Post-gene-time: Drug Discovery.* Military Medical Science Press, Beijing, pp. 17–20.

Liu CX (2004b). Significance of metabonomics in modern research of Chinese traditional and herbal drugs. *Chinese Trad Herbal Drugs* 35: 601–605.

Liu CX (2005a). History of application of medicinal plants in China. In: Yaniv Z and Bachrach U, ed. *Handbook of Medicinal Plants.* The Haworth Medical Press, New York. pp. 31–48.

Liu CX (2005b). Ethnopharmacology of traditional Chinese drugs from medicinal plants. In: Yaniv Z and Bachrach U ed. *Handbook of Medicinal Plants.*The Haworth Medical Press, New York. pp. 49–60.

Liu CX (2005c). Different perspectives and hot-points of studies on traditional Chinese medicines. *Acta Pharm Sin* 40: 395–401.

Liu CX (2005d). The understanding of drug metabolism and pharmacokinetics of traditional Chinese medicines *Asian J Drug Metabol Pharmacokinet* 5: 25–36.

Liu CX, Liu GS, Ji XJ (1979). Study on leukogenic effect of berbamine. *Chin Trad Herb Drugs* 10: 36–37.

Liu CX, Yaniv Z (2005). Research and development of new drugs originating from Chinese medicinal plants. In: Yaniv Z and Bachrach U, ed. *Handbook of Medicinal Plants.* The Haworth Medical Press, New York. pp. 61–96.

Liu CX, Xiao PG (1993). *An Introduction to Chinese Materia Medica.* Peking Union Medical College and Beijing Medical University Press, Beijing, pp. 246–283.

Liu CX, Xiao PG, Liu GS (1991). Study on plant resource, pharmacology and clinical therapy of berbamine. *Phytother Res* 5: 228–230.

Liu CX, Xiao PG (1992). *Chinese Medicinal Plants.* Tianjin Institute of Pharmaceutical Research, Tianjin, pp. 1–497.

Liu CX, Xiao PG (2001). Pharmacology, pharmacokinetics and therapeutics of active constituents from radix *Salviae miltirrhae. Asian J Drug Metabol Pharmacokinet* 1: 221–227.

Liu CX, Xiao PG (1992a). *An Introduction to Chinese Materia Medica.* Beijing Medical University & Peking Union Medical College Press, Beijing, pp. 1–36.

Liu CX, Xiao PG (1992b). *An Introduction to Chinese Materia Medica.* Peking Union Medical College and Beijing Medical University Press, Beijing, pp. 94–190.

Liu CX, Xiao PG, Li DP (2000). *Modern Research and Application of Chinese Medicinal Plants.* Hong Kong Medical Publishers, Hong Kong, pp. 1–100.

Liu CX, Xiao PG (1995). *Chinese Medicinal Plants.* Tianjin Pharmaceutical Research, Tianjin, pp. 1–256.

Liu CX, Li C, Lin DH, Song NN (2004). Significance of metabonomics in drug discovery and development. *Asian J Drug Metab Pharmacokinet* 4: 87–96.

Liu CX, Si DY, Xie HT, (2007). Challenges in research and development of traditional Chinese medicines. *Chin Clin Pharmacol Ther* 12: 1122–1129.

Liu WJ, Jiang JF, Ding J (2002). Down-regulation of telomerase activity via protein phosphatase 2A activation in salvicine-induced human leukemia HL-60 cell apoptosis. *Biochem Pharmacol* 64: 1677–1687.

Liu YM, Chen H, Zeng FD (2001). The advance in studies on pharmacokinetics of Ligustrazin in China. *Asian J Drug Metabol Pharmacokinet* 1: 217–220.

Lu R, Fan HR, Gao J, Zeng Y (2005). Effect of ginseng extract and ginsenosides on activity of cytochrome P450. *Asian J Drug Metabol Pharmacokinet* 5: 17–24.

Ma JZ, Zhao YC, Yin L *et al.* (1982). Studies on the effect of oleanolic acid on experimental liver injury. *Acta Pharm Sin* 17: 93–97.

Meng LH, Zhang JS, Ding J (2001). Salvicine, a novel DNA topoisomerase II inhibitor, exerting its effects by trapping enzyme–DNA cleavage complexes. *Biochem Pharmacol* 62: 733–741.

Meng LH, Zhang JS, Ding J (2001). DNA topoisomerase II as the primary cellular target for salvicine in *Saccharomyces cerevisiae. Acta Pharmacol Sin* 22: 741–746.

Meng LH, Ding J, (2001). Induction of bulk and c-myc P2 promoter-specific DNA damage by an anti-topoisomerase II agents salvicine is an early event leading to apoptosis in HL-60 cells. *Federation of European Biochermical Societies Letter* 501: 59–64.

Ministry of Health PR China (2002). *Concerning further standard administration on raw materials of health good* (No. 51, Appendix 1–3).

PRC Pharmacopoeia Committee (1953, 1963, 1977, 1985, 1990, 1995, 2000, 2005). *Pharmacopoeia of People's Republic of China.* People's Health Publishers, Beijing.

Qian MS (1998). Collection of the studies of Kanglaite injection against tumors. Zhejiang University Press, Hangzhou, pp. 214–229.

Qing C, Zhang JS, Ding J (1999). *In vitro* cytotoxicity of salvicine, a novel diterpenoid quinine. *Acta Pharmacol Sin* 20: 297–302.

Qing C, Jiang C, Zhang, JS, Ding J (2001). Induction of apoptosis in human leukemia K-562 and gastric cancenoma SGC-7901 cells by salvicine, a novel anticancer compound. *Anticancer Drugs* 12: 51–56.

Shen WJ (1998). *Collection of the studies of Kanglaite injection against tumors.* Zhejiang University Press, Hangzhou, pp. 198–203.

Shia SH, Shao BR, Ho YS, Yang YC (1962). Prophylatico-therapeutic studies of curcurbitine in *Schistosomiasis japonica* in mice. *Acta Pharm Sin* 9: 327–332.

State Food Drug Administration of China (SFDA). (2002). *Drug Registration Regulation.* Beijing: Chinese Pharmaceutical Science & Technology Press.

State Food Drug Administration of China (SFDA). (2002). *The Good Agricultural Practice for Chinese Crude Drugs* (GAP). Beijing, China, June 1 (2002).

Wang DD, Liu SQ, Chen YY *et al.* (1982). Studies on the active constituents of *Syringa oblata* Lindl. *Acta Pharm Sin* 17: 951–954.

Wang FP, Li Wang L, Yang JS *et al.* (2005). Reversal of P-glycoprotein-dependent resistance to vinblastine by newly synthesized bisbenzylisoquinoline alkaloids in mouse leukemia P388 cells. *Biol Pharmaceut Bull* 28: 1979–1982.

Wang LX, Lu LZ (1999). Study on the safety of Chinese herbs. *J Adverse React Drugs* (2): 88–91.

Wang ZG, Ren J (2002). Current status and function direction of Chinese herbal medicine. *Trend Pharm Sci* 23: 347–348.

Wang R, Zhang HY, Tang XC (2001). Huperzine A attenuates cognitive dysfunction and neuronal degeneration caused by beta-amyloid protein-(1–40) in rat. *Eur J Pharmcol* 421: 149–156.

Wang XR, Wang ZQ, Dong JG (1982). A new diterpene from Huang-hua-xiang-cha-cai (*Robdosia sculponeata*). *Chin Trad Herb Drugs* 13: 491–492.

Wei GL, Xiao SH, Lu R, Liu CX (2006). Pharmacokinetics of ZT-1 in experimental animals. *Drug Metab Rev* 37 (supp 2): 329.

Wei GL, Xiao SH, Lu R, Liu CX (2006). Simultaneous determination of ZT-1 and its metabolite huperzine A in plasma by high-performance liquid chromatography with ultraviolet detection. *J Chromatogr B* 830: 120–125.

World Health Organization (2000). WHO General Guidelines for Methodologies on Research and Evaluation of Traditional Medicine. WHO, Geneva, Switzerland, pp. 74.

World Health Organization (2004). WHO Guidelines on Good Agricultural and Collection Practices (GACP) for medicinal plants. WHO, Geneva, Switzerland, pp. 133.

Wu XJ, Lin YP, Song NN, Yuan YJ (2005). Application of principal component analysis for data process in metabonomic studies. *Asian J Drug Metab Pharmacokinet* 5: 287–294.

Wu SH (1964). Two cases with renal toxicity induced by *Aristolochia manshuriensis* Kom. *Jiangsu J Trad Chin Med* 5: 12–14.

Xiao PG, Fu SL (1986). Pharmacologically active substances of Chinese traditional and herbal medicines. *Herbs, Spices and Medicinal Plants.* Institute of Medicinal Plant Development, Beijing, pp. 49–103.

Xiao PG (1986). The role of traditional medicine in the primary health care system of China. *Econ Med Plant Res* 4: 17–26.

Xiao PG (1983). Recent developments on medicinal plants in China. *J Ethnopharmacol* 7: 95–100.

Xiao PG, Liu CX (1999). Immunostimulants in traditional Chinese medicine. In: Wagner H, ed. *Immunomodulatory Agents from Plants.* Birkhauser Verlag, Basel, pp. 325–356.

Xiao PG, Liu CX (2004). A re-understanding on the safety matters of Chinese herbal medicines. *Chin J Integr Med* 10: 242–245.

Xiao PG, Tong YY, Lou SR *et al.* (1982). Qian-cao (*Rubia cordifolia* L.). In: *Chinese Materia Medica* II. People's Health Publishers, Beijing, pp. 149–159.

Xiao SH, Wei GL, Liu CX, Wang FP (2004). Pharmacokinetics of bromotetrandrin (W198) in rats and beagle dogs. *Acta Pharm Sin* 39: 301–4.

Xiao SH, Wei GL, Liu CX, Wang FP (2005). Tissue distribution and excretion of bromotetrandrine in rats. *Acta Pharm Sin* 40: 453–456.

Xu RS, Zhao WM (2005). New drug research on basis of active compounds in traditional Chinese medicines. *Chin J Natur Med* 3: 322–327.

Xu Y, Hu ZB, Feng SC, Fan GJ (1979). Studies on the anti-tuberculosis principles from *Lysionotus pauciflora* Maxim. I. Isolation and identification of nevadensin. *Acta Pharm Sin* 14: 447–448.

Yang CM, Hou SX, Zhang ZR *et al.* (2001). Recent advance in metabolic chemistry of traditional Chinese medicine. *Asian J Drug Metabol Pharmacokinet* 1: 57–62.

Yang YX, Wang GY, Pan XC (2002). *List of Composition of Foods in China (2002).* Peking University Medical Press, Beijing, pp. 240–393.

Ye JS, Zhang HQ, Yuan CQ (1982). Isolation and identification of coumarin praeruption E from the root of Chinese drug *Peucedanum praeruptorum* Dunn. *Acta Pharm Sin* 17: 431–434.

Yeng HW, Kong YC, Lay WP, Cheng KF (1977). The structure and biological effect of leonurine, a uterotonic principle from Chinese drug I-mu-tsao. *Planta Med* 31: 51–56.

Yu SR, You SQ (1984). Anticonvulsant action of 3-n-butyphalide (Ag-1) and 3-n-butyl-4, 5-dihydrophthalide (Ag-2). *Acta Pharm Sin* 19: 566–570.

Yu SR, You SQ, Chen HY (1984). The pharmacological action of 3-n-butylphthalide (Ag-1). *Acta Pharm Sin* 19: 486–490.

Yu ZM, Lu AP, Wu P (2003). Thinking on the research of safety evaluation of Chinese herbs. *Clin J Basic Med Trad Chin Med* 9: 66–68.

Yuan DJ (1979). Clinical obsrvation on the effects of lactonin Coriae and tutin in the treatment of schizophrenia. *Chin J Neurol Psychiatr* 12: 196–200.

Yuan ST (2000). Thinking on the ascensive problems of Chinese drugs intoxication. *Chin J Clin Materia Medica* 25: 579–583.

Zangara A (2003). The psychopharmacology of huperzine A: an alkaloid with cognitive enhancing and neuroprotective properties of interest in the treatment of Alzheimer's disease. *Pharmacol Biochem Behav* 75: 675–685.

Zhang JS, Ding J, Tang Q *et al.* (1999). Synthesis and antitumor activity of novel diterpenequinone salvicine and the analogs. *Bioorg Med Chem Lett* 9: 2731–2736.

Zhang TM, Fong TC, Lue EH (1958). Studies of betadichroine, chloroguanide, cyclochloroquininde and baicalin on amebicides. *Acta Acad Med Wuhan* 1: 11–16.

Zhou YP, Fan LL, Zhang LY, Zeng GY (1978). The effect of higenamine on the cardiovascular system. *Nat Med J Chin* 58: 664–669.

Zhou JM, Yu ZQ, Cao Y *et al.* (1981). Active principles in Shehanqi. *Chin Trad Herb Drugs* 12: 99–107.

Zhou FJ (1979). Case report on toxicity induced by *Caulis Aristolochiae manshuriensis* (*Aristolochia manshuriensis* Kom). *J Bethune Med Univ* 5: 118–120.

Zhou FJ, Lu HW, Ye CF (1988). The renal toxicity induced by *Aristolochia manshuriensis* Kom. *Chin J Nephropt* 4: 223–224.

Zhu DY, Tang XC, Lin C *et al.* (1999). Huperzine, a derivative, their preparation and their use. *US Patent* 5929084 07/27/1999.

Zhu DY, Tang XC, Lin C *et al.* (2000). Huperzine, a derivative, their preparation and their use. *Chinese Patent* 95196884X, 0510/2000.

5

Traditional Chinese medicines: evaluation of botanical extracts and dietary supplements

Raymond Cooper, Tianan Jiang, Talash Anne Likimani and Ezra Bejar

Introduction

Although rich in folklore and used over many centuries, traditional Chinese medicine (TCM) has not been thoroughly examined using Western-developed biological criteria, nor has it been clinically evaluated in great detail outside of China and Asia. This is changing as more TCM plants are becoming accepted globally (Chen *et al.*, 2006; Wei *et al.*, 2006). In this review, several specific examples of TCM plants have been chosen that are gaining widespread interest in the wellness and medical arena and are now being sold as dietary or nutritional supplements worldwide. At least two of the top 10 selling botanical products are derived from TCM, including *Camellia sinensis*, green tea; *Panax ginseng,* ginseng, *Ginkgo biloba,* ginkgo, and *Allium sativum,* garlic (Blumenthal *et al.*, 2001).

These plants require different model systems to evaluate their therapeutic potential and are represented herein. Although each one has been well studied, there have been conflicting clinical data, suggesting a lack of specific activity or inappropriate preparation. We review several studies describing new mechanisms of action applied to each one of these botanicals, which may eventually lead to a positive clinical outcome or the potential for a better understanding of their respective modes of action.

Evidence-based approach

In many cases the exact chemical constituent and amount in the plant needed to give a defined and specific biological effect has yet to be verified. These then have to be limited to a biological effect that in turn is relevant to a therapeutic or nutritional target. This approach may be achieved by determining the structural analyses of natural compounds present in the selected botanical, followed by pharmacological testing, to identify biological fingerprints of the plant extracts and their effective concentration.

Various in-vitro/in-vivo bio-assays have been employed for evaluation of botanicals to determine the mechanism of their action and thereby to fix parameters of pharmacological, microbiological and allied standardisation methodology, leading to a more effective role in healthcare. These bioassays may include whole animal models, as well as organs, tissues, cells, receptors, enzymes or cell parts. Botanical extracts can only be declared pharmacologically active if a reliable correlation can be made between a measurable active principle and its declared medicinal effect. Clinical confirmation of pharmacological activity can only then be ascertained when unequivocal effects of standardised extracts are demonstrated in clinical trials (Awang and Bejar, 2001).

Green tea

There is an abundance of evidence linking specific molecular targets to green tea extracts (Cooper *et al.*, 2005a, b). This review provides further evidence that green tea, and specifically EGCg (epigallocatechin gallate), possesses more biological effects than solely as an antioxidant.

The major polyphenol, belonging to the family of catechins and found in green tea is (−)-EGCg, with lesser amounts of catechin (C), epicatechin (EC), gallocatechin (GC), gallocatechin gallate (GCG), epigallocatechin (EGC), and epicatechin gallate (ECG). These polyphenols are among the dietary factors that may play a role in cancer protection, and have recently been shown to have potent antioxidant and antitumour effects (Hara, 2001). Green tea polyphenols have been reported to protect in varying degrees against certain cancers, including colon, rectal, bladder (Kemberling *et al.*, 2003), breast (Seely *et al.*, 2005), stomach, pancreatic, lung, oesophageal and prostate (Adhami *et al.*, 2003).

Epidemiological observations

Anticancer effects for tea are indicated both from animal in-vivo studies and from human epidemiological observations (Imai *et al.*, 1997). Numerous studies were examined by Bushman (1998) to show an inverse association between tea consumption and cancer of the colon, urinary bladder, stomach, oesophagus, lung and pancreas. These studies are reviewed by Cooper *et al.* (2005b).

Studies have attempted to link green tea to antioxidant benefits including protection against the damage caused by cigarette smoke, pollution, stress, and other toxins (Mitscher, 1998; Benzie *et al.*, 1999). Further research from Palermo *et al.* (2003) suggested that the combination of EGCg and EGC in green tea may reduce the risk of cancer in smokers by shutting down in vitro the activity of the aryl hydrocarbon receptor known to activate cancer-activating genes. The fact that both EGCg and EGC shut down this receptor may demonstrate a different mechanism of action for green tea's anticancer benefits, and most likely the compounds act through many different pathways. These researchers indicated that green tea's inhibitory effects were present when levels of EGCg and EGC reached those typical in a cup of green tea. However, the metabolism will affect activity; therefore the in-vitro research may not be indicative of green tea's activity after ingestion.

Anticancer mechanisms of action

Various responses of specific cellular targets relating to cancer and EGCg have been recently reviewed (Cooper *et al.*, 2005b). Through in-vitro cell culture experiments and animal studies, many potential mechanisms have been proposed for the chemopreventive effect of green tea and/or EGCg (Lambert *et al.*, 2003). However, the exact mechanism(s) of anticarcinogenic activity remains to be found.

Researchers working with cancer cell lines have related the anticancer activity of EGCg to growth inhibition (Ahmad and Mukhtar, 1999; Morre *et al.*, 2000); and regulation of cell cycle progression and induction of apoptosis (Morre *et al.*, 2000) in place of a non-specific antioxidant function.

Published animal and in-vitro research shows that EGCg is protective against bladder cancer (Kemberling *et al.*, 2003). These researchers noted that EGCg inhibited the growth of bladder tumours both in vivo and in vitro with the AY-27 rat transitional cell cancer and the L1210 mouse leukaemia cell lines. When the cancer cell lines were exposed to increasing concentrations of EGCg for 30 min to 48 h, researchers noted both time- and dose-dependent responses. After 2 h, there was 100% cell death in the AY-27 cell line at concentrations greater than 100 mmol/L, and strong banding on the DNA ladder assay was observed with the mouse leukaemia cell line. The research group implanted tumours in the rats' bladders and either offered no treatment or injected 200 mmol/L of EGCg into the rats' bladders, 30 minutes after tumour implantation. After three weeks, the rats' bladders were analysed and 64% of the EGCg-treated animals had not developed tumours.

EGCg has been implicated in blocking DNA transcription of a number of genes in selective cancer cell lines. For example, in the human epidermal carcinoma cell line A431, EGCg inhibits both DNA and protein synthesis of the growth factor receptors: epidermal growth factor receptor (EGF-R), platelet-derived growth factor receptor (PDGF-R), and fibroblast growth factor receptor (FGF-R) (Liang *et al.*, 1997). EGCg has also been implicated in blocking transcription of nitric oxide (NO) synthase by inhibiting the binding of transcription factor NF-κB to the NO synthase promotor (Chan *et al.*, 1997; Lin and Lin, 1997). In the tumour cell line JB6, EGCg inhibits AP-1 transcriptional activity (Dong *et al.*, 1997). It also inhibits the activity of transcription factors AP-1 and NF-κB and the synthesis of nitric oxide (Yang *et al.*, 2001). In certain benign cell types, however, green tea can have different effects on AP-1-related activities (Ahmad *et al.*, 2000; Balasubramanian *et al.*, 2002). These results suggest that EGCg may prevent cancer at the level of gene transcription, i.e. by blocking the DNA synthesis of genes involved in signal transduction pathways. This has led to many other studies to look at the effect of EGCg on apoptosis, or programmed cell death.

Green tea has been shown to inhibit angiogenesis in both in-vitro proliferation studies and in-vivo angiogenesis assays. Researchers showed that green tea decreases the levels of two important angiogenic factors, VEGF (vascular endothelial growth factor), and bFGF as well as aFGF (basic and acidic fibroblast growth factor) in breast cancer (Sartippour *et al.*, 2004). Green tea polyphenols may cause reduced expression of proteins known to be associated with the metastatic spread of cancer cells, and contribute to minimising tumour development by governing the amount of vascular endothelial growth factor (VEGF) in the serum of the prostate cancer mouse model. By reducing the amount of VEGF, the polyphenols work to minimise nutrients flowing to, and supporting tumour growth. It has been shown that the polyphenols present in green tea help prevent the spread of prostate cancer by targeting molecular pathways that shut down the proliferation and spread of tumour cells, as well as inhibiting the growth of tumour-nurturing blood vessels.

Other studies suggest that one mechanism involves the suppression of interleukin (IL)-8 production by endothelial cells (Tang and Meydani, 2001). EGCg reduces urokinase (Jankun *et al.*, 1997), matrix metalloproteinases (MMP-2 and MMP-9) (Annabi *et al.*, 2002), and inhibits PDGF (platelet derived growth factor) signalling (Sachinidis *et al.*, 2000). Tumour necrosis factor (TNF)-α gene expression has been shown to be inhibited by EGCg (Yang *et al.*, 1998). It has also been demonstrated that EGCg, EGC and ECG inhibit cyclo-oxygenase (COX)-dependent arachidonic acid metabolism (Hong *et al.*, 2001).

Adhami *et al.* (2004) looked at the role of green tea polyphenols in modulating the insulin-like growth factor-1 (IGF-1)-driven molecular pathway in prostate tumour cells in a mouse model for human prostate cancer. They suggested that the IGF-I/IGFBP-3 signalling pathway is a prime pathway for green tea polyphenol-mediated inhibition of prostate cancer that limits the progression of cancer through inhibition of angiogenesis and metastasis.

In other postulated mechanisms, the effects of EGCg on the growth inhibition and induction of apoptosis in cancer cells has been studied extensively. A differential growth-inhibitory effect was reported in human colorectal cancer cells CaCo-2 (Salucci *et al.*, 2002), breast cancer cells Hs578T, and their non-cancer cell counterparts (Ahmad and Mukhtar, 1999), as well as HeLa (cervical carcinoma) and BT-20 mammary cancer and MCF-10A mammary non-cancer cells (Morré *et al.*, 2000). EGCg has been implicated in the growth arrest and subsequent induction of apoptosis following cell growth. Inhibition has also been shown in virally transformed fibroblast cells WI-38, human epidermal carcinoma cells A431, lung cancer tumour cells H611, prostate cancer cell lines LNCaP, PC-3, DU145, human carcinoma keratinocytes HaCaT, and mouse lymphoma cells LY-R (Yang *et al.*, 1998; Ahmad and Mukhtar, 1999). In studies where the apoptotic response was studied in cancer cells versus their non-cancer counterparts, e.g. human carcinoma keratinocytes (HaCaT versus normal human epidermal keratinocytes), the apoptotic response to EGCg was reported to be specific to the cancer cells (Ahmad *et al.*, 1997). A similar conclusion was reached for human breast cancer cells (Morré *et al.*, 2000).

It has been suggested that EGCg-induced apoptosis may result from either cell cycle arrest and/or H_2O_2 production (Ahmad *et al.*, 1997; Yang *et al.*, 1998). EGCg may be involved in the growth regulation of human epidermal carcinoma cells A431 by causing cell cycle arrest of the G0 to G1 phase (Ahmad *et al.*, 1997). In the EGCg-induced inhibition of human lung cancer cells, involvement of the tumour necrosis factor (TNF)-α pathway was suggested. Alternatively, the EGCg-induced apoptosis of the lung cancer tumour cells H611 was inhibited by catalase, suggesting that H_2O_2 production is a probable contributor to apoptosis (Yang *et al.*, 1998). Despite the abundance of evidence from these studies, the efficacy of EGCg as a single agent therapy for the prevention of cancer is still unclear. Moreover, the efficacy of EGCg as a therapeutic drug to treat or reverse cancer in a patient is unknown.

Inhibition of tNOX

A cell surface protein with NADH oxidase activity (tNOX), which exhibits protein disulfide-thiol interchange activity has been identified as the potential target for the anticancer action of green tea catechins and especially EGCg (Morré *et al.*, 2000). The expression of tNOX is restricted to cancer cells (Morré *et al.*, 1995) where it appears to represent an oncofetal antigen (Cho *et al.*, 2002). As a result of stable translation, tNOX, when expressed in COS cells or non-cancer mammary epithelial cells, increases both the growth rate and final cell size of the cells. With HeLa cells transfected with tNOX-directed antisense, a normal growth phenotype is restored and sensitivity to growth inhibition by EGCg is lost (Chueh *et al.*, 2004).

The cancer specificity of tNOX resides in expression of a tNOX protein splice variant that is uniquely both drug inhibited and associated with human cancer (Chueh *et al.*, 2002). It is absent from normal cells and tissues. Activity is correlated with cancer growth and, when blocked, cancer cells fail to enlarge following division and eventually die through apoptosis. Previous studies have utilised tNOX of cancer cell lines to model synergistic polyphenol compositions with utility in cancer prevention and/or treatment. EGCg is so far the safest and most effective polyphenol tNOX blocker found. EGCg blocks tNOX activity and growth of tumour cells without adverse effects on normal cells. The efficacy of EGCg can be enhanced 10-fold without effect on normal cells by combination with other non-gallate catechins such as (−)-epicatechin (EC) (Morré *et al.*, 2003). Furthermore, in animal studies, a catechin composition containing 40% EC, 58.5% ECG and 1.5% EGCg has been identified as being tenfold more efficacious than EGCg alone by evaluations using tNOX assays, growth of cells in culture and growth of transplanted mouse mammary tumours with the catechins administered intratumorally. Based on cell culture studies, a total catechin level surrounding the tumour in situ of 100 nmol/L would seem to be necessary to achieve growth stasis and to initiate apoptosis. Based on mean elimination half lives, the ratio of 1.7 : 5 : 1 for EGCg : EC : ECG is suggested.

Although there are significant amounts of data reporting on the cellular, subcellular biochemical and molecular responses to green and black tea, including signal transduction and telomere shortening (Yang, 2002), responses to EGCg are generally in the micro- or low millimolar ranges (in contrast to tNOX), suggesting these effects are neither cancer cell specific nor realistically attainable in tissue through dietary supplementation. In contrast, tNOX inhibition is the only biochemical parameter thus far reported where inhibitions are achieved at nanomolar concentrations of EGCg (EC_{50} of 5nmol/L) and where the dose response of inhibition of activity and inhibition of growth of cancer cells are correlated. This observation therefore suggests that tNOX is the primary target protein to explain cancer-cell-specific catechin inhibition of growth (Morre *et al.*, 2003).

Several studies in animals show promise of tea catechins as adjunct cancer therapy (Suganuma *et al.*,

1998; Sugiyama and Sadzuka, 1998). In preliminary human studies on patients (compassionate intervention) with severe head and neck carcinomas who were treated with a commercial preparation of a dietary supplement, Capsibiol-T (www.capsibiol-T.com), containing a mixture of decaffeinated green tea and red pepper (*Capsicum* sp.), the results to date indicate a positive role of this herbal mixture in clinical use. The use of Capsibiol-T as an adjunct with conventional cancer treatment was indicative of survival benefits both for cancer protection and for slowing the growth and metastatic spread of established cancers. This study (Fernandez and Ganzon, 2003) suggests a role of green tea as an aid for the prevention and control of cancer growth, metastasis and/or recurrence, and clearly warrants more clinical studies to determine a definitive role in cancer therapy.

Ginseng

Ginsenosides are the major active compounds of ginseng (*Panax ginseng*). In the various *Panax* species, more than 30 ginsenosides have been identified. The type, number and site of attachment of the sugars impart structural and functional variation among the ginsenosides (Attele *et al.*, 1999); and based on their structural differences, they can be classified into three categories (Liberti 1978).

Table 5.1 provides a listing of various pharmacological effects these ginseng compounds impart and several of these mechanisms are reviewed in detail below.

Ginsenoside variation and standardisation

Ginsenoside content is standardised to 1.5–7% (on average at 4%). Dosages used in clinical studies are typically around 200 mg a day of extract, equivalent to 0.5–2 g of dried root per day administered for 2–4 months.

The content and profile of ginsenosides differ between ginseng species and can differ among raw samples and commercial products of the same species (Vuksan, 2000). Asian ginseng (*Panax ginseng*) has a

Table 5.1 Biological effects of ginseng and its chemical constituents

Activity	Compounds responsible	References
Platelet inhibition	Various ginsenosides (Ro, Rg_1, and Rg_2) and polyacetylenes	Kuo *et al.*,1990
Antioxidant	Rg_1, Rb_1, Rd	Chang *et al.*, 1999; Kitts *et al.*, 2000; Yokozawa *et al.*, 2004
Cardiovascular protection	Rb_1	Zhan *et al.*, 1994; Zhou *et al.*, 2005
Angiogenesis (wound-healing)	Ginsenosides Re, Rg_1 (Rb_1 inhibits angiogenesis)	Huang *et al.*, 2005; Sengupta *et al.*, 2004
Nitric oxide release	Rb_1, Rg_1, Rg_3, polysaccharides	Kim *et al.*, 1992; Kang *et al.*, 1995; Chen, 1996; Kim *et al.*, 1999; Friedl *et al.*, 2001; Lu *et al.*, 2004
Antihypertensive	Rg_3	Kim *et al.*, 1999
Tumour inhibition	Polyacetylenes, polysaccharides, Rb_1, Rg_3, Rg_5	Helms *et al.*, 2004
Immunomodulation	Rg_1, Rg_3, polysaccharides	Joo *et al.*, 2005
Neuroprotection	Ginsenosides, Rb_1,Rg_1, Rg_3	Chen *et al.*, 2003; Bao *et al.*, 2005; Radad *et al.*, 2006
Memory enhancing	Rb_1, Rg_3, Rg_5/Rk_1	Rudarkewich *et al.*, 2001; Bao *et al.*, 2005
Antihyperglycaemic	Rb, Rc, Rd, Re, Rf, Rg_1, Rg_3, Rh_1	Sievenpiper *et al.* 2004; Xie *et al.*, 2002
Antiallergic	Rh_1, Rh_2	Friedl *et al.*, 2001; Park *et al.*, 2004

different ginsenoside profile than American ginseng (*Panax quinquefolius* L.). For the genus *Panax*, the pharmacologically active marker compounds are ginsensosides, while *P. quinquefolius* does not contain the ginsensoside Rf. Likewise, 24(R)-pseudoginsenoside F11 is specific to American ginseng. Thus, data from studies of *Panax ginseng* may not be applicable to other commercially available *Panax* species referred to by the general name ginseng. These include American ginseng (*Panax quinquefolius* L.), Japanese ginseng (*P. japonicus* CA Meyer) and Siberian ginseng (*Eleutherococcus senticosus* and *P. notoginseng*).

Among *Panax* species, significant variation exists in both the types and ratios of ginsensosides. The most abundant ginsensosides in *P. ginseng* are Rb_1 and Rg_1 which generally occur in a ratio from 1 to 3. For example, in *P. quinquefolius*, the $Rb_1 : Rg_1$ ratio is approximately 6 : 1; and Rb_1 and Rb_2 ginsenosides have been well documented to be higher and lower in concentration than those in *P. ginseng*. Variability in concentration suggests that standardisation is necessary for quality assurance (Cui *et al.*, 1996; Harkey *et al.*, 2001). However, it may be too simplistic to determine ginseng's biological activity by ginsenosides alone. For example, polysaccharides isolated from the aqueous extract of *Panax ginseng* root powder showed strong stimulation of inducible nitric oxide (NO) synthesis, whereas the fraction containing triterpenic ginsenosides does not show any stimulation of NO release (Friedl *et al.*, 2001). It seems questionable to qualify commercially available ginseng preparations solely via their ginsenoside content. Cell culture systems that provide activity-based tests could better serve as an effective means to provide specific predication about the overall effects.

Ratio of Rg_1 and Rb_1 and the yin and the yang

Ginsenosides are associated with the pharmacological activity of *Panax* species, yet, the two key ginsenosides, Rb_1 and Rg_1, may mechanistically exert opposing activity: Rg_1 is a weak stimulant of the central nervous system (which is considered to be 'yang', i.e. more stimulating and energising), whereas Rb_1 is a depressant of the central nervous system (which is considered to be more 'yin', i.e. more balanced, calming and less stimulating). The extract from *Panax ginseng*, which has a predominance of Rb_1, exerted a preventive effect in multiple cancer models (Yun *et al.*, 2001). For example, American ginseng has a lower ratio of ginsenoside Rg_1 to Rb_1 than Asian ginseng (Li, 1996), and is thus considered to be more 'yin' (i.e. more balanced and less stimulating) than Asian ginseng (Hobbs *et al.*, 1996). In contrast, *Sanqi ginseng* is considered the key ingredient for the treatment of trauma injuries and for promoting microcirculation (Lee *et al.*, 2000), which would be consistent with the proangiogenic activity of its predominant ginsenoside, Rg_1. There are reports of both wound-healing and antitumour effects of ginseng extract through opposing activities on the vascular system. Sengupta *et al.* (2004) demonstrated that the dominance of Rg_1 leads to angiogenesis, whereas Rb_1 exerts an opposing effect. Reconstituting an extract by adding Rg_1 and Rb_1 in a defined ratio could alter the angiogenic outcome. Thus the administration of an extract with a greater percentage of Rg_1 than Rb_1 might result in the induction of significant angiogenesis. In contrast, the overabundance of Rb_1 may only inhibit Rg_1-induced neovascularisation (Sengupta *et al.*, 2004).

In addition, Rb_1 and Rg_1 exert opposite effects on modulating the immune function and inflammation in a dose-dependent manner (Joo *et al.*, 2005). Whereas Rg_1 stimulated NO and pro-inflammatory cytokines (IL-1β, IL-6, and TNF-α), Rb_1 exerted a significant inhibitory effect on this pro-inflammatory repertoire. In addition, the genetic expression of bcl-2 and bax, both of which have been implicated in apoptosis, was regulated by treatment with Rb_1 and Rg_1. When combined treatment with equal doses of Rb_1 and Rg_1 was administered, Rb_1 significantly counteracted the stimulatory effects of Rg_1, as shown in a NO assay. The existence of opposing active principles in ginseng emphasises the importance of standardisation through compositional analysis, and the need for standardising herbal therapy.

Adaptogen and effects on exercise performance

Panax ginseng is considered a tonic or adaptogen that enhances physical performance, relieves fatigue, promotes vitality and increases resistance to stress

(Fulder, 1990, Tang *et al.*, 1992). Chinese traditional medicine considers ginseng to have beneficial effects on physical capacity, alertness, and power of concentration, especially in the elderly and those recovering from illness (Fulder, 1990, Tang *et al.*, 1992). It is also used by athletes to enhance their 'energy level' (Bahrke and Morgan, 2000).

Although the mechanism underlying the alleged ergogenicity of ginseng on physical performance has not been defined, theories include stimulation of the hypothalamic–pituitary–adrenal cortex axis and increased resistance to the stress of exercise, enhanced myocardial metabolism, increased haemoglobin levels, vasodilation, increased oxygen extraction by muscles, reduced oxidative stress, and improved mitochondrial metabolism in the muscle, all of which theoretically could enhance aerobic exercise performance (Kim *et al.*, 2005).

A careful study by Pieralisi *et al.* (1991), using a double-blind crossover design, indicated that ginseng significantly increased workload and oxygen uptake in normal subjects. At a fixed workload, ginseng decreased oxygen consumption, carbon dioxide production, and plasma lactate. Chinese ginseng improved maximal oxygen uptake (VO_{2max}), post-exercise recovery (heart rate lowered 6 beats/min for the 6 min after exercise), pectoral strength (by 22% as measured by a dynamometer), and quadriceps strength (by 18% as measured by dynamometer) (McNaughton *et al.*, 1989). Administration of ginseng or its components enhanced exercise endurance by altering fuel homeostasis during exercise, increased free fatty acid utilisation in preference over glucose for cellular energy demands in rats and mice (Bahrke and Morgan, 2000; Bucci, 2000). However, based on a review of the ergogenic properties of ginseng, most clinical trials investigating the value of *Panax ginseng* in enhancing physical performance have shown no clinical effect (Bahrke and Morgan, 2000). For example, two studies found no effects of ginseng on physical performance. The first study showed that 8 weeks of supplementation with a standardised ginseng extract of 200 mg a day failed to affect work performance and energy metabolism in a group of healthy women (Engels *et al.*, 1996). The second study, examined the effects of doses of 200 and 400 mg of standardised ginseng extract compared with a placebo, given to 36 healthy men and found no effect of ginseng at either dose on physiological or psychological parameters such as oxygen consumption, respiratory exchange ratio, minute ventilation, blood lactic acid concentrations, heart rate and perceived exertion (Engels *et al.*, 1997). In another small study 28 healthy, adult subjects were given a standardised ginseng extract for 21 days, but no ergogenic effects were found (Allen *et al.*, 1998).

An examination of available data reveals most of the variation in results arises from a dose–response and duration effect, differences between subjects' age, and the variability in the quality of the supplement and/or different methods of study. Properly controlled studies exhibiting statistically significant improvements in physical or psychomotor performance almost invariably used higher doses (usually standardised to ginsenoside content equivalent to 2 g dried root daily), longer durations of study (±8 week), and larger subject numbers, indicating greater statistical power (Buettner *et al.*, 2006). With lower doses, short durations, and small subject numbers, studies show no significant differences in performance, physiologic, or psychomotor measurements (Morris *et al.*, 1996; Engels and Wirth, 1997; Allen *et al.*, 1998).

Forgo *et al.* (1982) studied 120 subjects aged 30–60 years for 12 weeks in a double-blind study. Subjects were given either placebo or 200 mg/day of a standardised ginseng extract. Supplementation was associated with significantly reduced reaction times for those subjects aged 40–60 years but not for those aged 30–39 years. Men in this youngest group showed no significant effect from ginseng on pulmonary functions (vital capacity, forced expiratory volume, maximum expiratory flow, and maximum breathing capacity). Women aged 30–39 years and both sexes aged 40–60 years showed significant improvements in all four measurements of pulmonary function after 12 weeks of supplementation. No significant changes by age or sex were found for serum concentrations of luteinising hormone, testosterone or oestradiol. As with pulmonary function, subjective self-assessment showed significant improvements in women of all ages but only in men aged 40–60 years. Importantly, changes became significant after 6 weeks of supplementation and were more significant at 12 weeks, suggesting a slow-acting effect. Thus, studies lasting fewer than

12 weeks (Morris *et al.*, 1996; Engels and Wirth, 1997; Allen *et al.*, 1998) may not have been long enough to show a significant effect. For example, in a study with 31 healthy men who took 200 or 400 mg of extract daily for 8 weeks, no change in physiological or maximal exercise (Engels and Wirth, 1997) was found. In addition, there was no ergogenic effect on peak aerobic exercise performance following a 3-week supplementation period of 200 mg of 7% *Panax ginseng* in healthy young adults with moderate exercise capacities and unrestricted diets (Allen *et al.*, 1998).

Ginseng exhibits effective antioxidant, free-radical scavenging activity, and inhibits lipid peroxidation (Fu and Ji, 2003). Intense exercise may increase the production of free radicals or reactive oxygen species. A free radical prefers to steal electrons from the lipid membrane of a cell, initiating a free-radical attack on the cell known as lipid peroxidation. Kanter *et al.* (1988) have demonstrated that post-exercise plasma creatine kinase (CK) elevations may be related to an exercise-induced lipid peroxidation. Low physiological levels of NO could act as an antioxidant, protecting the muscle from any deleterious effect of exhaustive exercise (Perez *et al.*, 2002). NO production after a single bout of exercise may reflect a systemic inflammatory response to heavy exercise. In a recent study on rats, ginseng treatment (11 mg/kg) protected muscles from eccentric exercise injuries and reduced NO concentrations in vastus and rectus (Cabral de Oliveira *et al.*, 2005).

Hsu *et al.* (2005) reported that oral supplementation with American ginseng (400 mg per capsule, 4 capsules daily) containing 8.7% ginsenosides Rb1 for 4 weeks in 13 male volunteers (aged 23 years) significantly reduced the leakage of plasma CK during exercise, but did not enhance aerobic work capacity. The reduction of plasma CK may be due to the fact that ginseng is effective for decreasing skeletal muscle cell membrane damage, induced by exercise during an exhaustive treadmill run. Thus, under appropriate conditions, ginseng root extracts may increase muscular strength and aerobic work capacity. Requirements are:

- sufficient daily dose (≥2000 mg *P. ginseng* root powder or an equivalent amount of root extract with standardised ginsenoside content)
- sufficient duration for effects to develop (≥8 wk)
- sufficient intensity of physical or mental activity (especially in untrained or older subjects)(Bucci, 2000).

Ginseng may exert greater benefits for untrained or older (>40 years) subjects and does not appear to exert any acute effects on physical performance.

Role of nitric oxide

Studies have shown that ginseng and ginsenosides induce NO release, a primary vasodilator. Specifically in an animal model and in-vitro studies, ginseng causes vasorelaxation and prevents manifestations of oxygen free-radical injury by promoting release of NO by endothelial cells. Purified components of GS, Rb_1 and especially Rg_1, relax pulmonary vessels, and this effect is eliminated by nitro-L-arginine, an inhibitor of nitric oxide (NO) synthase (Chen *et al.*, 1996). In support of this proposal, Kim *et al.* (1992) found that conversion of [^{14}C]L-arginine to [^{14}C]L-citrulline in confluent bovine aortic endothelial cells in culture was enhanced significantly by ginseng and by Rg, but not by Rb. A single injection (intraperitoneal) of ginseng extract (200 mg/kg) increased the levels of nitrites, nitrates and cGMP in rat serum and urine (Han and Kim, 1996). These effects were reversed by inhibition of NO synthase and restored by L-arginine. Similar action was observed in the rat kidney, isolated glomeruli, and cortical tubules and the action was blocked by inhibition of NO synthase. Ginseng extract appears to stimulate NO production in the kidney and thus may protect against ischaemia by increasing renal blood flow (Han and Kim, 1996). Kang *et al.* (1995) found that addition of ginseng to a high-cholesterol diet fed to rabbits preserved most of the normal dilatation of preconstricted aortic rings in response to acetylcholine. Interestingly, ginseng did not change endothelium-dependent relaxation to acetylcholine in animals receiving a normal diet. The mechanism of this effect is unknown but could reflect enhanced NO production or some enhancement of the guanylate cyclase pathway. Therefore, it would be appropriate to determine whether ginsenoside affects expression of NO synthase and guanylyl cyclase genes.

Several observations suggest that release of NO by ginseng may underlie the antioxidant effect of the extract. Wink *et al.* (1993) showed that NO-releasing agents protected Chinese hamster lung fibroblasts (V79 cells) from oxy-radical damage caused by hypoxanthine/xanthine oxidase, implying that NO, even at low concentrations, need not be cytotoxic.

The study also assessed whether similar actions would be seen after digestion designed to mimic the pH exposure after oral ingestion. Both digested and undigested ginseng dilated preconstricted perfused lung and preserved acetylcholine dilation following free-radical injury (Rimar *et al.*, 1996). Ginsenosides Rg and Rb were much less effective vasodilators after similar digestion, suggesting that standardised extracts of ginseng may be more effective after oral administration than individual ginsenosides. It has been noted that ginsenosides from the protopanaxatriol group (e.g. Re and Rg), but not the protopanaxadiol group (e.g. Rb and Rc), enhanced the release of NO from endothelial cells (Kang, 1995). Kim *et al.* (1999) also showed that Rg_3 mediated endothelium-dependent relaxation through eNOs activation in rat arteries.

The relaxing blood vessels may contribute to the antifatigue and blood-pressure-lowering effects of ginseng. In a human study, a single administration of a ginseng water extract (500 mg/kg) increased NO levels in exhaled breath and concomitantly decreased mean blood pressure (Han *et al.*, 2005). Ginseng also improves the vascular endothelial dysfunction in patients with hypertension possibly through increasing synthesis of NO (Sung *et al.*, 2000). In some studies, total root extract was more effective than isolated ginsenosides. However, it appears that direct effects of ginseng on physical performance by enhancing the release of NO from endothelial cells in humans have not been conclusively linked.

Recent studies, therefore, suggest that some cardiovascular protection effects of ginseng may be explained by the enhanced presence of NO. Evidence has been offered that:

- ginseng enhances formation of citrulline from added arginine, implying enhanced synthesis of NO
- known inhibitors of NO synthase, including oxyhaemoglobin and substituted arginine derivatives, block both the action of ginseng on citrulline formation from arginine and Ach-induced vascular relaxation of preconstricted tissue
- when used, arginine reverses the action of NO synthase inhibitors
- when measured, tissue cGMP has been increased by ginseng
- some of the effects can be potentiated by the presence of arginine in ginseng extracts. It was found that 5mg/mL of a commercial ginseng extract may provide an average of 1 μmol/L arginine in the assays; this is enough to account for all inhibition of NO synthase (Bejar *et al.*, 2003).

Using a pulmonary model in which endothelial injury is caused by a variety of reduced oxygen species, the protective action of ginseng is shown. Ginsenoside (50 or 200 μg/mL) prevented these vascular effects and also reduced the pulmonary oedema that follows free-radical injury (Kim *et al.*, 1992). The latter effect was eliminated by 100 μmol/L nitro-L-arginine, an inhibitor of NO synthase. These data are consistent with the proposal that ginseng causes vasorelaxation and prevents manifestations of oxygen free-radical injury by promoting release of NO.

Effects on central nervous system

Recently, it has been shown that ginsenosides exert beneficial effects on ageing, central nervous system (CNS) disorders and neurodegenerative diseases in animal models (Bao *et al.*, 2005; Radad *et al.*, 2006). Rats treated orally with ginseng root extract (G115) 20 mg/kg per day for 3 days showed improved performance in behavioural tests designed to assess memory enhancement and retention. Ginseng also attenuated a pentylenetetrazole-induced decrease in rat brain monoamine oxidase activity, proposed as an endogenous marker for anxiety, confirming its tranquilising or anti-anxiety effect. In fact, actions of white and red ginseng after 5 days of treatment were comparable with those of diazepam (Bhattacharya and Mitra, 1991).

Some evidence is presented on the use of *Panax ginseng* and cognitive function. In one study, 112 healthy subjects over age 40 were given 400 mg of a standardised ginseng product or placebo for 8 weeks. Those taking the ginseng experienced improved reaction times and abstract thinking. No changes were seen in concentration, memory or subjective experience (Sorensen and Sonne, 1996). Results of two other small studies, each with about 30 young, healthy subjects who received 200 mg of a standardised ginseng product (G115 extract, Ginsana, Pharmaton) daily for 8 weeks, showed improvement in attention processing, auditory reaction time, social functioning and aspects of mental health (D'Angelo *et al.*, 1986; Ellis and Reddy, 2002). However, some of these effects, which were present at 4 weeks, disappeared by 8 weeks. Another small study of 20 healthy young subjects, who received a single dose of 400 mg ginseng extract found improvement in cognition, memory, speed of memory tasks and improvements in accuracy of memory tasks (Kennedy *et al.*, 2002). In another double-blind, placebo-controlled study, no effect on psychological wellbeing was found in 83 healthy subjects who took 200–400 mg a day of a standardised ginseng extract for 8 weeks (Cardinal *et al.*, 2001).

The mechanisms of ginseng's actions on the CNS are not entirely clear. A number of studies has shown that some ginsenosides can modulate the activities of various important neurotransmitters such as choline, serotonin, acetylcholine, dopamine and their precursors in the brain. The ginsenoside Rb_1 has been shown to prevent memory loss in rats caused by a cholinergic agent in rats. Ginsenosides Rb_1 and Rg_1 can modulate acetylcholine release and re-uptake and the number of choline uptake sites, especially in the hippocampus (Benishin *et al.*, 1992). They also increase choline acetyltransferase levels in rat brains (Salim *et al.*, 1997), indirectly leading to an increase in acetylcholine synthesis. Rb_1 increases the maximum velocity of choline re-uptake in the hippocampus and cortex of rat brain, involved in memory and learning function, suggesting that ginsenosides Rb1 may improve central cholinergic function in humans and thus may be used to treat memory deficit (Rudakewich, 2001).

Scientific evidence suggests ginseng extract acts as an unspecific inhibitor for monamine-noradrenaline (NET), dopamine (DET) and serotonin (SERT) transporters (Bao *et al.*, 2005; Radad *et al.*, 2006). This inhibition of the transporters would result in an increase in the concentration of neurotransmitters in the brain, which may be linked to a mild central stimulant effect. It has also been reported that ginsenosides increase dopamine and noradrenaline in the cerebral cortex (Itoh *et al.*, 1989), which may explain the favourable effects of ginseng extract upon attention, cognitive processing, integrated sensory motor function, and auditory reaction time in healthy subjects (D'Angelo *et al.*, 1986). It has been shown that certain ginsenosides inhibit dopamine uptake into rat synaptosomes (Tsang *et al.*, 1985) and consequently ginseng could potentially provide protection against MPP+ through blockade of its uptake by dopaminergic neurones (Van Kampen *et al.*, 2003). Accordingly, ginseng total saponins can modulate dopaminergic activity at both pre-synaptic and post-synaptic receptors; and they can block behavioural sensitisation induced by psychostimulants such as morphine, cocaine, methamphetamines and nicotine (Shim *et al.*, 2000; Radad *et al.*, 2006). Furthermore, it was found that ginseng increased serotonin in the cortex, the ginseng saponins raised the levels of biogenic amines in normal rat brain, and ginsenoside Rg_2 directly interacted with nicotinic receptor subtypes (Sala *et al.*, 2002).

Ginseng administration leads to regulation of γ-aminobutyric acid (GABA)-ergic transmission in animals (Kimura *et al.*, 1994; Choi *et al.*, 2003). $GABA_B$ receptor is widely distributed in the CNS; many receptors are presynaptic and inhibit the release of other neurotransmitters. $GABA_B$ also mediates long-lasting synaptic hyperpolarisation, which leads to attenuation of nerve conduction. Compounds that activate $GABA_B$ receptor function tend to be good analgesics, while baclofen is a specific agonist. Total ginseng saponins were found to decrease baclofen binding. Ginsenoside Rc has shown some interaction on GABA receptors, which are involved in mood regulation and pain relief. The concentration of ginsenoside Rc may be above 2% in many extracts containing a high 9% ginsenoside concentration (Bejar *et al.*, 2003). It has been reported that total saponin fraction (10 μg/mL) and all purified ginsenosides Rb_1, Rb_2, Rc, Re, Rf, and Rg_1 inhibited high specific binding at a single concentration of 100 μmol/L for the specific $[^3H]$muscimol. This binding reflects interaction with the $GABA_A$ agonist site of the $GABA_AR$. However, in contrast to

$GABA_AR$ reported results, not all ginsensoides, but only ginsenoside Rc, demonstrated inhibition at 100 μmol/L (Kimura *et al.*, 1994).

Ginsenosides Rg_3 (S) and Rg_5/Rk_1 have been shown to significantly reverse memory dysfunction (Bao *et al.*, 2005). Ginsenosides Rg_3(R), Rg_3(S) or Rg_5/Rk_1, when orally administered for 4 days, significantly ameliorated the memory impairment induced by the single oral administration of ethanol or intraperitoneal injection of scopolamine. These ginsenosides protect against the excito-toxic and oxidative stress-induced neuroneal cell damage in primary cultured rat cortical cells. Among the ginsenosides tested, the Rg_5/Rk_1 combination was the most effective and potent, suggesting Rg_5/Rk_1 and Rg_3(S) may have therapeutic potential for clinical management of memory loss.

More recent studies suggest the mechanisms by which ginseng improves cognitive performance may also be related to the glycemic properties of some *Panax* species (Reay *et al.*, 2005). In a double-blind, placebo-controlled, balanced crossover design study, 27 healthy young adults consumed capsules containing either ginseng (200 mg of extract G115) or a placebo and 30 minutes later a drink containing glucose or placebo. Both *Panax ginseng* and glucose enhanced the performance of a mental arithmetic task and ameliorated the increase in subjective feelings of mental fatigue experienced by participants, and cognitively demanding task performance. *Panax ginseng* caused a reduction in blood glucose levels 1 hour following consumption when ingested without glucose. These results confirm that *Panax ginseng* may possess gluco-regulatory properties and can enhance cognitive performance.

There are few reports concerning the effect of ginseng on other neurodegenerative diseases. For example, two reports suggest that ginseng and its components prevent neuronal loss in amyotrophic lateral sclerosis models, and *Ginseng radix* has also been used for treatment of Alzheimer's disease (Jiang *et al.*, 2000; Lee *et al.*, 2001).

Effects of cardiovascular protection

Cardiovascular effects of ginseng root and individual ginsenosides have been studied extensively. Many reports describe transient vasodilator actions, followed by vasoconstriction and increase in blood pressure. Several authors have implicated the adrenergic nervous system in the cardiovascular effects of ginseng (Zhang and Chen, 1987), and it was reported (Tachikawa *et al.*, 1995) that the panaxatriols, particularly Rg, reduced acetylcholine-evoked release of catecholamines from bovine adrenal chromaffin cells. Extrapolating from these data, the authors suggest that ginseng may reduce elevated circulating catecholamine concentrations associated with various forms of stress in humans. It has been suggested that these actions might reflect the interaction of ginseng with an endogenous vasoactive substance, and are associated with NO released from endothelial cells (see below) (Chen, 1996; Kim *et al.*, 1999; Friedl *et al.*, 2001; Radad *et al.*, 2006).

Ginsenoside Rb_1 bears various beneficial effects on the cardiovascular system. The treatment of rats with standardised ginseng extract (10 mg/mL of drinking water for 7 days) had cardioprotective effects that could be demonstrated in vivo (Maffei-Facino *et al.*, 1999). After treatment either with ginseng or water (as control), animals were exposed to hyperbaric hyperoxia (100% O_2; 2.5 atm [253.3 kPa] for 6 h). Hearts from G115-treated rats showed significantly lower coronary vasoconstriction in response to angiotensin II than control hearts. Endothelial function in aortic rings from ginseng-treated animals was preserved, as evidenced by normal relaxation in response to acetylcholine and a modest vasoconstriction after inhibition of NO synthase. Both observations imply protection of endothelial function from oxygen radical damage. Therefore, this study confirms and extends data of Kim *et al.* (1992) by establishing that oral administration of a standardised ginseng provides significant antioxidant action and may also stimulate NO synthase.

The cardioprotective action of ginseng against ischaemia–reperfusion injury has been reported in a study of patients undergoing cardiopulmonary bypass for mitral valve surgery (Zhan *et al.*, 1994). Among 30 patients studied, 11 received a normal cardioplegic solution (used to suspend cardiac action during phases of the surgical procedure), 11 received a solution with ginseng extract (0.6 to

1.2 mg/kg) and 8 received a solution containing ginsenosides in total and Rb (0.3 to 0.6 mg/kg). Cardiac performance was monitored by the oesophageal Doppler technique and also by morphometric analysis of samples of left ventricular myocardium. Total ginseng extract enhanced recovery of cardiac haemodynamic performance and significantly lowered mitochondrial swelling during the period of ischaemia. Interestingly, total root extract in these studies was more effective than the individual ginsenosides used. Unfortunately, the nature of the ginseng extract (type, extraction technique) is not stated. Nevertheless, this study is intriguing and awaits independent confirmation.

Homocysteine is an independent risk factor for cardiovascular disease by its multiple effects on vascular cells and thrombosis factors, which may be involved in oxidative stress mechanisms. Ginseng compounds have effects of vasorelaxation and antioxidation. Recent studies showed that ginsenoside Rb1 can effectively block homocysteine-induced dysfunction of endothelium-dependent vasorelaxation as well as superoxide anion production and endothelial nitric oxide synthase (eNOS) down-regulation (Ohashi *et al.*, 2005; Zhou *et al.*, 2005). The findings suggest that ginseng and its active constituents may have potential clinical applications in protecting the endothelium against homocysteine and superoxide-associated injuries. The study provides some new aspects of ginsenosides on cardiovascular disease prevention.

Effects on immune system and anti-inflammatory response

Ginseng may support a healthy immune system. A study with 227 healthy volunteers demonstrated that giving 100 mg daily of a standardised extract for a period of 12 weeks enhanced the effect of the influenza vaccine. Subjects who received ginseng had a lower incidence of influenza and common cold, high antibody titres and higher natural killer cell activity: all indicating an improvement in immune system response (Scaglione *et al.*, 1990). In a second study by the same research group, in 60 healthy volunteers 100 mg of standardised ginseng extract, given twice a day, improved a number of immune system response factors (chemotaxis, phagocytosis and increased white blood cell count) (Scaglione *et al.*, 1990). During a double-blind investigation, a standardised extract of ginseng root was given orally to volunteers, resulting in reduced susceptibility to infectious respiratory tract diseases (Scaglione *et al.*, 1996).

Macrophages constitute the first line of host defences in conferring immunity against infections. Macrophages are known to produce NO, and one of the most prominent functions of NO is its participation in antimicrobial and antiviral defence (Nathan *et al.*, 1991). iNOS inhibitors have been shown to exacerbate infectious diseases (Chan *et al.*, 1995), yet the enhancement of bacterial clearance in *Pseudomonas aeruginosa*-infected athymic rats by ginseng extract treatment has been shown (Song *et al.*, 1997). iNOS stimulation by *Panax ginseng* might contribute to a decreased susceptibility to infections because of an enhanced NO release. Aqueous extracts of *Panax ginseng* root directly enhance transcriptional activity of the iNOS promoter via transcription factor NF-κβ, leading to increased iNOS mRNA and protein levels (Friedl *et al.*, 2001).

A fraction from an aqueous extract of *Panax ginseng* root powder possesses stimulating activity completely attributed to the polysaccharide-containing fraction. The fraction containing triterpenic ginsenosides did not display any stimulation of NO release. Experiments with polysaccharides isolated from these aqueous extracts confirmed the stimulating activity of these substances on the inducible NO synthase. The effect of very high NO output at the highest concentration induced a phenomenon of negative feedback control of iNOS mRNA levels. Ginsenoside Rg1 increased the number of Th cells and induced an augmentation of the production of IL-1 by macrophages (Kenarova *et al.*, 1990); and enhanced the production of NO from interferon (IFN)-γ activated RAW cells (Fan *et al.*, 1995). In contrast, ginsenosides Rh1 and Rh2 inhibited NO production in LPS/IFN-γ treated macrophages (Park *et al.*, 1996). Ginsenoside Rg1 could enhance NO production and the expression of eNOS messenger RNA in TNF-α-stimulated human umbilical vein endothelial cells; and ginsenoside Rg1 regulates sets of genes in endothelial cells and protects endothelial cells from TNF-α activation (Lu *et al.*, 2004).

Panax ginseng with anti-inflammatory and anti-allergic actions

The root of *Panax ginseng* has been also reported to possess anti-inflammatory and anti-allergic actions. Park *et al.* (2004) reported the antiallergic activity of ginsenosides isolated from ginseng in vitro and in vivo on rat peritoneal mast cells and on IgE-induced passive cutaneous anaphylaxis in mice. Ginsenoside Rh_1 potently inhibited histamine release from rat peritoneal mast cells and the IgE-mediated anaphylaxis reaction in mice. Rh1 was also found to have a membrane-stabilising action. It also inhibited inducible nitric oxide synthase (iNOS) and cyclo-oxygenase-2 (COX-2) protein expression in RAW 264.7 cells, and the activation of the transcription factor, NF-κB, in nuclear fractions (Friedl *et al.*, 2001).

Effects on type 2 diabetes

The effects of *Panax ginseng* show promise for managing type 2 diabetes. In a study with 36 patients with newly diagnosed type 2 diabetes, 100 or 200 mg of a standardised ginseng extract for 8 weeks improved fasting blood sugar levels. The 200 mg dose also resulted in improved haemoglobin A1c values (a measurement of long-term blood sugar control) (Sotaniemi *et al.*, 1995). *Panax ginseng* (6 g/day for 6 weeks) also improved postprandial glycaemia and insulin sensitivity in type 2 diabetes (Vuksan *et al.*, 2000). American ginseng (3 g) decreased postprandial glycaemia acutely in healthy subjects and subjects with type 2 diabetes when taken orally (Sievenpiper *et al.*, 2004).

The mechanisms underlying improving blood glucose levels associated with ginseng extract and its major active components may be multifaceted. Firstly, ginseng extract may decrease food intake and reduce absorption of the source of carbohydrate (Attele *et al.*, 2002). Secondly, treatment with ginseng extract increased serum insulin levels (Kimura *et al.*, 1981), improved peripheral insulin sensitivity (Xie *et al.*, 2002), and stimulated cellular glucose uptake (Hasegawa *et al.*, 1994). Since ginsenosides are shown to release NO from vascular tissues (Chen, 1996), and NO is known to stimulate glucose-dependent secretion of insulin in rat islet cells (Spinas *et al.*, 1998), ginseng extract may affect glucose transport, which is mediated by NO and thus modulates NO-mediated insulin secretion (Roy *et al.*, 1998). Lastly, the antioxidant property of ginseng extract may be a significant mechanism of antidiabetic action.

Ginkgo

The constituents of the ginkgo leaf that are of primary interest are the phenolic and terpenoid compounds. For effectiveness, *Ginkgo biloba* extracts are recommended to be standardised to 24% ginkgo flavone glycosides and 6% terpene lactones (Stromgaard *et al.*, 2005). Generally, the ginkgolic acids are removed from ginkgo preparations.

The flavone glycosides neutralise free radicals and improve circulation by dilating small blood vessels, thereby believed to protect brain cells against damage by oxygen deprivation. The diterpene ginkgolides are believed to antagonise activities of inflammation and blood clotting associated with platelet-activating factor (Cooper, 2003; Nakanishi, 2005).

A combination of these chemical compounds and their actions are believed to be responsible for this herb's efficacy in improving blood circulation in the brain and application for use in slowing age-related cognitive decline. In a recent meta-analysis, researchers reviewed the efficacy and safety of *Ginkgo biloba* for the treatment of patients with dementia or cognitive decline. Thirty-three relevant clinical trials were selected for review and were all randomised, double-blind controlled studies (Birks and Evans, 2003). The daily dose of ginkgo extract used in these studies varied from 80 to 600 mg. All studies used a standardised extract containing 24% total flavone glycosides and 6% of ginkgolides. Treatment periods also varied from 3 to 52 weeks, with the majority being of 12 weeks' duration. Although most studies only reported the results of those who completed treatment, most studies indicated positive results compared with placebo. Several rating scales or tests were used to assess ginkgo's effect on cognition and included memory impairment, attention, concentration and speed of learning. In addition, the effect of ginkgo on activities of daily living and measures on mood and emotion were also studied in some cases. Results of this meta-analysis suggest that a daily dose of 80–200 mg of a standardised extract of ginkgo over a 12-week period has beneficial effects on cognition compared with a placebo.

Effects of ginkgo on memory and cognition

The effects of ginkgo on memory and cognition have also been studied in healthy subjects (no known cognitive decline). Kennedy *et al.* (2000) examined the effects of three doses of a standardised extract of ginkgo (120, 240 and 360 mg) vs placebo in a double-blind, placebo-controlled, crossover design study in healthy, young volunteers (age 19–24 years). Results indicated that ginkgo administration produced a number of significant time- and dose-specific changes in cognitive performance, especially noted in measurements of 'speed of attention' with doses of 240 and 360 mg (Kennedy *et al.*, 2000).

To demonstrate cognitive performance in healthy subjects, a large double-blind, placebo-controlled trial examined the effects of a standardised extract of ginkgo on neurological and memory processes of older, healthy adults. In this study 262 volunteers (male and female, 60 years and older) were randomised to receive 180 mg of ginkgo extract per day or a placebo for a duration of 6 weeks. Efficacy measures included a comparison of performance scores from baseline and 6 weeks on a series of standardised tests used to measure cognition and memory. Results indicated that the ginkgo treatment significantly improved tasks involving recall and recognition of visual and auditory material. Subjects taking ginkgo also reported subjective improvements in overall ability to remember compared with those taking a placebo (Mix and Crew, 2002).

Not all trials with healthy adult groups have resulted in positive effects. In a well-designed, 6-week, randomised, double-blind, placebo-controlled trial examining the effects of 120 mg of a standardised extract of ginkgo in 203 older men and women (60 and older), researchers found no effect of ginkgo treatment on measures of memory, attention and concentration using standardised neuropsychological tests. Limitations of this study may have impacted the results: the dose used was not high enough to elicit a response in healthy subjects or the duration of the study was too short at 6 weeks (Solomon *et al.*, 2002).

The main focus of the substantiated claims for a ginkgo extract at a 120 mg dose is centred on concentration and memory. These studies (Hofferberth *et al.*, 1989) all show significant improvements in memory and concentration versus placebo over 8–12-week periods of supplementation with *Gingko biloba* extract (GBE). Other cognitive function tests, mental performance tests, and psychometric exams, have also been utilised in clinical studies to show the effects of ginkgo. Three studies (Wesnes *et al.*, 1987; Rai *et al.*, 1991; Grässel, 1992), using either computer tests or exams, have independently shown significant improvements in memory and mental performance (speed in mental processing) versus placebo. Short-term effects of GBE have also been studied in normal, healthy volunteers, generally younger adults aged approximately 20–30 years. These studies have ranged from assessments conducted after 1–3 hours following acute (single-dose) ingestion of the product (Hindmarch, 1988). Furthermore, a 1995 double-blind crossover study out of New York compared GBE with two different Ginkgo extract products using computer electroencephalographic/brain-mapping techniques. GBE produced the most homogeneous CNS effects and was the only extract that could be classified as a cognitive activator (Itil and Martorano, 1995).

Ginkgo biloba has also been studied for its effectiveness as a treatment for Alzheimer's disease. The ginkgolides have long been promoted as memory-enhancing components and even demonstrated to inhibit or eliminate the deadly effects of amyloid peptides. Ginkgolide A and ginkgolide J are the two ginkgolides that were shown to exhibit activity, however, ginkgolide J is the least abundant ginkgolide (Nakanishi, 2005). The efficacy of ginkgo for this purpose was reviewed in a meta-analysis by Oken *et al.* (1998). A review of 50 articles resulted in only four studies that met researchers' inclusion criteria (clear diagnosis of Alzheimer's disease, clearly stated exclusion criteria, use of stated standardised extract of 24 or 25% ginkgo-flavone glycosides, 6% terpene lactones, randomised, placebo-controlled, double-blind study and at least one outcome measure to assess cognitive function). Of the four studies, a total of 212 subjects each received ginkgo (120 or 240 mg) or a placebo. The duration of these studies was 3–6 months and overall researchers concluded a significant effect of ginkgo treatment on objective measures of cognitive function in subjects with Alzheimer's. This translated into a 3% difference in the Alzheimer's disease assessment scale-cognitive subtest (Oken *et al.*, 1998).

Ginkgo and GABA

γ-Aminobutyric acid (GABA) is the major inhibitory amino acid neurotransmitter in the mammalian CNS and present in about 40% of all neurones. GABA protects brain cells by interfering with deleterious activity triggered during trauma or ageing. GABA effects are mediated through three different GABA receptors: $GABA_A$, $GABA_B$ and $GABA_C$. The $GABA_A$ receptor contains several sites of action referred to as the benzodiazepine, the GABA and the internal chloride channel sites. Drugs such as diazepam work by interacting in the benzodiazepine site, potentiating GABA activity, while the GABA and the chloride channel sites are considered targets for anticonvulsant medications.

Ginkgo extracts exhibit an interaction with benzodiazepine and $GABA_A$ agonist sites which may elicit an anti-anxiety effect. Bilobalide, one of the active constituents in Ginkgo, seems also to play a major role in GABA modulation in the brain (van Beek *et al.*, 1998). Ginkgo extract elicits antianxiety effects in a number of animal models and this has been observed in clinical trials.

Peripheral benzodiazepine receptor (stress regulation)

The peripheral benzodiazepine receptors (PBRs) were first described more than 20 years ago as benzodiazepine-binding sites in non-neuroneal tissue (Braestrup and Squires, 1977). Studies have demonstrated this mitochondrial receptor is implicated in regulating stress responses. Acute single forced swimming stress in rats is associated with a significant increase in PBR density in cerebral cortex, olfactory bulb, kidney, platelets, and lymphocytes (Novas *et al.*, 1987). The same increase is observed in animals subjected to acute noise levels. In clinical studies, platelet PBRs were assessed in psychiatric residents who were completing the written part of a board-certification examination in comparison with age- and sex-matched controls. The platelet PBR density was significantly elevated immediately after the examination and showed a trend toward a decrease to normal range 10 days later. Similar changes were detected in anxiety levels, as measured by the appropriate rating scale (Karp *et al.*, 1989). Thus, as shown in animal studies, acute stress in humans can lead to an increase in PBRs.

PBR is a key element in the formation of hormones transporting cholesterol essential for the synthesis of glucocorticoids. Research suggests that ginkgo decreases the levels of corticosterone by inhibiting production of PBR and the PBR channel itself. These findings may have an impact in a number of medical conditions such as panic disorder, post-traumatic stress disorder, and generalised anxiety disorder, where a large concentration of glucocorticoids has been found.

Research suggests that a standardised extract of ginkgo (761 EGb) and ginkgolides A and B decrease corticosterone levels by inhibiting production of PBR and the PBR channel itself (Amri *et al.*, 1996). The 761 EGb extract and the ginkgolides reduced ligand binding to PBR with very high affinity (K_d values were 1.9, 2.3 and 2.1 nmol/L respectively).

Garlic

The applicable part of garlic *Allium sativum* L. (Alliaceae) is the bulb and the pharmacological effects of garlic are attributed to allicin, ajoene and other organosulphur constituents such as *S*-allyl-L-cysteine.

A wide variation exists in the chemical composition of garlic products, reflecting differences in processing (Lawson, 1998). The constituent profile of garlic is unique and complex, being particularly rich in sulphur-containing compounds. The main constituents of garlic include cysteine sulphoxides (0.6% to 1.9%) of which the most abundant is alliin (*S*-allylcysteine sulphoxide) representing up to 14 mg/g fresh weight of cloves (Ueda *et al.* 1991; Mütsch-Eckner *et al.* 1992), followed by *S*-methyl analogue (methiin) which occurs in quantities of up to 2 mg/g, followed by *S*-trans-1-propenylcysteine sulphoxide (isoalliin) at about 0.5 mg/g (Koch and Lawson, 1996; Lawson *et al.*, 2005). The glutamylcysteines (0.5% to 1.6%) are represented by *S*-allyl and the *S*-trans-1-propenyl analogues which are the most abundant (Lawson *et al.*, 2005). Other organosulphur components include the scordinins, a family of structurally related compounds to the thioglyco-phosphopeptides (Kominato, 1969).

Garlic is also noted for its very high content of fructans or fructosans which account for up to 65% of its dry weight, total carbohydrate content can reach 77%. Free amino acids, of which arginine is the most prevalent, constitute 10–15 mg/g fresh weight in cloves (Ueda *et al.*, 1991). More detailed information about the chemical complexity in garlic preparations can be found elsewhere (Lawson *et al.*, 2005).

Numerous research papers describe the use of garlic as a cholesterol-lowering agent, and several as an immune-stimulating agent (Lawson *et al.*, 2005). Other activities such as antiatherosclerotic, antithrombotic, anticancer and antioxidant, as well as antimicrobial and detoxifying effects of garlic are well documented in the literature and beyond the scope of the present review (Lawson *et al.*, 2005).

Use of garlic in cardiovascular disease models

Garlic possesses pharmacological effects in a number of conditions including hypertension, hyperlipidaemia, prevention of coronary heart disease, as well as age-related vascular changes, atherosclerosis, reducing re-infarction and mortality rate post-myocardial infarction (World Health Organization, 1999).

A recent focus of attention is on the mechanism of action of how garlic lowers total cholesterol, low-density lipoproteins and triglycerides, and increases high-density lipoprotein cholesterol (Agarwal, 1998; Singh and Porter, 2006). There is substantial clinical evidence that shows the consumption of the equivalent of one half to one clove of garlic daily leads to a decrease of 9–12% in serum cholesterol and average decrease in serum triglycerides of about 13%. Over 50 clinical studies have been conducted on the lipid-lowering effects of garlic, at least 19 (including 1275 patients) have been included into two meta-analyses (Silagy and Neil, 1994) and are detailed elsewhere (Lawson *et al.*, 2005). Clearly various garlic preparations exhibit different antilipidaemic effects. In rodents oral and intraperitoneal administration of raw garlic (50–500 mg/kg) has a very significant effect in reducing glucose, cholesterol and triglycerides, whereas boiled garlic has little effect on these parameters (Thomson *et al.*, 2006).

In two separate studies, solvent-extracted garlic and sulphur compounds given to patients with hyperlipidaemia, lowered cholesterol levels and the researchers suggested the effects resembled those of HMG-CoA reductase inhibitors (Gebhardt and Beck, 1996).

One of the constituents in fresh garlic and solvent extracts is *S*-allyl-L-cysteine, which is also present in large amounts in aged garlic extract (AGE). This typically contains 19% of the *S*-allylcysteine found in the original cloves (Lawson, 1998). This compound is a potent inhibitor of hepatic cholesterol synthesis (Yeh and Liu, 2001). Recent research suggests the site of inhibition is downstream of lanosterol synthesis, as HMG CoA reductase does not appear to be affected (Singh and Porter, 2006).

Accumulation of methylsterols was detected by gas chromatography in cultured hepatoma cells treated with fresh garlic macerates, suggesting that 4a-methyl oxidase is the principal enzyme inhibited in cholesterol synthesis. It has been concluded that all garlic compounds sharing an allyl-disulphide, or allyl sulphydryl group appear to be inhibitors of the enzyme (Singh and Porter, 2006).

An additional benefit of allyl sulphides in garlic preparations is LDL oxidative prevention. Many compounds share this activity including *S*-allyl cysteine, *S*-allyl mercaptocysteine, alliin, allixin, and by *N*-acetyl-*S*-allyl cysteine, a metabolite of *S*-allyl cysteine (Lau, 2006).

For hypertension, garlic is thought to reduce blood pressure by two mechanisms:

- causing smooth muscle relaxation and vasodilation by activating production of endothelium-derived relaxation factor (EDRF, nitric oxide) (Pedraza-Chaverri *et al.*, 1998)
- inhibition of angiotensin-converting enzyme (ACE) (Sendl *et al.*, 1992), although the latter

effects have not been demonstrated conclusively in vivo and are not observed with all garlic preparations.

Garlic elicits vasodilator (antihypertensive) effects through activation of nitric oxide synthase (NOS) and thereby enhances the production of nitric oxide (NO). As noted earlier, NO is responsible for multiple functions in the body (see under ginseng). Garlic powder preparations also have been shown to possess strong affinity for NOS, although high concentrations of arginine may account for part of the effect when tested in vitro.

Garlic compounds have been shown to elicit ACE inhibition, particularly the γ-glutamyl cysteines (GGC) (Sendl *et al.*, 1992; Rahman and Lowe, 2006).

Antioxidant and immune-stimulating effects

AGE prevents endothelial cell depletion of glutathione and reduces levels of NO and peroxides in macrophages (Ide *et al.*, 1999). Although AGE preparations elicit some immune stimulation effects and enhance natural killer (NK) cell activity (Ishikawa *et al.*, 2006), other garlic preparations also support and enhance the immune function (Kyo *et al.*, 1999, 2001; Lamm and Riggs, 2001).

Comparison of the effects of garlic preparations to bacillus Calmette-Guérin (BCG) immunotherapy reveals many common mechanisms. These include stimulation of the proliferation of lymphocytes; enhancement of macrophage phagocytosis; increased infiltration of macrophages and lymphocytes into tumours transplanted into animals; induction of splenic hypertrophy; stimulation of cytotoxic enhancement of NK cell activity and lymphokine-activated killer cell activity (Lamm and Riggs, 2001).

Garlic powder demonstrated positive effects on the general immune system and phagocytosis. Oral administration (600 mg/day) of garlic powder for 3 months in a geriatric population increased the percentage of peripheral granulocytes able to effectively phagocytose *E. coli* in an ex vivo assay (Kyo *et al.*, 1999).

Allicin itself was shown to stimulate [^{3}H] thymidine incorporation in mouse splenocytes and enhance cell-mediated cytotoxicity in human peripheral mononuclear cells. The immune stimulatory effect of allicin appears to be mediated by redox-sensitive signalling of key regulatory proteins, such as activation of p21*ras*, which transduces a variety of extracellular signals regulating cell growth and differentiation. Allicin's immune-stimulatory properties may be responsible for some of the anticancer effects of garlic (Patya *et al.*, 2004), although the bioavailability of allicin and its rapid conversion to other compounds is now in question (Amagase, 2006).

Conclusions

In conclusion, it is clear that TCM is gaining wide acceptance beyond China and Asia. Today, as these medicines are being 'rediscovered', and are accepted by wider population groups, one challenge is to adapt modern scientific, biological and clinical standards. TCM favours a combination of several herbs to generate a putative clinical effect. This multiherb approach poses a challenge to manufacturing and to investigators seeking to identify the biological actives and substantiate a 'structure function' claim. There is, therefore, a need to carefully define a clinical trial paradigm that addresses structure function claims without sacrificing scientific rigour, and it is anticipated that more in vitro and in vivo pharmacology will be needed that links a biological response to an identified chemical signal. In this chapter, using select examples we have demonstrated the importance of linking such chemical signals to biological effects, leading to a therapeutic use, and this approach in turn may lead to better crafted, well-defined herbal extracts that demonstrate efficacy in clinical studies.

Acknowledgement

The author wishes to thank Chi Hee Kim for editorial help.

References

Adhami VM, Ahmad N, Mukhtar H (2003). Molecular targets for green tea in prostate cancer prevention. *J Nutrition* 133: 2417S–2424S.

Adhami VM, Siddiqui IA, Ahmad N, *et al.* (2004). Oral consumption of green tea polyphenols inhibits insulin-like growth factor-I-induced signaling in an autochthonous mouse model of prostate cancer. *Cancer Res* 64: 8715–8722.

Agarwal KC (1998). Therapeutic actions of garlic constituents. *Med Res Rev* 16: 111–124.

Ahmad N, Gupta S, Mukhtar H (2000). Green tea polyphenol epigallocatechin-3-gallate differentially modulates nuclear factor κB in cancer cells versus normal cells. *Archives Biochem Biophys* 376: 338–346.

Ahmad N, Mukhtar H (1999). Green tea polyphenols and cancer biologic mechanisms and practical implications. *Nutr Rev* 57: 78–83.

Allen JD, McLung J, Nelson AG, *et al.* (1998). Ginseng supplementation does not enhance healthy young adults' peak aerobic exercise performance. *J Am Coll Nutr* 17: 462–466.

Amagase H (2006). Clarifying the real bioactive constituents of garlic. *J Nutr* 136: 716S–772S.

Amri H, Ogwuegbu SO, Boujrad N, *et al.* (1996). In vivo regulation of peripheral-type benzodiazepine receptor and glucocorticoid synthesis by *Ginkgo biloba* extract EGb 761 and isolated ginkgolides. *Endocrinology* 137: 5707–5718.

Annabi B, Lachambre MP, Bousquet-Gagnon N *et al.* (2002). Green tea polyphenol (−)-epigallocatechin 3-gallate inhibits MMP-2 secretion and MT1–MMP-driven migration in glioblastoma cells. *Biochim Biophys Acta* 1542: 209–220.

Attele AS, Wu JA, Yuan CS (1999). Ginseng pharmacology: multiple constituents and multiple actions. *Biochem Pharmacol* 58: 1685–1693.

Attele AS, Zhou YP, Xie JT, *et al.* (2002). Antidiabetic effects of Panax ginseng berry extract and the identification of an effective component. *Diabetes* 51: 1851–1858.

Awang D, Bejar E (2001). Plant bioassays, the promise and the challenge. *J Herbs Spices Med Plants* 8: 1–5.

Bahrke MS, Morgan WR (2000). Evaluation of the ergogenic properties of ginseng: an update. *Sports Med* 29: 113–133.

Balasubramanian S, Efimova T, Eckert RL (2002). Green tea polyphenol stimulates a Ras, MEKK1, MEK3, and p38 cascade to increase activator protein 1 factor-dependent involucrin gene expression in normal human keratinocytes. *J Biochem* 277: 1828–1836.

Bao HY, Zhang J, Yeo SJ, *et al.* (2005). Memory enhancing and neuroprotective effects of selected ginsenosides. *Arch Pharmacol Res* 28: 335–342.

Benishin CG (1992). Actions of ginsenoside Rb1 on choline uptake in central cholinergic nerve endings. *Neurochem Int* 21: 1–5.

Benzie IF, Szeto YT, Strain JJ, *et al.* (1999). Consumption of green tea causes rapid increase in plasma antioxidant power in humans. *Nutr Cancer* 34: 83–87.

Berova N, Jaracz S, Kim SR, *et al.* (2003). Bioorganic Studies on Ginkgolides http://www.columbia.edu/cu/chemistry/groups/nakanishi/ginkgo.html.

Bhattacharya SK, Mitra SK (1991). Anxiolytic activity of Panax ginseng roots: an experimental study. *J Ethnopharmacol* 34: 87–92.

Birks J, Grimley EJ (2004). Ginkgo biloba for cognitive impairment and dementia (Cochrane Review). In: *The Cochrane Library*, Issue 1. John Wiley & Sons, Ltd., Chichester, UK.

Blumenthal M (1998). German Federal Institute for Drugs and Medical Devices. Commission E. *The Complete German Commission E monographs: therapeutic guide to herbal medicines.* American Botanical Council, Austin, Texas.

Blumenthal M, Brinckmann J, Dinda K, *et al.* (2001). *The ABC Clinical Guide to Herbs.* Austin, Texas, American Botanical Council, pp. 335–349.

Braestrup C, Squires RF (1977). Specific benzodiazepine receptors in rat brain characterized by high affinity [3H] diazepam binding. *Proc Nat Acad Sci* 74: 3805–3809.

Buettner C, Yeh GY, Phillips RS, *et al.* (2006). Systematic review of the effects of ginseng on cardiovascular risk factors. *Ann Pharmacother* 40: 83–95.

Cabral de Oliveira AC, Perez AC, Prieto JG, *et al.* (2005). Protection of Panax ginseng in injured muscles after eccentric exercise. *J Ethnopharmacol* 92: 211–214.

Cardinal BJ, Engels HJ (2001). Ginseng does not enhance psychological well-being in healthy, young adults: results of a double-blind, placebo-controlled, randomized clinical trial. *J Am Diet Assoc* 101: 655–660.

Chan J, Tanaka K, Carroll D, *et al.* (1995). Effects of nitric oxide synthase inhibitors on murine infection with *Mycobacterium tuberculosis. Infect Immun* 63: 736–740.

Chan MM, Fong D, Ho CT, Huang HI (1997). Inhibition of inducible nitric oxide synthase gene expression and enzyme activity by epigallocatechin gallate, a natural product from green tea. *Biochem Pharmacol* 54: 1281–1286.

Chen X, (1996). Cardiovascular protection by ginsenosides and their nitric oxide releasing action. *Clin Exp Pharmacol Physiol* 23: 728–732.

Chen X, Wu T, Liu G (2006). Chinese medicinal herbs for influenza; a systematic review. *J Altern Complement Med* 12: 171–180.

Chen XC, Zhu YG, Zhu LA, *et al.* (2003). Ginsenoside Rg1 attenuates dopamine-induced apoptosis in PC12 cells by suppressing oxidative stress. *Eur J Pharmacol* 473: 1–7.

Chen ZM, Yu YM (1994). Tea. In: Arntzen C J, Ritter E M eds. *Encyclopedia of Agricultural Science.* Academic Press, San Diego, pp. 281–288.

Cho NM, Chueh PJ, Kim C, *et al.* (2002). A monoclonal antibody to a circulating form of a drug-responsive hydroquinone (NADH) oxidase from sera of cancer patients. *Cancer Immunol Immunother* 51: 121–129.

Choi SE, Choi S, Lee JH, *et al.* (2003). Effects of ginsenosides on GABA(A) receptor channels expressed in *Xenopus* oocytes. *Arch Pharmacol Res* 26: 28–33.

Chueh PJ, Morré DM, Morré DJ (2002). A site-directed mutagenesis analysis of tNOX functional domains. *Biochim Biophys Acta* 1594: 74–83.

Chueh PJ, Wu LY, Morré DM, Morré DJ (2004). tNOX is both necessary and sufficient as a cellular target for the anticancer actions of capsaicin and the green tea catechin (−)-epigallocatechin gallate. *Biofactors* 20: 237–241.

Cooper R (2003). Gin(kgo) and tonic – with a twist! *J Altern Complement Med* 9: 599–601.

Cooper R, Morré DJ, Morré DM (2005a). Medicinal benefits of green tea. Part I: review of non cancer health benefits. *J Altern Complement Med* 11: 521–528.

Cooper R, Morré DJ, Morré DM (2005b). Medicinal benefits of green tea. Part II: review of anti cancer properties. *J Altern Complement Med* 11: 639–652.

Cui JF, Garle M, Bjorkhem I, Eneroth P (1996). Determination of aglycones of ginsenosides in ginseng preparations sold in Sweden and in urine samples from Swedish athletes consuming ginseng. *Scand J Clin Lab Invest* 56: 151–160.

D'Angelo L, Grimaldi R, Caravaggi M, *et al.* (1986). A double-blind, placebo-controlled clinical study on the effect of a standardized ginseng extract on psychomotor performance in healthy volunteers. *J Ethnopharmacol* 16: 15–22.

Ellis JM, Reddy P (2002). Effects of *Panax ginseng* on quality of life. *Ann Pharmacother* 36: 375–379.

Engels HJ, Said JM, Wirth JC (1996). Failure of chronic ginseng supplementation to affect work performance and energy metabolism in healthy adult females. *Nutr Res* 16: 1295–1305.

Engels HJ, Wirth JC (1997). No ergogenic effects of ginseng (*Panax ginseng* C.A. Meyer) during graded maximal aerobic exercise. *J Am Diet Assoc* 97: 1110–1115.

Fan ZH, Isobe K, Kiuchi K, Nakashima I (1995). Enhancement of nitric oxide production from activated macrophages by a purified form of ginsenoside (Rg1). *Am J Chin Med* 23: 279–287.

Farnsworth NR (1990). The role of ethnopharmacology in drug development. In: *Bioactive Compounds from Plants*. Eds. DJ Chadwick and J Marsh. Ciba Foundation Symposium 154. Wiley, Chichester, UK.

Fernandez R, Ganzon D (2003). Use of green tea-capsicum supplement (capsibiol-T) as adjuvant cancer treatment: case study reports. *Philippine J Otolaryngol Head Neck Surg* 18: 171–177.

Forgo I, Kirchdorfer AM (1982). The effect of different ginsenoside concentrations on physical work capacity. *Notabene Med* 12: 721–727.

Friedl R, Moeslinger T, Kopp B, Spieckermann PG (2001). Stimulation of nitric oxide synthesis by the aqueous extract of *Panax ginseng* root in RAW 264.7 cells. *Br J Pharmacol* 134: 1663–1670.

Fu Y, Ji LL (2003). Chronic ginseng consumption attenuates age-associated oxidative stress in rats. *J Nutr* 133: 3603–3609.

Fulder SJ (1990). *The Book of Ginseng*. Healing Arts Press, Rochester, VT.

Gebhardt R, Beck H (1996). Differential inhibitory effects of garlic-derived organosulfur compounds on cholesterol biosynthesis in primary rat hepatocyte cultures. *Lipids* 31: 1269–1276.

Grässel E (1992). Effect of *Ginkgo biloba* extract on mental performance. Double-blind study using computerized measurement conditions in patients with cerebral insufficiency. *Fortschr Med* 110: 73–78.

Gupta S, Ahmad N, Nieminen AL, *et al.* (2000). Growth inhibition, cell-cycle dysregulation and induction of apoptosis by green tea constituent (−)-epigallocatechin-3-gallate in androgen-sensitive and androgen-insensitive human prostate carcinoma cells. *Toxicol Appl Pharmacol* 164: 82–90.

Han K, Shin IC, Choi KJ, *et al.* (2005). Korea red ginseng water extract increases nitric oxide concentrations in exhaled breath. *Nitric Oxide* 12: 159–162.

Han SW, Kim H (1996). Ginsenosides stimulate endogenous production of nitric oxide in rat kidney. *Int J Biochem Cell Biol* 28: 573–580.

Hara Y (2001). *Green Tea: Health Benefits and Applications*. Marcel Dekker Inc., New York.

Harkey MR, Henderson GL, Gershwin ME, *et al.* (2001). Variability in commercial ginseng products: an analysis of 25 preparations. *Am J Clin Nutr* 73: 1101–1106.

Helms S (2004). Cancer prevention and therapeutics: *Panax ginseng*. *Altern Med Rev* 9: 259–274.

Hindmarch I (1986). Activity of *Ginkgo biloba* on short-term memory. *Presse Med* 15: 1592–1594.

Hobbs C (1996). *Ginseng, the Energy Herb*. Interweave Press, Inc, Loveland, CO.

Hofferberth B (1989). Influence of GBE on neurophysiological and psychometric measurements. *Arzneimittelforschung* 39: 918–922.

Hong J, Smith TJ, Ho CT, *et al.* (2001). Effects of purified green and black tea polyphenols on cyclooxygenase- and lipooxygenase-dependent metabolism of arachidonic acid in human colon mucosa and colon tumor tissues. *Biochem Pharmacol* 62: 1175–1183.

Hsu CC, Ho MC, Lin LC, *et al.* (2005). American ginseng supplementation attenuates creatine kinase level induced by submaximal exercise in human beings. *World J Gastroenterol* 11: 5327–5331.

Huang YC, Chen CT, Chen SC, *et al.* (2005). A natural compound (ginsenoside Re) isolated from *Panax ginseng* as a novel angiogenic agent for tissue regeneration. *Pharm Res* 22: 636–646.

Ide N, Lau BH (1999). Aged garlic extract attenuates intracellular oxidative stress. *Phytomedicine* 6: 125–131.

Imai K, Suga K, Nakachi K (1997). Cancer-preventive effects of drinking green tea among a Japanese population. *Prev Med* 6: 769–775.

Ishikawa H, Saeki T, Otani T *et al.* (2006). Aged garlic extract prevents a decline of NK cell number and activity in patients with advanced cancer. *J Nutr* 136: 816S–820S.

Itil T, Martorano D (1995). Natural substances in psychiatry (*Ginkgo biloba* in dementia). *Psychopharmacol Bull* 31: 147–158.

Itoh T, Zang YF, Murai S, Saito H (1989). Effects of *Panax ginseng* root on the vertical and horizontal motor activities and on brain monoamine-related substances in mice. *Planta Med* 55: 429–433.

Jiang F, DeSilva S, Turnbull J (2000). Beneficial effect of ginseng root in SOD-1 (G93A) transgenic mice. *J Neurol Sci* 180: 52–54.

Joo SS, Won TJ, Lee I (2005). Reciprocal activity of ginsenosides in the production of proinflammatory repertoire, and their potential roles in neuroprotection in vivo. *Planta Med* 715: 476–481.

Kang SY, Schini-Kerth VB, Kim ND (1995). Ginsenosides of the protopanaxatriol group cause endothelium-dependent relaxation in the rat aorta. *Life Sci* 56: 1577–1586.

Kanter MM, Lesmes GR, Kaminsky LA, *et al.* (1988). Serum creatine kinase and lactate dehydrogenase changes following an eighty kilometer race. Relationship to lipid peroxidation. *Eur J Appl Physiol Occup Physiol* 57: 60–63.

Karp L, Weizman A, Tyano S, Gavish M (1989). Examination stress, platelet peripheral benzodiazepine binding sites, and plasma hormone levels. *Life Sci* 44: 1077–1082.

Kemberling JL, Hampton JA, Keck RW, *et al.* (2003). Inhibition of bladder tumor growth by the green tea derivative epigallocatechin-3-gallate. *J Urol* 170: 773–776.

Kenarova B, Neychev H, Hadjiivanova C, Petkov VD (1990). Immunomodulating activity of ginsenoside Rg1 from *Panax ginseng*. *Jap J Pharmacol* 54: 447–454.

Kim ND, Kang SY, Kim MJ, *et al.* (1999). The ginsenoside Rg3 evokes endothelium-independent relaxation in rat aortic rings: role of K+ channels. *Eur J Pharmacol* 367: 51–57.

Kim SH, Park KS, Chang MJ, Sung JH (2005). Effects of *Panax ginseng* extract on exercise-induced oxidative stress. *J Sports Med Phys Fitness* 45: 178–182.

Kimura M, Waki I, Chujo T, *et al.* (1981). Effects of hypoglycemic components in ginseng radix on blood insulin level in alloxan diabetic mice and on insulin release from perfused rat pancreas. *J Pharmacobiodynam* 4: 410–417.

Kimura T, Saunders PA, Kim HS, *et al.*(1994). Interactions of ginsenosides with ligand-bindings of GABA(A) and GABA(B) receptors. *Gen Pharmacol* 25: 193–199.

Kominato K (1969). Studies on biological active component in garlic (*Allium scorodoprasm* L. or *Allium sativum*). I. Thioglycoside. *Chem Pharm Bull* 17: 2193–2197.

Kuo SC, Teng CM, Lee JC, *et al.* (1990). Antiplatelet components in *Panax ginseng*. *Planta Med* 56: 164–167.

Kyo E, Uda N, Kasuga S, *et al.* (1999). Garlic as an immunostimulant. In: *Immunomodulatory agents from plants*. Ed E. Wagner. Verlag, Basel, Switzerland.

Kyo E, Uda N, Kasuga S, Itakura Y (2001). Immunomodulatory effects of aged garlic extract. *J Nutr* 131: 1075S–1079S.

Lambert JD, Yang CS (2003). Mechanisms of cancer prevention by tea constituents. *J Nutr* 133: 3262S–3267S.

Lamm DL, Riggs DR (2001). Enhanced immunocompetence by garlic: role in bladder cancer and other malignancies. *J Nutr* 131: 1067S–1070S.

Lau BH (2006). Suppression of LDL oxidation by garlic compounds is a possible mechanism of cardiovascular health benefit. *J Nutr* 136: 765S–768S.

Lawson LD (1998). Garlic: a review of its medicinal effects and indicated active compounds. In: *Phytomedicines of Europe: Chemistry and Biological Activity.* Eds LD Lawson and R Bauer. American Chemical Society Books, Washington (DC), pp. 176–209.

Lawson LD, Upton R, Graff A, *et al.* (2005). Garlic bulb, *Allium sativum*, analytical, quality control, and therapeutic monograph. In: *American Herbal Pharmacopoeia and Therapeutic Compendium*, Eds. R Upton, A. Graff and D. Swisher. Santa Cruz, CA.

Lee K, Wang H, Itokawa H, Morris-Natschke SL (2000). Current perspective on Chinese medicines and dietary supplements in China, Japan, and the United States. *J Food Drug Anal* 8: 219–228.

Lee TF, Shiao YJ, Chen CF, Wang LC (2001). Effect of ginseng saponins on beta-amyloid-suppressed acetylcholine release from rat hippocampal slices. *Planta Med* 67: 634–637.

Li TSC, Mazza G, Cottrell AC, Gao L (1996). Ginsenosides in roots and leaves of American ginseng. *J Agric Food Chem* 44: 717–720.

Liang YC, Lin-shiau SY, Chen CF, Lin JK (1997). Suppression of extracellular signals and cell proliferation through EGF receptor binding by (−)-epigallocatechin gallate in human A431 epidermoid carcinoma cells. *J Cell Biochem* 67: 55–65.

Liberti LE, Der Marderosian A (1978). Evaluation of commercial ginseng products. *J Pharm Sci* 67: 1487–1489.

Lin YL, Lin JK (1997). (−)-Epigallocatechin-3-gallate blocks the induction of nitric oxide synthase by down-regulating lipopolysaccharide-induced activity of transcription factor nuclear factor kappa-B. *Mol Pharmacol* 52: 465–472.

Lu JP, Ma ZC, Yang J, *et al.* (2004). Ginsenoside Rg1-induced alterations in gene expression in TNF-alpha stimulated endothelial cells. *Chin Med J* 117: 871–876.

Maffei-Facino R, Carini M, Aldini G, *et al.* (1999). *Panax ginseng* administration in the rat prevents myocardial ischemia-reperfusion damage induced by hyperbaric oxygen: evidence for an antioxidant intervention. *Planta Med* 65: 614–619.

McKenna DJ, Jones K, Hughes K (2002). Green tea and garlic. In: *Botanical Medicines: the desk reference for major herbal supplements*, 2nd edn. Eds. DJ McKenna, K Jones and K Hughes. Haworth Press, New York, pp. 375–409, 597–656.

McNaughton L, Egan G, Caelli G (1989). A comparison of Chinese and Russian ginseng as ergogenic aids to improve various facets of physical fitness. *Int Clin Nutr Rev* 90: 32–35.

Mitscher LA (1998). *The Green Tea Book*. Avery Publishing Group, Garden City Park, New York.

Mix JA, Crew WD (2002). A double-blind, placebo-controlled, randomized trail of *Ginkgo biloba* extract EGb761 in a sample of cognitively intact older adults: neuropsychological findings. *Hum Psychopharmacol* 17: 267–277.

Morré DJ, Bridge A, Wu LY, Morré DM (2000). Epigallocatechin gallate inhibits preferentially the NADH oxidase and growth of transformed cells in culture. *Biochem Pharmacol* 60: 937–946.

Morré DJ, Chueh P, Morré DM (1995). Capsaicin inhibits preferentially the NADH oxidase and growth of transformed cells in culture. *Proc Nat Acad Sci* 92: 1821–1835.

Morré DJ, Morré DM, Sun H, *et al.* (2003). Tea catechin synergies in inhibition of cancer cell proliferation and of cancer cell-specific ECTO-NOX activity. *Basic Clin Pharmacol Toxic* 92: 234–241.

Morris AC, Jacobs I, McLellan TM, *et al.* (1996). No ergogenic effect of ginseng ingestion. *Int J Sports Nutr* 6: 263–271.

Mütsch-Eckner M, Sticher O, Meier B (1992). Reversed-phase high-performance liquid chromatography of S-alk(en)yl L-cysteine derivatives in *Allium sativum* including the determination of (+)-S-allyl-L-cysteine sulfoxide, -glutamyl-S-allyl-L-cysteine and -glutamyl-S-(trans-1–propenyl)-L-cysteine. *J Chromatogr* 625: 183–190.

Nakanishi K (2005). Terpene trilactones from *Ginkgo biloba*: from ancient times to the 21st century. *Bioorg Med Chem* 13: 4987–5000.

Nathan CF, Hibbs JB (1991). Role of nitric oxide synthesis in macrophage antimicrobial activity. *Curr Opin Immunol* 3: 65–70.

Novas ML, Medina JH, Calvo D, De Robertis E (1987). Increase of peripheral type benzodiazepine binding sites in kidney and olfactory bulb in acutely stressed rats. *Eur J Pharmacol* 135: 243–246.

Oken BA, Storzback DM, Kaye JA (1998). The efficacy of *Ginkgo biloba* on cognitive function in Alzheimer's disease. *Arch Neurol* 55: 1409–1415.

Palermo CM, Hernando JIM, Dertinger SD, *et al.* (2003). Identification of potential aryl hydrocarbon receptor antagonists in green tea. *Chem Res Toxicol* 16: 865–872.

Park EK, Choo MK, Han MJ, *et al.* (2004). Ginsenoside Rh1 possesses antiallergic and anti-inflammatory activities. *Int Arch Allergy Immunol* 133: 113–120.

Park YC, Lee CH, Kang HS, *et al.* (1996). Ginsenoside-Rh1 and Rh2 inhibit the induction of nitric oxide synthesis in murine peritoneal macrophages. *Biochem Mol Biol Int* 40: 751–757.

Patya M, Zahalka MA, Vanichkin A, *et al.*(2004). Allicin stimulates lymphocytes and elicits an antitumor effect: a possible role of p21*ras*. *Int Immunol* 16: 275–281.

Pedraza-Chaverri J, Tapia E, Medina-Campos ON, *et al.* (1998). Garlic prevents hypertension induced by chronic inhibition of nitric oxide synthesis. *Life Sci* 62: 71–77.

Perez AC, de Oliveira CC, Prieto JG, *et al.* (2002). Quantitative assessment of nitric oxide in rat skeletal muscle and plasma after exercise. *Eur J Appl Physiol* 88: 189–191.

Pieralisi G, Ripari P, Vecchiet L (1991). Effects of a standardized ginseng extract combined with dimethylaminoethanol bitartrate, vitamins, minerals, and trace elements on physical performance during exercise. *Clin Ther* 13: 373–382.

Radad K, Gille G, Liu L, Rausch WD (2006). Use of ginseng in medicine with emphasis on neurodegenerative disorders. *J Pharmacol Sci* 100: 175–186.

Rahman K, Lowe GM (2006). Garlic and cardiovascular disease: a critical review. *J Nutr* 136: 736S–740S.

Rai GS, Shovlin C, Wesnes KA (1991). A double-blind placebo-controlled study of *Ginkgo biloba* extract in elderly patients with mild to moderate memory impairment. *Curr Med Res Opin* 12: 350–355.

Reay JL, Kennedy DO, Scholey AB (2005). Single doses of *Panax ginseng* (G115) reduce blood glucose levels and improve cognitive performance during sustained mental activity. *J Psychopharmacol* 19: 357–365.

Rimar S, Lee-Mengel M, Gillis CN (1996). Pulmonary protective and vasodilator effects of a standardized *Panax ginseng* preparation following artificial gastric digestion. *Pulm Pharmacol* 9: 205–209.

Roy D, Perreault M, Marette A (1998). Insulin stimulation of glucose uptake in skeletal muscles and adipose tissues in vivo is NO dependent. *Am J Physiol* 274: E692–E699.

Rudakewich M, Ba F, Benishin CG (2001). Neurotrophic and neuroprotective actions of ginsenosides Rb1 and Rg1. *Planta Med* 67: 533–537.

Sachinidis A, Seul C, Seewald S, *et al.* (2000). Green tea compounds inhibit tyrosine phosphorylation of PDGF B-receptor and transformation of A172 human glioblastoma. *FEBS Letters* 471: 51–55.

Sala F, Mulet J, Choi S, *et al.* (2002). Effects of ginsenoside Rg2 on human neuronal nicotinic acetylcholine receptors. *J Pharmacol Exp Ther* 301: 1052–1059.

Salim KN, McEwen BS, Chao HM (1997). Ginsenoside Rb1 regulates ChAT, NGF and trkA mRNA expression in the rat brain. *Mol Brain Res* 47: 177–182.

Salucci M, Stivala LA, Maiani G, *et al.* (2002). Flavonoids uptake and their effect on cell cycle of human colon adenocarcinoma cells (Caco2). *Br J Cancer* 55: 1645–1651.

Sartippour MR, Heber D, Henning S, *et al.* (2004). cDNA microarray analysis of endothelial cells in response to green tea reveals a suppressive phenotype. *Int J Oncol* 25: 193–202.

Scaglione F, Cattaneo G, Alessandria M, Cogo R (1996). Efficacy and safety of the standardized Ginseng extract G115 for potentiating vaccination against the influenza syndrome and protection against the common cold. *Drugs Exp Clin Res* 22: 65–72.

Scaglione F, Ferrara F, Dugnani S, *et al.* (1990). Immunomodulatory effects of two extracts of *Panax ginseng* C.A. Meyer. *Drugs Exp Clin Res* 16: 537–542.

Scholey AB, Kennedy DO (2002). Acute dose dependent cognitive effects of *Ginkgo biloba*, *Panax ginseng*, and their combination in healthy young volunteers: differential interactions with cognitive demand. *Hum Psychopharmacol* 17: 35–44.

Seely DE, Mills EJ, Wu P, *et al.* (2005). The effects of green tea consumption on incidence of breast cancer and recurrence of breast cancer: A systematic review and meta-analysis. *Integr Cancer Ther* 4: 144–155.

Sendl A, Elbl G, Steinke B, *et al.* (1992). Comparative pharmacological investigations of *Allium ursinum* and *Allium sativum*. *Planta Med* 58: 1–7.

Sengupta S, Toh SA, Sellers LA, *et al.* (2004). Modulating angiogenesis: the yin and the yang in ginseng. *Circulation* 110: 1219–1225.

Shim I, Javaid JI, Kim SE (2000). Effect of ginseng total saponin on extracellular dopamine release elicited by local infusion of nicotine into the striatum of freely moving rats. *Planta Med* 66: 705–708.

Sievenpiper JL, Arnason JT, Vidgen E, *et al.* (2004). A systematic quantitative analysis of the literature of the high variability in ginseng (*Panax* spp.): should ginseng be trusted in diabetes? *Diabetes Care* 27: 839–840.

Silagy C, Neil A (1994). Garlic as a lipid lowering agent – a meta-analysis. *J R Coll Physicians Lond* 28: 39–45.

Singh DK, Porter TD (2006). Inhibition of sterol 4α-methyl oxidase is the principal mechanism by which garlic decreases cholesterol synthesis. *J Nutr* 136: 759S–764S.

Solomon DR, Adams F, Silver A, *et al.* (2002). Ginkgo for memory enhancement: a randomized, controlled trial. *JAMA* 288: 835–840.

Song ZJ, Johansen HK, Faber V, Hoiby N (1997). Ginseng treatment enhances bacterial clearance and decreases lung pathology in athymic rats with chronic *P. aeruginosa* pneumonia. *APMIS* 105: 438–444.

Sorensen H, Sonne J (1996). A double-masked study of the effects of ginseng on cognitive functions. *Curr Ther Res Clin Exp* 57: 959–968.

Sotaniemi EA, Haapakoski E, Rautio A (1995). Ginseng therapy in non-insulin-dependent diabetic patients. *Diabetes Care* 18: 1373–1375.

Spinas GA, Laffranchi R, Francoys I, *et al.* (1998). The early phase of glucose-stimulated insulin secretion requires nitric oxide. *Diabetologia* 41: 292–299.

Stromgaard K, Vogensen SB, Nakanishi K (2005). Ginkgo biloba. In: *Encyclopedia of Dietary Supplements*, Eds. PM Coates, MR Blackman and GM Cragg. Marcel Dekker Inc, NY, pp. 249–257.

Suganuma M, Okabe S, Oniyama M, *et al.* (1998). Wide distribution of [3H](−)-epigallocatechin gallate, a cancer preventive tea polyphenol, in mouse tissue. *Carcinogenesis* 19: 1771–1776.

Sugiyama T, Sadzuka T (1998). Enhancing effect of green tea compounds on the antitumor activity of adriamycin against M5076 ovarian sarcomas. *Cancer Letters* 133: 19–26.

Sung J, Han KH, Zo JH, *et al.* (2000). Effects of red ginseng upon vascular endothelial function in patients with essential hypertension. *Am J Chin Med* 28: 205–216.

Tachikawa E, Kudo K, Kashimoto T, Takahashi E (1995). Ginseng saponins reduce acetylcholine-evoked Nat influx and catecholamine secretion in bovine adrenal chromaffin cells. *J Pharmacol Exp Ther* 273: 629–636.

Tang FY, Meydani M (2001). Green tea catechins and vitamin E inhibit angiogenesis of human microvascular endothelial cells through suppression of IL-8 production. *Nutr Cancer* 41: 119–125.

Tang W, Eisenbrand G (1992). *Panax ginseng*. In: *Chinese Drugs of Plant Origin*, Ed. CA Myer. Springer, London, pp. 711–737.

Thomson M, Al-Qattan KK, Bordia T, Ali M (2006). Including garlic in the diet may help lower blood glucose, cholesterol and triglycerides. *J Nutr* 136: 800S–802S.

Tsang D, Yeung HW, Tso WW, Peck H (1985). Ginseng saponins: influence on neurotransmitter uptake in rat brain synaptosomes. *Planta Med* 3: 221–224.

Ueda Y, Kawajiri H, Miyamura N, Miyajima R (1991). Content of some sulfur-containing components and free amino acids in various strains of garlic. *Nippon Shokuhin Kogyo Gakkaishi* (*J Jap Soc Food Sci Technol*) 38: 429–434.

Van Kampen J, Robertson H, Hagg T, Drobitch R (2003). Neuroprotective actions of the ginseng extract G115 in two rodent models of Parkinson's disease. *Exp Neurol* 184: 21–29.

Vuksan V, Stavro MP, Sievenpiper JL, *et al.* (2000). American ginseng improves glycemia in individuals with normal glucose tolerance: effect of dose and time escalation. *J Am Coll Nutr* 19: 738–744.

Wei J, Ni J, Wu T, *et al.* (2006). A systematic review of Chinese medicinal herbs for acute bronchitis. *J Altern Complement Med* 12: 159–169.

Weisburger JH (1997). Tea and health: a historical perspective. *Cancer Lett* 114: 315–317.

Wink DA, Hanbauer I, Krishna MC, *et al.* (1993). Nitric oxide protects against cellular damage and cytotoxicity from reactive oxygen species. *Proc Nat Acad Sci* 90: 9813–9817.

World Health Organization (1999). *WHO Monographs on Selected Medicinal Plants*. Geneva, Switzerland.

Xie JT, Aung HH, Wu JA, *et al.* (2002). Effects of American ginseng berry extract on blood glucose levels in ob/ob mice. *Am J Chin Med* 30: 187–194.

Yang CS, Yang GY, Landau JM, *et al.* (1998). Tea and tea polyphenols inhibit cell hyperproliferation, lung tumorigenesis, and tumor progression. *Exp Lung Res* 24: 629–639.

Yang CS, Maliaka P, Meng X (2002). Inhibition of carcinogenesis by tea. *Annu Rev Pharmacol Toxicol* 42: 25–54.

Yang F, Oz HS, Barve S, *et al.* (2001). The green tea polyphenol (−)-epigallocatechin-3-gallate blocks nuclear factor –kB activation by inhibiting 1kB kinase activity in the intestinal epithelial cell line IEC-6. *Mol Pharmacol* 60: 528–533.

Yang GY, Liao J, Kim K, *et al.* (1998). Inhibition of growth and induction of apoptosis in human cancer cell lines by tea polyphenols. *Carcinogenesis* 19: 611–616.

Yao GK, Chen PF (1995). *Tea Drinking and Health*. Shanghai Culture Publishers, Shanghai, pp. 6–7.

Yeh YY, Liu L (2001). Cholesterol-lowering effect of garlic extracts and organosulfur compounds: human and animal studies. *J Nutr* 131: 989S–993S.

Yokozawa T, Satoh A, Cho EJ (2004). Ginsenoside-Rd attenuates oxidative damage related to aging in senescence-accelerated mice. *J Pharm Pharmacol* 56: 107–113.

Yun TK, Choi SY, Yun HY (2001). Epidemiological study on cancer prevention by ginseng: are all kinds of cancers preventable by ginseng? *J Korean Med Sci* 16: S19–S27.

Zhan Y, Xu XH, Jiang YP (1994). Effects of ginsenosides on myocardial ischemia/reperfusion damage in open-heart surgery patients. *Med J China* 74: 626–628.

Zhang FL, Chen X (1987). Effects of ginsenosides on sympathetic neurotransmitter release in pithed rats. *Acta Pharmacol Sin* 8: 217–220.

Zhou W, Chai H, Lin PH, *et al.* (2005). Ginsenoside Rb1 blocks homocysteine-induced endothelial dysfunction in porcine coronary arteries. *J Vasc Surg* 41: 861–868.

6

Synergy and polyvalence: paradigms to explain the activity of herbal products

Peter J Houghton

Introduction

The terms *synergy* and *polyvalence* are often used to explain the effects of the many constituents found in herbal medicinal products and their extracts, particularly where it is difficult to distinguish the 'active ingredient'.

The concept of 'active ingredient' has been useful in elucidating the chemical basis for the biological effect of a large number of medicinal and poisonous plants. Many naturally occurring compounds such as atropine, morphine, digoxin, quinine and menthol, originally taken as part of the complex mixture occurring in a solvent extract or distilled oil, now have extensive clinical use as single compounds since they give a pharmacological effect similar to that given by an extract from the plant in which they occur. It would be true to say that, to a large extent, over the last 100 years 'orthodox' 'Western' medicine has valued plants only as a source of such potent compounds, whose activity could be clearly demonstrated at low doses. Any drug discovery from natural sources carried out by the pharmaceutical industry is still very much based on this paradigm.

However, there were many medicinal plant species from which active ingredients could not be isolated and/or gave no immediately obvious effects when their extracts were tested pharmacologically. These extracts consisted of complex mixtures of many different compounds and were either dismissed as inactive, with anecdotal reports of activity being explained by the placebo effect, or they declined in use because of difficulties in analysis, standardisation or making 'user-friendly' dosage forms. It is only in the past three decades that this group of plants has re-emerged in the developed world, arousing interest from the general public as alternatives to orthodox medicines or as complementary products used to maintain health or treat aspects of diseases in which orthodox medication has had only limited success. As well as the mainly European and North American herbal substances that have enjoyed this renaissance, there is now a vast array of medicinal plants from other parts of the world, many of which have become globalised and become significant items of commerce. This increase in commerce and public use has stimulated much scientific and clinical interest and one aspect of research that has been generated is to explain the effects seen in terms of ingredients detected which, on their own as single compounds, have relatively weak activity. Such explanations are often couched in terms of synergy and polyvalence, but the meaning of these terms is often not fully understood, with consequent confusion in their use.

For example, synergy is often stated to occur when an extract of a plant gives a greater (or safer) response than an equivalent dose of the compound considered to be the 'active' one. An example of this is the much improved antispastic effect shown by cannabis extract compared with an equivalent dose of tetrahydrocannabinol (Baker *et al.*, 2000; Williamson, 2001). However, in such an instance, it might well be that other active compounds are present, some as yet undiscovered. In whole organism or tissue studies, other compounds present may be active against a range of targets, all contributing to the observed effect. In this instance it is polyvalence, rather than synergy, which is occurring, and this topic is discussed below.

Another situation sometimes explained by synergy is the loss of activity seen when an active crude extract is fractionated and the resulting fractions, when tested for the same activity, do not show an enhanced effect, e.g. the loss of cytotoxic activity seen when extracts of *Kigelia pinnata* were fractionated (Houghton, 2000). The explanation given in such circumstances is that activity is reduced because two compounds, which act together synergistically, have been separated into two discrete fractions. However, it should be always borne in mind that the loss may be due to the 'actives' having decomposed during the fractionation process or that they have become bound to one of the materials used, e.g. the stationary phase in chromatography.

This chapter aims to define synergy and polyvalence, discuss ways in which they can be assessed and quantified and give some examples of herbal medicinal products where these processes have been shown to occur.

Synergy

Definition

The literal meaning of synergy is 'working together' but a useful definition is 'an effect seen by a combination of substances that is greater than would have been expected from a consideration of individual contributions' (Heinrich *et al.*, 2004). More precise definitions, incorporating mathematical considerations, have been discussed by Berenbaum (1989), who favoured the use of isoboles (see below) in determining synergy, since these are concerned with the effect and not with the mechanisms involved. Synergy as applied to herbal products has been discussed well in seminal papers by Williamson (2001; 2002), who also included the attenuation of toxicity or adverse effects seen with a mixture compared with one of its constituents. Synergy in the present chapter is used in a 'positive' sense, i.e. an increase in effect greater than that predicted, but it should not be forgotten that an unexpected decrease in activity, sometimes called 'negative synergy' or 'antagonism' may also occur, particularly in some interactions between orthodox medication and some herbal products (Barnes *et al.*, 2002).

In the case of the pharmacological or clinical effects of herbal material, two types of synergy are observed. In one case the activity of an active compound, or extract, is increased in the presence of another compound or extract which, on its own, has no effect in the system under test at the concentrations used. This has been demonstrated for the flavonoids present in *Artemisia annua*, source of the antimalarial drug artemisinin, which at 5 μmol/L, well below their IC50 value of about 25 μmol/L, gave rise to a three- to fivefold reduction in the IC_{50} value of artemisinin when they were added to the in-vitro antiplasmodial test used (Chiung-Sheue Chen Liu *et al.*, 1992).

The more common situation is when all compounds concerned have activity but, in combination, this is much greater than expected. This is exemplified by the reduction in platelet aggregation observed for the total mixture of ginkgolides from *Ginkgo biloba* L., as opposed to that given by individual compounds, because of their activity as platelet-activating factor antagonists (Williamson, 2002).

In some traditional medicine systems, mixtures of plants are used rather than one species and so the situation is even more complex, although the same concepts of synergy apply, i.e. the mixture of the two (or more) species gives a better activity than either species on its own. This has been demonstrated for a mixture of extracts of *Salvia chamelaegnea* Berg. and *Leonotis leonorus* (L.) R.Br. against Gram-positive bacteria (Kamatou *et al.*, 2006). This mixture was used traditionally in South Africa against infections.

Measurement of synergy: use of isoboles and isobolograms

Various mathematical models have been used to describe and determine synergism (Berenbaum, 1989) but the use of isobolograms is the method that is reckoned to be the best and has been used in recent publications. Although many researchers use the method without considering the mathematics involved, proof of the validity of the method was given by Berenbaum (1989) and this has provided a sound basis for its use.

The *isobole* method is applicable under most conditions and, since it is the ultimate effect which is the factor used in the measurement, it is independent of the mechanisms of action involved. The isobole is a curve, constructed by plotting coordinates consisting of values representing the *fractional effect* for each of two components. The fractional effect is the ratio of the 'effect' caused by the two compounds in combination to that of one of the compounds alone. The effect is a measure of activity, e.g. minimum inhibitory concentration (MIC) for antibacterial and antifungal compounds, concentration giving 50% inhibition (IC_{50}) for enzyme studies or studies on cytotoxicity, 50% binding coefficient for receptor-binding studies.

The fractional effect (FE) of two compounds (or extracts) X and Y for antibacterial studies, in terms of their MIC for bacterial growth, can be expressed as follows (Schelz *et al.*, 2006):

$$FE^X = \frac{MIC_{(X \text{ with } Y)}}{MIC_{(X \text{ alone})}}$$

$$FE^Y = \frac{MIC_{(Y \text{ with } X)}}{MIC_{(Y \text{ alone})}}.$$

The sum of the two fractional effects is known as the FE index and is the correlation between the two test substances. Different authors interpret the FE index in different ways. According to Berenbaum (1989) synergism is said to occur if the FE index is ≤ 1.0, if 1.0, an additive effect is reckoned to occur, and antagonism if the FE is greater than 1.0. Schelz (2006), however, stated that if the FE index is ≤ 0.5, the effect is synergistic; if >0.5 to 1.0, the effect is additive, if >1.0 to 4.0 it is indifferent and if ≥ 4.0 the effect of the two substances is antagonistic.

If FE^X and FE^Y are calculated for a series of the two compounds in different ratios, then an isobologram (Figure 6.1) can be constructed using the two values as coordinates to express the FE index for each combination of the two compounds. If no synergism exists, the coordinate points form a straight line but, if synergism exists, the points occur between the straight line and the origin in a concave shape, whereas if they are 'outside' the straight line, and give a convex curve, antagonism exists. Note that for a set of different mixtures of the same compounds, not all the combinations may give the same effect, i.e. some may show synergy while others may not.

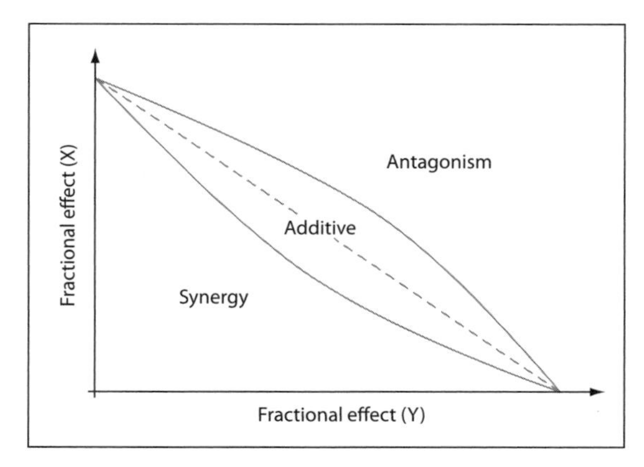

Figure 6.1 Isobologram to show areas of synergy and antagonism.

This is exemplified in Table 6.1 in data for the antibacterial activity (expressed as MIC) of volatile (X) and non-volatile (Y) fractions from the South African herb *Tarchonanthus camphoratus* L. (Asteraceae) (Van Vuuren, 2007). The data are plotted as an isobologram in Figure 6.2. The mixtures consisting of concentration ratios 12.8 : 3.2, 11.2 : 4.8, 9.6 : 6.4 and 8.0 : 8.0 all show synergism as shown by their being in a concave distribution in Figure 6.2. The 14.4 : 1.6 mixture shows an additive effect while the 6.4 : 9.6, 4.8 : 11.2, 3.2 : 12.8, 1.6 : 14.4 mixtures all show antagonism since they are 'outside' the straight line, representing a mere additive response. These set of results demonstrate the point noted above; that some concentration ratios may display synergy while others do not. Such a situation demonstrates how complicated it is to try to predict the activity of a herbal extract where relative concentrations of compounds may vary widely between batches or chemical races of the plant.

Polyvalence

Polyvalence can be defined as the range of biological activities that an extract may exhibit which contribute to the overall effect observed clinically or in vivo. It is often confused with synergism but the distinction lies in the fact that synergism is strictly concerned with only one pharmacological function, rather than a range of activities resulting in an overall effect. As mentioned above for synergy, Williamson (2001) discussed the role played by polyvalence in the scientific evidence for the claims often made for herbal traditional medicines, that the overall effect is greater, and sometimes different, than might be predicted from the activities of the individual components.

It is unusual for a disease to be due to, or to be corrected by, a single factor, so it is unlikely that one compound alone would successfully treat the disease in the patient, even when the disease and its cause are unequivocally certain. This 'silver bullet' concept, which has driven the drug discovery process for the past 100 years, is now increasingly viewed as inadequate in many clinical situations (Walker, 2007). As a result, in orthodox Western medicine, a cocktail of drugs is now commonly employed against diseases such as HIV infection and cancer. A similar situation arises in the treatment of a disease such as hypertension, where symptoms may be reduced by using a diuretic or beta-blocker, but other drugs have to be employed to compensate for their side-effects, e.g. potassium supplements are given to overcome the hypokalaemia induced by diuretics. Similarly antiemetics are commonly given as part of the regimen in cancer chemotherapy.

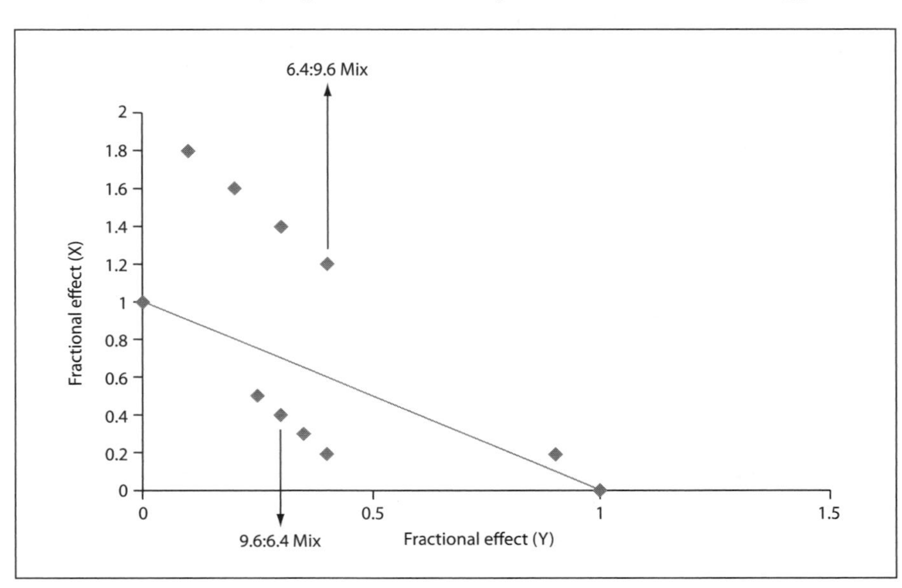

Figure 6.2 Isobologram to demonstrate synergy, additive and antagonistic antibacterial effects with different ratios of volatile and non-volatile fractions of the South African herb *Tarchonanthus camphoratus* L.

Table 6.1 Data for antibacterial activity (minimum inhibitory concentration, MIC) against *Escherichia coli* for different ratios of volatile (X) and non-volatile (Y) fractions from the South African herb *Tarchonanthus camphoratus* L.

Concentration (mg/mL)		MIC (mg/mL)		Fractional effect*		FE index
X	Y	X	Y	FEX	FEY	
16	0	8.0	–	1	–	
14.4	1.6	7.2	0.8	0.90	0.20	1.1
12.8	3.2	3.2	0.8	0.40	0.20	0.6
11.2	4.8	2.8	1.2	0.35	0.30	0.65
9.6	6.4	2.4	1.6	0.30	0.40	0.7
8.0	8.0	2.0	2.0	0.25	0.50	0.75
6.4	9.6	3.2	4.8	0.40	1.20	1.6
4.8	11.2	2.4	5.6	0.30	1.40	1.7
3.2	12.8	1.6	6.4	0.20	1.60	1.8
1.6	14.4	0.8	7.2	0.10	1.80	1.9
0	16	–	4	–	1	

*In this instance the FE is calculated as follows:

$$FE^{X} = \frac{MIC(X\ with\ Y)}{MIC(X\ alone)}$$

$$FE^{Y} = \frac{MIC(Y\ with\ X)}{MIC(Y\ alone).}$$

Worked example for 9.6 : 6.4 ratio mixture:

$$FE^{X} = \frac{2.4}{8} = 0.3$$

$$FE^{X} = \frac{1.6}{4} = 0.4$$

A similar situation can be seen in many different traditional systems where herbs are used. In some systems, e.g. TCM and Ayurvedic medicine, such adjuvant herbs are clearly recognised and classified. Thus, in a Chinese prescription of, say, ten different herbs, one is recognised as providing the major activity, i.e. ‘the monarch’, while two or three others have a similar activity, i.e. ‘the ministers’, one or more others are included to aid absorption and delivery to the site of action, i.e. ‘the guides’ and the fourth group is chiefly utilised because they reduce unwanted side-effects caused by the major active herbs, i.e. ‘the assistants’ (Xue *et al.*, 2003).

In many traditions however, such differentiation has not been codified, and knowledge is pragmatic or empirical. The need for a herbal plant to be collected at a specific time of year, or processed in a particular way, may be associated with a high level of the actives, but may also coincide with the presence (or absence) of other compounds that affect the activity. Even where such matters are of little concern, pharmacological and biochemical research over the past 30 years has increasingly shown that most herbs have several types of constituents and a corresponding range of biological effects. It is too simplistic to talk about a herb having one ‘active ingredient’ and one ‘activity’. The spectrum of activities, i.e. the polyvalence and the variety of compounds responsible for the effects seen are discussed in the following paragraphs.

Polyvalence can be due to the following:

- A variety of types of chemical compound is present, each type having a different biological effect.
- Compounds of one particular chemical type are present which have more than one biological effect relevant to treating the disease and/or improving the health of the patient.
- Compounds are present, which do not affect the cause or symptoms of the disease itself, but which modify the side-effects, absorption, distribution, metabolism and excretion of active constituents.

Each of these three points is considered in more detail below.

A variety of types of chemical compound being present

The leaves and flowers of many *Buddleja* species throughout the world are used to treat wounds and inflamed tissues (Houghton, 1984). In a study on some Chinese species of *Buddleja*, compounds extracted from the leaves of *B. asiatica* and flowers of *B. officinalis* were tested for their inhibitory effects on eicosanoid synthesis, a key part of the inflammatory process (Liao *et al.*, 1999). Four major types of compounds, triterpenes, phenylethanoids, flavonoids and carotenoid glycosides were found to be present in the extracts. The triterpene δ-amyrone, the flavonoid aglycone acacetin and the carotenoid glycoside crocetin displayed inhibition of cycloxygenase, while acacetin also inhibited lipoxygenase. These results suggested that an aqueous extract or poultice of the plant material, which is likely to contain these compounds, and is the form used traditionally, might well include anti-inflammatory effects as part of its portfolio of properties that would help wounds to heal.

Another example of polyvalence is the widely used anxiolytic and sleep-promoting herb valerian (*Valeriana officinalis*). This contains sesquiterpenes such as valerenic acid, which appear to inhibit γ-aminobutyric acid (GABA) breakdown, thus causing a net increase of this CNS-depressant neurotransmitter (Riedel *et al.*, 1982); the monoterpenes known as valepotriates which relax smooth muscle (Wagner and Jurcic, 1979); large amounts of free GABA, which might bind to the GABA receptors (Santos *et al.*, 1994); lignans, e.g. 1-hydroxypinoresinol, which inhibit binding of serotonin to receptors (Bodesheim and Hölzl, 1997); and flavonoids, e.g. 6-methylapigenin, which have been shown to bind to benzodiazepine receptors (Wasowski *et al.*, 2002). All of these effects contribute to depression of CNS activity and to overall relaxation, thus aiding reduction in anxiety and promoting the onset of sleep (Houghton, 1989).

Ginkgo (the leaves of *Ginkgo biloba* L.) is an ancient Chinese medicinal plant which is now widely sold throughout the world to preserve good memory and cognitive function (Barnes *et al.*, 2007). Clinical studies have given a considerable evidence base to its efficacy, which is generally ascribed to an improved blood flow in the microcirculation of the CNS and a concomitant reduction in damage caused by reactive oxygen species associated with ischaemia. Ginkgo contains flavonoids such as ginkgetin which are neuroprotective because of their antioxidant and anti-inflammatory activities (Kang *et al.*, 2005), the diterpenoid ginkgolides, which are potent anticoagulants because of their ability to inhibit platelet aggregation, thereby increasing blood flow (Braquet *et al.*, 1991) and the sesquiterpene biolobalide which has antioxidant properties (Joyeux *et al.*, 1995). In addition, the ginkgolides are antioxidant as well as anticoagulant (Joyeux *et al.*, 1995). All of these properties would increase blood flow and protect against oxidative damage.

St John's Wort (*Hypericum perforatum L.*) contains a variety of compounds and work still needs to be done to fully ascertain the roles played by each. Its major use in modern phytotherapeutics is for treating mild-to-moderate depression. Extensive research into the compounds responsible for this has revealed that this herb is a good example of polyvalent complexity. It contains the naphthodianthrone hypericin, prenylated phloroglucinols (e.g. hyperforin) and flavonoids. Hyperforin has been shown to inhibit serotonin re-uptake, an activity common to synthetic antidepressants such as fluoxetine (Prozac) (Chatterjee *et al.*, 1998), while there is evidence that hypericin inhibits binding to some subtypes of dopamine receptors (Butterveck *et al.*, 2002).

Compounds of one particular type with more than one biological effect

An interesting example of polyvalency being due to the same group of compounds having different effects, all of which might contribute to the treatment of a disease, is afforded by the tanshinone diterpenes present in *Salvia miltiorrhiza*. This herb is used extensively in TCM and has been investigated as potentially useful in Alzheimer's disease. The tanshinones were shown to have acetylcholinesterase inhibitory activity (Ren *et al.*, 2004), but are also potent cyclo-oxygenase inhibitors and therefore likely to have anti-inflammatory properties, thought to be associated with a reduction in incidence of Alzheimer's disease (Paulus and Bauer, 1999). It should be noted that the tanshinones have some antioxidant effects, as have the group of compounds known as salvianolic acids, e.g. salvianolic acid B 16, which are also present in *S. miltiorrhiza* (Du *et al.*, 2000), and such antioxidants are thought to play a part in reducing the incidence of Alzheimer's disease (Maxwell, 1995).

European *Salvia* species have been investigated for possible use in Alzheimer's disease, based on traditional usage for poor memory in old age. The oil of *S. lavandulaefolia* has acetylcholinesterase-inhibitory effects because of the monoterpenes (Perry *et al.*, 2001), but also some anti-inflammatory and antioxidant action (Perry *et al.*, 2002; Houghton *et al.*, 2007a).

The phenylpropanoid compounds from south-eastern Asian species of *Alpinia* also display at least two activities that support their traditional uses for prevention or treatment of cancer. Some of these compounds, especially 1′-acetoxychavicol, display direct cytotoxic activity against cancer cell lines (Lee and Houghton, 2005). However, they also up-regulate the cell's self-defence systems, the increased production of the antioxidant glutathione (GSH) and the up-regulation of glutathione-*S*-transferase (GST), an enzyme involved in phase 2 metabolism and removal of reactive oxygen species and other harmful compounds. Using in vitro methods for detecting these activities, it has been shown that five species from Malaysia showed activity in at least one of the bioassays, the two most active being *Alpinia officinarum* and *A. galanga,* with 1′-acetoxychavicol being found to be the most active compound (Houghton *et al.*, 2007b).

Compounds present that modify the pharmacokinetics of active constituents

Pharmacokinetics is the term used to describe the absorption, metabolism and excretion of chemical substances in the body. These aspects are well-researched for single chemical entity pharmaceuticals since the data have to be presented for registration of the drug. Deviation from the norm can be due to genetic factors in the patient, e.g. 'fast' and 'slow' metabolisers, dietary factors and interactions with other medication. The same factors can apply with herbal products, but an extra dimension can occur because the plant material or extracts used can, in themselves, contain substances that modify the pharmacokinetics of the 'actives' present.

If the herbal material is taken orally, which is the most common situation, absorption occurs across the wall of the gastrointestinal (GI) tract. This can be slowed down if the plant contains a large amount of polysaccharide polymers, a factor exploited in the use of guar gum in diabetes to reduce the absorption rate of glucose. The presence of high levels of tannins can also reduce the rate of absorption. A more rapid effect is noted with coffee than tea, even though a cup of each contains about the same amount of caffeine, because tea contains high levels of tannins which reduce absorption and provide a slower increase in caffeine levels in the blood by complexing with the caffeine (Heinrich *et al.*, 2004).

It has been shown that some hot spices, e.g. black pepper *Piper nigrum* and ginger *Zingiber officinale*, increase the transfer of many chemical substances across the gastrointestinal wall and it is of interest that black pepper is not only used as a drug in Ayurvedic medicine in its own right, but is also often added to mixtures containing other drugs (Atal *et al.*, 1981). Piperine, the major constituent of black pepper, has been shown to affect the uptake of several conventional drugs in humans (Bano *et al.*, 1991).

Once absorbed, the plasma levels of any drug are affected by its metabolism and excretion. Metabolism chiefly takes place in the liver, especially by the group of enzymes known as cytochrome P450

(CYP), of which many sub-types exist. If these are up-regulated, plasma levels of active substances decrease more rapidly than might be expected, whereas the reverse may be seen if the enzymes are inhibited or the liver cells damaged in some way. Both effects have been noted with plant constituents, e.g. St John's wort (*Hypericum perforatum*) is known to up-regulate CYP4A, leading to loss in efficacy of a wide range of drugs such as the immunosuppressant cyclosporin, the anti-HIV drugs and the contraceptive steroids (Mannel, 2004), while the furanocoumarins present in grapefruit juice are thought to be responsible for the high levels of the cardiotoxic antihistamine terfenadine which have had serious effects in some patients (Barnes *et al.*, 2007). Most of the concern which has arisen over these effects has come from herb–drug interaction studies, but it should not be forgotten that the types of compounds affecting metabolism may coexist in a herb with the actives, or be constituents of a herb added to the 'active' according to a herbal prescription.

In addition, the constituents of a herb may not be very active per se, but may need to be metabolised to more active forms by gut or liver enzymes. This is true for many of the laxative herbs containing anthracene-derivative glycosides and it has been demonstrated that the activity of senna (*Cassia acutifolia, Cassia angustifolia*) is due to rheins formed by the activity of intestinal bacteria (Kobashi *et al.*, 1980). Many flavonoids are probably also metabolised by gut bacteria but it should also be remembered that the CYP enzymes in the liver may also act as conversion agents from the 'prodrug' form found naturally to more active metabolites. Other compounds present in a particular plant, or another plant when the herbal substance is given in a mixture, may affect the enzyme activity of gut bacteria or liver enzymes, and consequently also the conversion process.

The duration of activity of a particular herb is also affected by the excretion which occurs in the urine through the kidneys, or by sweating. Reduced absorption might also take place if gastric transit time is decreased due to any laxative effect. If the glomerular filtration through the kidneys is increased due to a diuretic effect, then levels will drop rapidly and the same result will be obtained if sweating increases due to changes in temperature regulation or increased blood flow to the skin. It should be noted that, in European herbal treatment, increased diuresis and/or sweating is a major approach in eliminating 'toxins' from the body to restore health, so it would not be surprising to find herbs used which exert these effects, but which would also decrease the time over which the herb constituents reach effective levels in the blood. A recent review (Wright *et al.*, 2007) has highlighted the large number of diuretic herbs in use, which must be seen as potential modifiers of pharmacological activity.

Polyvalency and testing of herbal extracts for activity

If polyvalency occurs, it should be noted that the use of only one bioassay for in vitro testing for clinically relevant activity should be treated with great caution, since this approach is usually much too reductionist (Houghton *et al.*, 2007a). In cases of polyvalence, a battery of bioassays covering different aspects of the condition should be used, to elucidate a greater range of possible activities that could explain traditional usage. This must certainly be the case when a specific disease is diagnosed because of its presenting symptoms, but where these may be caused by a variety of factors. It would not be unusual to find that two different herbs, used for the same condition, have differing portfolios of activities.

Conclusions

Plant material or herbal extracts display much chemical complexity and it is only recently that advances in analytical procedures, coupled with sensitive bioassays, have allowed some teasing out of the factors that contribute to any overall effect. The interaction with such a complex mixture with the complicated array of biochemical pathways and other physiological processes, that exist in a delicate balance to maintain a healthy state in the human body, is a challenge for systems biology. The use of its approaches and techniques in seeking to understand what happens when a herb is taken is in its infancy but it appears likely that a greater understanding and demonstration of synergy and polyvalence in herbal extracts will be a feature of research in the next few years.

References

Atal CK, Zutshi U, Rao PG (1981). Scientific evidence on the role of Ayurvedic herbals on bioavailability of drugs. *J Ethnopharmacol* 4: 229–232.

Baker D, Pryce G, Croxford JL *et al.* (2000). Cannabinoids control spasticity and tremor in an animal model of multiple sclerosis. *Nature* 404: 84–87.

Bano G, Raina RK, Zutshi U *et al.* (1991). Effect of piperine on bioavailability and pharmacokinetics of propanolol and theophylline in healthy volunteers. *Eur. J Clin. Pharmacol* 41: 615–617.

Barnes J, Anderson LA, Phillipson JD (2002). *Herbal Medicines: a guide for healthcare professionals,* 2nd edn. Pharmaceutical Press, London, pp. 497–501.

Barnes J, Anderson LA, Phillipson JD (2007a). *Herbal Medicines: a guide for healthcare professionals,* 3rd edn. Pharmaceutical Press, London, pp. 299–314.

Barnes J, Anderson LA, Phillipson JD (2007b). *Herbal Medicines: a guide for healthcare professionals,* 3rd edn. Pharmaceutical Press, London, p. 613.

Berenbaum MC (1989). What is synergy? *Pharmacol Rev* 41: 93–141.

Bodesheim U, Hölzl J (1997). Isolierung, Strukturaufklärung und Radiorezeptorassays von Alkaloiden und Lignanen aus *Valeriana officinalis* L. *Pharmazie* 52: 387–391.

Braquet P, Esanu A, Buisine E *et al.* (1991). Recent progress in ginkgolide research. *Med Res Rev* 11: 295–355.

Butterveck V (2002). In vitro receptor screening of pure constituents of St John's wort reveals novel interactions with a number of GPCRs. *Psychopharmacology* 162: 193–202.

Chatterjee SS (1998). Hyperforin as a possible anti-depressant component of hypericum extracts. *Life Sci* 63: 499–510.

Chiung-Sheue Chen Liu K, Yang S-L, Roberts MF *et al.* (1992). Antimalarial activity of *Artemisia annua* flavonoids from whole plants and cell cultures. *Plant Cell Reports* 11: 637–640.

Du GH, Qiu Y, Zhang JT (2000). Salvianolic acid B protects the memory functions against transient cerebral ischemia in mice. *J Asian Nat Prod Res* 2: 145–152.

Heinrich M, Barnes J, Gibbons S, Williamson EM (2004). *Fundamentals of Pharmacognosy and Phytotherapy.* Churchill Livingstone, London, p. 161.

Houghton PJ(1984). Ethnopharmacology of some *Buddleja* species. *J Ethnopharmacol* 11: 293–308.

Houghton PJ (1999). The scientific basis for the reputed activity of Valerian. *J Pharm Pharmacol* 51: 505–512.

Houghton PJ (2000). Use of small scale bioassays in the discovery of novel drugs from natural sources. *Phytother Res* 14: 419–423.

Houghton PJ, Howes M-J, Lee CC, Steventon G (2007a). Uses and abuses of in vitro tests in ethnopharmacology: Visualising an elephant. *J Ethnopharmacol* 110: 391–400.

Houghton PJ, Fang R, Techatanawat I *et al.* (2007b). The Sulphorhodamine (SRB) assay and other approaches to testing plant extracts and derived compounds for activities related to reputed anticancer activity. *Methods* 42: 377–387.

Joyeux M, Lobstein A, Anton R, Mortier F (1995). Comparative antilipoperoxidative, antinecrotic and scavenging properties of terpenes and biflavones from Ginkgo and some flavonoids. *Planta Med* 61: 126–129.

Kamatou GPP, Viljoen AM, van Vuuren SF, van Zyl RL (2006). *In vitro* evidence of antimicrobial synergy between *Salvia chamelaeagnea* and *Leonotis leonurus. S Afr J Bot* 72: 634–636.

Kang SS, Lee JY, Choi YK *et al.* (2005). Neuroprotective effects of naturally occurring biflavonoids. *Bioorg Med Chem Lett* 15: 3588–3591.

Kobashi K, Nishimura T, Kusaka M, *et al.* (1980). Metabolism of sennosides by human intestinal bacteria. *Planta Med* 40: 225–236.

Lee CC, Houghton PJ (2005). Cytotoxicity of plants from Malaysia and Thailand used traditionally to treat cancer. *J Ethnopharmacol* 100: 237–243.

Mannel M (2004). Drug interactions with St John's Wort. *Drug Saf* 27: 773–797.

Maxwell SJ (1995). Prospects for the use of anti-oxidant therapies. *Drugs* 49: 345.

Perry NSL, Houghton PJ, Theobald AE *et al.* (2000). In-vitro inhibition of human erythrocyte acetylcholine esterase by *Salvia lavandulaefolia* essential oil and constituent terpenes. *J Pharm Pharmacol* 52: 895–902.

Perry NSL, Houghton PJ, Sampson J *et al.* (2001). In-vitro activity *of S. lavandulaefolia* (Spanish sage) relevant to treatment of Alzheimer's disease. *J Pharm Pharmacol* 53: 1347–1356.

Riedel E, Hansel R, Ehrke G (1982). Hemmung des γ-Aminobuttersaureabbaus durch Valerensaurederivate. *Planta Med* 46: 219–220.

Santos MS, Ferreira F, Faro C *et al.* (1994). The amount of GABA present in aqueous extracts of valerian is sufficient to account for [^{3}H]GABA release in synaptosomes. *Planta Med* 60: 2475–2476.

Savelev S, Okello E, Perry NSL *et al.* (2003). Synergistic and antagonistic interactions of anticholinesterase terpenoids in *Salvia lavandulaefolia* essential oil. *Pharmacol Biochem Behav* 75: 669–675.

Schelz Z, Molmar J, Hohmann J (2006). Antimicrobial and antiplasmid activities of essential oils. *Fitoterapia* 77: 279–285.

Van Vuuren SF (2007). *The Antimicrobial Activity and Essential Oil Composition of Medicinal Aromatic Plants Used in African Traditional Healing.* PhD thesis, University of Witswatersrand, Johannesburg, South Africa, pp. 100–102.

Wagner H, Jurcic K (1979). Uber die spasmolytische Wirkung des Baldrians. *Planta Med* 37: 84–86.

Walker M (2007). Drug evaluation in the 21st century. *Pharm J* 279 (supp.): B8.

Wasowski C, Marder M, Viola H *et al.* (2002). Isolation and identification of 6-methylapigenin, a competitive ligand for the brain GABA(A) receptors, from *Valeriana wallichii. Planta Med* 68: 934–936.

Williamson EM (2001). Synergy and other interactions in phytomedicines. *Phytomedicine* 8: 401–409.

Williamson EM (2002). Synergy in relation to the pharmacological action of phytomedicinals. In: *Trease and Evans Pharmacognosy,* Ed. WC Evans. W.B. Saunders, Edinburgh, UK, pp. 49–54.

Wright CI, Van-Buren L, Kroner CI *et al.* (2007). Herbal medicines as diuretics: A review of the scientific evidence. *J Ethnopharmacol* 114: 1–31.

Xue CC, O'Brien K (2003). Modalities in Chinese Medicine. In: *A Comprehensive Guide to Chinese Medicine*, Ed PC Leung. World Scientific Publishing, Singapore, p. 25.

7

From clinical evidence to mechanism of action: the development of standardised phytomedicines

Bhushan Patwardhan, Gulam Nabi Qazi and Ashok Vaidya

Introduction

In traditional medicine research, clinical experiences, observations or available data are starting points, whereas in 'conventional' 'Western' drug research, they come at the end of the drug discovery process. Thus, the first type of drug discovery follows a *reverse pharmacology* path (Vaidya *et al.*, 2001; Vaidya, 2006), which is the subject of this chapter.

Whenever any botanicals or phytomedicines are used in medicinal preparations, issues related to their quality assurance remain vitally important. It is important to ensure that any processing is in accordance with current good manufacturing procedures for herbal products (Verpoorte *et al.*, 2003). To understand various processes involved in a journey from clinical evidence to mechanism of action, it is important to know the various approaches involved in the development of phytomedicines and strategies of their therapeutic applications. Some of the important strategies include systems biology and reverse pharmacology approaches.

Systems biology approach

Traditional medicines have been developed through real-life experiences and direct observations on people with diseases, and represent highly complex biological systems. The typical conventional drug discovery pipeline includes preclinical studies on animal models and cell and tissue screens involving high-throughput assays. However, the numbers of new chemical/molecular entities that are approved are declining (Butcher *et al.*, 2004). This situation calls for critical assessment of the current reductionist strategies, where only new chemical entities are valued as potential new drugs and molecular biological technology is primarily used for defining molecular targets and for creating new miniaturised screening tests. Such reductionism, where a whole organism is broken down in to groups of cells, subcells, molecules and molecular interactions undermines the importance of the system as a whole. While interacting with each other, macromolecules form complex networks organised into systems with properties that extend beyond individual functions. When multiple cell types and diverse pathways contribute to the disease, a single molecule may not be effective in the modulation of multiple targets and such conditions require combination therapy. Modern medicine has also developed combinations of drugs for addressing more than one therapeutic target (Morphy *et al.*, 2004).

Systems biology attempts to provide predictive models of behaviour of such molecular systems to identify such functional interactions (Gannon, 2005). and is aptly summarised as follows: 'Compared with the analytical procedure of classical science with resolution into component elements and one-way or linear causality as basic category, the investigation of organised wholes of many variables requires new categories of interaction, transaction, organisation, teleology' (Ludwig von Bertalanffy, 1968).

A systems approach or 'science of wholeness' is actually central to the philosophy of several traditional medicine systems, particularly Ayurveda. Herbal extracts represent the 'combinatorial chemistry of nature' with a vast array of chemical compounds that can deal with multiple targets simultaneously, leading to synergistic and/or polyvalence systems effects.

Earlier drugs were created within the confines of a chemical paradigm of medicine and drug therapy but now the entry of a new informational paradigm into medicine can be seen, which is most prominently represented by *proteomics* and *metabonomics*. Metabonomics is a systems approach for studying in-vivo metabolic profiles, which promises to provide information on drug toxicity, disease processes and gene function at several stages in the drug development process. It uses spectroscopic methods, e.g. nuclear magnetic resonance, liquid chromatography mass spectroscopy and gas chromatography mass spectroscopy for identifying and characterising certain metabolic changes in humans, then integrating the data outcome by bioinformatics software to create a metabolic profile for a single individual. Such integration of data types will also pave the way to understanding the relationships between gene function and metabolic control in health and disease. Systems biology thus offers the computational integration of data generated by the suite of genetic, transcriptomic, proteomic and metabonomic platforms to understand function through different levels of biomolecular organisation. This offers exciting new prospects for determining the causes of human disease and finding possible cures. Certainly the judicious use of '-omics' data should give new insights and opportunities for the drug discovery process and for understanding drug toxicology.

This paradigm will bring two important changes in the therapy of diseases. Firstly, science will be able to study complex genomes and their functionality in complex organisms such as humans. Therefore, results from these studies no longer have to be translated into the context of medicine as they are already within this context. Secondly, drug therapy which used to be largely based on symptomatic relief, will now aim at targets emerging from the system that are closer to the causes of diseases. Therapeutic progress, which used to be indirect, conjectural and coincidental, is about to become more directed, definitive and intentional. The holistic approach to health differs from that of the conventional medicinal approach in that it takes into account the whole patient, rather than just focusing on the symptoms or the affected organ, so medicines are usually customised to an individual constitution. Traditional knowledge-driven drug development can follow a reverse pharmacology path and reduce time and cost of development.

Reverse pharmacology approach

A new chemical entity travels a path from laboratories to clinics, involving target identification, lead identification, lead optimisation, preclinical studies and then the four phases of clinical trials, which takes a long time, e.g. the average time from synthesis to approval of a new-drug application has increased significantly, from an average 7.9 years in the 1960s to 12.8 years in the 1990s. The drug development process is becoming more and more complex and capital intensive, and companies remain 'target rich' but 'lead poor', with lead discovery as a greater bottleneck. In such a situation, industrialisation of the drug development process is underway.

Although high-throughput screening and combinatorial chemical synthesis are being explored with high hopes, general experience points to the fact that in most companies, the investments in these technologies have not reaped the rewards in new lead discovery that were expected. Despite technological advances, genomics and bioinformatics predictions, the number of new molecular (chemical and biological) entities has actually dropped since the year 2002 to fewer than 20 per year. Approaches such as reverse pharmacology might help in reducing three major bottlenecks of costs, time and toxicity (Figure 7.1).

Reverse pharmacology, as an academic discipline, can be perceived to consist of three phases:

- robust documentation of clinical observations of the biodynamic effects of standardised Ayurvedic drugs by meticulous record keeping
- exploratory studies for tolerability, drug interactions, dose-range findings in ambulant patients with defined subsets of the disease and paraclinical studies in relevant in-vitro and in-vivo models to evaluate the target activity
- experimental studies, basic and clinical, at several levels of biological organisation, to identify and validate the reverse pharmacological correlates of Ayurvedic drug safety and efficacy (von Bertalanffy, 1968).

Such a creative research endeavour requires excellent teamwork by multisystem and multidisciplinary experts. Reverse pharmacology, for drug development, has been highly productive, and cost-effective too, in the recent past. Molecules such as the curcuminoids, reserpine and digoxin have emerged through knowledge of traditional medicines. The reverse pharmacology approach is cost-effective, as it travels back from clinical evidence so the cost of clinical trials, which is an expensive task, is reduced. Globally, this approach has now generated greater interest in Ayurveda and pharmacology. The scope of reverse pharmacology is to understand the mechanisms of action, at multiple levels of biology and to optimise safety, efficacy and acceptability of the leads

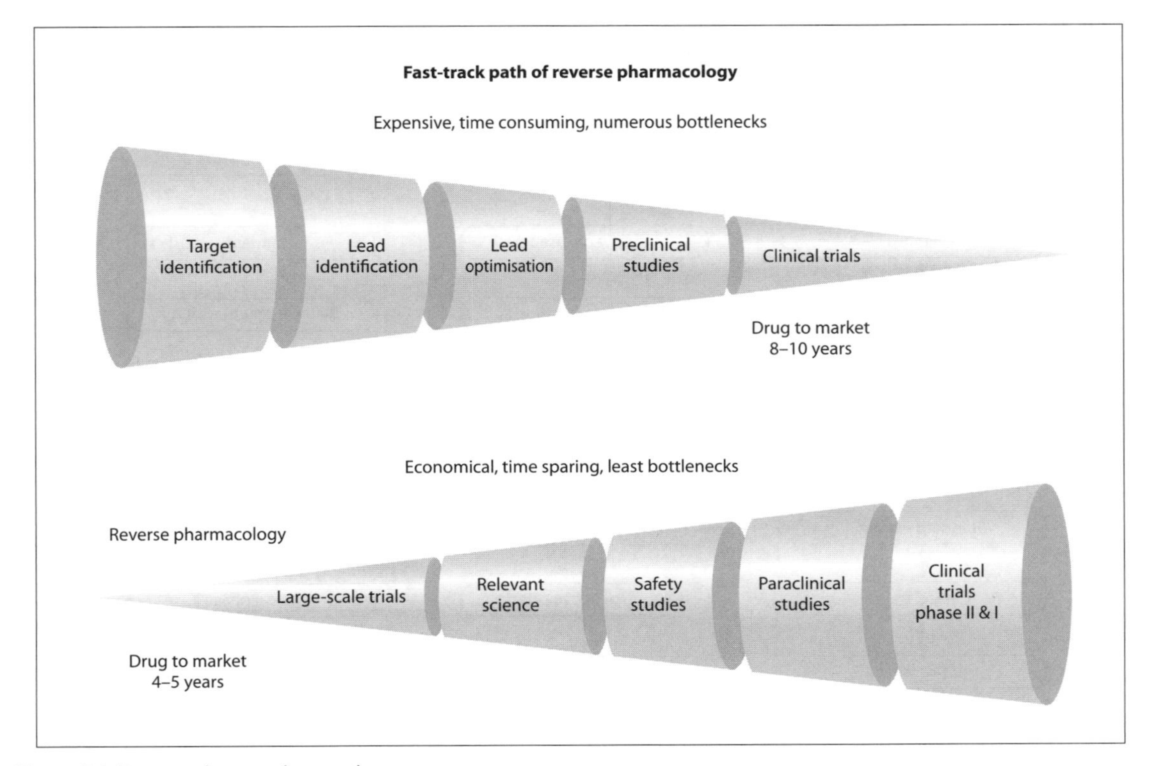

Figure 7.1 Reverse pharmacology path.

in natural products, based on relevant science. In this approach, the candidate drug travels a reverse path from clinic to laboratory rather than the classic laboratory to clinic path.

Drug development for phytomedicines

The future drug discovery and development particularly based on phytomedicines will be more often based on intent rather than coincidence. Proper bioprospecting of medicinal sources will still remain an important factor. However, despite the call from the US Food and Drug Administration (FDA) for an increase in science-based drug development and the recognition within the industry of the productivity challenges, there is only sporadic activity directly in line with the systems thinking presented here. Proof-of-principle studies are currently being undertaken, but no critical path success has yet emerged. From a cost–benefit point of view, the full incorporation of systems thinking into the pharmaceutical value chain will substantially increase the cost in the short term. The implementation of such a new concept over the entire process can only take place gradually, given the existing infrastructures that might need to be changed, the current development pipelines and the regulatory constraints. The analytical platforms necessary to undertake systems approaches are not inexpensive, nor trivial, to implement. Furthermore, the effort to establish quality-controlled methods to acquire, store, integrate and interpret datasets from different analytical platforms is substantial and the task of obtaining high-quality biological samples from animal and clinical studies consumes much time and human resources. The current need of the industry is a cost-effective, fast-track approach for drug development (Morphy *et al.*, 2004). Based on traditional experiences, drug development for herbal drugs can follow the different paths explained in Figure 7.2.

There are four estabished routes:

- The ethnomedicine path is based on observing the field use of the plants and then standardising it for the activity, e.g. tubocurarine isolated from curare – commonly known as South American arrow poison.
- Another adopted path is screening of the extracts in selected models, isolation of the active principles and then production of a modern

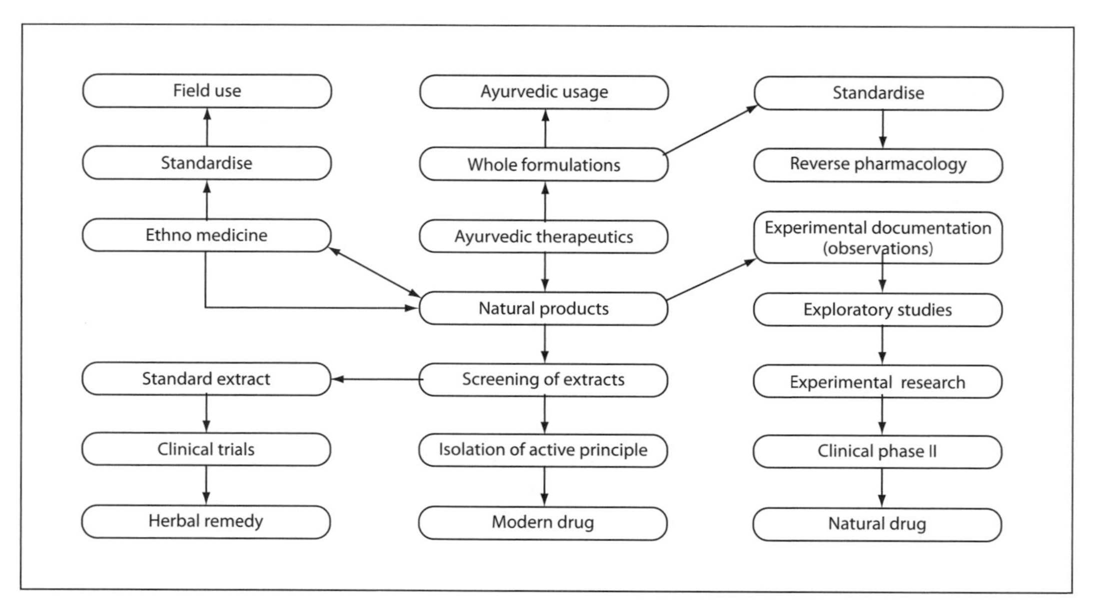

Figure 7.2 R&D paths for natural products.

drug, which enters a preclinical and clinical phase, e.g. isolation of reserpine from *Rauwolfia serpentina*.

- The third path is the herbal product path of the screening of extract in models and then testing the extract for its efficacy and safety in a clinical set up, e.g. *Ganoderma lucidum* and *Hypericum perforatum*.
- The fourth path is the holistic path using the formulation mentioned in classic texts of Ayurveda and other herbal systems and then evaluating its efficacy through pharmacoepidemological studies, e.g. chavanprash, which is an Ayurvedic preparation used from ancient times for cough, cold and healthy living.

All the above paths are explored for years together and have yielded important medicines. Despite all these established approaches the contribution to the development of mainstream drugs remained limited, as major pharmaceutical companies refrained from taking this field seriously. In addition, although botanical medications continue to be produced in every country, the clinical efficacy of these has usually not been evaluated and the composition of these complex mixtures was only crudely analysed.

Mechanisms of action

Actual human use is the ultimate 'model' and in-depth investigation of the effects of drugs and the nature of disease progression is becoming ever more feasible because of advances in clinical biomarkers. Combining the reverse pharmacology and systems biology approaches, the process of drug discovery and development can be greatly facilitated. We need to adopt such innovative approaches, models and designs in studying human subjects for establishing proof of concept and mechanisms of action of phytomedicines. Some of the case studies emerging from this approach are discussed in the next section.

Case studies

Rauwolfia serpentina (Sarpagandha)

Sen and Bose (1931) not only showed the antihypertensive effects of sarpagandha but they were also astute clinicians to note certain side-effects such as parkinsonism, depression, gynaecomastia, acid-peptic symptoms, etc. It was only recently that a Nobel prize in medicine and physiology was given to those who validated and explained the actions by mechanistic correlates. As a spin-off from the side-effects of *Rauwolfia serpentina*, several new drugs were developed i.e. L-dopa, antidepressants, bromoergocriptine, and H_2-receptor blockers (Patwardhan *et al.*, 1990; Devi *et al.*, 1992). The alkaloids of *Rauwolfia serpentina*, reserpine and ajmalcine, have served as research tools in many experiments (Patwardhan *et al.*, 1990; Devi *et al.*, 1992).

There are still some unanswered questions, e.g. does reserpine have more incidences of depression and/or extrapyramidal side-effects than the standardised extract of the plant? It has been proposed that it might be worthwhile to apply combinatorial chemical methods for reserpine derivatives, which do not cross the blood–brain barrier, so that depression is avoided as a side-effect. The uptake of noradrenaline by isolated chromaffin granules, by inhibition of ATP–Mg^2-dependent mechanism has to be studied afresh at the transcriptional level. The *kapha-vatashamak* (anti-inflammatory) properties of the plant described in Ayurveda also requires investigation. Although reserpine has been withdrawn globally from most markets, the extracts of the plant are still used as Ayurvedic drugs. There is a need to conduct pharmacovigilance on Sarpagandha Ghanavati, which is the traditional preparation made from *R. serpentina*.

Picrorrhiza kurroa (Kutki)

The late Vaidya Zandu Bhattji has popularised Arogyawardhani, a traditional Ayurvedic formula used by itself or in conjunction with herbal products/supplements for the treatment of jaundice. A double-blind trial with Arogyawardhani Kutki and placebo was conducted in viral hepatitis (Vaidya *et al.*, 1996; Patwardhan *et al.*, 2006) and significant hepatoprotective effects were observed for Kutki, either in Arogyawardhani or as a single plant. Later, picrosides, constituents of Kutki, were also tested in vivo and in vitro and found to be active (Druker *et al.*, 2003; Faivre *et al.*, 2006). Significant antioxidant as well as hydrocholeritic effects were noted for Kutki. The effects of hepatoprotection in carbon tetrachloride and galactosamine models are considered to be the pharmacological correlates of clinical actions

(Kerr *et al.*, 2004). However, there is a need to study at the cellular and molecular levels how the water outflow in the biliary microcanaliculae is enhanced. The Central Drug Research Institute in India has now developed a cucurbitacin-free extract of *P. kurroa* (Picroliv), which is now in Phase III trials. The plant also inhibits passive cutaneous anaphylaxis, as shown by Mahajani (Mahajani *et al.*, 1977).

Commiphora wightii (guggulu)

Guggulu is a major Ayurvedic drug and is used widely in diverse formulations. A monograph of all the major citations has been published (Vaidya, 2006). The hypolipidaemic effects of guggulu were primarily discovered through the reverse pharmacology approach. Antarkar, Satyavati, and Nityanand have carried out an extensive study on the hypolipidaemic effect of guggulu (Antarkar *et al.*, 1984; Satyavati, 1988). The product had been already marketed and widely used but the antiarthritic effects of guggulu in the clinic have been relatively less investigated. Sizeable experimental and reverse pharmacological studies with standardised guggulu preparations have been carried out (Nityanand *et al.*, 1989). Phase I study, long-term and large-dose ambulant studies have been conducted and the ongoing studies at cellular and molecular levels have helped in evolving pharmacological correlates of clinically shown actions. The side-effects of guggulu have also been documented, but the mechanisms of toxicity are yet to be studied. Guggulu can offer a platform for technological innovations in pharmaceutics, pharmacodynamics and pharmacokinetics. The use of guggulu as a *homadravya* (sacrificial incense) in *Shantikarma* (sacrificial use) is currently being evaluated for the antimicrobial effects of the volatiles. Topical formulations of guggulu demand unique dermato-pharmacological reverse correlates. The statement found in the literature on different properties of fresh and aged guggulu needs additional clinical investigations – empirical and exploratory. Use of Ayurvedic therapeutics in the context of modern medicine will give us many more insights into the newer targets in the disease pathogenesis and effects of the drugs. Blending the ancient wisdom and the modern science opens up existing fields where both can benefit mutually by adopting each others' techniques.

Ayurveda: a rich source of phytomedicines

Combining the strengths of the knowledge base of traditional systems such as Ayurveda with the dramatic power of combinatorial sciences and high-throughput screening will help in the generation of structure–activity data. Ayurvedic knowledge and investigational results can provide new functional leads to reduce time, money and toxicity – the three main hurdles in drug development. These records are particularly valuable, since effectively these medicines have been tested for thousands of years on people. Efforts are underway to establish a pharmaco-epidemiological evidence base regarding safety and practice of Ayurvedic medicines.

Development of standardised herbal formulations is underway as an initiative of the Council for Scientific and Industrial Research (CSIR) New Millennium Indian Technology Leadership Initiative (NMITLI). Randomised, controlled clinical trials for diabetes, rheumatoid and osteoarthritis, hepatoprotectives, and many other disorders have reasonably established clinical efficacy. A review of some exemplary evidence-based researches and approaches has now resulted in wider acceptance of Ayurvedic medicines. Thus the Ayurvedic knowledge database allows drug researchers to start from a well-tested and safe botanical material. With Ayurveda, the normal drug discovery course of 'laboratories to clinics' actually becomes from 'clinics to laboratories' – a true reverse pharmacology approach.

Globally, there is a positive trend towards holistic health, integrative sciences, systems biology approaches in drug discovery and therapeutics that has remained one of the unique features of Ayurveda. A golden triangle consisting of Ayurveda, modern medicine and science will converge to form a real discovery 'engine' that can result in newer, safer, cheaper and effective therapies. It will be in the interests of pharmaceutical companies, researchers and ultimately the global community to respect the traditions and build on their knowledge and investigational wisdom.

Currently, many pharmaceutical companies and research organisations have demonstrated renewed interest in investigating higher plants as sources for new lead structures and also for the development of standardised phytomedicines with reasonable efficacy, safety and quality (Brevoort, 1995; Subramoniam, 2001; Awang, 2007).

CSIR NMITLI herbal drug development

This initiative is the largest public/private partnership effort within the research and development domain in India. An Ayurveda-based herbal drug development project under CSIR NMITLI has a component of osteoarthritis and rheumatoid arthritis. Research partners for this project include:

- Interdisciplinary School of Health Sciences, University of Pune, Pune
- Indian Institute of Integrated Medicine, Jammu (formerly known as RRL–J)
- National Botanical Research Institute, Lucknow
- Agharkar Research Institute and Interactive Research School for Health Affairs, Pune
- Swami Prakashananda Ayurveda Research Center and KEM Hospital, Mumbai
- Nizam Institute of Medical Sciences, Hyderabad
- All India Institute of Medical Sciences, New Delhi and Center for Rheumatic Diseases, Pune.

The project involved industry partners including:

- Arya Vaidya Shala Kottakal
- Arya Vaidya Pharmacy, Coimbtore
- Dabur, Nicholas Piramal
- Natural Remedies, Bangalore
- Zandu Pharmaceuticals.

The following is a case study of standardised phytomedicine drug development and summary of the drug development process of a 4-year project on drug development for treatment of osteoarthritis.

Case study of standardised phytomedicine drug development for osteoarthritis treatment

Following several rounds of national level consultation of Ayurvedic physicians and scholars, a few drugs were short-listed. These drugs entered a parallel track of open-label observational studies by selected Ayurvedic physicians called *vaidyas* and rapid animal pharmacology studies. This led to two platforms of drug formulations. This was followed by a randomised, placebo-controlled, seven-limb, multicentric clinical trial where five formulations were tested with glucosamine as the positive control. Two formulations, which performed statistically better than placebo and glucosamine were then taken up for further studies.

Quality, safety, activity and mechanistics

The quality of crude drugs, extracts and formulations was monitored using chemistry, manufacturing and control guidelines of the US FDA. In-vitro studies using suitable cell and tissue culture models on these formulations revealed significant chondroprotection (proteoglycan release, nitric oxide release, aggrecan release and hyaluronidase inhibition as markers) in explant models of OA cartilage damage. In animal pharmacology these formulations demonstrated moderate analgesic and anti-inflammatory activities in both acute and chronic models. There was reasonable evidence for synergistic activity in the formulation as compared with single drugs. The formulations were found to be safe as per the guidelines set out by the Organisation for Economic Co-operation and Development, and were devoid of any significant genotoxicity or mutagenic activity in a micronucleus test.

Exploratory studies

A systematic dosing study was undertaken on the best formulation and the entire data, including observational, exploratory clinical trials, dosing studies, in-vitro and animal pharmacology, were collated for detailed discussions, assessment and analysis by experts. The team realised the need to further augment any analgesic effect, especially for use in osteoarthritis patients. After detailed study, discussions and evidence, one more ingredient was added to the best formulation. Thus two formulations (one with three ingredients and another with four) were finalised and taken for manufacture for the final, randomised clinical trial of equivalence.

Product development

A platform approach was adopted where base formulation based on traditional knowledge was used, followed by optimisation by adding other ingredients to obtain synergistic activity. All the formulations prepared for clinical trials were manufactured and labelled generally in accordance with US FDA guidance to industry for botanical drugs. Most of the required tests were performed during the entire process starting from passport data of raw material, botanical identification, chemical quality by spectroscopy and chromatography and molecular (DNA fingerprinting) standardisation to establish stability and pharmacopoeia standards of finished product. Necessary documentation was maintained for review, records or regulatory needs.

All extracts used in formulations were standardised with respect to their marker compounds. Shunthi (*Zingiber officinale*) hydro-alcoholic extract was standardised with respect to 6-gingerol, 8-gingerol, 10-gingerol, 6-shogaol and total gingerols. Salai guggul (*Boswellia serrata*) hydroalcoholic extract was standardised with respect to total boswellic acid percentage, boswellic acid (α + β), α-boswellic acid, β-boswellic acid, α-acetyl-boswellic acid, β-acetyl-boswellic acid, 11-keto-β-boswellic acid, acetyl-11-keto-β-boswellic acid and acetyl-boswellic acid (α + β). Amla (*Phyllanthus emblica*) extract was standardised with respect to total tannin as tannic acid and gallic acid. Guduchi (*Tinospora cordifolia*) extract was standardised with respect to the marker compound tinosporoside.

Clinical studies

The Phase 3 multicentric clinical trial was initiated on 12 January 2006 and involved four reputable centres, which followed a common protocol. This 24-week, randomised, clinical trial of equivalence using glucosamine and celecoxib for comparison, involved 300 patients and was statistically sufficiently powered. The evaluation parameters include clinical assessment as per American College of Rheumatology criteria and most of the critical markers (urinary CTX-II, serum cytokines (interleukin (IL)-1β, IL-6 and tumour necrosis factor (TNF)-α), serum matrix metalloproteinase (MMP)-1 and 3, serum hyaluronic acid) were measured in the laboratory. Knee radiographs have been done for 160 patients at baseline and at the completion using a validated, digitised image-analysis system to measure the changes in the width of the femorotibial joint space, as a surrogate marker for cartilage. This trial has demonstrated statistically significant equivalence of Ayurvedic test formulations with celecoxib and glucosamine. An Indian patent describing the innovative process, formulation and use has been filed by CSIR.

The CSIR NMITLI Herbal Drug Development project provides one of the best examples of systems and reverse pharmacology, where traditional knowledge as clinical evidence was used for developing a standardised phytomedicine. Here all the modern methodology was adopted for scientific investigation to establish an evidence base. The good laboratory practices and good clinical practices guidelines were followed and the US FDA Herbal Drug Guidance was adhered to. At the end of 5 years, this project successfully completed Phase 3 trials and is now ready with a complete dossier for investigational new drug and new-drug application submissions (Chopra and Patwardhan, 2007).

Conclusions

In short, newer approaches based on systems biology and reverse pharmacology are useful to develop standardised phytomedicines. Since most of the botanical materials have actually been in clinical use for a considerable time, there are reasonably high safety expectations. While well-controlled clinical studies may be undertaken to establish a sufficient evidence base, mechanistic studies can be undertaken simultaneously. This parallel processing shortens the drug discovery and development period considerably, resulting in time and money savings.

Acknowledgements

We thank Amrutesh Puranik and Prajakta Kulkarni for their help.

References

Antarkar DS, Pande R, Athavale AV (1984). Phase I tolerability study of Yogaraj-guggulu – a popular Ayurvedic drug. *J Postgrad Med* 30: 111–115.

Awang DVC (2007). Standardisation of herbal medicinal products. *ISHC Acta Horticult* 629: XXVI.

Beuth J(1997). Clinical relevance of immunoactive mistletoe lectin-I. *Anticancer Drugs* 8: S53–55.

Brekhman IL, Dardimov IV (1969). New substances of plant origin which increase non-specific resistance. *Annu Rev Pharmacol* 21: 419–426.

Brevoort P (1995). The U.S. botanical market. An overview. *Herbgram* 36: 49–59.

Butcher EC, Berg EL, Kunkel EJ, (2004). Systems biology in drug discovery. *Nature Biotechnol* 22(10): 1253–1259.

Calixto JB (2000). Efficacy, safety, quality control, marketing and regulatory guigelines for herbal medicines (phytotherapeutic agents). *Braz J Med Biol Res* 33: 179–189.

Chopra Arvind Patwardhan Bhushan (2007). *Indo–US Symposium on Botanicals.* University of Mississippi and IIIM, Jammu, November 12–14, 2007, New Delhi.

Devi PU, Sharada AC, Solomon EF, Kamath MS (1992). In vivo growth inhibitory effect of *Withania somnifera* (Ashwagandha) on a transplantable mouse tumor, Sarcoma 180. *Indian J Exp Biol* 30 169–172.

Dickson M, Gagnon JP (2004). The cost of new drug discovery and development. *Discov Med* 4: 172–179.

Druker BJ, David A (2003). Karnofsky Award Lecture. Imatini as a paradigm of targeted therapies. *J Clin Oncol* 21: 239s–245s.

Elsasser-Beile U, Leiber C, Wolf P *et al.* (2005). Adjuvant intravesical treatment of superficial bladder cancer with a standardized mistletoe extract. *J Urol* 174: 76–9.

Faivre S, Djelloul S, Raymond E (2006). New paradigms in anticancer therapy: targeting multiple signaling pathways with kinase inhibitors. *Semin Oncol* 33: 407–420.

Gannon F (2005). Welcome to molecular systems biology. *EMBO Report* 6: 291.

Gillis NC (2001). Biomedical science and herbal medicine: a reluctant but necessary alliance. *FASEB Newslett* 34: 23.

WHO (1996). *Good Manufacturing Practices: supplementary guidelines for manufacture of herbal medicinal products.* In: WHO expert committee on specifications for pharmaceutical preparations, 34th report. Geneva, World Health Organization, 1996, Annex 8 (WHO technical Series, no 863), 134–139.

Huber R, Rostock M, Goedl R, *et al.* (2005). Mistletoe treatment induces GM-CSF and IL-5 production by PBMC and increases blood granulocyte and eosinophil counts: a placebo controlled randomized study in healthy subjects. *Eur J Med Res* 18: 10: 411–418.

Kerr DJ, La Thangue NB (2004). Signal transduction blockade and cancer: combination therapy or multi-targeted inhibitors? *Ann Oncol* 15: 1727–1729.

Kim JY, Germolee DR, Luster MI, (1990). *Panax ginseng* as a potential immunomodulator; studies in mice. *Immunopharmacol Immunotoxicol* 12(2): 257–276.

Mahajani SS, Kulkarni RD (1977). Effect of disodium cromoglycate and *Picrorhiza kurroa* root powder on sensitivity of guinea pigs to histamine and sympathomimetic amines. *Int Arch Allergy Appl Immunol* 53: 137–144.

Morphy RK, Rankovic C (2004). From magic bullets to designed multiple ligands. *Drug Discov Today* 9: 641–651.

Nityanand S, Srivastava JS, Asthana OP (1989). Clinical trials with gugulipid, a new hypolipidaemic agent. *J Assoc Physicians India* 37: 323–328.

Patwardhan B (2000). Ayurveda, the designer medicine: review of ethnopharmacology and bioprospecting research. *Indian Drugs* 37: 213–227.

Patwardhan B, Patwardhan A (2006). Traditional Medicine: Modern Approach for Affordable Global Health. *Report for World Health Organization's Commission on Intellectual Property Innovation & Public Health, Ancient Science of Life*, Supplement to Silver Jubilee issue, Jan–July (2006).

Patwardhan B, Kalbag D, Patki PS, Nagasampagi BA (1990). Search of immunoregulatory agents – A review. *Indian Drugs* 28 (2): 56–63.

Patwardhan B, Vaidya A, Chorghade M (2004). Ayurveda and natural products drug discovery. *Curr Sci* 86: 789–799.

Patwardhan B, Warude D, Pushpangadan P, Bhatt N (2005). Ayurveda and traditional Chinese medicine: a comparative overview. *Evid Based Complement Altern Med* 2: 465–473.

Rege NN (1999). Adaptogenic properties of six Rasayana herbs in Ayurvedic Medicine. *Phytother Res* 13: 275–291.

Salaman CR, (1989). Immunomodulators and feeding regulation; a humoral link between the immune and nervous systems. *Brain Behav Immun* 3: 193–213.

Satyavati GV (1988). Gum guggul (Commiphora mukul) – the success story of an ancient insight leading to a modern discovery. *Indian J Med Res* 87: 327–335.

Sen G, Bose KC (1931). Rauwolfia serpentina, a new Indian drug for insanity and high blood pressure. *Indian Med Wld* 2: 194.

Siegel RK (1979). Ginseng abuse syndrome – problems with the Panacea. *JAMA* 241: 1614–1615.

Subramoniam A (2001). The problems of prospects of plant drug research in India: Pharmacological evaluation of ecotypes in herbal drug development. *Indian J Pharmacol* 33: 145–146.

Vaidya AB, Antarkar DS, Doshi JC *et al.* (1996). *Picrorhiza kurroa* (kutki) Royle ex Benth as a hepatoprotective agent – experimental and clinical studies. *J Postgrad Med* 42: 105–108.

Vaidya ADB (2006). Reverse pharmacological correlates of Ayurvedic drug actions. *Indian J Pharmacol* 38: 311–315.

Vaidya ADB, Vaidya RA, Nagaral SI (2001). Ayurveda and a different level of evidence: From Lord Macaulay to Lord Walton (1835–2001 AD). *J Assoc Physicians India* 49: 534–537 and Approach Paper, *New Millennimum Indian Technology Leadership Initiative Herbal Drug Development Program*, CSIR New Delhi (2002).

Verpoorte R, Mukherjee P (2003). GMP for Botanicals, Business Horizons, New Delhi, India.

von Bertalanffy L (1968). *General System Theory: foundations, development, applications.* New York: George Braziller.

Wang Z, Zheng Q, Liu K, Li G, Zheng R (2006). Ginsenoside Rh(2) enhances antitumour activity and decreases genotoxic effect of cyclophosphamide. *Basic Clin Pharmacol Toxicol* 98: 411–415.

Wang CZ, Luo X, Zhang B *et al.* (2006). Notoginseng enhances anti-cancer effect of 5-fluorouracil on human colorectal cancer cells. *Cancer Chemother Pharmacol* 60: 69–79.

Yu S, Zhang Y (1995). Effect of *Achyranthes bidenta* polysaccharide (ABP) on antitumor activity and immune function of S-180 bearing mice. *Chung Hua Chung Liu Tsa Chih (China)* 17: 275–278.

Part 2

Pharmacological evaluation for some therapeutic areas

8

Herbal medicines for functional gastrointestinal disorders: study methods for quality, safety and efficacy

Vietla S Rao

Introduction

Gastrointestinal complaints rank among the most frequent reasons why people seek medical advice. The most common functional gastrointestinal disorders (FGIDs) seen in clinical practice are functional dyspepsia (FD) and irritable bowel syndrome (IBS), characterised by recurrent episodes of gastrointestinal symptoms, in the absence of structural lesions that explain symptoms. While symptoms of epigastric pain, bloating, nausea, belching, early satiety and heartburn are predominant in FD (Holtmann *et al.*, 2006), abdominal discomfort, bloating and disturbed patterns of defecation (constipation, diarrhoea or constipation/diarrhoea) are common in patients with IBS (Brandt *et al.*, 2005). FGIDs reduce the health-related quality of life and account for an increased healthcare burden (Talley and Vakil, 2005). The pathogenesis of FGIDs is probably multifactorial, genetic and environmental factors are thought to contribute to alterations in visceral sensory function, motility, bacterial overgrowth and central nervous system processing (Drossman, 2005). Inflammation is considered a risk factor for the development of both functional dyspepsia and IBS (Thornley *et al.*, 2001; Dunlop *et al.*, 2003; Hall *et al.*, 2003). Currently, the existing therapies to treat multiple symptoms of FGIDs are suboptimal, associated with restricted therapeutic potential and new agents are awaited that would improve global IBS symptoms (Tack *et al.*, 2006a,b). A wide variety of treatments have been used to manage FGIDs and include *Helicobacter pylori* eradication, antacids, mucosal protectants, antisecretory agents, prokinetics, antidepressants and visceral analgesics. The fact that no single available therapy consistently provides relief to the majority of the patients validates the heterogeneity of these disorders. The emerging therapies are largely aimed to normalise pain perception and gastrointestinal motor and reflux function.

The therapy of functional gastrointestinal disorders is one of the domains of phytotherapeutic treatments. Traditionally, plants with a high tannin content, showing astringent properties, were particularly valued to treat diarrhoea and dysentery whereas bitter, aromatic and bitter-aromatic plants were especially employed to treat gastrointestinal cramps and pain. Investigations on traditionally used plants have resulted in the isolation, and chemical and pharmacological characterisation of many different types of compounds. Most of these agents are helpful to prevent or arrest the progression, rather than to treat disease. Further, they exhibit pleotropic actions and therefore may serve as important leads for developing novel therapies for the treatment of FGIDs.

So far, relatively few herbal medicines have been evaluated scientifically to prove their safety, potential benefits and effectiveness in gastrointestinal disorders (Table 8.1) (Rösch *et al.*, 2002; Holtmann *et al.*, 2004; Liu *et al.*, 2006). This chapter specifically deals with the evaluation methods for the development of quality herbal medicines intended to be useful in FGIDs.

Functional dyspepsia

Functional dyspepsia is a clinical syndrome, whose origin is unknown, defined by chronic or recurrent pain or discomfort in the upper abdomen. On the basis of the Rome III diagnostic criteria for functional gastrointestinal disorders, patients who suffer from FD in the absence of any organic disease are categorised as having postprandial distress syndrome or epigastric pain syndrome for at least 3 months (Drossman, 2006; Tack *et al.*, 2006a). About 15–30% of adult patients suffer from various different functional dyspeptic conditions. Several pathophysiological mechanisms are involved in FD, including visceral hypersensitivity, both in the stomach and the duodenum, impaired gastric accommodation, antral overdistention, delayed gastric emptying and abnormal duodenojejunal motility (Kleibeuker and Thijs, 2004). Induction of gastric hypersensitivity by acid in the stomach seems to be important in a subset of patients. Many drugs can induce dyspepsia as a gastrointestinal side-effect, the major cause being the use of nonsteroidal anti-inflammatory drugs (NSAIDs) for arthritis and chemotherapeutic agents in cancer. Studies also suggest a possible link with G-protein polymorphisms in dyspepsia.

Currently, functional dyspepsia is classified into ulcer-like dyspepsia, dysmotility-like dyspepsia and non-specific dyspepsia, in which symptoms do not clearly fit into any of the above categories. While antacids, H_2-receptor antagonists and proton-pump inhibitors are useful in ulcer-like dyspepsia, prokinetic agents are more effective in dysmotility-like dyspepsia. Most therapies for patients with FD are intended to normalise pain perception and gastrointestinal motor and reflex function. Serotonin is the key mediator of gut function in relation to gastrointestinal motility, secretion and sensation of pain. There is limited evidence that the 5-hydroxytryptamine 5-HT_3 antagonist alosetron has potential efficacy in functional dyspepsia, perhaps via visceral analgesic effects (Talley *et al.*, 2001). Animal studies also suggest that acid can induce serotonin release from enterochromaffin cells in the duodenum, which may in turn activate 5-HT_3 receptors and alter visceral sensation. Acid in the duodenum can also induce fundic relaxation (Lee *et al.*, 2004). Thus, the interaction between acid and 5-HT_3 receptor antagonism is of interest in functional dyspepsia. A number of compounds may have visceral analgesic effects in the upper gastrointestinal tract, including 5-HT_3 antagonists and 5-HT_4 agonists. Approximately 25% of patients with functional dyspepsia have slow gastric emptying, and perhaps 10% have accelerated gastric emptying (Talley *et al.*, 1999). It is, therefore, important to avoid the use of prokinetic therapy in patients who have accelerated gastric emptying, as presumably this would worsen symptoms (Talley *et al.*, 2006).

No standard therapy is currently available for FD. From ancient times, bitter herbal drugs have played a role in the therapy of patients with dyspeptic symptoms. Studies point out that different plant-derived extracts and their constituents can give gastro/cytoprotection through several mechanisms (Table 8.1). Flavonoids are highly gastroprotective probably due to enhancement of the release of nitric oxide and neuropeptides, such as calcitonin gene-related peptide, released from sensory afferent nerves, which increase gastric microcirculation. These appear to stimulate, at even very small concentrations, the secretion of the stomach as well as the digestive glands and strengthen the smooth musculature of the digestive tract. Bitter substances are often combined with essential oils, which act primarily as spasmolytics and analgesics and possess anti-*Helicobacter pylori* effects. They exert anti-inflammatory action by:

Table 8.1 Experimental studies on traditional herbs used in gastrointestinal disorders

Name	Part used	Use	Constituents	Study type	Results	Reference
STW 5 Iberogast® (herbal formula)	Ethanolic extracts of 9 plants	Functional dyspepsia (FD) and IBS	Methionine-like sulphur-compounds	Animal studies	Diminished binding affinity of 5-HT(4), muscarinic M(3), and opioid receptors in vitro	Simmen *et al.*, 2006
Artichoke (*Cynara scolymus* L.)	Leaf extract	IBS	Caffeoylquinic acids and flavonoids	Animal studies	Protected animals from gastric ulceration	Jimenez-Escrig *et al.*, 2003; Emendorfer *et al.*, 2005
N-095 (crude drug containing red ginseng, polygala root, saffron, antelope horn and aloe wood)	Dried powder	Combat stress	Multicomponents	Experimental studies in rats	Prevented gastric ulceration — induced by restraint and water-immersion stress	Inoue *et al.*, 2005
Baishouwu (Chinese herbal drug)	Dried root tubers of 3 plants	Gastric diseases	Multicomponents	Experimental studies in rats	Offered gastroprotection against ethanol and indometacin-induced gastric lesions	Shan *et al.*, 2006
Turmeric (*Curcuma longa* L.)	Rhizome extract	Ulcer and non-ulcer dyspepsia	Curcumin (diferuloyl methane)	Animal studies in vivo and anti-*H. pylori* in vitro	Demonstrated antiulcer, anti-inflammatory, anticancer and analgesic effects	Mahady *et al.*, 2002; Kim *et al.*, 2005; Aggarwal *et al.*, 2007
Peppermint (*Mentha piperita* L.)	Leaf essential oil	Gastroprotective use	Menthol and menthonin	Animal studies	Antimicrobial, antispasmodic, antioxidant and analgesic effects	McKay and Blumberg, 2006
Anise (*Pimpinella anisum* L.)	Seed aqueous suspension	Gastroprotective use in Arab medicine	Volatiles	In vivo experimental ulceration in rats and anti-*H.pylori* in vitro	Gastroprotection against necrotising agents and indometacin	Mahady *et al.*, 2005; Al Moflehm *et al.*, 2007
Cardamom (*Elettaria cardamomum* Maton.)	Crude methanolic extract and fractions	Gastroprotective use in Unani medicine	Terpenes and phenolic compounds	Experimental ulceration in rats	Gastroprotection against ethanol and aspirin-induced injury	Jamal *et al.*, 2006
Fenugreek (*Trigonella foenum graecum*)	Aqueous extract of seed and gel fraction	Gastric complaints	Steroidal saponins and alkaloids	Rat study	Prevents ethanol-induced gastric lesions	Pandian *et al.*, 2002

(*continued overleaf*)

Table 8.1 *(continued)*

Name	Part used	Use	Constituents	Study type	Results	Reference
Myrrh (*Commiphora molmol* Engl.)	Aqueous suspension of oleo-gum-resin	Gastroprotective use in Arab medicine	Furanoeudesma-1,3-dien and linderstrene	Experimental ulceration in rats	Gastroprotection against necrotising agents and indometacin	Al-Harbi *et al.*, 1997
Sangre de grado (*Croton urucurana* var. genuinus and related species)	Red sap from trunk wood of *C. urucurana*	Gastric ulcer and diarrhoea	Proantocyanidins, taspine	Experimental study in rats and guinea-pigs	Antiulcer, antidiarrhoeal and visceral antinociceptive effects	Miller *et al.*, 2000; Tran *et al.*, 2006; Rao *et al.*, 2007
Copaiba oil (*Copaifera langs dorffii* Desf.) and related species)	Oleo-resin from trunk wood	Gastrointestinal disorders	Volatiles and diterpenes that include kaurenoic acid	In vivo experimental studies with rats	Antiulcer, wound healing and anti-inflammatory effects	Paiva *et al.*, 1998; 2002; 2004a; 2004b
Aroeira (*Myracrodruon urundeuva* Engl.)	Aqueous extract from stem bark	Traditional use in gastric dyspepsia, and diarrhoea	Tannins and Chalcones	Experimental studies with rats and guinea-pigs	Gastroprotection against ethanol, stress and histamine-induced lesions; acetic acid-induced colitis	Rao *et al.*, 1987; Menezes and Rao, 1988
Monkey puzzle (*Araucaria araucana* Mol.)	Resin	Mapuche Amerindians use to treat ulcers	Labdane diterpenes and lignans	Experimental studies with mice	Gastroprotection against ethanol-HCl-induced lesions	Schmeda-Hirschmann *et al.*, 2005
Macela (*Egletes viscosa* L.)	Ethanolic extract of flower buds and flavonoid, ternatin	Gastric dyspepsia, diarrhoea and constipation	Volatiles, flavonoid (ternatin) and diterpenes (centipedic acid and 12-acetoxy hawtriwaic acid)	Animal studies	Antiulcer, antidiarrhoeal and anti-inflammatory effects	Rao *et al.*, 1997; Guedes *et al.*, 2002; Rao *et al.*, 2003
Tsubaki (*Camellia japonica* L.)	Methanolic extract of flower buds	Blood vomiting and stomach ache	Camelliosides	Experimental studies in rats	Decreased the ethanol and indometacin-evoked gastric ulceration	Yoshikawa *et al.*, 2007
Mango (*Mangifera indica* L.)	Aqueous decoction of mango flowers	Gastrointestinal disorders and arthralgias	Xanthone (mangiferin), flavonoids and triterpenes	Acute and subacute models of gastric ulceration in rodents	Decreased the acetic acid, ethanol and stress-induced gastric ulceration	Lima *et al.*, 2006
Grape-seed (*Vitis vinifera* L.)	Seed extract	Gastroprotection	Proanthocyanidins	Animal models of gastric ulceration	Decreased the ethanol, stress, and indometacin-induced gastric ulceration	Brzozowski *et al.*, 2005

Table 8.1 *(continued)*

Name	Part used	Use	Constituents	Study type	Results	Reference
Karela (*Momordia charantia* L.)	Dried powdered fruits	Traditionally used in diabetes and for healing of peptic ulcer	Triterpenes and glycosides, karavilagenins and karavilosides	Animal models of gastric ulceration	Reduced ulceration	Gurbiz *et al.*, 2000
Almécega (*Protium heptaphyllum* March.)	Resin from the trunk wood	Traditionally used remedy in gastrointestinal disorders	Volatiles and triterpenes (alpha- and beta-amyrin)	Animal studies	Antiulcer, visceral antinociceptive and anti-inflammatory effects of α- and β-amyrin	Oliveira *et al.*, 2004a; 2004b; 2005;
Coptis (*Coptis Chinensis* Franch.)	Root extract	Traditionally used remedy in gastrointestinal disorders	Alkaloids (10% berberine)	Animal studies	Inhibits ulcer formation and acid secretion	Li *et al.*, 2005
Bone setter (*Cissus quadrangularis* L.)	Methanolic extract	Traditionally used for fracture healing	Vitamin C and β- carotene	Rat study	Prevents indometacin-induced ulceration	Jainu *et al.*, 2006
Red sanders (*Pterocarpus santalinus* L.)	Ethanolic extract	Traditional herbal drug for wound healing	3-keto-oleanane	Rat gastric ulceration model in vivo and anti-H. pylori in vitro	Cytoprotection antioxidant, anti-*H. pylori* and antiulcer effects	Narayan *et al.*, 2005; 2007

STW 5 is composed of ethanolic extracts from nine plants (Ibera Amara Totalis, Angelicae Radix, Cardui Mariae Fructus, Carvi Fructus, Chelidonii Herba, Liquiritae Radix, Marticariae Flos, Melissae Folium, Menthae Piperitae Folium). N-095 is a mixture of red ginseng, polygala root, saffron, antelope horn and aloe wood.

Sangre de grado is derived from several *Croton* species (*Croton dracanoides, C. palanostigma, C. lecheleri, C. urucurana*).

Baishouwu is an appellative name of dried root tubers from three Asclepiadaceae plants: *Cynanchum auriculatum* Royle ex Wight, *Cynanchum bungei* Decne and *Cynoctonum wilfordii Maxim*.

- suppressing the neutrophil/cytokine cascade in the gastrointestinal tract
- promoting tissue repair through expression of various growth factors
- exhibiting antioxidant activity, scavenging reactive oxygen species
- inhibiting cytochome P450 2F1 activity, producing antinecrotic and anticarcinogenic activities.

However, experimental studies have aimed mostly to validate the traditional use of plants in gastrointestinal disease, but no attempt has been made to verify their potential in FD.

Irritable bowel syndrome

IBS is a potentially debilitating condition characterised by abdominal discomfort, bloating, and disturbed patterns of defecation with a lower health-related quality of life (Chang, 2004). According to Rome III criteria, IBS is defined as recurrent abdominal pain or discomfort for at least 3 days per month (Talley *et al.*, 1999). It affects approximately 15–30% of the general population. The prevalence is equally divided among three subtypes: IBS with constipation, IBS with diarrhoea, and IBS with alternating constipation/diarrhoea (Brandt *et al.*, 2005).

Conventional therapy includes the use of bulk laxatives and stool softeners for constipation, antimotility drugs for diarrhoea, and antispasmodics, antimuscarinics and antidepressants for pain and spasm (Maxwell *et al.*, 1997). Chronic constipation is a very common disorder, and the goals in treating such patients are to improve the patient's symptoms and to restore normal bowel function, aiming to achieve at least three bowel movements per week. Serotonin plays a prominent role in chronic constipation, since it affects the intestinal motility, fluid secretion and sensation through activation of receptors present in enterochromaffin cells (Gershon and Tack, 2007).

The only FDA-approved agents for chronic idiopathic constipation are tegaserod ($5\text{-}HT_3$ agonist) and lubiprostone, a type 2 chloride-channel activator, which both represent real therapeutic advances in the management of these patients (Ambizas and Ginzburg, 2007). Lubiprostone draws chloride, sodium, and water into the lumen of the gut enhancing fluid secretion and facilitating increased motility and colonic transit. Lubiprostone, although significantly better than placebo in improving symptoms of constipation severity, stool consistency, straining, and abdominal discomfort, has been shown to be associated with adverse events such as nausea (30.2%), diarrhoea (19.2%) and distention (9.3%) (Johanson and Ueno, 2007). However, patients are refractory to these agents in the presence of pelvic floor dyssynergia, leaving the option for therapy with a prokinetic agent, fibre or a laxative. Thus, there is an overall dissatisfaction with traditional treatment options from patients and physicians.

Clinical studies with herbals in functional gastrointestinal disorders

In the recent past, a few controlled clinical studies were carried out with phytotherapeutic combinations (i.e. combinations of various plant/herbal extracts with a number of different active ingredients) which showed superiority over the placebo treatments (see Table 8.2). However, randomised controlled trial (RCTs) data supporting the efficacy of these treatments in patients with FGIDs are still lacking (Liu *et al.*, 2006). RCTs indicated that peppermint oil could be efficacious for symptom relief in IBS and meta-analysis confirmed this (Pittler and Ernst, 1998). Placebo-controlled RCTs demonstrated the clinical efficacy and safety of a polyherbal preparation, STW 5 (Iberogast, Enzymatic Therapy Inc.) for the treatment of both FD and patients with IBS. The pharmacological effects, as well as the therapeutic effectiveness, tolerability, and toxicity, of Iberogast were experimentally and clinically recorded and documented (Saller *et al.*, 2002; Pilichiewicz *et al.*, 2007). These studies indicated that Iberogast promotes gastric relaxation and stimulates antral motility. Tong-xie-ning, a standard Chinese traditional herbal formula, and Padma Lax, a Tibetan herbal medicine, showed significant improvement of global symptoms in FGID, when compared with placebo treatment (Liu *et al.*, 2006). An RCT assessing artichoke leaf extract in 247 patients with FD demonstrated a significant improvement in both overall symptoms and disease-specific quality of life compared with placebo (Holtmann *et al.*, 2003).

Studies on curcumin (diferuoylmethane), an ingredient of turmeric (*Curcuma longa*) demonstrated improvement in healing of peptic ulcer and symptoms in non-ulcer dyspepsia but not in IBS (Prucksunand *et al.*, 2001). Capsaicin, the active ingredient of another spice, red chilli pepper, has been evaluated in small RCTs, which yielded conflicting results in patients with FD. While one study reported significant improvement in overall symptoms, epigastric pain, fullness and nausea compared with placebo (Bortolotti *et al.*, 2002), an earlier placebo-controlled crossover trial was unable to show significant improvements in postprandial dyspepsia scores with capsaicin (Rodriguez-Stanley *et al.*, 2000).

The combination of extracts of different plants appears to be advantageous to treat FGIDs compared with conventional chemically well-defined drugs. Nevertheless, several issues regarding herbal products deserve mention. Based on current evidence, the scientific validity of the use of many of these commercial natural products in FGIDs is severely limited, with quality control and regulatory issues continuing to be a concern. The available trials almost all suffer from significant methodological flaws making the results difficult to interpret. Although the short-term use appears relatively safe, the long-term safety of these agents has not been established. Further, because these natural products are not regulated as pharmaceuticals, questions regarding agent purity and potency could be raised.

Safety and efficacy issues

The quality of herb used and its chemical constitution is fundamental to understanding the product's intended use and factors affecting its safety. It is the chemical constituents that are the basis for the pharmacological activity of a herbal product, and consequently for the therapeutic efficacy. Use of validated, reliable, and relevant methods for efficacy/toxicity studies with regulatory strategies are essential to create a stronger evidence base on the safety, efficacy and quality of the herbal products for FGIDs.

Evaluation of herbal medicines: preclinical studies

Preclinical assays are essential to guarantee the safety and efficacy of natural products in FGIDs. The pathophysiology of FGID is not firmly established, and is characterised by recurrent episodes of gastrointestinal symptoms with no structural alterations. Visceral hypersensitivity, disordered gastrointestinal motility and secretion are presently considered key mechanisms underlying FGID symptoms. Therefore, pharmacological studies with new herbal products for efficacy and safety assessment are carried out using in-vitro and in-vivo experimental models that helped define basic mechanisms of FD and IBS symptoms. Animal testing should follow the ethical considerations and the approval of the Institutional Committee on the Use of Animals for experimentation.

In-vitro and animal testing

The emerging therapies for FGIDs are largely aimed at normalising pain perception and gastrointestinal motor and reflux function. *Helicobacter pylori* infection, NSAID consumption and severe physical stress are associated with FGID. For this reason, the most common pharmacological properties determined in the evaluation of drugs effective for FGID are the anti-*Helicobacter*, cytoprotection, visceral analgesic, spasmolytic, antisecretory, antidiarrhoeal and prokinetic effects. The requirement for each one of these studies include experimental animals (two species, one rodent and another non-rodent, 6–8 per group), appropriate controls (negative and positive), and product evaluation at three dose levels.

H. pylori may induce gastritis and chronic dyspepsia (functional non-ulcer dyspepsia or gastroduodenal ulcer) in humans. Mongolian gerbils or BALB/c mice infected with *H. pylori* are often used as animal models to screen test compounds for their efficacy in reducing the extent of gastric ulceration or inflammation. Although these animals demonstrate gastric ulceration, virtually no gastritis is seen in the antrum of infected animals, but this is, however, the hallmark of human infection (Lee, 2000). The anti-*H. pylori* activity of a test drug can be assessed through in-vitro studies employing rat gastric epithelial cell cultures and *H. pylori* isolates from gastric

Table 8.2 Clinical studies with herbal medicinals in gastrointestinal functional disorders

Name	Part used	Use	Constituents	Study type	Results	Reference
STW 5 Iberogast ® (herbal formula)	Ethanolic extracts of 9 plants	FD and IBS	Methionine like sulphur-compounds	Placebo-controlled RCT	Improved gastrointestinal symptom-severity score	Madisch *et al.*, (2004); Rösch *et al.*, 2006; von Arnim *et al.* (2007)
Carmint	Total extracts of 3 plants	IBS	(E)-2-dodecenal, eugenol, menthol and L-carvone	Pilot clinical study	Reduced the severity and frequency of abdominal pain/ discomfort	Vejdani *et al.*, 2006
Tong-xie-ning (TCM-herbal formula)	Dried extract of four herbs	Diarrhoea-predominant IBS	Complex compound containing paeoniflorin	Placebo-controlled RCT	Reduced symptom severity	Wang *et al.*, 2006
Hange-koboku-to (HKT, Kampoo medicine)	Dried mixture of 5 crude herbs	FD	Magnorol, konokiol, perillaldehyde, 6-gingerol, 6-shogaol	Open clinical study	Improves delayed gastric emptying (prokinetic effect)	Oikawa *et al.*, 2005
Padma Lax (Tibetan herbal medicine)	Dried extract from 10 plants	Constipation-predominant IBS	Multicomponent	Double-blind randomised pilot study	Reduced symptom severity	Sallon *et al.*, 2002
Artichoke (*Cynara scolymus* L.)	Leaf extract	Dyspepsia and IBS	Caffeoylquinic acids and flavonoids	Open clinical study	Amelioration of global symptoms and improvement in QOL score	Marakis *et al.*, 2002; Bundy *et al.*, 2004b
Peppermint (*Mentha piperita* L.)	Leaf essential oil	IBS	Menthol and menthonin	Double-blind RCT	Smooth muscle relaxation; analgesia	Pittler and Ernst, 1998
Turmeric (*Curcuma longa* L.)	Rhizome extract	IBS; ulcer and non-ulcer dyspepsia	Curcumin (diferuloyl methane)	Placebo-controlled RCT	Improved healing of peptic ulcer and of non-ulcer dyspepsia but not of IBS	Bundy *et al.*, 2004a; Pruksunand *et al.*, 2001; Brinkhaus *et al.*, 2005

Table 8.2 (*continued*)

Name	Part used	Use	Constituents	Study type	Results	Reference
Red pepper (*Capsicum annuum* ssp.)	Powder	FD	Capsaicin	Placebo-controlled RCT	60% Reduction of symptom score	Bortolotti *et al.*, 2002
Mangava-brava (*Lafoensia pacari* St Hil.)	Methanolic extract	Used in gastric ulcer and inflammatory conditions	Ellagic acid	Double-blind RCT against *H. pylori*	Well tolerated and patients were symptom-free in an 8-week trial	Da Mota Menezes *et al.*, 2006

STW 5 is composed of ethanolic extracts from nine plants (Ibera Amara Totalis, Angelicae Radix, Cardui Mariae Fructus, Carvi Fructus, Chelidonii Herba, Liquiritae Radix, Marticariae Flos, Melissae Folium, Menthae Piperitae Folium).

Carmint contains total extracts from three plants (*Melissa officinalis, Mentha spicata* and *Coriandrum sativum*).

Tong-xie-ning consists of dried substances of *Paeonia lactiflora* Pali. (root), *Atractylodes macrocephala* Koidz. (rhizome), *Citrus reticulata* Blanco. (unripe exocarp) and *Allium macrostemon* Bge. (bulb).

HKT is a composite of five crude herbs: Pinelliae Tuber, Hoelen, Magnoliae Cortex, Perillae Herba and Zingiberis Rhizoma.

Padma Lax is composed of Aloes, Calumba, Cascara, Myrobalan, Condurango, Elecampane, Frangula, Gentian, Pepper and Nux vomica.

IBS = irritable bowel syndrome; FD = functional dyspepsia; RCT = randomised, controlled trial; QOL = quality of life.

mucosal biopsy patients. The minimum inhibitory concentration value of test drug is first established against *H. pylori* and then *H. pylori* is co-cultivated with rat gastric epithelial cells in the presence/absence of test drug at its minimum inhibitory concentration. A reduction in the activity of urease, a normal appearance of the epithelial cells on electron microscopic examination, a decrease in lipid peroxidation and lactate dehydrogenase suggests the possible anti-*H. pylori* activity of PS (Narayan *et al.*, 2007).

Gastric cytoprotection can be evaluated using rat/mouse/guinea pig models of gastric lesions induced by absolute ethanol, indometacin, histamine and immobilisation stress (Robert *et al.*, 1979; Paiva *et al.*, 1995; Trevithick *et al.*, 1995) and, to elucidate the physiological mechanism, effects of herbal products on mucus secretion, acid secretion (pylorus-ligated animals), glutathione reserve, mucosal blood flow and gastric emptying time are analysed (Gronbech and Lacy, 1995; Rao *et al.*, 1997; Paiva *et al.*, 1998). In addition, to understand the pharmacological mechanism underlying the gastroprotection, the role of capsaicin-sensitive fibres, endogenous prostaglandins and nitric oxide may be verified, using capsaicin-desensitisation procedure, and/or analysis of prostaglandins by ELISA and nitrite/nitrate by Griess reaction or indirectly by the use of nitric oxide synthase inhibitors (Brzozowski *et al.*, 2005).

Visceral hyperalgesis is a characteristic feature of FD and IBS. Visceral antihyperalgesic effects of herbals can be examined using animal models of nociception induced by intracolonic administration of mustard or capsaicin. These chemicals evoke both inflammatory and non-inflammatory pain through sensitisation of neurones at the peripheral and/or central sites, involving several neuropeptides and a great variety of inflammatory mediators. They serve as valuable tools in assessing gut pain and to study the possible mechanism (Oliveira *et al.*, 2005; Maia *et al.*, 2006).

Spasmolytic and antidiarrhoeal properties of test compounds can be assessed in well-established models such as the USSING-chamber, a pharmacological model for diarrhoea, and the isolated guinea pig ileum, a model for modulatory effects on ileum contraction. The inhibitory effect observed in these models provides ex-vivo evidence for the spasmolytic and antidiarrhoeal activities of herbal products (Heinrich *et al.*, 2005). Several studies have investigated abnormalities of serotonin signalling in IBS. Decreased post-prandial serotonin plasma levels have been reported to occur in constipation-predominant IBS, and increased plasma levels have been reported to occur in diarrhoea-predominant IBS (Atkinson *et al.*, 2006).

To verify the potential usefulness of herbals in diarrhoea-prone IBS, in-vivo testing could be carried out in mice on castor oil- or croton oil-induced diarrhoea, cholera toxin-induced intestinal secretion and on gastrointestinal transit induced by 5-HTP (Gurgel *et al.*, 2001; Pascual *et al.*, 2002), using alosetron, an antagonist for 5-HT_3 receptors and a known agent effective for diarrhoea-predominant IBS as a positive control. Further, morphine-induced gastrointestinal delay in mice may be used as a model to test the compound's likely use in constipation-predominant IBS, using tegaserod, a 5-HT_4 receptor agonist, as a positive control. Tegaserod is a known prokinetic agent that speeds small-bowel transit and right-colon transit in IBS, reducing symptoms of constipation, pain and bloating (Mertz, 2005).

Safety pharmacology

Clinical assessment of the gastrointestinal tract is often limited to measurements of transit time and observations of vomiting or diarrhoea. In-vitro functional human tissue assays can be performed to measure a vast range of toxic effects of drugs under investigation, at the level of the organ, cell or even gene and these assays are considered an important adjunct to routine safety pharmacology tests (Harrison *et al.*, 2004; Hillier and Bunton, 2007). The cytotoxicity of new compounds can be determined by the MTT reduction assay using human lung fibroblasts (MRC-5) (Schmeda-Hirschmann *et al.*, 2005). These models are rapid, less expensive and reveal mechanisms of action. The data obtained serve as signals of potential harmful effects in humans and are often superior to extrapolation from animals. The heart is a frequent site of toxicity of pharmaceutical compounds in humans, and, when developing a new drug, it is critical to conduct a thorough preclinical evaluation of its possible adverse effects on cardiac structure and function. Changes in cardiac morphology such as myocardial necrosis, hypertrophy or valvulopathy are assessed in laboratory animals. The potential proarrhythmic risk of new drugs is a major subject of concern and needs to be fully addressed before treatment of volunteers or patients takes place. The recommended tests to detect most arrythmic drugs were to determine the effects on cardiac ion channels, in particular I(Kr) potassium channel antagonism in vitro and prolongation of the QT interval, assessed in vivo, in telemetred dogs (Hanton, 2007).

In-vivo animal safety data serve as important signal generators and in some cases, may stand alone as indicators of unreasonable risks. These include acute toxicity, and long-term toxicity, reproduction toxicity, genotoxicity and carcinogenicity studies. Knowledge of an ingredient's pharmacokinetics and in-vivo metabolism will allow most appropriate interpretation of relevancy of the dose/concentration used in the in-vitro tests. Evidence of abnormalities from laboratory animal studies can be indicative of potential harm to humans.

Acute toxicity testing involves the study of toxic effects after a single (oral/parenteral) administration of the test compound with the objective to classify the substance associated on the basis of acute toxicity, identification of target involved in the acute toxic effect (signs: time of appearance, progression and reversibility), and to establish the dose intervals that may be of relevance to other toxicological studies. A long-term toxicity study (4–12 weeks) involves the repeated doses of the test substance, aimed to determine the maximum tolerable dose, the highest dose that does not result in toxic effects and the mechanism underlying the toxic effects in vivo by means of biochemical, behavioural and histopathological studies. Genotoxicity and carcinogenesis studies are important because several medicinal plants contain substances such as pyrrolizidine alkaloids, flavonoids, phorbol esters, etc., which can cause mutagenic effects. The Ames test using *Salmonella typhimurium* strains and the CHO (Chinese hamster ovary) chromosomal aberration test are the two most commonly used methods for the evaluation of genetic mutation and chromosome damage (Maron and Ames, 1983; Cavalcante *et al.*, 2006).

Evaluation of herbal medicines: controlled clinical trials

The choice of primary endpoint for a clinical trial is to demonstrate the efficacy of a therapeutic agent. The Rome III Committee recommends two types of measures to assess the efficacy of new treatments for IBS and FD:

- binary endpoints addressing the construct of relief (that is, adequate relief and satisfactory relief)
- an integrative symptom questionnaire that addresses the change in severity of a representative group of symptoms of IBS (that is, the IBS Severity Scale).

The current evidence suggests that at present, adequate relief should be recognised by regulatory authorities as an acceptable primary endpoint in clinical trials. This analysis also suggests that data from individual clinical trials should be pooled and undergo meta-analysis, and that prospective studies should be considered to further characterise the performance of available endpoints as outcome measures in pharmacotherapeutic trials (Camilleri *et al.*, 2007). Literature search reveals that few well-controlled, double-blind (placebo-controlled) trials have been carried out with herbal medicines (see Table 8.2). Meta-analyses of reviews published reveal several discrepancies, and these are mostly due to:

- lack of standardisation and quality control of the herbal drugs used in clinical trials
- use of different dosages of herbal medicines
- inadequate randomisation in most studies, and patients not properly selected
- numbers of patients in most trials insufficient for the attainment of statistical significance
- difficulties in establishing appropriate placebos because of the tastes, aromas, etc.
- wide variations in the duration of treatments using herbal medicines.

A few herbal products, e.g. STW 5 (Iberogast), Artichoke, Carmint, Tong-xie-ning (Chinese herbal formula), Hange-koboku-to (Kampoo medicine), and Padma Lax (Tibetan herbal medicine) have been evaluated in clinical trials, but they still have the difficulties mentioned above and need additional, well-controlled and appropriate randomised clinical trials to prove their efficacy.

To assess the efficacy of new herbals in FGIDs, a double-blind, randomised, placebo-controlled, parallel group trial remains the preferred design. Investigators should include as broad a spectrum of patients as possible and should report recruitment strategies, inclusion/exclusion criteria, and attrition data. The primary analysis should be based on the proportion of patients in each treatment arm who satisfy a prespecified clinically meaningful change in a patient-reported symptom-improvement measure. Such measures of improvement are psychometrically validated subjective global assessments or a change from baseline in validated symptom guidelines and include an analysis of harms data and secondary outcome measures to support severity questionnaire. Data analysis should address all patients enrolled, using an intention-to-treat principle. Reporting of results should follow the Consolidated Standards for Reporting Trials or explain the primary outcome. Trials should be registered in a public location, prior to initiation, and should be reported even if the results are negative or inconclusive (Irvine *et al.*, 2006).

Conclusions

No standard therapy is currently available for FGIDs such as FD and IBS, which are characterised by multiple symptoms associated with disordered gut function. There is limited evidence for the efficacy, safety and tolerability of currently available conventional therapies and it may be that, with traditional herbal therapies, patients may respond better in symptom improvement because of their multicomponent nature with different active constituents having pleotropic actions. However, herbal medicinals should undergo the same procedures as conventional drugs and should not be considered differently because they are of natural origin. Preclinical studies on very many herbal extracts and their active constituents demonstrated interesting pharmacological properties relevant to FD and IBS, but only few of them were taken to clinical trials with limited success. Future studies should address their effectiveness and safety in patients with FGIDs by the double-blind, randomised, placebo-controlled, parallel-group trial study design. The safety and their quality should be ensured through greater pharmacovigilance studies and by governmental regulatory mechanisms. To provide uniform quality of raw material, emphasis must be laid on domestication, production and biotechnological studies and genetic improvement of medicinal plants to provide uniform and high-quality raw material.

References

Aggarwal BB, Sundaram C, Malani N, Ichikawa H (2007). Curcumin: the Indian solid gold. *Adv Exp Med Biol* 595: 1–75.

Al-Harbi MM, Qureshi S, Raza M, Ahmed MM, Afzalm M, Shah AH (1997). Gastric antiulcer and cytoprotective effect of Commiphora molmol in rats. *J Ethnopharmacol* 55: 141–150.

Al Moflehm IA, Alhaider AA, Mossa JS, Al-Soohaibani MO, Rafatullah S (2007). Aqueous suspension of anise "Pimpinella anisum" protects rats against chemically induced gastric ulcers. *World J Gastroenterol* 13: 1112–1118.

Ambizas EM, Ginzburg R (2007). Lubiprostone: a chloride channel activator for treatment of chronic constipation. *Ann Pharmacol Ther* 41: 957–964.

Atkinson W, Lockhart S, Whorwell PJ *et al.* (2006). Altered 5-hydroxytryptamine signaling in patients with constipation- and diarrhea-predominant irritable bowel syndrome. *Gastroenterology* 130: 34–43.

Bortolotti M, Coccia G, Grossi G, Miglioli M (2002). The treatment of functional dyspepsia with red pepper. *Aliment Pharmacol Ther* 16: 1075–1082.

Brandt L, Schoenfeld P, Prather C *et al.* (2005). American College of Gastroenterology Functional Gastrointestinal Disorders Task Force. An evidence based approach to the management of chronic constipation in North America. *Am J Gastroenterol* 100: S1–S21.

Brinkhaus B, Hentschel C, Von Keudell C *et al.* (2005). Herbal medicine with curcuma and fumitory in the treatment of irritable bowel syndrome: a randomized, placebo-controlled, double-blind clinical trial. *Scand J Gastroenterol* 40: 936–943.

Brzozowski T, Konturek PC, Drozdowicz D *et al.* (2005). Grapefruit-seed extract attenuates ethanol- and stress-induced gastric lesions via activation of prostaglandin, nitric oxide and sensory nerve pathways. *World J Gastroenterol* 11: 6450–6458.

Bundy R, Walker AF, Middleton RW, Booth J (2004a). Turmeric extract may improve irritable bowel syndrome symptomology in otherwise healthy adults: a pilot study. *J Altern Complement Med* 10: 1015–1018.

Bundy R, Walker AF, Middleton RW, Marakis G (2004b). Artichoke leaf extract reduces symptoms of irritable bowel syndrome and improves quality of life in otherwise healthy volunteers suffering from concomitant dyspepsia: a subset analysis. *J Altern Complement Med* 10: 667–669.

Camilleri M, Mangel AW, Fehnel SE *et al.* (2007). Primary endpoints for irritable bowel syndrome trials: a review of performance of endpoints. *Clin Gastroenterol Hepatol* 5: 534–540.

Cavalcanti BC, Costa-Lotufo LV, Moraes MO *et al.* (2006). Genotoxicity evaluation of kaurenoic acid, a bioactive diterpenoid present in Copaiba oil. *Food Chem Toxicol* 44: 388–392.

Chang L (2004). Review article: Epidemiology and quality of life in functional gastrointestinal disorders. *Aliment Pharmacol Ther* 20 (supp. 7): 31–39.

Da Mota Menezes V, Atallah AN, Lapa AJ *et al.* (2006). Assessing the therapeutic use of *Lafoensia pacari* St. Hil. extract (mangava-brava) in the eradication of *Helicobacter pylori*: double-blind randomized clinical trial. *Helicobacter* 11: 188–195.

Drossman DA (2005). What does the future hold for irritable bowel syndrome and the functional gastrointestinal disorders? *J Clin Gastroenterol* 39 (5 Suppl): S251–256.

Drossman DA (2006). Rome III: the new criteria. *Chin J Dig Dis* 7: 181–185.

Dunlop SP, Jenkins D, Neal KR, Spiller RC (2003). Relative importance of enterochromaffin cell hyperplasia, anxiety, and depression in postinfectious IBS. *Gastroenterology* 125: 1651–1659.

Emendörfer F, Bellato F, Noldin VF *et al.* (2005). Evaluation of the relaxant action of some Brazilian medicinal plants in isolated guinea-pig ileum and rat duodenum. *J Pharm Pharm Sci* 8: 63–68.

Gershon MD, Tack J (2007). The serotonin signaling system: from basic understanding to drug development for functional GI disorders. *Gastroenterology* 132: 397–414.

Gronbech JE, Lacy ER (1995). Role of gastric blood flow in impaired defense and repair of aged rat stomachs. *Am J Physiol-Gastroenterol Liver Physiol* 32: 737–744.

Guedes MM, Cunha AN, Silveira ER, Rao VS (2002). Antinociceptive and gastroprotective effects of diterpenes from the flower buds of *Egletes viscosa*. *Planta Med* 68: 1044–1046.

Gürbüz I, Akyüz C, Yeşilada E, Sener B (2000). Anti-ulcerogenic effect of *Momordica charantia* L. fruits on various ulcer models in rats. *J Ethnopharmacol* 71: 77–82.

Gurgel LA, Silva RM, Santos FA *et al.* (2001). Studies on the antidiarrhoeal effect of dragon's blood from *Croton urucurana*. *Phytother Res* 15: 319–322.

Hall W, Buckley M, Crotty P, O'Morain CA (2003). Gastric mucosal mast cells are increased in *Helicobacter pylori*-negative functional dyspepsia. *Clin Gastroenterol Hepatol* 1: 363–369.

Hanton G (2007). Preclinical cardiac safety assessment of drugs. *Drugs R D* 8: 213–28.

Harrison AP, Erlwanger KH, Elbrønd VS *et al.* (2004). Gastrointestinal-tract models and techniques for use in safety pharmacology. *J Pharmacol Toxicol Methods* 49: 187–199.

Heinrich M, Heneka B, Ankli A *et al.* (2005). Spasmolytic and antidiarrhoeal properties of the Yucatec Mayan medicinal plant Casimiroa tetrameria. *J Pharm Pharmacol* 57: 1081–1085.

Hillier C, Bunton D (2007). Functional human tissue assays. *Drug Discov Today* 12: 382–388.

Holtmann G, Adam B, Vinson B (2004). Evidence-based medicine and phytotherapy for functional dyspepsia and irritable bowel syndrome: a systematic analysis of evidence for the herbal preparation Iberogast. *Wien Med Wochenschr* 154: 528–534.

Holtmann G, Talley NJ, Liebregts T *et al.* (2006). A placebo-controlled trial of itopride in functional dyspepsia. *N Engl J Med* 355: 429.

Holtmann G, Adam B, Haag S, *et al.* (2003). Efficacy of artichoke leaf extract in the treatment of patients with functional dyspepsia: a six-week placebo-controlled, double-blind, multicentre trial. *Aliment Pharmacol Ther* 18: 1099–1105.

Inoue E, Shimizu Y, Shoji M *et al.* (2005). Pharmacological properties of N-095, a drug containing red ginseng, polygala root, saffron, antelope horn and aloe wood. *Am J Chin Med* 33: 49–60.

Jainu M, Vijai Mohan K, Shyamala Devi CS (2006). Gastroprotective effect of *Cissus quadrangularis* extract in rats with experimentally induced ulcer. *Indian J Med Res* 123: 799–806.

Jiménez-Escrig A, Dragsted LO, Daneshvar B *et al.* (2003). In vitro antioxidant activities of edible artichoke (*Cynara scolymus* L.) and effect on biomarkers of antioxidants in rats. *J Agric Food Chem* 51: 5540–5545.

Johanson JF, Ueno R (2007). Lubiprostone, a locally acting chloride channel activator, in adult patients with chronic constipation: a double-blind, placebo-controlled, dose-ranging study to evaluate efficacy and safety. *Aliment Pharmacol Ther* 25: 1351–1361.

Kim DC, Kim SH, Choi BH *et al.* (2005). Curcuma longa extract protects against gastric ulcers by blocking H2 histamine receptors. *Biol Pharm Bull* 28: 2220–2224.

Kleibeuker JH, Thijs JC (2004). Functional dyspepsia. *Curr Opin Gastroenterol* 20: 546–550.

Koretz RL, Rotblatt M (2004). Complementary and alternative medicine in gastroenterology: the good, the bad, and the ugly. *Clin Gastroenterol Hepatol* 2: 957–967.

Lee A (2000). Animal models of gastroduodenal ulcer disease. *Baill Clin Gastroenterol* 14: 75–96.

Li B, Shang JC, Zhou QX (2005). Study of total alkaloids from Rhizoma Coptis Chinensis on experimental gastric ulcers. *Chin J Integr Med* 11: 217–221.

Lima ZP, Severi JA, Pellizzon CH *et al.* (2006). Can the aqueous decoction of mango flowers be used as an antiulcer agent? *J Ethnopharmacol* 106: 29–37.

Liu JP, Yang M, Lium YX *et al.* (2006). Herbal medicines for treatment of irritable bowel syndrome. *Cochrane Database Syst Rev* 25: CD004116.

Madisch A, Holtmann G, Plein K *et al.* (2004). Treatment of irritable bowel syndrome with herbal preparations: results of a double-blind, randomized, placebo-controlled, multi-centre trial. *Aliment Pharmacol Ther* 19: 271–279.

Mahady GB, Pendland SL, Yun G *et al.* (2002). Turmeric (*Curcuma longa*) and curcumin inhibit the growth of *Helicobacter pylori*, a group 1 carcinogen. *Anticancer Res* 22: 4179–4181.

Mahady GB, Pendland SL, Stoia A *et al.* (2005). In vitro susceptibility of *Helicobacter pylori* to botanical extracts used traditionally for the treatment of gastrointestinal disorders. *Phytother Res* 19: 988–991.

Maia JL, Lima-Junior RC, Melo CM *et al.* (2006). Oleanolic acid, a pentacyclic triterpene attenuates capsaicin-induced nociception in mice: possible mechanisms. *Pharmacol Res* 54: 282–286.

Marakis G, Walker AF, Middleton RW *et al.* (2002). Artichoke leaf extract reduces mild dyspepsia in an open study. *Phytomedicine* 9: 694–699.

Maxwell PR, Mendall MA, Kumar D (1997). Irritable bowel syndrome. *Lancet* 350: 1691–1695.

McKay DL, Blumberg JB (2006). A review of the bioactivity and potential health benefits of peppermint tea (*Mentha piperita* L.). *Phytother Res* 20: 619–633.

Menezes AM, Rao VS (1988). Effect of *Astronium urundeuva* (aroeira) on gastrointestinal transit in mice. *Braz J Med Biol Res* 21: 531–533.

Mertz H (2005). Psychotherapeutics and serotonin agonists and antagonists. *J Clin Gastroenterol* 39 (supp. 3): S247–250.

Miller MJS, Macnaughton WK, Zhang XJ *et al.* (2000). Treatment of gastric ulcers and diarrhea with the Amazonian herbal medicine sangre de grado. *Am J Physiol Gastrointest Liver Physiol* 279: G192–G200.

Narayan S, Devi RS, Srinivasan P *et al.* (2005). *Pterocarpus santalinus*: a traditional herbal drug as a protectant against ibuprofen induced gastric ulcers. *Phytother Res* 19: 958–962.

Narayan S, Veeraraghavan M, Devi CS (2007). *Pterocarpus santalinus*: an in vitro study on its anti-*Helicobacter pylori* effect. *Phytother Res* 21: 190–193.

Oikawa T, Ito G, Koyama H *et al.* (2005). Prokinetic effect of a Kampo medicine, Hange-koboku-to (Banxia-houpo-tang), on patients with functional dyspepsia. *Phytomedicine* 12: 730–734.

Oliveira FA, Vieira-Ju-acutenior GM, Chaves HM *et al.* (2004a). Gastroprotective and anti-inflammatory effects of resin from *Protium heptaphyllum* in mice and rats. *Pharmacol Res* 49: 105–111.

Oliveira FA, Vieira-Júenior GM, Chaves HM *et al.* (2004b). Gastroprotective effect of the mixture of alpha- and beta-amyrin from *Protium heptaphyllum*: role of capsaicin-sensitive primary afferent neurons. *Planta Med* 70: 780–782.

Oliveira FA, Costa CL, Chaves HM *et al.* (2005). Attenuation of capsaicin-induced acute and visceral nociceptive pain by alpha- and beta-amyrin, a triterpene mixture isolated from *Protium heptaphyllum* resin in mice. *Life Sci* 77: 2942–2952.

Paiva LA, Rao VS, Gramosa NV, Silveira ER (1998). Gastroprotective effect of *Copaifera langsdorffii* oleoresin on experimental gastric ulcer models in rats. *J Ethnopharmacol* 62: 73–78.

Paiva LA, de Alencar Cunha KM, Santos FA *et al.* (2002). Investigation on the wound healing activity of oleoresin from *Copaifera langsdorffii* in rats. *Phytother Res* 16: 73–78.

Paiva LA, Gurgel LA, Campos AR *et al.* (2004a). Attenuation ischemia/reperfusion-induced intestinal injury by oleo-resin from *Copaifera langsdorffii* in rats. *Life Sci* 75: 19781–19787.

Paiva LA, Gurgel LA, De Sousa ET *et al.* (2004b). Protective effect of *Copaifera langsdorffii* oleo-resin against acetic acid-induced colitis in rats. *J Ethnopharmacol* 93: 51–56.

Pandian RS, Anuradha CV, Viswanathan P (2002). Gastroprotective effect of fenugreek seeds (*Trigonella foenum graecum*) on experimental gastric ulcer in rats. *J Ethnopharmacol* 81: 393–397.

Pascual D, Alsasua A, Goicoechea C, Martin MI (2002). The involvement of 5-HT3 and 5-HT4 receptors in two models of gastrointestinal transit in mice. *Neurosci Lett* 326: 165–166.

Petrovick PR, Marques LC, De Paula IC (1999). New rules for phytopharmaceutical drug registration in Brazil. *J Ethnopharmacol* 66: 51–55.

Pilichiewicz AN, Horowitz M, Russo A *et al.* (2007). Effects of Iberogast on proximal gastric volume, antropyloroduodenal motility and gastric emptying in healthy men. *Am J Gastroenterol* 102: 1276–1283.

Pittler MH, Ernst E (1998). Peppermint oil for irritable bowel syndrome: a critical review and metaanalysis. *Am J Gastroenterol* 93: II31–II35.

Pruksunand C, Indrasukhare B, Leechochawalit M, Hungspreugs K (2001). Phase II clinical trial on effect of the long turmeric (*Curcuma longa* Linn) on healing of peptic ulcer. *Southeast Asian J Trop Med Public Health* 12: 208–215.

Rao VS, Viana GS, Menezes AM, Gadelha MG (1987). Studies on the anti-ulcerogenic activity of *Astronium urundeuva* Engl. II. Aqueous extract. *Braz J Med Biol Res* 20: 803–805.

Rao VS, Santos FA, Sobreira TT *et al.* (1997). Investigations on the gastroprotective and antidiarrhoeal properties of ternatin, a tetramethoxyflavone from *Egletes viscosa*. Planta. Med 63: 146–149.

Rao VS, Paiva LA, Souza MF *et al.* (2003). Ternatin, an anti-inflammatory flavonoid, inhibits thioglycollate-elicited rat peritoneal neutrophil accumulation and LPS-activated nitric oxide production in murine macrophages. *Planta Med* 69: 851–853.

Robert A, Nezamis JE, Lancaster C (1979). Cytoprotection by prostaglandins in rats: prevention of gastric necrosis produced by alcohol, HCl, hypertonic NaCl, and thermal injury. *Gastroenterology* 77: G395–G402.

Rodriguez-Stanley S, Collings KL, Robinson M *et al.* (2000). The effects of capsaicin on reflux, gastric emptying and dyspepsia. *Aliment Pharmacol Ther* 14: 129–134.

Rösch W, Vinson B, Sassin I (2002). A randomised clinical trial comparing the efficacy of a herbal preparation STW 5 with the prokinetic drug cisapride in patients with dysmotility type of functional dyspepsia. *Z Gastroenterol* 40: 401–408.

Rösch W, Liebregts T, Gundermann KJ, Vinson B, Holtmann G (2006). Phytotherapy for functional dyspepsia: a review of the clinical evidence for the herbal preparation STW 5. *Phytomedicine* 13 (supp. 5): 114–121.

Saller R, Iten F, Reichling J (2001). Dyspeptic pain and phytotherapy–a review of traditional and modern herbal drugs. *Forsch Komplement Klass Naturheilkd* 8: 263–273.

Saller R, Pfister-Hotz G, Iten F, Melzer J, Reichling J (2002). Iberogast: a modern phytotherapeutic combined herbal drug for the treatment of functional disorders of the gastrointestinal tract (dyspepsia, irritable bowel syndrome)–from phytomedicine to "evidence based phytotherapy." A systematic review. *Forsch Komplement Klass Naturheilkd* 9(supp. 1): 1–20.

Sallon S, Ben-Arye E, Davidson R, Shapiro H, Ginsberg G, Ligumsky M (2002). A novel treatment for constipation-predominant irritable bowel syndrome using Padma Lax, a Tibetan herbal formula. *Digestion* 65: 161–171.

Schmeda-Hirschmann G, Astudillo L, Rodríguez J, Theoduloz C, Yáñez T (2005). Gastroprotective effect of the Mapuche crude drug Araucaria araucana resin and its main constituents. *J Ethnopharmacol* 101: 271–276.

Shan L, Liu RH, Shen YH *et al.* (2006). Gastroprotective effect of a traditional Chinese herbal drug "Baishouwu" on experimental gastric lesions in rats. *J Ethnopharmacol* 107(3): 89–94.

Simmen U, Kelber O, Okpanyi SN *et al.* (2006). Binding of STW 5 (Iberogast) and its components to intestinal 5-HT, muscarinic M3, and opioid receptors. *Phytomedicine* 13 (supp. 5): 51–55.

Tack J, Talley NJ, Camilleri M *et al.* (2006a). Functional gastroduodenal disorders. *Gastroenterology* 130: 1466–1479.

Tack J, Fried M, Houghton LA *et al.* (2006b). Systematic review: the efficacy of treatments for irritable bowel syndrome – a European perspective. *Aliment Pharmacol Ther* 24: 183–205.

Talley NJ, Van Zanten SV, Saez LR *et al.* (2001). A dose-ranging, placebo-controlled, randomized trial of alosetron in patients with functional dyspepsia. *Aliment Pharmacol Ther* 15: 525–537.

Talley NJ, Vakil N (2005). Guidelines for the management of dyspepsia. *Am J Gastroenterol* 100: 2324–2337.

Talley NJ, Locke GR, Lahr BD *et al.* (2006). Functional dyspepsia, delayed gastric emptying and impaired quality of life. *Gut* 55: 933–939.

Talley NJ, Stanghellini V, Heading RC *et al.* (1999). Functional gastroduodenal disorders. *Gut* 45 (supp. 2): II37–II42.

Thompson WG, Longstreth GF, Drossman DA *et al.* (1999). Functional bowel disorders and functional abdominal pain. *Gut* 45 (supp. 2): II43–II47.

Thompson CJ, Ernst. E (2002). Systematic review: herbal medicinal products for non-ulcer dyspepsia. *Aliment Pharmacol Ther* 16: 1689–1699.

Thornley JP, Jenkins D, Neal K *et al.* (2001). Relationship of *Campylobacter* toxigenicity *in vitro* to the development of postinfectious irritable bowel syndrome. *J Infect Dis* 184: 606–609.

Tran CD, Butler RN, Miller MJS (2006). The role of Amazonian herbal medicine Sangre de Grado in *Helicobacter pylori* infection and its association with metallothionein expression. *Helicobacter* 11: 134–135.

Trevithick MA, Oakley I, Clayton NM, Strong P (1995). Non-steroidal anti-inflammatory drug-induced gastric damage in experimental animals – underlying pathological mechanisms. *Gen Pharmacol* 26: 1455–1459.

Vejdani R, Shalmani HR, Mir-Fattahi M *et al.* (2006). The efficacy of an herbal medicine, Carmint, on the relief of abdominal pain and bloating in patients with irritable bowel syndrome: a pilot study. *Dig Dis Sci* 51: 1501–1517.

Von Arnim U, Peitz U, Vinson B *et al.* (2007). STW 5, a phytopharmacon for patients with functional dyspepsia: results of a multicenter, placebo-controlled double-blind study. *Am J Gastroenterol* 102: 1268–1275.

Wang G, Li TQ, Wang L, Xia Q *et al.* (2006). Tong-xie-ning, a Chinese herbal formula, in treatment of diarrhea-predominant irritable bowel syndrome: a prospective, randomized, double-blind, placebo-controlled trial. *Chin Med J* 119: 2114–2119.

Yoshikawa M, Morikawa T, Asao Y *et al.* (2007). Medicinal flowers. XV. The structures of noroleanane- and oleanane-type triterpene oligoglycosides with gastroprotective and platelet aggregation activities from flower buds of *Camellia japonica*. *Chem Pharm Bull (Tokyo)* 55: 606–612.

9

Therapy and prevention of hepatocellular carcinoma using herbal drugs

KC Preethi, KB Harikumar and Ramadasan Kuttan

Introduction

Cancer is a condition characterised by the uncontrolled growth and spread of abnormal cells, causing their massive aggregation producing either tumours or dispersal in the vascular system such as blood and lymph. Owing to a deviation from normal genetic makeup, cancer cells acquire immortality and a capability to evade apoptosis, non-responsiveness to anti-growth signals, self-sufficiency in growth factors, the ability to metastasise and to form new blood vessels that can supply nutrition and oxygen to the growing tissues. The transformation of normal to cancer cell occurs through accumulation of a series of genetic alterations or mutations, especially of oncogenes.

Carcinogenesis

There are many aetiological factors leading to cancer through a multistep process called carcinogenesis, which involves initiation, promotion, progression and malignant conversion. Mutation in a single cell initiates clonal expansion to form a premalignant lesion. These initiated cells will have resistance to cytotoxicity, defects in maturation, escape from senescence and have altered dependence on growth factors and hormones. Tumour promotion involves activation of cell surface receptors, activation/inhibition of cytosolic enzymes and nuclear transcription factors, stimulation of proliferation and inhibition of apoptotic cell death. Progression is accelerated by additional exposure to genotoxic agents and it is due to genetic instability and nonrandom sequential chromosomal aberrations. Malignant conversion involves multifocal change in premalignant lesions. There will be up-regulation of transcriptional activity and expression of modified cell surface molecules, gene amplification, alterations in cell-cycle regulatory genes, secreted proteases and methylation of DNA. All these changes facilitate migration and invasion.

Inhibition of carcinogenesis

As the progression of carcinogenesis is through a multistep pathway, there are many possible intervention sites inhibiting this progression. The procarcinogen can be detoxified and eliminated from the system. The conversion of procarcinogen to ultimate carcinogen is through multiple mechanisms including metabolic activation by enzymes. These mechanisms can be inhibited by blocking those enzymes involved in the activation step and several natural compounds of plant origin are reported as blocking agents in the chemoprevention of cancer, including flavonoids, ellagic acid and sulforaphane. These either block the conversion of carcinogen to ultimate carcinogen, or prevent the action of active metabolites on the normal cell. They may also alter carcinogen metabolism, enhance carcinogen detoxification, scavenge electrophiles and reactive oxygen species or enhance DNA repair.

The conversion of normal cells from preneoplastic cells to neoplastic cells takes several years, either by a second exposure to the carcinogen or promoting agent and accumulation of genetic variations. These steps can be inhibited by compounds such as curcumin, resveratrol, carotenoids, retinoids and genistein, which inhibit the malignant transformation of initiated cells by scavenging reactive oxygen species, altering gene expression, decreasing inflammation, suppressing proliferation, inducing differentiation, encouraging apoptosis, enhancing immunity or inhibiting angiogenesis and metastasis.

Several chemopreventive phytochemicals have been shown to interfere with the cell-cycle regulatory pathways, qualifying them as potential therapeutic agents. Some are powerful inhibitors of growth factor receptors, including epidermal growth factor receptor (EGFR), and a variety of flavonoids are inhibitory, e.g. apigenin, luteolin, quercetin, catechin, epigallocatechin gallate, hesperitin, anthocyanins, genistein, with potential use in preventive anticancer treatment. Some phytochemicals undergoing clinical trials in the inhibition of carcinogenesis are given in Table 9.1.

Table 9.1 Selected ongoing Phase I and II cancer prevention trials sponsored by the US National Cancer Institute

Target organ	Agent
Phase I trials	
Breast	Soy isoflavones
Colon	Curcumin
Prostate	Lycopene (3 trials); Soy isoflavones
Skin	Epigallocatechin gallate
Phase II trials	
Anogenital warts, human papillomavirus, HIV	Indole-3-carbinol
Cervix	9-*cis*-Retinoic acid
Prostate	Soy (dietary); soy isoflavones

Hepatocellular carcinoma

Hepatocellular carcinoma (HCC) is the most common primary malignant tumour of the liver and is the fifth most common cancer in the world, ranking fourth in annual mortality rates. An estimated 564 000 new cases of HCC are diagnosed each year, with the highest incidence in eastern and southeastern Asia, some of the western Pacific islands and sub-Saharan Africa. Men are affected four to eight times more often than women and the incidence generally increases with increasing age, although there is a definite shift towards a younger age distribution in black African and ethnic Chinese populations.

Aetiological factors

There are some well-documented aetiological associations of HCC. The aetiological association between hepatitis-B virus (HBV) and HCC is well established. Chronic HBV infection is the leading risk factor and it has been estimated that 53% of cases worldwide are related to HBV. Malignant transformation occurs after a long period of chronic liver disease, frequently associated with cirrhosis. Chronic inflammation of the liver, continuous cell death and consequent cell proliferation might increase the occurrence of genetic alterations and risk of cancer. The long-term expression of regulator gene product of the X-gene and large envelope proteins (LHBs) are thought to play a major role in tumorigenesis. This viral oncoprotein behaves as a transcriptional transactivator, which activates oncogenes, cytokines and growth factors. A direct role of the virus through integration of viral DNA directly to host genome has also been hypothesised that may enhance chromosomal instability, large inverted duplications, deletions, amplifications or chromosomal translocations which lead to the activation of oncogenic pathways.

Chronic HCV (hepatitis C virus) infection is also associated with HCC. The HCC incidence rate in patients with HCV-related cirrhosis is about 3.7%.

Chemical carcinogens which are linked to HCC include nitrites, hydrocarbons, solvents, organochlorine pesticides, primary metals and polychlorinated biphenyls. Of all the chemicals linked to HCC, ethanol is the most important one that leads to HCC. Overconsumption of alcohol is one of the leading causes of liver cirrhosis which makes the patient more susceptible to HBV and HCV infection.

Aflatoxins produced by the fungi, *Aspergillus flavus* and *A. parasiticus* have also been linked to HCC. These fungal species grow on grains, peanuts and other food products and are the most common cause of food spoilage. These fungi also produce aflatoxins, aflatoxin B1 being the most hepatotoxic and chronic exposure to these mycotoxins will lead to HCC.

Some congenital conditions also lead to development of HCC. Genetic diseases such as haemochromatosis, Wilson's disease, hereditary tyrosinaemia, type I glycogen storage disease and porphyria, have all been linked to a high incidence of HCC.

Symptoms and markers

The symptoms related to the early stages of HCC are poor. When HCC presents with clinical symptoms, the tumour is usually advanced and there are few therapeutic options. The current effective treatments available are only applicable in a relatively small proportion of early stage cases.

Serum α-fetoprotein is a useful tumour marker for the detection and monitoring of HCC development, but gives false-negatives in about 40% of patients. Serum γ-glutamyl transpeptidase (GGT) is frequently overexpressed in cancer cells. GGT activity is a sensitive marker of hepatobiliary disorders, exhibiting tissue-specific expressions under various physiological and pathological conditions. Other enzymes that are increased in the blood during HCC include alkaline phosphatase, alanine transaminase and aspartate transaminase, but they are non-specific.

The overexpression of transforming growth factor (TGF)-β1 and TGF-β1 messenger RNA is seen in most patients with HCC. The level of insulin-like growth factor (IGF)-II and IGF-II mRNA is also overexpressed in HCC. The analysis of telomerase activity in combination with α-fetoprotein increases the accuracy of HCC diagnosis to about 93%.

Even though tumours present limitations for cytogenetic analysis, there are some reports of cytogenetic analysis of HCC. They include chromosome 1p abnormalities and 8q amplification. Molecular studies have demonstrated frequent loss of heterozygosity on 1p, 4q, 8p, 11p, 13q, 16q and 17p and amplification of 8q areas in HCC.

Models

Rodents are usually studied as models of hepatic carcinogenesis. Many chemicals induce liver cancer in rodents since their livers are very sensitive to chemical carcinogens. Thus, a single experimental protocol can be used to understand the mechanisms of a number of carcinogens. The low cost of rodents and their potential for genetic studies and manipulation are also attributes. Apart from this, a fairly extensive understanding of liver biology has made rodent HCC a popular model. Other models used for HCC study include hamsters and other non-primates.

The chemicals used to study the initiation of HCC include nitrosamines, aromatic amines, vinyl chloride, polycyclic aromatic hydrocarbons, heterocyclic amines, aflatoxin and tamoxifen. The promoters which are used after initiation include phenobarbital, dioxin and polychlorinated biphenyl. The mechanism of action of these chemical carcinogens is combination with DNA to form adducts, either by direct binding to DNA, or after enzymatic activation in the liver to produce the carcinogen. Some agents that produce hepatic carcinogenesis are discussed below.

Polycyclic aromatic hydrocarbons

Polycyclic aromatic hydrocarbons require metabolic activation to elicit their detrimental effect, e.g. benzo(a)pyrene is enzymatically activated to the 7,8-dihydrodiol, which induces both somatic mutations in crucial genes through DNA binding and subsequent outgrowth of irreversibly transformed cells.

Aryl amines/amides

In rodents these compounds induce tumours in the liver, e.g. acetamido-fluorine undergoes *N*-hydroxylation in liver cells. Additional tumour-promoting activities of acetamido-fluorine include the triggering of adaptive responses in mitochondria permeability transition pores and Bcl-2 production levels that increase resistance to apoptosis.

Alcohol

The mechanism of ethanol-induced cancer is closely related to its metabolism. Acetaldehyde, the end-product of ethanol metabolism, is the causative agent of cancer in chronic conditions. Oxidative stress and cirrhosis are important factors in ethanol-induced HCC.

Nitrosamines

These are the most widely used chemical carcinogen for animal experiments. *N'*-nitrosodiethylamine (NDEA) is metabolised in the liver and its ethyl radical product is responsible for induction of HCC. This radical attacks the DNA and produces genetic changes which result in carcinogenesis. It also produces the conversion of certain proto-oncogenes to oncogenes.

Azo dyes

Para-dimethylaminoazobenzene (*p*-DAB) is metabolised to monoaminoazobenzene by *N*-demethylation and subsequently to aminoazobenzene or to *N*-hydroxy-*N*-methyl-4-aminoazobenzene. Covalent bindings of these metabolites with DNA are major carcinogenic factors.

Aflatoxins

Aflatoxins are highly mutagenic and are metabolised by cytochrome p450 to their epoxides, which results in formation of DNA adducts with the guanine N7, thus causing carcinogenicity.

Treatment

If detected early, suitable curative treatments include surgical resection, liver transplantation and percutaneous ablation. In patients with advanced stage of HCC, transarterial chemoembolisation has been proved to improve survival in selected candidates. Other therapeutic modalities such as intra-arterial chemotherapy and internal radiation offer promising results but have not been shown to improve survival. As HCC is usually chemoresistant, cytotoxic drugs are poorly tolerated in cirrhotic patients so many of the known anticancer agents, e.g. tamoxifen, octreotide, interferon, fail to produce any benefit in HCC patients. Promising results have been obtained with agents targeting receptor tyrosine kinase pathways. Since HCC is dependent on angiogenesis, molecules targeting the angiogenesis are currently under investigation. BAY 43-9006, which inhibits multiple pathways, mainly Raf kinase and VEGF, has been undergoing Phase II and III trials and has shown a partial response in a patient with advanced HCC (Strumberg *et al.*, 2005).

The presence of unlimited chemical molecules, with diverse mechanisms, present in herbal drugs makes them interesting starting points in the search for newer drugs for cancer treatment.

Natural templates for treatment

The plant kingdom produces many potent pharmacologically active components, several of which have provided promising results to combat various diseases. Possible uses of herbal drugs in cancer are illustrated in Figure 9.1.

The chemical basis of some anticancer plants has been elucidated and some are now used clinically. Plant extracts and their constituents which show significant activity against hepatic cancer are described in more detail below.

Curcuma longa *(turmeric)*

The rhizome of *C. longa* (Zingiberaceae) is described as an anti-inflammatory agent in Ayurveda and is widely used in foods and as a medicine thoughout India and other Asian countries as a treatment for liver disorders, including cancer. The most-studied ingredient in the rhizome is curcumin but several

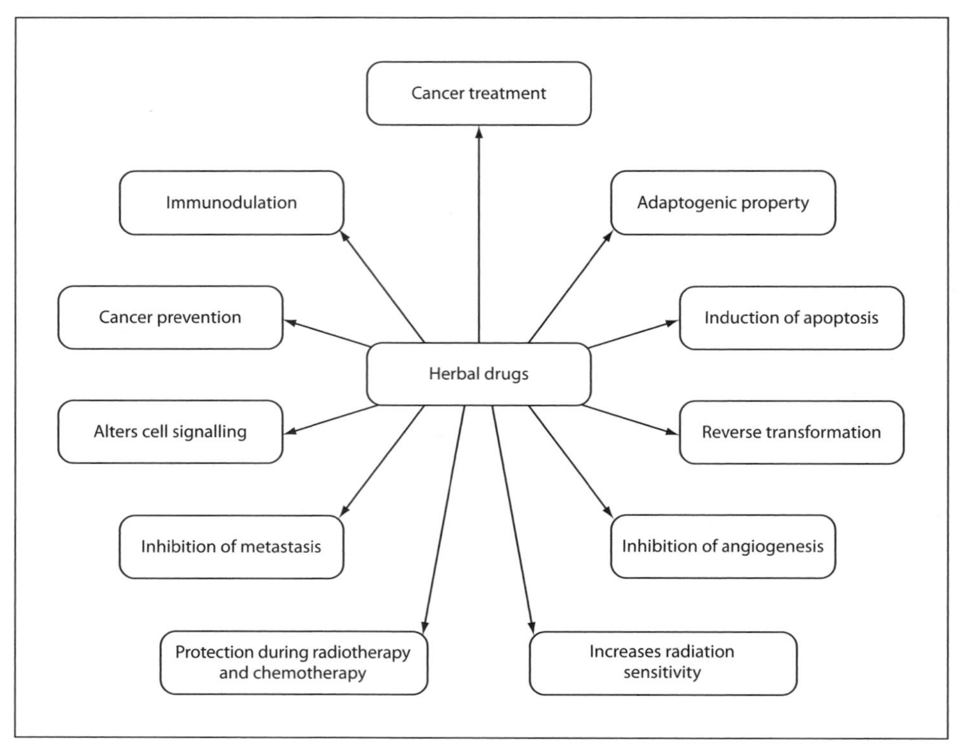

Figure 9.1 Potential uses of herbal drugs in cancer treatment.

related compounds are present such as demethoxy-curcumin and bidemethoxycurcumin.

Curcumin treatment has been reported to reduce tumour incidence and inhibit the liver inflammation and hyperplasia in *N*-nitrosodiethylamine-induced liver-cancer-bearing animals (Chuang *et al.*, 2000). The chemopreventive effect of turmeric and curcumin against diethylnitrosamine-induced and phenobarbital-promoted hepatocarcinogenesis has been reported (Sreepriya and Bali, 2005). Curcumin also suppressed diethylnitrosamine-induced development of altered hepatic foci in rat liver (Shukla and Arora, 2003). The number of γ-GT positive foci induced by aflatoxin B1 was found to be reduced by curcumin treatment (Soni *et al.*, 1997). Curcumin significantly protected the liver from oxidative stress-induced damage during chemically induced hepatocarcinogenesis in rats (Sreepriya and Bali, 2006).

In a patient study, Curcuma aromatic oil showed a positive effect in treating primary liver cancer with longer survival time and myelosuppression (Cheng *et al.*, 2001). Curcumin treatment reduced the tumour incidence by inhibiting angiogenesis through down-regulating cyclo-oxygenase 2 and vascular endothelial growth factor in HepG2 cells (Yosungneon *et al.*, 2006). It was reported that curcumin induces mitochondrial and nuclear DNA damage, thereby inducing apoptosis through caspase 3 and 9 activation. Curcumin also suppressed intrahepatic metastasis mediated by the inhibition of MMP-9 and through alteration of cytoskeletal organisation. In-vitro studies showed that the production of p21(ras) was inhibited by curcumin. It also inhibited transcription factor NF-κB and *IAP* gene expression (Aggarwal *et al.*, 2007). External curcumin application has been tried as a palliative therapy for cancerous skin lesions (Kuttan *et al.*, 1987). Clinical trials (Phase I and II) of curcumin are being carried out in several hospitals to find out its therapeutic role against colon cancer, pancreatic cancer, hepatocellular cancinoma and multiple myeloma (Goel *et al.*, 2008). Curcumin was found to be non-toxic at doses up to 12 g/day in patients.

Silybum marianum *(milk thistle)*

The active ingredients present in *S. marianum* (Compositae) are the flavonolignans silymarin and silybinin. Silymarin has been proposed as a promising chemotherapeutic adjuvant for the treatment of liver cancer. *N′*-nitrosodiethylamine-induced hepatocellular carcinoma was found to be inhibited by silymarin by modulating antioxidant defence status in rats (Ramakrishnan *et al.*, 2006). Silybin was found to inhibit the growth of Hep3B and HepG2 cells by G1 arrest. The apoptosis-inducing property of silybin has been shown to be through decreasing cyclin D1, cyclin D3, cyclin E and cyclin dependent kinases 2 and 4 (Varghese *et al.*, 2005). Silymarin can suppress the proliferation of a variety of tumour cells through cell cycle arrest at the G1/S-phase, induction of cyclin-dependent kinase inhibitors (such as p15, p21 and p27), down-regulation of anti-apoptotic gene products (e.g. Bcl-2 and Bcl-xL), inhibition of cell-survival kinases (AKT, PKC and MAPK) and inhibition of inflammatory transcription factors (e.g. NF-κβ). Silymarin can also down-regulate gene products involved in the proliferation of tumour cells (cyclin D1, EGFR, COX-2, TGF-beta, IGF-IR), invasion (MMP-9), angiogenesis (VEGF) and metastasis (adhesion molecules). The anti-inflammatory effects of silymarin are mediated through suppression of NF-κB-regulated gene products, including COX-2, LOX, inducible iNOS, TNF and IL-1 (Aggarwal *et al.*, 2006). Treatment of patients with hepatitis B or C infection with silymarin seemed to be effective, although no effect in decreasing viral load was found (Mayer *et al.*, 2005).

Camellia sinensis *(tea)*

Constituents of *C. sinensis* (Theaceae) include flavonols, e.g. myricetin, kaempferol and quercetin; as well as caffeine and proanthocyanidins such as epigallocatechin gallate. Green tea was observed to have protective effect on liver cancer in population-based studies (Mu *et al.*, 2003).

In multidose NDEA-induced HCC followed by carbon tetrachloride injection and partial heptoectomy studies, it was found that treatment with tea polyphenols and pigment showed significant reduction in number and area of GST-positive foci, which is a proliferative indicator of precancerous liver lesions by immunohistochemistry (Gong *et al.*, 1999). Green tea was reported to exert antiproliferative activity towards hepatoma cells. Green tea was also reported to possess chemopreventive activity against nitrosamine-initiated hepatocellular carcinoma (Cao *et al.*, 1996). It was found that the production of p21(WAF1/CIP1) was significantly induced and that of cyclin D1 and cyclin-dependent kinase 4 were inhibited in tea-treated animals (Jia *et al.*, 2002). Tea catechins, black tea extract and oolong tea extract are also reported to inhibit hepatocellular carcinoma (Matsumoto *et al.*, 1996).

Allium sativum *(garlic)*

The bulbs of *Allium sativum* (Alliaceae) have been described as useful against inflammation and tumours in Ayurveda. The anticarcinogenic activity of whole garlic (Samaranayake *et al.*, 2000), as well as its isolated ingredients (Singh *et al.*,1996), against NDEA-induced hepatocellular carcinoma in animals is well documented. Aged garlic extract inhibited the development of putative lesions in rat hepatocarcinogenesis involving a slowing in the proliferation rate of liver cells after partial hepatoectomy (Uda *et al.*, 2006). Garlic powder inhibited the formation of preneoplastic foci during hepatocarcinogenesis initiated by diethylnitrosamine through suppression of CYP2E1 (Park *et al.*, 2002). The organosulphur compounds isolated from garlic are highly active against liver cancer. There was a decrease in the number of preneoplastic, GST-positive foci of the liver and also a down-regulation of IGF-I and iNOS mRNA expression in the liver of organosulphur-treated animals which were induced with 2-amino-3,8-dimethylimidazo [4–5-f] quinoxaline (Ogawa *et al.*, 2006). The protective effect of diallylsulphide isolated from garlic against HCC was reported by Singh *et al.* (2004). *S*-allyl-cysteine, an organosulphur compound, showed inhibition of tumour incidence and lipid peroxidation in NDEA-induced hepatic cancer animals with simultaneous elevation in antioxidants (Sunderasen and Subramanian, 2003).

Benzo(a)pyrene-induced cancer was found to be inhibited by garlic constituents such as diallylsulphide (DAS), diallyldisulphide (DADS) and diallyltrisulphide (DATS). Diallylsulphide prevented DNA adducts induced by the carcinogen, thereby preventing the initiation of oestrogen-induced cancer (Green *et al.*, 2003). Allylthiopyridazine derivatives induced apoptosis in Sk-Hep-1 cells through a caspase-3-dependent mechanism and this also contributes to their chemopreventive function (Jung *et al.*, 2001). The antiproliferative property of aqueous garlic extract was studied in HepG2 cells and it was found that these compounds induced a p53/p21-dependent cell cycle arrest in G2/M phase and apoptosis through activation of c-Jun-NH (2) terminal kinase (JNK)/c-Jun phosphorylative cascade (De Martino *et al.*, 2006). DAS, DADS and DATS also caused G2/M phase arrest in human liver tumour cells (Wu *et al.*, 2004).

Emblica officinalis *Gaertn. (emblica)*

The extract of fruits of *E. officinalis* (Euphorbiaceae) was reported to give chemoprotection against chemically induced carcinogenesis (Jeena *et al.*, 1999). The fruits are rich in polyphenolic compounds such as gallic acid, tannic acid, emblicanin A and B and ellagitannins. Polyphenolic compounds, such as epigallocatechin gallate, found in tea are also present in *E. officinalis*. Because of the presence of these compounds, emblica extract has been shown to possess significant antioxidant activity and is also antimutagenic (Jeena *et al.*, 1997), inhibiting DNA adducts produced by benzo(a)pyrene (Jeena *et al.*, 1998). The polyphenolic fraction of *E. officinalis* was found to modulate NDEA-induced hepatic cancer in rats (Jeena *et al.*, 1998). In-vitro experiments showed that it inhibited DNA topoisomerase I in *Saccharomyces cerevisiae* mutant cell culture and also inhibited the activity of cdc25 tyrosine phosphatase (Jeena *et al.*, 2001).

Phyllanthus amarus

The fresh root of *P. amarus* (Euphorbiaceae) is said to be an excellent remedy for jaundice. The components present in *P. amarus* are lignans, e.g. phyllanthin; tannins, e.g. phyllanthusiin D3, amariin and amarulone; alkaloids, e.g. ent-norsecurinine, diarylbutanes; and neolignans, e.g. phyllnirurin. A variety of hydrolysable tannins purified from *P. amarus* were reported to be potent inhibitors of rat liver cyclic AMP-dependent protein kinase catalytic subunit (Polya *et al.*, 1995). *P. amarus* extract was reported to significantly inhibit NDEA-induced hepatocarcinogenesis in rats in a dose-dependent manner (Jeena *et al.*, 1999). In another study the lifespan of rats bearing NDEA-induced hepatocellular carcinoma was found to be significantly increased by the treatment with *P. amarus* (Rajeshkumar and Kuttan, 2000), from 33 weeks to 52 weeks. *P. amarus* extract has been shown to have antiviral activity against hepatitis B virus (Yeh *et al.*, 1993). In a patient study, it was found that approximately 60% of the carriers of HBV lost the virus within 1 month of *Phyllanthus amarus* treatment (Blumberg *et al.*, 1990).

Picrorhiza kurroa *(kutki)*

The root/rhizomes of *Picrorhiza kurroa* (Scrophulariaceae) are used in Ayurveda against jaundice. The components present in the root include the glycosides picrorhizin and kutkin, and sterols. Picroliv, an iridoid glycoside mixture prepared from this plant, contains equal concentrations of picroside and kutkoside as well as vanillic acid and sterols. Amelioration of NDEA-induced hepatocellular carcinoma was seen in animals treated with *P. kurroa* extract, and there was a significant reduction in the levels of drug-metabolising enzymes such as glutathione-*S*-transferase (GST) and aniline hydroxylase (AH) (Jeena *et al.*, 1999). Liver morphology and histopathology also revealed the protective effect of the extract against chemical carcinogenesis. Picroliv was found to inhibit HCC (Rajeshkumar and Kuttan, 2000) and was also reported to possess protective effect against 1,2-dimethylhydrazine-induced HCC in animals (Rajeshkumar and Kuttan, 2003). Picroliv significantly down-regulated transcription factor AP1 and thereby decreased the level of *c-fos* mRNA as well as c-jun and c-fos proteins in liver tissue (Seth *et al.*, 2003). This would indicate a base for their potential anti-HCC activity.

Semecarpus anacardium *(marking nut)*

The rind of the fruit of *S. anacardium* (Anacardiaceae) is used in Ayurvedic medicine against inflammatory diseases. The active ingredient is usually reckoned as anacardic acid. *S. anacardium* nut extract affords anticancer activity by enhancing both phase I and phase II enzymes and it has been proposed that the anticancer activity may be mediated through the induction of hepatic biotransformation enzymes (Premalatha and Sachidanandam, 2000). It was found to modulate the carcinogenic effect of aflatoxin by enhancing antioxidant capacity in the system (Premalatha and Sachidanandam, 1999).

Andrographis paniculata *(creat)*

The root of *Andrographis paniculata* (Acanthaceae) is used in both Ayurvedic and Chinese medicine. The component present is a diterpene lactone andrographolide. The roots also contain a variety of compounds including the sesquiterpene andrographolide. The effectiveness of *A. paniculata* was found to be through modulating hepatic and extrahepatic carcinogen-metabolising enzymes and antioxidant status (Trivedi and Rawal, 2001). *A. paniculata* extract and andrographolide stimulated CTL production through enhanced secretion of IL-2 and IFN-γ by T cells and thereby inhibited the tumour growth (Sheeja and Kuttan, 2007a). The species has been reported to modulate the immune response through enhancing natural killer (NK) cell activity and antibody-dependent cell-mediated cytotoxicity and antibody-dependent complement mediated cytotoxicity in tumour-bearing animals (Sheeja and Kuttan, 2007b).

Glycine max *(soybean)*

G. max (Papilionaceae) contains isoflavone glycosides genistein and diadzin as active principles but certain saponin constituents were also found to be biologically active. The administration of 30% soybean to the rat diet was found to have protective effect against hepatocarcinogenesis induced by DL-ethionone (Aiad *et al.*, 2004). There was a 92.7% increase in lifespan in rats with primary liver cancer when treated with doxorubicin encapsulated with soybean-derived sterylglycoside mixture when compared with free doxorubicin (Shimizu *et al.*, 1998). Genistein was found to inhibit diethylnitrosamine-induced and phenobarbital-promoted HCC (Lee *et al.*, 1995). Genistein has been reported to inhibit lung metastasis in animals (Menon *et al.*, 1998). Genistein was found to inhibit cell proliferation and induced apoptosis through caspase-3 induction and caspase-2 activation (Chodon *et al.*, 2007). In another study apoptosis was induced by genistein in Hep 3B cells through initiating endoplasmic reticular stress relevant regulators including m-calpain, GADD 153, GRP 78 and caspase-12 (Yeh *et al.*, 2007).

Panax ginseng *(ginseng)*

P. ginseng (Araliaceae) root (white and red) is extensively used in traditional Chinese medicine against various diseases. Ginseng contains polysaccharides and saponins, those known as ginsenosides are commonly considered to be the active constituents. The incidence of liver tumour development was lower in animals treated with red ginseng extract, and the average number of tumours per mouse was significantly reduced in the treated group (Li and Wu, 1991). White ginseng was also found to possess anticarcinogenic properties both in vitro and in vivo (Nishino *et al.*, 2001). In another study, red ginseng was found to possess both preventive as well as curative properties against diethylamine-induced hepatic cancers in rats (Wu *et al.*, 2001).

Terminalia arjuna *(arjuna bark)*

T. arjuna (Combretaceae) bark is extensively used against tumours in Ayurvedic medicine. *T. arjuna* was reported to possess chemopreventive activity in NDEA-induced HCC-bearing animals (Sivalokanathan *et al.*, 2005). In another study, diethylnitrosamine-induced HCC was inhibited by *T. arjuna* bark extract through modulating the antioxidant status in tumour-bearing animals (Sivalokanathan *et al.*, 2006). The ingredients of *T. arjuna* bark include flavonoids, e.g. arjunone, arjunolone and luteolin; phenols, e.g. gallic acid and ellagic acid; and terpenoids, e.g. oleanolic acid. The antitumour potential of luteolin and triterpenoids has been reported, while phenolic ingredients have significant chemopreventive activity.

Other plants

Bauhinia variegata and *B. racemosa* were reported to ameliorate NDEA-induced HCC in rats through modulation of antioxidant enzymes. Chemopreventive potential of extracts from *Tamarix gallica, Paullina cupana, Butea monosperma, Lygodium flexuosum, Indigofera aspalathoides, Apium graveolens, Solanum trilobatum, Ardisia compressa, Calotropis procera, Amaranthus gageticus, Astragalus membranaceus, Beta vulgaris, Cymbopogon citrates, Asteracantha longifolia, Trianthema portulacastrum* etc. has been reported in hepatic cancer models in animals.

Conclusions

There is no really effective treatment for hepatocellular carcinoma and so it stands high in global cause of mortality. Chronic hepatitis and lifestyle-induced oxidative stress are the major factors associated with hepatic cancer. It is detected in the later stages in many patients, and the current treatment modalities fail to keep the disease under control. Plants and plant-derived compounds have been found to be effective against hepatic cancer in animal models and through a few clinical studies. The antiviral and free-radical scavenging activities of the plant-derived constituents in many cases have proven to be beneficial. Many of the compounds, e.g. curcumin, are in the process of being testing in clinical trials and are giving promising results, while explorations for newer compounds are still progressing.

References

Aggarwal BB, Surh YJ, Shishodia S, eds (2007). *The Molecular Targets and Therapeutic Uses of Curcumin in Health and Disease. Advances in Experimental Medicine and Biology.* London: Springer Inc.

Aggarwal R, Aggarwal C, Ichikawa H, *et al.* (2006). Anticancer potential of silymarin: from bench to bed side. *Anticancer Res* 26: 4457–4498.

Aiad F, El-Gamal B, Al-Meer J, *et al.* (2004). Protective effect of soybean against hepatocarcinogenesis induced by DL-ethionine. *J Biochem Mol Biol* 37: 370–375.

Blumberg BS, Millman I, Venkateswaran PS, *et al.* (1990). Hepatitis B virus and primary hepatocellular carcinoma: treatment of HBV carriers with *Phyllanthus amarus. Vaccine* 8 (supp.): S86–S92.

Cao J, Xu Y, Chen J, Klaunig JE (1996). Chemopreventive effects of green and black tea on pulmonary and hepatic carcinogenesis. *Fundam Appl Toxicol* 29: 244–250.

Cheng JH, Chang G, Wu WY (2001). A controlled clinical study between hepatic arterial infusion with embolized curcuma aromatic oil and chemical drugs in treating primary liver cancer. *Zhongguo Zhong Xi Yi Jie He Za Zhi* 21: 165–167.

Chodon D, Banu SM, Padmavathi R, Sakthisekaran D (2007). Inhibition of cell proliferation and induction of apoptosis by genistein in experimental hepatocellular carcinoma. *Mol Cell Biochem* 297: 73–80.

Chuang SE, Cheng AL, Lin JK, *et al.* (2000). Inhibition by curcumin of diethylnitrosamine-induced hepatic hyperplasia, inflammation, cellular gene products and cell cycle related proteins in rats. *Food Chem Toxicol* 38: 991–995.

De Martino A, Filomeni G, Aquilano K, Ciriolo MR, *et al.* (2006). Effects of water garlic extracts on cell cycle and availability of HepG2 hepatoma cells. *J Nutr Biochem* 17: 742–749.

Goel A, Kunnumakkara AB, Aggarwal BB (2008). Curcumin as "curecumin": from kitchen to clinic. *Biochem Pharmacol* 75: 787–809.

Gong Y, Han C, Chen J (1999). Inhibitory effects of tea polyphenols and tea pigments on liver precancerous lesions in rats. *Wei Sheng Yan Jiu* 28: 294–296.

Green M, Thomas R, Gued L, *et al.* (2003). Inhibition of DES induced DNA adducts by diallyl sulphide: implications in liver cancer prevention. *Oncol Rep* 10: 767–771.

Jeena KJ, Kuttan G, Josely G, *et al.* (1997). Antimutagenic and anticarcinogenic activity of *Emblica officinalis* Gaertn. *J Clin Biochem Nutr* 22: 171–176.

Jeena KJ, Kuttan R, Bhattacharya RK (1998). Effect of *Emblica officinalis* extract on hepatocarcinogenesis and carcinogen metabolism. *J Clin Biochem Nutr* 25: 31–39.

Jeena KJ, Joy KL, Kuttan R (1999). Effect of *Emblica officinalis, Phyllanthus amarus* and *Picrorrhiza kurroa* on N-nitrosodiethylamine induced hepatocarcinogenesis. *Cancer Lett* 136: 11–16.

Jeena KJ, Kuttan G, Kuttan R (2001). Antitumor activity of *Emblica officinalis. J Ethnopharmacol* 75: 65–69.

Jia X, Han C, Chen J (2002). Effects of tea on preneoplastic lesions and cell cycle regulators in rat liver. *Cancer Epidemiol Biomarkers Prev* 11: 1663–1667.

Jung MY, Kwon SK, Moon A (2001). Chemopreventive allylthiopyridazine derivatives induce apoptosis in SK-Hep-1 hepatocarcinoma cells through a caspase-3-dependent mechanism. *Eur J Cancer* 16: 2104–2110.

Kuttan R, Sudheeran PC, Joseph CD (1987). Turmeric and curcumin as topical agents in cancer therapy. *Tumori* 73: 29–31.

Lee KW, Wang HJ, Murphy PA, *et al.* (1995). Soybean isoflavone extract suppresses early but not later promotion of hepatocarcinogenesis by phenobarbital in female rat liver. *Nutr Cancer* 24: 267–278.

Li X, Wu XG (1991). Effects of ginseng on hepatocellular carcinoma in rats induced by diethylnitrosamine – a further study. *J Tongji Med Univ* 11: 73–80.

Matsumoto N, Kohri T, Okushio K, *et al.* (1996). Inhibitory effects of tea catechins, black tea and oolong tea extract on hepatocarcinogenesis. *Jpn J Cancer Res* 87: 1034–1038.

Mayer KE, Myers RP, Lee SS (2005). Silymarin treatment of viral hepatitis: a systemic review. *J Viral Hepatitis* 12: 559–567.

Menon LG, Kuttan R, Nair MG, *et al.* (1998). Effect of isoflavones genistein and daidzein in the inhibition of lung metastasis in mice induced by B16F-10 melanoma cells. *Nutr Cancer* 30: 74–77.

Mu LN, Zhou XF, Ding BG, *et al.* (2003). Study on the protective effect of green tea on gastric, liver and esophageal cancers. *Zhonghua Yu Fang Yi Xue za Zhi* 37: 171–173.

Nishino H, Tokuda H, Ii T, Takemura M, *et al.* (2001). Cancer chemoprevention by ginseng in mouse liver and other organs. *J Korean Med Sci* 16 (supp.) S66–S69.

Ogawa NM, Wanibuchi H, Morimura K, *et al.* (2006). N-acetylcysteine and S-methylcysteine inhibit MeIQx rat hepatocarcinogenesis in the post-initiation stage. *Carcinogenesis* 27: 982–988.

Park KA, Kweons S, Choi H (2002). Anticarcinogenic effect and modification of cyt.P450 2E1 by dietary garlic powder in diethylnitrosamine initiated rat hepatocarcinogenesis. *J Biochem Mol Biol* 35: 615–622.

Polya GM, Wang BH, Foo LY (1995). Inhibition of signal regulated protein kinases by plant derived hydrolysable tannins. *Phytochemistry* 38: 307–314.

Premalatha B, Sachdanandam P (1999). *Semecarpus anacardium* L. nut extract administration induces the in vivo antioxidant defence system in aflatoxin B1 mediated hepatocellular carcinoma. *J Ethnopharmacol* 66: 131–139.

Premalatha B, Sachdanandam P (2000). Potency of *Semecarpus anacardium* Linn. Nut milk against aflatoxin B1 induced hepatocarcinogenesis: reflection on microsomal biotransformation enzymes. *Pharmacol Res* 42(2)b: 161–166.

Rajeshkumar NV, Kuttan R (2000a). *Phyllanthus amarus* extract administration increases the life span of rats with hepatocellular carcinoma. *J Ethnopharmacol* 73: 215–219.

Rajeshkumar NV, Kuttan R (2000b). Inhibition of N-nitrosodiethylamine induced hepatocarcinogenesis by Picroliv. *J Exp Clin Cancer Res* 19: 459–465.

Rajeshkumar NV, Kuttan R (2003). Modulation of carcinogenic response and antioxidant enzymes of rats administered with 1, 2-dimethylhydrazine by Picroliv. *Cancer Lett* 191: 137–143.

Ramakrishnan G, Raghavendran HR, Vinodhkumar R, *et al.* (2006). Suppression of N-nitrosodiethylamine induced hepatocarcinogenesis by silymarin in rats. *Chem Biol Interact* 161: 104–114.

Samaranayake MD, Wickramasinghe SM, Angunawela P, *et al.* (2000). Inhibition of chemically induced liver carcinogenesis in wistar rats by garlic (allium sativum). *Phytother Res* 14: 564–567.

Seth P, Sundar SV, Seth RK, *et al.* (2003). Picroliv modulates antioxidant status and down regulates AP1 transcription factor after hemorrhage and resuscitation. *Shock* 19: 169–175.

Sheeja K, Kuttan G (2007a). Activation of cytotoxic T lymphocyte responses and attenuation of tumor growth in vivo by *Andrographis paniculata* extract and andrographolide. *Immunopharmacol Immunotoxicol* 29: 81–93.

Sheeja K, Kuttan G (2007b). Modulation of natural killer cell activity, antibody dependent cellular cytotoxicity and antibody dependent complement mediated cytotoxicity by andrographolide in normal and Ehrlich ascites carcinoma bearing mice. *Integr Cancer Ther* 6: 66–73.

Shimizu K, Qi XR, Maitani Y, *et al.* (1998). Targeting of soybean derived sterylglucoside liposomes to liver tumors in rat and mouse models. *Biol Pharm Bull* 21: 741–746.

Shukla Y, Arora A (2003). Suppression of altered hepatic foci development by curcumin in wistar rats. *Nutr Cancer* 45: 53–59.

Singh A, Arora A, Shukla Y (2004). Modulation of altered hepatic foci induction by diallyl sulphide in wistar rats. *Eur J Cancer Prev* 13: 263–269.

Singh SV, Mohan RR, Agarwal R, *et al.* (1996). Novel anticarcinogenic activity of an organosulfide from garlic: Inhibition of H-ras oncogenes transformed tumor growth in vivo by diallyldisufide is associated with inhibition of p21H-ras processing. *Biochem Biophys Res Commun* 225: 660–665.

Sivalokanathan S, Ilayaraja M, Balasubramanian MP (2005). Efficacy of *Terminalia arjuna* (Roxb.) on N-nitrosodiethylamine induced hepatocellular carcinoma in rats. *Indian J Exp Biol* 43: 264–267.

Sivalokanathan S, Ilayaraja M, Balasubramanian MP (2006). Antioxidant activity of *Terminalia arjuna* bark extract on N-nitrosodiethylamine induced hepatocellular carcinoma in rats. *Mol Cell Biochem* 281: 87–93.

Soni KB, Lahiri M, Chackradeo P, *et al.* (1997). Protective effect of food additives on aflatoxin-induced mutagenicity and hepatocarcinogenicity. *Cancer Lett* 115: 129–133.

Sreepriya M, Bali G (2005). Chemopreventive effects of embelin and curcumin against N-nitrosodiethylamine/phenobarbital induced hepatocarcinogenesis in wistar rats. *Fitoterapia* 76: 549–555.

Sreepriya M, Bali G (2006). Effects of administration of embelin and curcumin on lipid peroxidation, hepatic glutathione antioxidant defense and hematopoietic system during N-nitrosodiethylamine/phenobarbital induced hepatocarcinogenesis in wistar rats. *Mol Cell Biochem* 284: 49–55.

Strumberg D, Richly H, Hilger RA, *et al.* (2005). Phase I clinical and pharmacokinetic study of the novel Raf kinase and vascular endothelial growth factor recetor inhibitor BAY 43-9006 in patients with advanced refractory solid tumors. *J Clin Oncol* 23: 965–972.

Sundaresan S, Subramanian P (2003). S-allylcysteine inhibits circulatory lipid peroxidation and promotes antioxidants in N-nitrosodiethylamine induced carcinogenesis. *Pol J Pharmacol* 55: 37–42.

Trivedi NP, Rawal UM (2001). Hepatoprotective and antioxidant property of *Andrographis paniculata* (Nees) in BHC induced liver damage in mice. *Indian J Exp Biol* 39: 41–46.

Uda N, Kashimoto N, Sumioka I, *et al.* (2006). Aged garlic extract inhibits development of putative preneoplastic lesions in rat hepatocarcinogenesis. *J Nutr* 136 (supp. 3): 855S–860S.

Varghese L, Aggarwal C, Tyagi A, *et al.* (2005). Silibinin efficacy against human hepatocellular carcinoma. *Clin Cancer Res* 11: 8441–8448.

Wu CC, Chung JG, Tsai SJ, *et al.* (2004). Differential effects of allyl sulphides from garlic essential oil on cell cycle regulation in human liver tumor cells. *Food Chem Toxicol* 42: 1937–1947.

Wu XG, Zhu DH, Li (2001). Anticarcinogenic effect of red ginseng on the development of liver cancer induced by diethylnitrosamine in rats. *J Korean Med Sci* 16 (supp.): S61–S65.

Yeh SF, Hong CY, Huang YL, *et al.* (1993). Effect of an extract from *Phyllanthus amarus* on hepatitis B surface antigen gene expression in human hepatoma cells. *Antiviral Res* 20: 185–192.

Yeh TC, Chiang PC, Li TK, *et al.* (2007). Genistein induces apoptosis in human hepatocellular carcinoma via interaction of endoplasmic reticulum stress and mitochondrial insult. *Biochem Pharmacol* 73: 782–792.

Yosurgnoen P, Wirachwong P, Bhattarakosol P, *et al.* (2006). Effects of curcumin on tumor angiogenesis and biomarkers, COX-2 and VEGF, in hepatocellular carcinoma cell-implanted nude mice. *Clin Hemorheol Microcirc* 34: 109–115.

10

Testing of herbal products used to treat infections

José-Luis Ríos

Antimicrobial activity

Introduction

Infectious diseases are one of the greatest causes of mortality around the world, specifically in the underdeveloped regions of Asia and Africa. As a consequence of globalisation and the migratory movements of the population from the developing world to the more developed countries, some of the infectious pathologies that had been partially controlled are now causing renewed problems because of their acquired resistance to known antibiotics. For this reason, research into new anti-infectious compounds is a subject of intense interest for the scientific community. Careful in-vitro biological evaluation is essential for quantifying and understanding the basis of the antibacterial activity of new compounds as it provides preliminary indications and evaluations of therapeutic potential, helps assess the likelihood for the development of bacterial resistance, guides chemical refinement and even assists in subsequent stages of appraisal for any new antibacterial drug (O'Neill and Chopra, 2004).

The search for novel antimicrobial agents includes researchers interested in medicinal plants and their isolated compounds. Myriad studies have been published, but they are usually carried out according to different criteria and with different methodologies. Recently, Ríos and Recio (2005) reviewed the most relevant papers published on this subject and observed that even the objectives varied; so general criteria must be established for studying the antimicrobial activity of extracts and derived compounds. Most important is the definition of common parameters such as the type of plant material used, the techniques employed, the growth medium used, and the microorganisms tested (Cos *et al.*, 2005).

Selection of experimental conditions

Scientific criteria should be used in the selection of the plant material. In preference to random criteria, the selection of plants should be made from an ethnopharmacological perspective. All the species tested should be perfectly described and identified; this must include the specifics of collection, i.e. location, season, date, and time of day. The use of commercial samples should be limited to cases of standardised extracts or defined phytomedicines (Ríos and Recio, 2005). While research on the antimicrobial activity of medicinal plants is quite common, standardised criteria for studying this activity are often lacking. For testing the antimicrobial activity of medicinal plant extracts, several factors must be considered, one factor being the selection of the appropriate solvent. This is especially important in cases in which folk medicine makes use of a water infusion of the medicinal plant whereas the plant extract used for research purposes is often a non-polar organic extract. Eloff (1998) favours the use of an acetone extract. The selection of the microorganism to be tested should also be a high priority. Thus, to test the activity of a medicinal plant used against urinary infections, strains of Gram-negative bacteria are essential, whereas for testing the anti-acne effect of a plant extract, a series of Gram-positive bacteria are preferable. Finally the preparation of samples in an appropriate sterile atmosphere along with a standard way of expressing the results are essential for evaluating the data in a correct and comprehensive fashion.

Selection of the solvent and extraction system

The appropriate selection of the extraction solvent is important for establishing the potential activity of a medicinal plant. Plant extracts are usually prepared by maceration or percolation of either fresh plants or dried, powdered plants and can be performed with water or organic solvents (Vanden Berghe and Vlietinck, 1991). The plant material may be extracted with one solvent and then fractionated with solvents of different polarity. This is a good way of detecting minor active compounds that are present in the preliminary extract, albeit in minor quantities and was the methodology used by Ríos *et al.* (1987) and Recio *et al.* (1989), which employed a sequential extraction with two solvents of different polarity, e.g. chloroform and methanol, and then tested each separately, finding clear differences between the activities of extracts obtained from the same source. Other authors have established a selective protocol of extraction to study the differences between extracts obtained in different ways. Nostro *et al.* (2000) suspended the powdered drug in water, adjusted the mixture to pH 2.0 and incubated it at 37°C for 30 min in a water bath. The mixture was then neutralised to pH 7.0, filtered, extracted with diethyl ether and concentrated to dryness, and finally the remaining aqueous extract was lyophilised, and then all the extracts were tested. Thongson *et al.* (2004) determined the influence of the extraction system on antimicrobial activity. They compared the effects of both conventional and high-intensity ultrasound-assisted solvent-extraction. The conventional system consisted of an extraction of the sample (10 g) with the solvent (mixtures of isopropanol-hexane, 100 mL) in an orbital shaker for 24 h at room temperature. The high-intensity ultrasound system consisted of the extraction of the same quantity of the sample, but this time the sample was sonicated in an ice-bath for 5 min with a 20 kHz ultrasonic generator connected to a half inch transducer at an ultrasonic intensity of 6.8 W/cm. All the extracts were filtered/sterilised using a 0.45 μm filter.

Culture media

The composition of the growth medium can also influence the activity of the tested extracts or compounds. Thus, when Ross *et al.* (2001) reported the effects of garlic powder and garlic oil, the antimicrobial activity of garlic oil was found to be greater in media lacking tryptone or cysteine, which led to the hypothesis that the effects may involve sulphydryl reactivity.

Mueller-Hinton agar is probably the universal culture media for testing the antimicrobial activity of medicinal plant extracts. Certain microorganisms, including *Candida albicans* or *Mycobacterium phlei*, can be studied in a non-selective medium; however, if a preliminary study of these microorganisms is of interest, a specific medium should be used (Villar *et al.*, 1987). Depending on the microorganism, the culture medium could be supplemented, for example with defibrinated sheep's blood for *Streptococcus pneumoniae* and *Streptococcus pyogenes* (Rojas *et al.*, 2001) or yeast extract for *Lysteria monocytogenes* (Thongson *et al.*, 2004). Diagnostic sensitivity test agar (Vanden Berghe and Vlietinck, 1991), heart infusion broth (Hammer *et al.*, 1996; 1999), tryptone soya agar (Nostro *et al.*, 2000) and Mueller-Hinton broth (Bylka *et al.*, 2004) can all be used for bacteria, whereas Sabouraud dextrose agar (Nostro *et al.*, 2000) and Sabouraud chloramphenicol broth (Bylka *et al.*, 2004) are better for mycetes and Sabouraud liquid medium is best used for yeasts (Nostro *et al.*, 2000).

Selection of microorganisms

American type culture collection (ATCC) or similar standard microorganisms are commonly used in studies on antimicrobial activity. A correct selection of type strains is essential for subsequent comparison of results obtained from different groups, not to mention the fact that it is the only possible way to obtain reproducible results. However, it is not a guarantee for secure and exact screening if different precautions have not been taken (Vanden Berghe and Vlietinck, 1991). When the possible treatment of an infectious disease is the subject of the research, it is recommendable to carry out subsequent experiments with the isolated clinical pathogen (Hammer *et al.*, 1996; Thongson *et al.*, 2004). A correct selection of Gram-positive and Gram-negative bacteria for the preliminary screening is basic for such studies. For example, *Staphylococcus aureus* and/or *Streptococcus pyogenes* as aerobic Gram-positive cocci, *Bacillus cereus* as an aerobic Gram-positive spore-forming bacillus, *Escherichia coli* and *Pseudomonas aeruginosa* as aerobic Gram-negative bacilli, *Klebsiella pheumoniae* as a facultatively anaerobic Gram-negative bacillus. In addition, some Gram-positive acid-fast bacteria (*Mycobacterium phlei* or *M. fortuitum*) and some types of yeast (*Candida albicans*) can be tested in a standard medium. The use of species such as *Campylobacter fetus*, *Chlamydia trachomatis* or *Neisseria gonorrhoeae*, however, requires enriched or specific media (Vanden Berghe and Vlietinck, 1991).

Authors sometimes test antimicrobial compounds against a specific disease or infection. For example, dental caries are known to develop because of an increase in strongly acidogenic and aciduric Gram-positive bacteria, while common forms of periodontal disease are linked to the presence of anaerobic Gram-negative bacteria in subgingival plaque. In this context, Tichy and Novak (1998) evaluated the feasibility of screening for antibacterial agents from plants against three representative oral streptococci. Depending on the indicator microorganisms used, the screening assay could target additional pathogens including other streptococci (group A and B, and pneumococci) along with periodontal pathogens. In general, however, authors screen the activity of plant extracts or essential oils with no comparative criteria, which creates a problem when results from different studies are to be compared. Thus, when Hammer *et al.* (1996) studied the effect of tea tree oil on commensal skin flora, they selected a wide range of clinically isolated microorganisms, including different skin pathogens, but still insisted on the necessity of an in-vivo study to establish the proper value of this oil. However, most other researchers, when testing medicinal plants used in folk medicine against specific pathologies, only screen the activity against a standard strain without selecting any specific microorganisms implicated in the disease (Rojas *et al.*, 2001; Ram *et al.*, 2004).

Preparation of samples

A common flaw in many papers is to claim positive activity for excessively high concentrations. For testing the antimicrobial activity of plant extracts, concentrations higher than 1 mg/mL for extracts or 100 μg/mL for isolated compounds should be avoided, whereas the presence of activity is very interesting in the case of concentrations below 100 μg/mL for extracts and 10 μg/mL for isolated compounds (Ríos and Recio, 2005).

Another problem is the possibility of contaminating the samples during manipulation, thereby causing the final results to be erroneous. The sterilisation of plant extracts by autoclaving or other strenuous methods should be avoided and even the use of membrane-filtration may absorb many antimicrobial agents on the filter material itself (Vanden Berghe and Vlietinck, 1991). To avoid this problem, some authors use methanol as solvent in the agar dilution method, because it is not toxic at a final concentration of 2% (0.2 mL in 10 mL) and it additionally acts as an antiseptic agent. Moreover, aerobic organisms do not develop well on solid agar and since the occasional contaminating culture on the surface of the agar can be easily recognised, it poses no problem (Ríos *et al.*, 1988).

Different solvents or emulsifiers can be used, including dimethyl sulphoxide (DMSO), alcohols, acetone and glycerol, but in all cases a blank should be prepared containing only the solvent in the same quantity present in the testing compounds (Vanden Berghe and Vlietinck, 1991). When water or physiological saline are used as solvent, the final pH should be tested, and the range of analysis should be between 6.0 and 8.0. This is due to the fact that the pH of compounds in dilutions may also modify the results, as can sometimes be observed with ionisable compounds such as phenolics or alkaloids. The influence of pH on the different effects of neutral essential oil has already been described. Thus, for example, anise oil exhibited higher antifungal activity at pH 4.8 than at 6.8, while the oil of *Cedrus deodara* Loud. was most active at pH 9 (Janssen *et al.*, 1987). For essential oils the use of an adequate solvent is important. An optimised broth dilution method, using 0.02% Tween 80 to emulsify the oils, was developed and shown to be the most accurate method for testing the antimicrobial activity of the hydrophobic and viscous essential oils (Hood *et al.*, 2003).

Expression of results

Depending on the methods used for studying the activity, the results should be expressed in various forms, e.g. as the growth inhibition index, which is calculated as the ratio of the growth of the control with no test sample to that of a test sample. They can also be given as the minimal concentration that restrains the growth of the microorganisms or the minimal lethal concentration against the microorganisms. In a preliminary screening with an agar dilution method, a selection of positive (+) and negative (−) or (0) values could be interesting for determining whether the extract totally inhibited (+) or had no effect (−) or (0) on the growth of the selected bacteria at the concentration assayed.

Usually, 1 mg/mL is a good initial concentration; subsequent dilutions can then be tested when positive activity has been observed. Dilutions of 100, 50, 25 μg/mL and lower should be tested to determine the minimum inhibitory concentration (MIC), which should be expressed as μg of extract per mL of culture medium that totally inhibited the microorganism growth. MIC values higher than 100 μg/mL should be of no interest for plant extracts. For liquid samples, such as essential oils, the expression *maximal inhibitory dilution* (MID) is more appropriate.

When the potency of a compound as an antimicrobial agent is evident, other factors should be considered, including the bactericidal or bacteriostatic effect, along with determination of the minimum bactericidal concentration (MBC). For this purpose, a liquid dilution method is recommended, since high dilutions of plant extracts are not a problem in an aqueous liquid medium. To determine the bactericidal or bacteriostatic effect, growth curves of the microorganism in the presence of the test compound or extract should be calculated. While use of an automated system is convenient, it is not essential. In the first case, a series of sample dilutions are measured in parallel against a predetermined concentration of microorganisms during a period of 20 h and the results are expressed as the logarithms of the delta optical density plotted against time, which indicates changes in the biomass in the growth chambers (Villar *et al.*, 1987). The other method for establishing a possible bacteriostatic effect is by making a subculture of the tube that exhibited inhibition in an agar plate or liquid medium. The growth of colonies is indicative of a bacteriostatic effect whereas the absence of growth indicates a bactericidal effect (Ríos *et al.*, 1988).

Antimicrobial test methods

As seen above, many factors, including considerations such as solubility, can give rise to problems in studies on the antimicrobial activity of medicinal plants and their extracts. In contrast, research into the activity of antibiotics or isolated natural products minimises this problem with respect to the situation of non-polar extracts such as essential oils, acetogenins or terpenoids.

The various methodologies that have been employed in such studies in the past must be examined more closely. For non-polar extracts, for example, the use of diffusion techniques seems to be inadequate, although many reports have been published in which these techniques were used, so we propose the use of solid dilution techniques for studying plant extracts or non-polar compounds. Only when a very small sample amount is available is the use of diffusion techniques possibly more appropriate (Ríos and Recio, 2005). Janssen *et al.* (1987) concluded that the results are difficult to compare as the test methods differed so widely. They went on to propose that in future the strain number of the tested microorganism, the composition of the essential oil, and the conditions under which it was obtained be included as an integral part of the report. In 2003, Kalemba and Kunicka reviewed the methods commonly used for the evaluation of the antibacterial and antifungal activities of essential oils to draw conclusions about the factors that influence the in-vitro antimicrobial activity of essential oils and their mechanisms of action. They included an overview of the susceptibility of human and food-borne bacteria and fungi towards different essential oils and their constituents.

Diffusion methods

Agar diffusion techniques are widely used to assay plant extracts for antimicrobial activity, but there are problems associated with this technique, which entails a reservoir containing the plant extract to be tested being brought into contact with the inoculated medium. After incubation, the diameter around the reservoir (hole, cylinder or disc) is measured. This method is good for preliminary testing, allowing rapid selection of active extracts. However, even though the determination of the MIC of an extract by means of agar diffusion methods is frequent in this kind of study, it is inadequate for comparing the results obtained from different studies and the solvent used for dissolving the extract sometimes modifies the response, e.g. the use of a particular solvent may actually cause a non-polar compound to show up as a false negative. As a result, findings can only be compared when the substances all have similar characteristics and when all the conditions are the same. Examples of this kind of study include the research of Nostro *et al.* (2000), Ogundipe *et al.* (2000) and Unal *et al.* (2001).

When using any of the three systems, it is always necessary to sterilise the sample. While the cylinder and the paper disc methods are both adequate for assaying water-soluble extracts, the hole-plate is the only suitable method for testing aqueous suspensions of non-water-soluble plant extracts. When samples are introduced into the recipient, it is generally recommendable to carry out a pre-incubation at 4°C to facilitate the diffusion but when the cylinder or disc methods are used with samples comprising aqueous suspensions of non-water-soluble extracts, the pre-incubation should be carried out at 25°C to avoid the precipitation of insoluble compounds. Finally, plates should be incubated at 37°C for 18, 24 or 36 h, depending on the microorganism being tested. The diffusion methods are good for determining the sensitivity of different microorganisms to an extract, but the comparison of data inhibition halos obtained thereby is not appropriate for determining the potency of a compound or for comparing it with antibiotic standards, which are only valid for testing water-soluble antibiotics.

One modification, the so-called microatmosphere method, could be applied to the study of the antimicrobial activity of essential oil in the vapour phase. In this method, a disc moistened with essential oil is attached to the lid of a Petri dish, which is then inverted and incubated. The results are presented either as the diameter of the zone of microorganism growth inhibition or as the minimal inhibitory quantity (MIQ) of essential oil that totally inhibits the growth of microorganisms (Kalemba and Kunicka, 2003).

Dilution methods

In the classic dilution method (liquid), samples are mixed with an adequate culture medium that has previously been inoculated with the targeted microorganism. The suspension is incubated and the growth is then measured by turbidimetry and compared with a control that does not contain any sample. This is a good method to use with isolated compounds, especially those that are soluble in water. Moreover, it is the best method for determining the potency of an agent after calculating the MIC of the sample that completely inhibited the growth of the microorganism. However, the low solubility of plant extracts, especially those obtained with non-polar solvents such as hexane or dichloromethane, often hampers such tests of their activity.

There is also a microdilution technique that makes use of a 96-well microplate (Figure 10.1) and in which bacterial growth is detected by turbidimetry (Kalemba and Kunicka, 2003) or tetrazolium salts (Eloff, 1998). Liquid cultures containing different concentrations of the samples are placed in a 96-well, flat-bottom, polystyrene microtitre test plate and, after incubation, the plates are vigorously shaken on a vibrating platform and immediately scanned with a multiscan photometer. As the emulsion can interfere with the endpoint reading, indicators could be used to avoid this problem.

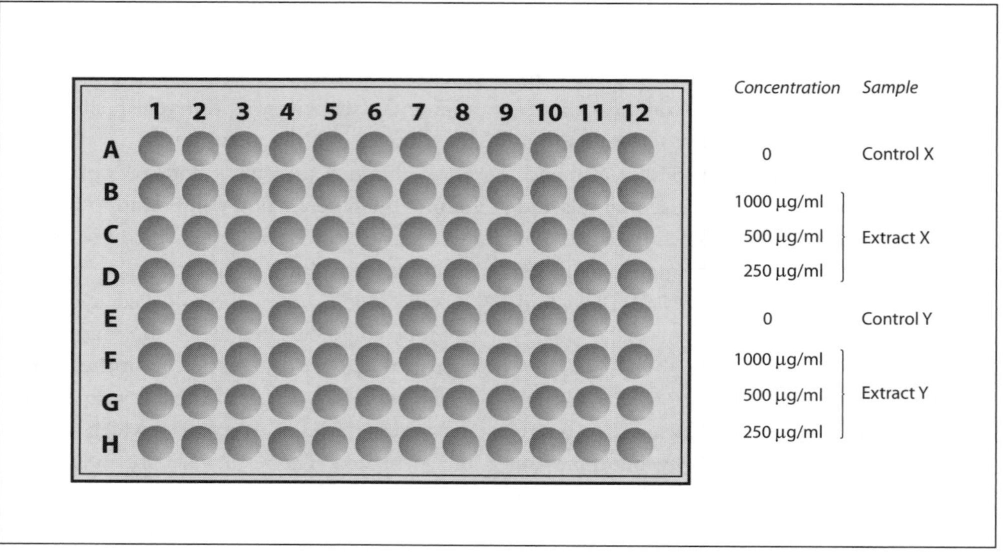

Figure 10.1 Scheme of an agar dilution method for plant extracts by a microtitre plate. In the well series 1–12, 12 different microorganisms are inoculated. Row A is the control and has no actual sample, but merely contains the vehicle used for the other samples. Rows B, C and D are in decreasing concentrations of one test sample (X). Row E should be the control of F, G and H, in which a second test sample (Y) is introduced at different concentrations.

Kalemba and Kunicka (2003) propose the use of a bioimpedimetric method for studying antimicrobial activity. The method is based on the correlation between the altered electrical parameters of the growth culture and the number of cells regarded as a colony forming unit (CFU)/mL. In this method the analysis time is shorter than that of usual detection systems.

The method has been shown to give reproducible results; furthermore, it requires only 10–25 μL of extract to determine the MICs, it distinguishes between cidal and static effects, and it also provides a permanent record of the results. In addition, this technique is 32 times more sensitive than usual agar diffusion techniques and is not sensitive to the culture age of the test organism up to 24 h. In a similar vein, micro-scale assays are useful for testing natural components available only in low quantities. This was demonstrated by Barreteau *et al.* (2004), who examined a rapid method that used microplates for the evaluation of antimicrobial substances and then validated their results using five food-borne pathogens. The assay required only a small amount of product and was convenient for determining correlations between the bacterial growth inhibition and the concentrations of the antimicrobial substances. The dilution methods are the best for determining the MIC and the MBC of a plant extract in the case of good solubility, and especially from isolated natural products.

In the agar dilution method, incorporation of the plant extract into the agar is carried out prior to solidification, making it possible to test a series of microorganisms in the same plate. For this reason, it is probably the best system for assaying antimicrobial activity in a quick and safe fashion. The agar dilution method is thus useful for establishing the spectrum of an extract because, if a multipoint inoculation system is used, it is possible to inoculate up to 21 strains in the same 10 mL plate (Figure 10.2).

Bioautographic methods

Bioautography, described by Betina in 1973, is not only a good method for studying antimicrobial activity, but has also proven to be useful for the detection of new active compounds in plant extracts. The method facilitates the detection of growth inhibition of cultures directly in thin-layer chromatograms of the extract by spraying with a broth culture containing the microorganisms (Navarro *et al.*, 1998). The three

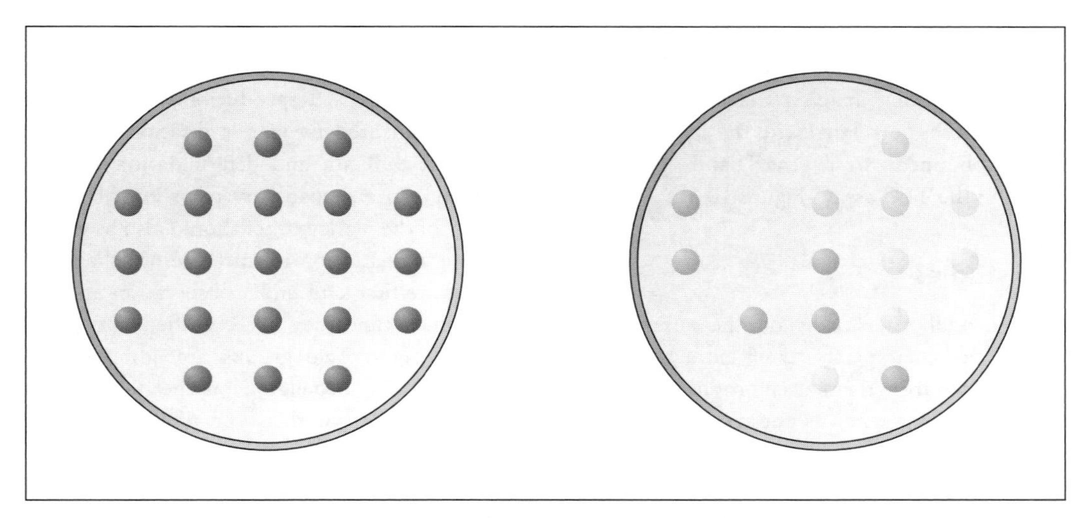

Figure 10.2 Multipoint inoculation in an agar plate previously prepared with a dilution of plant extract in agar. Positive activity is considered only when there is total inhibition of growth.

basic bioautographic methods are the contact, the direct and the immersion bioautographies. The first method is based on the diffusion of separated compounds by means of thin-layer chromatography (TLC). The developed TLC plate is carefully dried to remove the resident mobile phase and then it is placed on the surface of a large nutrient agar plate inoculated with sensitive microorganisms. After 15–30 min, the TLC plates are removed and the agar plate is incubated at an appropriate temperature until the growing microorganisms are visible on the surface and the zones of inhibition are clearly visible. Inhibition zones can be made more conspicuous by using dehydrogenase indicators (Ríos *et al.*, 1988) or *p*-iodonitrotetrazolium violet (Nostro *et al.*, 2000). The effectiveness of the method depends on the diffusion capacity of the compounds to be separated during chromatography.

In direct bioautography, the developed TLC plates are carefully dried for complete removal of the solvents and then overlaid with agar that has been seeded with an overnight culture of the test microorganism, then incubated and viewed as explained below (Nostro *et al.*, 2000). This is the most widely used method because no diffusion is required, which eliminates the problems of the contact method, but it has its own limitations. The most relevant of these is the necessity of the conditions of a well-equipped microbiology laboratory. Furthermore, it is not appropriate for studying pathological microorganisms.

The third bioautographic method is both more appropriate for non-specialised microbiological laboratories and more secure for the study of pathological agents. This method involves the introduction of the previously developed TLC plate in a Petri dish, but only after the mobile phase has been totally removed. The TLC plate is then covered with Mueller-Hinton agar at 50°C in a uniform fashion to keep the silica gel layer from sliding. After solidification, the Petri dishes are refrigerated at 4°C for 4 h to obtain a better diffusion of the principles from the plate toward the surface of the agar. Afterwards, the plates are seeded with an overnight culture of the microorganism previously detected as sensitive, and the plates are then incubated at 37°C for 24 h (Ríos *et al.*, 1988). The inhibition halos can be observed in different ways. They can be directly detected either after the observation of the inhibition bands (Figure 10.3), or after being sprayed with an aqueous solution of *p*-iodonitrotetrazolium violet (2 mg/mL), which turns a yellow colour in the areas of inhibition. The spots are then compared with the related spots on the reference TLC plate that has been developed in parallel (Nostro *et al.*, 2000). However, Ríos *et al.* (1988) proposed an even simpler method, which involves first developing a plate as bands, viewing it under ultraviolet light and using a pencil to mark all the bands with the corresponding RF. Different strips are then cut longitudinally, and each strip is then stained with a different phytochemical reagent. When the assay is finished, the inhibition halos can then be located in relationship to the bands in the strips. In this analysis the active principle (band) can thus be correlated with the specific phytochemicals obtained from the band previously developed in the TLC assay (Figure 10.3).

In-vivo studies

As mentioned above, studies on the antimicrobial activity of medicinal plants, their extracts and the products isolated from them often produce misleading results. Since their potency as antimicrobial agents is generally low, when the compounds are tested in vivo, the previously reported results are often not accurate. For this reason, complementary in-vivo studies that are carried out to corroborate the initial findings should be of great interest.

For in-vivo tests, male Swiss mice weighing 18–20 g are generally the animals of choice. Prior to the assays, they should be maintained under standard conditions at 21 ± 1°C and 50–60% relative humidity, with a photoperiod of 14 : 10 h of semi-darkness, with water and a solid diet ad libitum. The test strain must also be selected with care. For example, Sarkar *et al.* (2003) for testing a synthetic product chose to work with *Salmonella typhimurium* NCTC 74, the virulence of which had been heightened by passing the test strain repeatedly among various mice. The lethal dose-50 (LD50) of the passage strain corresponding to 0.95×10^9 colony forming units (CFU) per mouse suspended in 0.5 mL nutrient broth served as the challenge dose for all groups of animals. Reproducibility of the challenge dose was ensured by standardisation of its optical density at 640 nm and determination of the CFU count in nutrient agar. Any prior knowledge of the toxicity of the plant extract should also be considered for its administration to mice. Before challenge, the animals are first kept under observation up to 100 h, after which time they are classified into groups in separate cages. Two groups are administered two different doses, depending on the possible toxicity and the LD50. For this type of screening, a good reference dose would be 100 and 300 mg/kg for extracts, or 50 and 100 mg/kg for pure compounds. After 3 h, the groups are challenged with the microorganisms; in the example given above, the median lethal dose of the passage strain corresponded to 0.95×10^9 CFU per mouse suspended in 0.5 mL in the case of *S. typhimurium* NCTC 74 (Sarkar *et al.*, 2003). A control group is also injected with the same bacterial strain, but with 0.1 mL sterile saline instead of extract. The protective capacity of the extract is determined by recording the mortality of the mice in the different groups tested up to 100 h of treatment. A parallel experiment could be run to obtain heart blood, livers and spleens aseptically. Once removed, these would then be aseptically homogenised, after which the CFU counts of the individual organs can be determined separately. The latter experiment could be realised at different hours

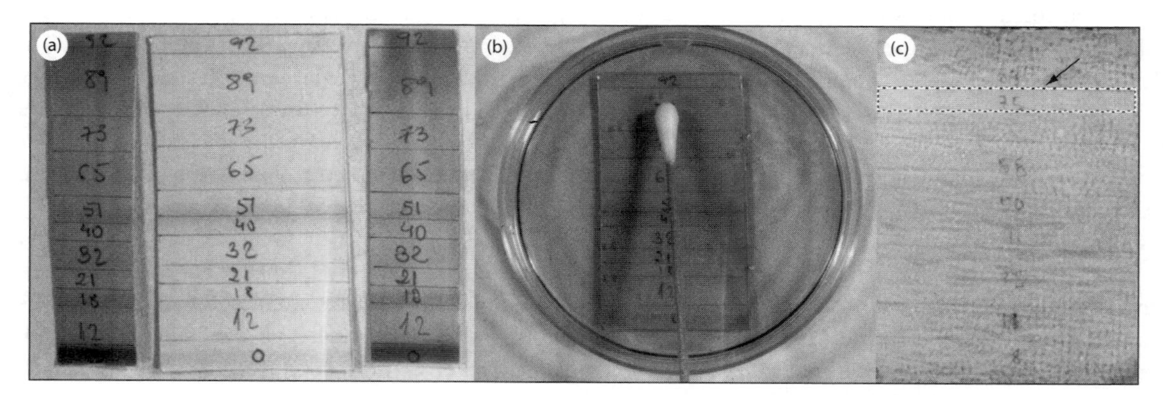

Figure 10.3 Immersion bioautography. (a) The developed TLC plate is dried and the different bands are marked under ultraviolet light. Various strips are cut longitudinally. Each strip is stained with different reagents to determine the phytochemicals present. (b) The central body is deposited in a Petri dish, covered with agar, seeded and incubated. Inhibition bands are observed. (c) Example of an inhibition band observed over the RF × 100 band at 75 (arrow).

after the challenge. In all the cases, an appropriate statistical analysis should be carried out.

Unfortunately, only a small number of papers describe in-vivo studies with plant extract or natural products. One such study is that of Ohno *et al.* (2003), who investigated the antimicrobial effects of essential oils against *Helicobacter pylori* and demonstrated that lemongrass has the highest activity. They went on to study its effect on an in-vivo experimental model, demonstrating its activity in 10% of the infected mice. Moreover, they showed that even after 10 passages it did not produce resistance whereas the bacteria acquired resistance against the antibiotic used as standard in the experiment. Using female mice, Talwar *et al.* (2000) demonstrated the activity of several polyherbal formulations against various sexually transmitted pathogens such as *Neisseria gonorrhoeae* and *Candida albicans*, including strains resistant to standard antibiotics. Both formulations prevented lesions and vaginal transmission when applied intravaginally before inoculation of the pathogen.

Using a porcine model, Mertz *et al.* (2003) studied various topical antimicrobial agents and dressings on colonised wounds. This method could be of interest for studying the topical antimicrobial activity of different plant extracts or isolated compounds. For a model representing a clinical wound infection, the researchers included inoculated wounds that were subsequently covered with a polyurethane film for a minimum of 48 h, which allowed the bacteria to form firmly attached aggregates of microcolonies on the wound bed, thereby facilitating the investigation of the efficacy of the antimicrobial agents.

Takahata *et al.* (1999) used an in-vivo therapeutic efficacy test for experimental systemic infections and experimental pneumonia. For the former they used *Staphylococcus aureus* CR-3 and *S. aureus* CRCP-9 prepared from an overnight culture on heart infusion agar at 37°C and suspended in saline to give a final concentration of approximately 10^8 CFU/mL. The inocula were obtained by means of a 10-fold dilution in saline containing 5% gastric mucin. Intraperitoneal injection of 0.5 mL of 4.0×10^7 to 10.4×10^7 CFU/mL induced systemic infections. One hour after infection, the antimicrobial agents, which were suspended and diluted in 0.5% methylcellulose, were administered orally or subcutaneously. The total number of surviving mice at day 7 after challenge was recorded, the 50% effective dose (ED50) and confidence limits were determined, and the significance of the differences between groups was estimated with the Probit method. For the latter study, a clinically isolated *Streptococcus pneumoniae* strain was used to induce experimental pneumonia in mice. The bacteria from overnight cultures on a heart infusion agar plate containing 5% sheep's blood at 37 °C were suspended in brain–heart infusion broth to give a final concentration of 10^8 CFU/mL. After 10-fold dilution in the same medium, this suspension was shake-cultured at 37°C for 4 h. The inocula were obtained with a 100-fold dilution in brain–heart infusion broth. Finally, experimental pneumonia was induced in ether-anaesthetised mice by means of intratracheal injection of 0.05 mL of the suspension. Oral or subcutaneous administration of the extract three times a day (at intervals of 4 h) over 3 days was started 20 h after the challenge. The total number of mice surviving at day 10 after challenge was recorded, the ED50 and the confidence limits were determined, and the significance of the differences between groups was estimated with the Probit method.

Determining the MIC of plant extracts and natural products

In the course of their work on plant extracts, Sarkar *et al.* (2003) developed an effective method for determining the MIC of active extracts and isolated compounds. For broth dilutions, 0.1 mL of a standardised suspension of the strain (10^6 CFU/mL) is added each to a series of tubes containing a range of the extract at concentrations of 0 (control) and 10–1000 μ/mL in Mueller-Hinton broth. For pure isolated compounds, the concentrations will be 0 (control) and then range from 0.1 to 50 μg/mL. The tubes are incubated at 37°C for 24 h and examined for visible growth after vortexing the tubes gently.

For agar dilutions, the sample could be added at the same concentrations into melted nutrient agar and poured in Petri dishes. The microorganism cultures, which have been grown in peptone water overnight, are then spot-inoculated on the nutrient agar plates such that each inoculum contains 2×10^6

CFU. The plates are incubated at 37°C, examined after 24 h and, if necessary, incubated for another 72 h. The lowest concentration of extract in a tube (or plate) that failed to show any visible macroscopic growth is considered to be the MIC. This procedure should be performed in duplicate for each organism.

Recent studies on antimicrobial activity of medicinal plants

Recently, Ríos and Recio (2005) reviewed the latest papers published on the antimicrobial activity of medicinal plants and their extracts. Upon closer examination, they found that studies on the activity of isolated compounds comprised 65% of the publications whereas the study of medicinal plants used in specific countries or regions of the world represented only 17% of all the papers on this general topic. A third group of papers consisted of specific studies of the activity of a plant or principle against a definite pathological microorganism, such as *Candida albicans*, *Helicobacter pylori* or enterohaemorrhagic *Escherichia coli.*

One example of this kind of paper is the study by Thongson *et al.* (2005) on the potential antimicrobial activity of extracts and essential oils of spices from Thailand against five strains of *Listeria monocytogenes* and four strains of *Salmonella enterica* ssp. *enterica* serovar *Typhimurium* DT104. Various interesting and complementary studies have also been carried out to demonstrate the antimicrobial activity in vitro of the ethanolic extract of propolis against *Staphylococcus aureus* (Lu *et al.*, 2005) and against 94 *Helicobacter pylori* strains (Boyanova *et al.*, 2005). Moreover, Oksuz *et al.* (2005) determined in vivo the synergistic activity between ciprofloxacin and propolis in the treatment of experimental *Staphylococcus aureus* keratitis. As a final consideration, when the antimicrobial activity of medicinal plants is demonstrated both in vitro and in vivo, corroboration of the effect through clinical trials is of great interest. Thus, Aksoy *et al.* (2006) recently demonstrated the antimicrobial activity of mastic gum against *Streptococcus mutans* by means of a disc diffusion method in vitro and then performed clinical studies on 25 periodontally healthy volunteers.

Martin and Ernst (2003a) reviewed different clinical trials for bacterial infections and conclude that no clinical efficacy was demonstrated by the herbal medicines tested.

Isolated natural products from active plant extracts

Different studies have established the antimicrobial activity of isolated compounds such as alkaloids (Klausmeyer *et al.*, 2004), flavonoids (Sohn *et al.*, 2004), sesquiterpene lactones (Lin *et al.*, 2003), diterpenes (El-Seedi *et al.*, 2002), triterpenes (Katerere *et al.*, 2003), or naphthoquinones (Machado *et al.*, 2003), among others. Some of these studies have focused on concrete pathological microorganisms, for example *Candida albicans* (Duarte *et al.*, 2005), *Helicobacter pylori* (O'Gara *et al.*, 2000), enterohaemorrhagic *Escherichia coli* (Voravuthikunchai *et al.*, 2004), sexually transmitted diseases (Tshikalange *et al.*, 2005) including *Neisseria gonorrhoeae* (Shokeen *et al.*, 2005), bacteria resistant to known antibiotics such as *Staphylococcus aureus*, which is resistant to methicillin (Machado *et al.*, 2003), or vancomycin-resistant enterococci (Fukai *et al.*, 2004), as well as multi-drug resistant bacteria such as *Salmonella typhi* (Rani and Khullar, 2004). It should be noted that in some of these studies, the active principles themselves were not actually isolated. Recently, there has been a resurgence of interest in essential oils because they are perceived to be natural alternatives to chemical biocides and, in some applications, antibacterial and antifungal agents. Thus, studies have examined the useful effects of essential oils, such as that from *Cinnamomum osmophloeum* Kaneh., oregano and peppermint (Wallace, 2004).

To date, few reports focus on the mechanism of action of these active compounds. Cushnie and Lamb (2005) reviewed the antimicrobial activity of different phenolics, and cited that the activity of quercetin is partially attributable to inhibition of DNA gyrase while sophoraflavone G and (−)-epigallocatechin gallate inhibit cytoplasmic membrane function. In addition, licochalcones A and C inhibit energy metabolism, and ellagitannins produce destabilisation of the cytoplasmic membrane, permeabilisation of the plasma membrane, inhibition of extracellular microbial enzymes, direct action on microbial metabolism, deprivation of the substrates required for microbial growth and inhibition of adherence of bacteria to epithelial cells, which is a prerequisite for colonisation and infection in many pathogens (Puupponen-Pimia *et al.*, 2004).

In their work, Lin *et al.* (2005) have opened new perspectives for studying natural products as antimicrobial agents. While the potency of natural products is not high with respect to antibiotics or chemotherapeutics, natural products such as flavonoids could exert synergistic effects when administered together with antibiotics that have a high level of microbial resistance. Thus, although the flavonol myricetin was shown to inhibit extended-spectrum β-lactamase-producing *Klebsiella pneumoniae* isolates only at a high MIC, it exhibited significant synergistic activity against these bacteria in combinations with either amoxicillin/clavulanate, ampicillin/sulbactam or cefoxitin, thereby increasing the number of isolates susceptible to these antibiotics. Moreover, galangin showed activity against 4-quinolone-resistant strains of *Staphylococcus aureus*. This is of interest for future research since, although galangin interferes with the type II topoisomerase enzymes, there is no cross resistance between the flavonoid and the 4-quinolones (Cushnie and Lamb, 2006).

Another interesting effect of ethyl gallate and other alkyl gallates on β-lactam susceptibility in methicillin-resistant and methicillin-sensitive strains of *Staphylococcus aureus* has been demonstrated, namely the fact that these natural products seem to intensify the antibiotic effect and the synergistic activity of β-lactams by means of a highly specific mechanism, since no significant changes were observed in the potency of the other classes of antibiotics tested. These results support the possible use of these principles together with known antibiotics to increase their potency and avoid undesirable side-effects (Shibata *et al.*, 2005). Another study reports on the effect of 5′-methoxyhydnocarpin, a compound isolated from chaulmoogra oil, on the activity of berberine. While 5′-methoxyhydnocarpin exhibited no antimicrobial activity on its own, it greatly enhanced the action of berberine against *Staphylococcus aureus*. The level of accumulation of berberine in the cells was seen to increase sharply in the presence of 5′-methoxyhydnocarpin, which indicates that this natural product effectively disables the bacterial resistance mechanism against berberine since this alkaloid is otherwise readily extruded by multidrug-resistant strains of the human pathogen *Staphylococcus aureus* (Stermitz *et al.*, 2000).

Antifungal assays for higher plants and natural products

Within the field of natural product research, one of the most relevant areas is that of testing the toxicity of various compounds against human and plant fungal diseases. Of the former, the most commonly studied are athlete's foot, aspergillosis, actinomycosis, histoplasmosis and coccidioidomycosis while the most commonly researched plant fungal diseases include potato late blight, tobacco blue mould and hop downy mildew. Other fungal diseases of note may also affect animals (Paxton, 1991).

When investigating new antifungal compounds of natural origin, several factors must be taken into account. Obviously, the search for new antifungal compounds with no negative effects for animals and humans is of extreme interest but there is also a need for new fungicides that can be used for other purposes, e.g. preservation of food, wood and cloth (Paxton, 1991). While the former is a primary concern for public health, the economic implications of the latter research field cannot be denied.

Common testing methods

There are various experimental protocols for testing antifungal activity; however, the most common screening procedures are the agar tube dilution assay and direct bioautography. Other more specific methods include the in-vivo protocols for studying various epidermal pathogens.

Agar dilution assay

Many fungi can be tested by means of this protocol (Atta-ur-Rahman *et al.*, 2001), but the researcher must take all necessary precautions when testing human pathogenic fungi, such as species of *Epidermophyton*, *Tricophyton*, *Microsporum*, *Pseudallescheria* and *Candida*, among others. For such testing, Sabouraud dextrose agar is the most adequate medium and samples should be dissolved in DMSO. The most commonly used standard antifungal drugs are amphotericin-B and ketoconazole.

The procedure is as follows: first, Sabouraud dextrose agar is prepared and autoclaved at 121°C for 15 min. The tubes are then cooled to room temperature. Next, test samples that have been dissolved in DMSO at different concentrations are inoculated with a piece of inoculum measuring 4 mm in diameter which has been removed from a 7-day-old culture of the fungus to be tested. The tubes containing the cultures are then incubated at optimum temperature and humidity. The cultures are examined both during incubation and after growth has been completed; the test tubes with no visible microorganism growth are taken to represent the MIC of the test sample, expressed in μg/mL.

Direct bioautography method

This protocol (Atta-ur-Rahman *et al.*, 2001) is carried out in the same way as when testing for antibacterial activity, i.e. the TLC plates are developed and all volatile solvents are eliminated, after examination under ultraviolet light, the plates are sprayed with a conidial suspension of test microorganisms. Here the researcher must take care not to let the plates become too wet. The chromatograms are then incubated in a moist atmosphere for 2–3 days at 25°C. The inhibition zones that are subsequently visualised indicate the activity of fungitoxic products against the tested microorganisms. An additional TLC developed in parallel could serve to clarify the nature of the toxic compounds in question.

Special considerations for carrying out bioassays

When carrying out a bioassay, several practical aspects should be taken into account to avoid mistakes and ensure valid results. For example, both the chemical reactivity of the active compounds and the purity of the test compounds should be known. In the case of extracts, their exact nature and the solvent with which they were obtained should be clearly defined; many times the elimination of reactive substances may be necessary to avoid false-positive results. In addition, the time frame of the experiment may generate substances other than the original; for example, hydrolysis, oxidation or reaction between compounds in mixtures is frequent in cases in which an aqueous medium is used. Moreover, changes in growth stages, mutation of the test organism and contamination of the culture may also occur, causing confusion in the interpretation of the results. Changes in pH caused by the nature of the test compound and even the composition of the medium could also affect the results. Finally, it is important to remember that the natural environment in which fungicides develop their function is usually different from that of the bioassay (Paxton, 1991).

Some relevant results

Many antifungal extracts and compounds have been tested to date. Of these, the most promising are the phytoalexins, compounds with a relatively low toxicity against mammals, but with a broad spectrum against pathogenic fungi. This family of compounds is thus a good source of potential new agents. The compounds themselves are generally of low molecular weight and are synthesised and accumulated in the plants after infection by fungi; however, as with other kinds of biological analysis, the in-vivo effectiveness is difficult to estimate from in-vitro assays. For this reason, many researchers use animals to study the activity in vivo after screening the compounds with in-vitro methods. For instance, *Microsporum lanosum* infections have been induced in dogs, cats and rabbits, *Trichophyton mentagrophytes* in guinea pigs and humans and *Candida albicans* in dogs, mice, guinea pigs, rabbits and humans (Paxton, 1991).

Of all the natural products studied for antifungal activity, essential oils are the phytochemical group which holds the most interest for researchers. For example, when Helal *et al.* (2006) studied the essential oil from *Cymbopogon citratus* L. against *Aspergillus niger*, they demonstrated that the mycelial growth was completely inhibited after fumigation or upon contact with the oil. Subsequent microscopic studies showed that after treatment with the essential oil, *A. niger* hyphae underwent structural modifications, including plasma membrane disruption and reorganisation of the mitochondrial structure.

Other authors have used different experimental protocols. For instance, Inouye *et al.* (2006) studied the activity of six essential oils against *Trichophyton mentagrophytes* using a closed box and the oil vapours. The vapours of oregano, perilla, tea tree and lavender oils all killed the mycelia after only a short time while the vapours of clove and geranium oils required overnight exposure to exert any activity. The vapour of oregano oil was found to induce lysis of the mycelia and cell-wall damage in a dose- and time-dependent manner, causing rupture and peeling of the cell wall (Inouye *et al.*, 2006).

The antifungal properties of the essential oil of *Melaleuca alternifolia* Cheel (tea tree oil) have been tested against vaginal candidiasis. To date, however, there are no in-vivo data which unequivocally support the in-vitro results, especially with regard to the antifungal action of the oil's constituents. Mondello *et al.* (2006) assayed the in-vitro and in-vivo anti-*Candida* activity of terpinen-4-ol and 1,8-cineole on oophorectomised, pseudo-oestrous rats undergoing the oestrogen treatment used for experimental vaginal infection with fluconazole- and itraconazole-susceptible or -resistant strains of *C. albicans*. The in-vitro MIC90 values were 0.06% (v/v) for terpinen-4-ol and 4% (v/v) for 1,8-cineole, regardless of the susceptibility or resistance of the strains to fluconazole and itraconazole. In this particular model of infection, terpinen-4-ol was as active as tea tree oil in accelerating the clearance from the vagina of all *Candida* strains examined.

While mostly volatile compounds from essential oils have been found to be active, non-volatile principles have also been recorded as being antifungal agents. For example, Kuiate *et al.* (2007) tested an extract of *Syzygium jambos* (L.) Alston and the contained triterpenes, e.g. friedelin, betulinic acid and lupeol, along with two semisynthetic derivatives, for their antidermatophytic action against *Microsporum audouinii*, *Trichophyton mentagrophytes* and *T. soudanense*. Betulinic acid and the derivative friedelolactone were found to be the most active compounds, while the most sensitive fungi were *T. soudanense* and *T. mentagrophytes*.

Products of animal origin, such as propolis, may also be of interest as antifungal agents. Oliveira *et al.* (2006) tested the in-vitro activity of propolis extract against 67 yeasts isolated from onychomycosis in different patients. The yeasts in question included *Candida parapsilosis*, *C. tropicalis*, *C. albicans* and other species, all of which were inhibited by the propolis extract. *Trichosporon* spp. proved to be the most sensitive species, with *C. tropicalis* being the most resistant. The authors went on to propose the use of propolis as an option in the treatment of onychomycosis because it is a natural, low-cost, non-toxic product with proven antifungal activity.

While the activity of plant extracts and natural products should be previously tested in vitro, in-vivo studies and clinical trials are essential for determining their possible use in humans as therapeutic drugs. For example, when a hexane extract from aerial parts of *Ageratina pichinchensis* (H.B. and K.) R.M. King and H. Rob., a plant which has been used for generations in traditional Mexican medicine for the treatment of superficial mycosis, was tested in vitro, it was found to be effective against *Candida albicans*, *Aspergillium niger*, *Trichophyton mentagrophytes* and *T. rubrum*. To validate its clinical use, Romero-Cerecero *et al.* (2006) conducted a double-blind pilot study to compare the effectiveness and tolerability of the crude extract of *Ageratina pichinchensis* with that of ketoconazole in patients with the clinical and mycological diagnosis of tinea pedis. All patients underwent a weekly mycological examination for 4 weeks to gauge the therapeutic effects. At the end of the 4 weeks, therapeutic success had been achieved in 80% of the experimental cases (using cream containing 10% standardised extract) and in 72% of the control cases (with a cream containing 2% ketoconazole).

Martin and Ernst (2004) reviewed some clinical trials for fungal infections and concluded that herbal remedies require further investigation in rigorous clinical trials.

Other assays for higher plants and natural products

While assays for compounds with antiviral and antiparasitic effects, including antimalarial, amoebicidal, molluscicidal, cercaricidal, schistosomicidal and piscicidal activities, are also relevant, their specificity and number put them beyond the scope of the present chapter. Still, it is worth noting that the most relevant methods have been reviewed by Vanden Berghe and Vlietinck (1991) and Atta-Ur-Rahman *et al.* (2001) for antiviral methods, and Phillipson (1991) and Marston and Hostettmann (1991) for antiparasitic methods. Other interesting reviews in this area include those conducted by Vlietinck *et al.*

(1998), Jassim and Naji (2003), and Martin and Ernst (2003b) for antiviral medicinal compounds, Keene *et al.*, (1986), Mott (1987), Marston *et al.* (1993), Di Stasi (1995), Whitfield (1996), de Luna *et al.* (2005), Kapoor and Kumar (2005), Biot and Chibale (2006), and Taylor and Berridge (2006) for antiparasitic medicinal plants.

References

Aksoy A, Duran N, Koksal F (2006). In vitro and in vivo antimicrobial effects of mastic chewing gum against *Streptococcus mutans* and mutans streptococci. *Arch Oral Biol* 51: 476–481.

Atta-ur-Rahman Choudhary MI, Thomsen WJ (2001). *Bioassay Techniques for Drug Development*. Harwood Academic Publishers, Amsterdam, pp. 14–27.

Barreteau H, Mandoukou L, Adt I *et al.* (2004). A rapid method for determining the antimicrobial activity of novel natural molecules. *J Food Prot* 67: 1961–1964.

Betina V (1973). Bioautography in paper and thin-layer chromatography and its scope in the antibiotic field. *J Chromatogr* 78: 41–51.

Biot C, Chibale K (2006). Novel approaches to antimalarial drug discovery. *Infect Disord Drug Targets* 6: 173–204.

Boyanova L, Gergova G, Nikolov R *et al.* (2005). Activity of Bulgarian propolis against 94 *Helicobacter pylori* strains in vitro by agar-well diffusion, agar dilution and disc diffusion methods. *J Med Microbiol* 54: 481–483.

Bylka W, Szaufer-Hajdrych M, Matlawska I, Goslinska O (2004). Antimicrobial activity of isocytisoside and extracts of *Aquilegia vulgaris* L. *Letters Appl Microbiol* 39: 93–97.

Cos P, Vlietinck AJ, Vanden Berghe D (2005). Anti-infective potential of natural products: how to develop a stronger in vitro 'proof of concept'. *J Ethnopharmacol* 106: 290–302.

Cushnie TP, Lamb AJ (2005). Antimicrobial activity of flavonoids. *Int J Antimicrob Agents* 26: 343–356.

Cushnie TP, Lamb AJ (2006). Assessment of the antibacterial activity of galangin against 4-quinolone resistant strains of *Staphylococcus aureus*. *Phytomedicine* 13: 187–191.

de Luna J, dos Santos AF, de Lima MR *et al.* (2005). A study of the larvicidal and molluscicidal activities of some medicinal plants from northeast Brazil. *J Ethnopharmacol* 97: 199–206.

Di Stasi LC (1995). Amoebicidal compounds from medicinal plants. *Parasitologia* 37: 29–39.

Duarte MC, Figueira GM, Sartoratto A *et al.* (2005). Anti-*Candida* activity of Brazilian medicinal plants. *J Ethnopharmacol* 97: 305–311.

El-Seedi HR, Sata N, Torssell KB *et al.* (2002). New labdene diterpenes from *Eupatorium glutinosum*. *J Nat Prod* 65: 728–729.

Eloff JN (1998). A sensitive and quick microplate method to determine the minimal inhibitory concentration of plant extracts for bacteria. *Planta Med* 64: 711–713.

Fukai T, Oku Y, Hano Y, Terada S (2004). Antimicrobial activities of hydrophobic 2-arylbenzofurans and an isoflavone against vancomycin-resistant enterococci and methicillin-resistant *Staphylococcus aureus*. *Planta Med* 70: 685–687.

Hammer KA, Carson CF, Riley TV (1996). Susceptibility of transient and commensal skin flora to the essential oil of *Melaleuca alternifolia* (tea tree oil). *Am J Infect Control* 24: 186–189.

Hammer KA, Carson CF, Riley TV (1999). Antimicrobial activity of essential oils and other plant extracts. *J Appl Microbiol* 86: 958–990.

Helal GA, Sarhan MM, Abu Shahla AN, Abou El-Khair EK (2006). Effects of *Cymbopogon citratus* L. essential oil on the growth, lipid content and morphogenesis of *Aspergillus niger* ML2-strain. *J Basic Microbiol* 46: 456–469.

Hood JR, Wilkinson JM, Cavanagh HMA (2003). Evaluation of common antibacterial screening methods utilized in essential oil research. *J Essential Oil Res* 15: 428–433.

Inouye S, Nishiyama Y, Uchida K *et al.* (2006). The vapor activity of oregano, perilla, tea tree, lavender, clove, and geranium oils against a *Trichophyton mentagrophytes* in a closed box. *J Infect Chemother* 12: 349–354.

Janssen AM, Scheffer JJC, Baerheim Svendsen A (1987). Antimicrobial activity of essential oils: a 1976–1986 literature review. Aspects of the test methods. *Planta Med* 53: 395–398.

Jassim SA, Naji MA (2003). Novel antiviral agents: a medicinal plant perspective. *J Appl Microbiol* 95: 412–427.

Kalemba D, Kunicka A (2003). Antibacterial and antifungal properties of essential oils. *Curr Med Chem* 10: 813–829.

Kapoor VK, Kumar K (2005). Recent advances in the search for newer antimalarial agents. *Prog Med Chem* 43: 189–237.

Katerere DR, Gray AI, Nash RJ, Waigh RD (2003). Antimicrobial activity of pentacyclic triterpenes isolated from African Combretaceae. *Phytochemistry* 63: 81–88.

Keene AT, Harris A, Phillipson JD, Warhurst DC (1986). In vitro amoebicidal testing of natural products; part I. Methodology. *Planta Med* 52: 278–285.

Klausmeyer P, Chmurny GN, McCloud TG *et al.* (2004). A novel antimicrobial indolizinium alkaloid from *Aniba panurensis*. *J Nat Prod* 67: 1732–1735.

Kuiate JR, Mouokeu S, Wabo HK, Tane P (2007). Antidermatophytic triterpenoids from *Syzygium jambos* (L.) Alston (Myrtaceae). *Phytother Res* 21: 149–152.

Lin F, Hasegawa M, Kodama O (2003). Purification and identification of antimicrobial sesquiterpene lactones from yacon (*Smallanthus sonchifolius*) leaves. *Biosci Biotechnol Biochem* 67: 2154–2159.

Lin RD, Chin YP, Lee MH (2005). Antimicrobial activity of antibiotics in combination with natural flavonoids against clinical extended-spectrum β-lactamase (ESBL)-producing *Klebsiella pneumoniae*. *Phytother Res* 19: 612–617.

Lu LC, Chen YW, Chou CC (2005). Antibacterial activity of propolis against *Staphylococcus aureus*. *Int J Food Microbiol* 102: 213–220.

Machado TB, Pinto AV, Pinto MC *et al.* (2003). In vitro activity of Brazilian medicinal plants, naturally occurring naphthoquinones and their analogues, against methicillin-resistant *Staphylococcus aureus*. *Int J Antimicrob Agents* 21: 279–284.

Marston A, Hostettmann K (1991). Assays for molluscicidal, cercaricidal, schistosomicidal and piscicidal activities. In: *Methods in Plant Biochemistry*, Ed. K. Hostettmann, vol. 6, Academic Press, London, pp. 153–178.

Marston A, Maillard M, Hostettmann K (1993). Search for antifungal, molluscicidal and larvicidal compounds from African medicinal plants. *J Ethnopharmacol* 38: 215–223.

Martin KW, Ernst E (2003a). Herbal medicines for treatment of bacterial infections: a review of controlled clinical trials. *J Antimicrob Chemother* 51: 241–246.

Martin KW, Ernst E (2003b). Antiviral agents from plants and herbs: a systematic review. *Antivir Ther* 8: 77–90.

Martin KW, Ernst E (2004). Herbal medicines for treatment of fungal infections: a systematic review of controlled clinical trials. *Mycoses* 47: 87–92.

Mertz PM, Davis SC, Cazzaniga AL *et al.* (2003). Barrier and antimicrobial properties of 2-octyl cyanoacrylate derived wound treatment films. *J Cutan Med Surgery* 7: 1–12.

Mondello F, De Bernardis F, Girolamo A *et al.* (2006). In vivo activity of terpinen-4-ol, the main bioactive component of *Melaleuca alternifolia* Cheel (tea tree) oil against azole-susceptible and -resistant human pathogenic *Candida* species. *BMC Infect Dis* 6: 158 (doi: 10.1186/1471-2334-6-158).

Mott KE *Plant molluscicides* (1987). John Wiley and Sons, Chichester, pp. 1–323.

Navarro V, Rojas G, Delgado G, Lozoya (1998). Antimicrobial compounds detected in *Bocconia arborea* extracts by a direct bioautographic method. *Arch Med Res* 29: 191–194.

Nostro A, Germano-grave, MP, D'Angelo V *et al.* (2000). Extraction methods and bioautography for evaluation of medicinal plant antimicrobial activity. *Lett Appl Microbiol* 30: 379–384.

O'Gara EA, Hill DJ, Maslin DJ (2000). Activities of garlic oil, garlic powder, and their diallyl constituents against *Helicobacter pylori*. *Appl Environ Microbiol* 66: 2269–2273.

Ogundipe OO, Moody JO, Fakeye TO, Ladipo OB (2000). Antimicrobial activity of *Mallotus oppositifolium* extractives. *Afr J Med Med Sci* 29: 281–283.

Ohno T, Kita M, Yamaoka Y *et al.* (2003). Antimicrobial activity of essential oils against *Helicobacter pylori*. *Helicobacter* 8: 207–215.

Oksuz H, Duran N, Tamer C *et al.* (2005). Effect of propolis in the treatment of experimental *Staphylococcus aureus* keratitis in rabbits. *Ophthal Res* 37: 328–334.

Oliveira AC, Shinobu CS, Longhini R *et al.* (2006). Antifungal activity of propolis extract against yeasts isolated from onychomycosis lesions. *Mem Inst Oswaldo Cruz* 101: 493–497 (Erratum in: *Mem Inst Oswaldo Cruz* 101: following 696).

O'Neill AJ, Chopra I (2004). Preclinical evaluation of novel antibacterial agents by microbiological and molecular techniques. *Expert Opin Investig Drugs* 13: 1045–1063.

Paxton JD (1991). Assays for antifungal activity. In: *Methods in Plant Biochemistry*, Ed. K. Hostettmann, vol. 6, Academic Press, London, pp. 33–46.

Phillipson JD (1991). Assays for antimalarial and amoebicidal activities. In: *Methods in Plant Biochemistry*, Ed. K. Hostettmann, vol. 6, Academic Press, London, pp. 135–152.

Puupponen-Pimia R, Nohynek L, Alakomi HL *et al.* (2004). Bioactive berry compounds – novel tools against human pathogens. *Appl Microbiol Biotechnol* 67: 8–18.

Ram AJ, Bhakshu LM, Raju RRV (2004). In vitro antimicrobial activity of certain medicinal plants from Eastern Ghats, India, used for skin diseases. *J Ethnopharmacol* 90: 353–357.

Rani P, Khullar N (2004). Antimicrobial evaluation of some medicinal plants for their anti-enteric potential against multi-drug resistant *Salmonella typhi*. *Phytother Res* 18: 670–673.

Recio MC, Ríos JL, Villar A (1989). Antimicrobial activity of selected plants employed in the Spanish Mediterranean area. Part II. *Phytother Res* 3: 77–80.

Ríos JL, Recio MC (2005). Medicinal plants and antimicrobial activity. *J Ethnopharmacol* 100: 80–84.

Ríos JL, Recio MC, Villar A (1987). Antimicrobial activity of selected plants employed in the Spanish Mediterranean area. *J Ethnopharmacol* 21: 139–152.

Ríos JL, Recio MC, Villar A (1988). Screening methods for natural products with antimicrobial activity: A review of the literature. *J Ethnopharmacol* 23: 127–149.

Rojas G, Lévaro J, Tortoriello J, Navarro V (2001). Antimicrobial evaluation of certain plants used in Mexican traditional medicine for the treatment of respiratory diseases. *J Ethnopharmacol* 74: 97–101.

Romero-Cerecero O, Rojas G, Navarro *et al.* (2006). Effectiveness and tolerability of a standardized extract from *Ageratina pichinchensis* on patients with tinea pedis: an explorative pilot study controlled with ketoconazole. *Planta Med* 72: 1257–1261.

Ross ZM, O'Gara EA, Hill DJ *et al.* (2001). Antimicrobial properties of garlic oil against human enteric bacteria: evaluation of methodologies and comparisons with garlic oil sulfides and garlic powder. *Appl Environ Microbiol* 67: 475–480.

Sarkar A, Kumar KA, Dutta NK *et al.* (2003). Evaluation of *in vitro* and *in vivo* antibacterial activity of dobutamine hydrochloride. *Indian J Med Microbiol* 21: 172–178.

Shibata H, Kondo K, Katsuyama R *et al.* (2005). Alkyl gallates, intensifiers of beta-lactam susceptibility in methicillin-resistant *Staphylococcus aureus*. *Antimicrob Agents Chemother* 49: 549–555.

Shokeen P, Ray K, Bala M, Tandon V (2005). Preliminary studies on activity of *Ocimum sanctum*, *Drynaria quercifolia*, and *Annona squamosa* against *Neisseria gonorrhoeae*. *Sex Transm Dis* 32: 106–111.

Sohn HY, Son KH, Kwon CS, Kwon GS, Kang SS (2004). Antimicrobial and cytotoxic activity of 18 prenylated flavonoids isolated from medicinal plants: *Morus alba* L., *Morus mongolica* Schneider, *Broussnetia papyrifera* (L.) Vent, *Sophora flavescens* Ait and *Echinosophora koreensis* Nakai. *Phytomedicine* 11: 666–672.

Stermitz FR, Lorenz P, Tawara JN *et al.* (2000). Synergy in a medicinal plant: antimicrobial action of berberine potentiated by 5'-methoxyhydnocarpin, a multidrug pump inhibitor. *Proc Natl Acad Sci USA* 97: 1433–1437.

Takahata M, Mitsuyama J, Yamashiro Y *et al.* (1999). In vitro and in vivo antimicrobial activities of T-3811ME, a novel des-F(6)-quinolone. *Antimicrob Agents Chemother* 43: 1077–1084.

Talwar GP, Raghuvanshi P, Mishra R *et al.* (2000). Polyherbal formulations with wide spectrum antimicrobial activity against reproductive tract infections and sexually transmitted pathogens. *Am J Reprod Immunol* 43: 144–151.

Taylor S, Berridge V (2006). Medicinal plants and malaria: an historical case study of research at the London School of Hygiene and Tropical Medicine in the twentieth century. *Trans R Soc Trop Med Hyg* 100: 707–714.

Thongson C, Davidson PM, Mahakarnchanakul W *et al.* (2004). Antimicrobial activity of ultrasound-assisted solvent-extracted spices. *Lett Appl Microbiol* 39: 401–406.

Thongson C, Davidson PM, Mahakarnchanakul W *et al.* (2005). Antimicrobial effect of Thai spices against *Listeria monocytogenes* and *Salmonella typhimurium* DT104. *J Food Prot* 68: 2054–2058.

Tichy J, Novak J (1998). Extraction, assay, and analysis of antimicrobials from plants with activity against dental pathogens (*Streptococcus* sp.). *J Altern Complement Med* 4: 39–47.

Tshikalange TE, Meyer JJ, Hussein AA (2005). Antimicrobial activity, toxicity and the isolation of a bioactive compound from plants used to treat sexually transmitted diseases. *J Ethnopharmacol* 96: 515–519.

Unal R, Fleming HP, McFeeters RF *et al.* (2001). Novel quantitative assays for estimating the antimicrobial activity of fresh garlic juice. *J Food Prot* 64: 189–194.

Vanden Berghe DA, Vlietinck AJ (1991). Screening methods for antibacterial and antiviral agents from higher plants. In: *Methods in Plant Biochemistry*, Ed. K. Hostettmann, vol. 6, Academic Press, London, pp. 47–69.

Villar A, Mares M, Ri-acuteos JL *et al.* (1987). Antimicrobial activity of benzylisoquinoline alkaloids. *Pharmazie* 42: 248–250.

Vlietinck AJ, De Bruyne T, Apers S, Pieters LA (1998). Plant-derived leading compounds for chemotherapy of human immunodeficiency virus (HIV) infection. *Planta Med* 64: 97–109.

Voravuthikunchai S, Lortheeranuwat A, Jeeju W *et al.* (2004). Effective medicinal plants against enterohaemorrhagic *Escherichia coli* O157: H7. *J Ethnopharmacol* 94: 49–54.

Wallace RJ (2004). Antimicrobial properties of plant secondary metabolites. *Proc Nutr Soc* 63: 621–629.

Whitfield PJ (1996). Novel anthelmintic compounds and molluscicides from medicinal plants. *Trans R Soc Trop Med Hyg*. 90: 596–600.

11

Natural products research in *Helicobacter pylori* infections

Christine M Slover, Bolanle A Adeniyi, Brian J Doyle, Tracie Locklear, Larry H Danziger and Gail B Mahady

Introduction

Epidemiology and clinical syndromes

Helicobacter pylori (HP) is a Gram-negative spiral or helical-shaped, aerobic bacillus that colonises the gastric epithelial surface, and can withstand the stomach's environment by microaerophilic growth capability and high urease activity (IARC Working Group, 1994; Moss and Sood, 2003). *Helicobacter pylori* is considered to be one of the most significant discoveries in the field of gastroenterology of the 20th century (Graham, 1989). HP-induced gastritis has been associated with duodenal ulcer disease, peptic ulcer disease, gastric carcinoma, primary gastric B-cell lymphoma, ischaemic heart disease and hyperemesis gravidarum (Graham, 1989; Goodwin, 1997; Frigo *et al.*, 1998; Laine and Fendrick, 1998; Lindsberg and Grau, 2003).

Current statistics indicate that as much as one-half of the world's population is infected with HP (World Health Organization, 2003). The infection begins early in childhood via the faecal–oral route, and transmission appears to be from person to person. *Helicobacter* infections are more prevalent in developing countries because of poor sanitation, overcrowded living conditions and a lack of clean water supplies (Graham, 1989). Gastritis, the most common finding of HP infections, has one salient feature, an acute or chronic inflammation of the gastric mucosa (Owen, 2003). Individuals infected with HP are predisposed to duodenal ulcer and gastric mucosa-associated lymphoid tissue (MALT) lymphoma caused by a persistent superficial gastritis. Atrophic gastritis predisposes patients to gastric ulcer and adenocarcinoma (Owen, 2003).

Infection with HP is now also accepted as the primary cause of peptic ulcer disease (Graham, 1989). In the United States, 4–5 million people have peptic ulcer disease, and the economic consequences are responsible for approximately $3–4 billion in annual healthcare costs (Isenberg, 2003). The situation in many developing countries is even more dramatic, as HP infections, peptic ulcer disease and gastric cancer are major causes of morbidity, mortality and healthcare expenditures (Frenck and Clemens, 2003). The prevalence of HP infection among children in parts of the developing world exceeds 90% by 5 years of age, e.g. in Ethiopia, HP infection is acquired early in life, with 60% of 4-year-olds being infected, and almost 100% of 12-year-olds (Lindkvist *et al.*, 1996). In addition to the above HP-induced findings, the infection in the developing world appears to be linked with chronic diarrhoea, malnutrition and impaired growth in children (Frenck and Clemens, 2003), as well as a predisposition to other enteric infections, including typhoid fever and cholera.

The treatment of HP has become increasingly more difficult because of the frequency of antibiotic resistance and recurrence after successful treatment. In Peru, the recurrence rate of the infection is as high as 73% even after successful eradication (Ramirez-Ramos *et al.*, 1997). In this instance recurrence is not attributed to antibiotic resistance, but to reinfection of patients. In the United States, resistant HP is also of concern; the *Helicobacter pylori* Antimicrobial Resistance Monitoring Program (HARP) is a multi-centre US network that tracks HP patterns of resistance. HARP recently reported that 34% of 347 HP isolates tested were resistant to one or more antibiotics commonly used to treat HP infections (Duck *et al.*, 2004). In the US most antibiotic resistance is associated with metronidazole and clarithromycin, both standard treatment options for HP. Thus, antibiotic resistance and high reinfection rates strongly argue for the development of new therapeutic modalities to prevent and treat HP infections worldwide.

Natural products in HP research (in-vitro data)

In most developing countries, plant-based medicines are commonly used to treat gastrointestinal ailments, including gastritis, peptic ulcer disease and diarrhoea (Bhamarapravati *et al.*, 2003). Thus, considering the strong association between these conditions and HP infections, it should not be surprising that some plant-based medicines would have activity against HP in vitro.

The first investigation of the in-vitro efficacy of plant extracts against HP was published in 1991 (Cassel-Beraud, 1991). This group reported that extracts of 13 Malagasy medicinal plants were effective against a number of clinical strains of HP in vitro. In 1996, Fabry and coworkers reported that a number of east African medicinal plant extracts had inhibitory effects on the growth of HP in vitro (Fabry *et al.*, 1996). One plant, *Terminalia spinosa* was reported to be the most active, with a minimum inhibitory concentration (MIC) range of 62.5–500 μg/mL. Extracts of *Thymus vulgaris* (aqueous extract) and *Cinnamonum zeylanicum* (alcohol extract) were also reported to inhibit the growth of the bacterium at concentrations of 3.5 mg/mL (Tabak *et al.*, 1996).

In 1997, investigators discovered that common food plants such as garlic, soybean and fresh vegetables may be protective against HP infections (Shinchi *et al.*, 1997; Sivam *et al.*, 1997). An aqueous extract of garlic (*Allium sativum*) inhibited the growth of HP strains at concentrations of 40 μg/mL (Sivam *et al.*, 1997) and MICs of 8–32 μg/mL for garlic oil against several HP strains were reported (O'Gara *et al.*, 2000).

Rabdosia trichocarpa, a traditional remedy for gastric and stomachic complaints in Japan, also inhibits the growth of HP in vitro, because of a diterpene trichorabdal A (Kadota *et al.*, 1997). In 1999, the anti-HP effects of seven Turkish plant extracts, used in folk medicine for the treatment of gastric ailments including peptic ulcers, were reported (Yesilada *et al.*, 1999). Extracts of the flowers of *Cistus laurifolius*, cones of *Cedrus libani*, aerial parts of *Centaurea solstitialis* ssp. *solstitialis*, fruits of *Momordica charantia*, aerial parts of *Sambucus ebulus*, and flowering herbs of *Hypericum perforatum* were active with a MIC range of between 1.95 and 250 μg/mL. In 2003, a screening of 20 plant extracts from Thailand used to treat gastrointestinal ailments reported that over 50% of the plant species tested had anti-HP activity (Bhamarapravati *et al.*, 2003). Methanol extracts of *Myristica fragrans* (aril) inhibited the growth of all HP strains with a MIC of 12.5 μg/mL; extracts from *Barringtonia acutangula* (leaf) and *Kaempferia galanga* (rhizome) had a MIC of 25 μg/mL; *Cassia grandis* (leaf), *Cleome viscosa* (leaf), *Myristica fragrans* (leaf) and *Syzygium aromaticum* (leaf) had MICs of 50 μg/mL. Extracts with a MIC of 100 μg/mL included *Pouzolzia pentandra* (leaf), *Cycas siamensis* (leaf), *Litsea elliptica* (leaf) and *Melaleuca quinquenervia* (leaf) (Bhamarapravati *et al.*, 2003).

Ginger root (*Zingiber officinale*), a plant well known worldwide to treat gastrointestinal ailments, also has activity against HP (Mahady *et al.*, 2003a). Methanol extracts of ginger rhizome inhibited the growth of 19 HP strains in vitro with a MIC range of 6.25–50 μg/mL. The 6-, 8- and 10-gingerols all had varying degrees of activity, with a MIC range of 0.78 to 12.5 μg/mL and interestingly had significant activity against the *CagA* cancer-causing strains (Mahady *et al.*, 2003a). Curcumin, a polyphenolic constituent isolated from turmeric (*Curcuma longa*), and a methanol extract of the dried, powdered turmeric rhizome were both active against 19 strains of HP, including five *CagA* strains. The MIC range was 6.25–50 μg/mL (Mahady *et al.*, 2002). In addition, red wine extract (*Vitis vinifera*) and resveratrol inhibited the growth of HP in vitro (Mahady and Pendland, 2000; Mahady *et al.*, 2003b). Resveratrol, a stilbene present in red wine had a MIC of 25 μg/mL, while the red wine extract had a MIC range of 25–50 μg/mL (Mahady and Pendland, 2000). Interestingly, resveratrol was more active against *CagA* strains of HP than *CagA*− strains (Mahady *et al.*, 2003b).

Two indigenous American plants, *Sanguinaria canadensis* and *Hydrastis canadensis*, used traditionally by the Native American Indians for the treatment of gastrointestinal ailments, have also been shown to be active against HP (Mahady *et al.*, 2003c). Methanol extracts of the rhizome or suspension cell cultures of *S. canadensis* had a MIC range of 12.5–50.0 μg/mL. Three isoquinoline alkaloids were identified in the active fraction. Sanguinarine and chelerythrine, two benzophenanthridine alkaloids, inhibited the growth of the HP, with a MIC of 50 and 100 μg/mL, respectively. Protopine, an alkaloid, also inhibited the growth of bacterium, with a MIC of 100 μg/mL. A crude methanol extract of *H. canadensis* rhizomes was very active, with a MIC of 12.5 μg/mL (range 0.78 to 25 μg/mL). Two isoquinoline alkaloids, berberine and β-hydrastine, were identified as the active constituents, and having a MIC of 12.5 and 100.0 μg/mL, respectively (Mahady *et al.*, 2003c).

The in-vitro susceptibility of 15 HP strains to natural products that had a history of traditional use in the treatment of GI disorders was recently assessed (Mahady *et al.*, 2005). Methanol extracts of *Myristica fragrans* (seed) had a MIC of 12.5 μg/mL and *Rosmarinus officinalis* (rosemary leaf) had a MIC of 25 μg/mL. Methanol extracts of botanicals with a MIC of 50 μg/mL included *Achillea millefolium* (aerial parts), *Foeniculum vulgare* (seed), *Passiflora incarnata* (aerial parts), *Origanum majorana* (herb) and a (1 : 1) combination of *Curcuma longa* (root) and ginger rhizome. Botanical extracts with a MIC of 100 μg/mL included *Carum carvi* (seed), *Elettaria cardamomum* (seed), *Gentiana lutea* (roots), *Juniper communis* (berry), *Lavandula angustifolia* (flowers), *Melissa officinalis* (leaves), *Mentha piperita* (leaves) and *Pimpinella anisum* (seed). Methanol extracts of *Matricaria recutita* (flowers) and *Ginkgo biloba* (leaves) had a MIC of 100 μg/mL (Mahady *et al.*, 2005). A traditional medicine from Iceland, the lichen *Cetaria islandica*, also used to treat gastrointestinal ailments has anti-HP activity (Ingolfsdottir *et al.*, 1997). Protolichesterinic acid, an aliphatic α-methylene-γ-lactone, was identified as one of the active constituents. The MIC range of protolichesterinic acid, in free as well as salt form, was 16–64 μg/mL.

The antibacterial activity of Gosyuyu, a crude extract from the fruit of *Evodia rutaecarpa*, a Chinese herbal medicine, has also been tested for activity against HP in vitro (Hamasaki *et al.*, 2000). Two compounds were identified as the active constituents and were the quinolone alkaloids, 1-methyl-2-[(Z)-8-tridecenyl]-4-(1H)-quinolone and 1-methyl-2-[(Z)-7-tridecenyl]-4-(1H)-quinolone. The MIC of these compounds against reference strains and clinically isolated HP strains was <0.05 μg/mL, similar to that of amoxicillin and clarithromycin (Hamasaki *et al.*, 2000). Finally, in a recent report, screening of 70 medicinal plants from Greece, led to the discovery of a number of plants with anti-HP activity. Extracts of *Anthemis melanolepis, Cerastium candidissimum, Chamomilla recutita, Conyza albida, Dittrichia viscosa, Origanum vulgare* and *Stachys alopecuros* were active against one standard strain and 15 clinical isolates of HP (Stamatis *et al.*, 2003).

In addition to antibacterial activity, tea (*Camellia sinensis*) and rosemary (*Rosmarinus officinalis* L.) extracts inhibit HP urease in vitro. Green tea extract showed the strongest inhibition of HP urease, with a MIC of 13 μg/mL. Active principles were identified as catechins, with the hydroxyl group of 5′ position appearing important for urease inhibition (Matsubara *et al.*, 2003).

In-vivo data

The in-vivo model of choice for HP infections is the Mongolian gerbil model developed by Japanese researchers (Hirayama *et al.*, 1996a,b). This model was a major advancement and has accelerated investigations of the anti-HP activities of natural products. A number of botanical extracts have been tested in this animal model and have been shown to have significant activity. For example, treatment of HP-inoculated Mongolian gerbils with green tea extract in drinking water at concentrations of 500, 1000 and 2000 ppm for 6 weeks, suppressed gastritis and HP load in a dose-dependent manner (Matsubara *et al.*, 2003). The effect of a garlic extract on HP-induced gastritis in this model has also been reported. Garlic extract was fed to gerbils, in rations, at doses of 1%, 2% and 4% in the diet from four hours after HP inoculation until the end of a 6-week experiment. Administration of the garlic extract to these animals reduced HP-induced gastritis in a dose-dependent manner, and was statistically significant at a dose of 4% garlic extract. However, HP bacterial load was not altered by the garlic extract treatment (Iimuro *et al.*, 2002).

The effect of tryptanthrin and kaempferol, two compounds isolated from *Polygonum tinctorium* were assessed in HP-infected Mongolian gerbils. The gerbils were inoculated with HP strain ATCC 43504, and after 4 weeks, the infected gerbils were treated with tryptanthrin and/or kaempferol, by gastric lavage, twice a day for 10 days. The results demonstrated that administration of tryptanthrin and/or kaempferol significantly reduced bacterial load in the gerbils' stomachs (Kataoka *et al.*, 2001).

Clinical data

In terms of human studies, four clinical trials were found that tested the efficacy of natural products for the eradication of HP. Two of the studies tested different preparations of garlic bulbs (*Allium sativum*), one tested an extract of cinnamon, and one tested the efficacy of cranberry juice. In the first study, a group of 20 HP-infected patients suffering from dyspeptic complaints for more than 2 months were treated for 2 weeks with capsules containing an oil macerate of garlic (275 mg, three times a day) (Martin and Ernst, 2003). Garlic alone was compared with the combination of garlic and omeprazole (20 mg, twice a day) for the eradication of HP. All subjects underwent endoscopy prior to and 1 month after the completion of treatment. The presence of HP was confirmed by urease tests and microscopy of biopsy specimens. Symptom scores were recorded pre- and post-treatment as was the degree of gastritis, evaluated by histological examination. Garlic alone and in combination with omeprazole did not result in the elimination of HP, change gastritis severity or significantly change symptom scores (garlic only group 9.2 ± 1.55 versus 8.7 ± 1.70, combination group 9.0 ± 1.49 versus 8.5 ± 1.51) (Martin and Ernst, 2003). This study has several design flaws: it was not randomised, likely not patient-blinded and had a small sample size.

In the second clinical trial, preparations of fresh garlic or capsaicin-containing peppers were tested for their ability to reduce the bacterial load and symptoms in a crossover trial involving 12 individuals infected with HP (Graham *et al.*, 1999). Mexican-style meals including the test substances were given to subjects three times daily. Test subjects participated in a minimum of 3 study days including positive and negative control days and one experimental ingredient study day. During each test meal subjects received one intervention: garlic (10 sliced cloves), capsaicin (six freshly sliced jalapeno peppers), two bismuth subsalicylate tablets (Pepto-Bismol, positive control) or no meal additions (negative control). Urea breath tests were performed prior to the first meal of the day, prior to the evening meal and then the next morning. Ten subjects received garlic, six received jalapenos and 11 received bismuth. There was no significant effect on urease levels pre- and post-intervention in the garlic or jalapenos groups (28.5 versus 39.8 and 43.7 versus 46.6, respectively; $P > 0.8$). There was however a significant reduction in urease levels after subjects received bismuth (55.8 versus 14.3; $P < 0.001$). Two subjects reported severe nausea and diarrhoea after eating meals containing jalapenos. Seventy per cent of subjects who received garlic reported taste disturbances and body odour. Some of the limitations of this study included small sample size and lack of randomisation (Mahady and Pendland, 1999; Martin and Ernst, 2003).

A pilot study tested the effectiveness of treatment with an extract of cinnamon (*Cinnamonum cassia*) in subjects who were undergoing gastroscopy and had a positive urea breath test for HP (Nir *et al.*, 2000). Thirty-two subjects were randomised in a 2 : 1 ratio of study group to control group, but 7 were eventually excluded from the final analysis. Fifteen subjects (11 women, 4 men) received 40 mg of cinnamon extract twice daily and eight subjects (7 women, 1 man) received placebo for 4 weeks. Urea breath tests were repeated at the end of the 4-week study period. Both increased and decreased urea breath test values were reported in both groups, but overall mean values showed no significant changes (study group: 22.1 versus 24.4; control group: 23.9 versus 25.9). Cinnamon extract was well tolerated by the majority of patients. Three patients reported clinical improvement of dyspepsia during treatment (Nir *et al.*, 2000). This trial had a better design overall, but the sample size was still small, increasing the likelihood of type II error (Martin and Ernst, 2003).

The final clinical trial was a prospective, double-blind, randomised placebo-controlled trial to evaluate the efficacy of cranberry juice in treating HP (Zhang *et al.*, 2005). Subjects with positive urea breath tests were randomised to receive either two 250 mL cranberry juice boxes (Ocean Spray, Inc.) daily or a look-alike placebo beverage that simulated the taste of cranberry juice. Duration of treatment was 90 days. A total of 225 subjects were randomised; 112 received placebo (control group) and 113 received cranberry juice (treatment group). Several subjects either withdrew or were excluded from final analysis leaving only 92 in the control group and 97 in the treatment group. Efficacy was evaluated by repeat urea breath tests at 35 and 90 days. Urea breath tests were negative for 14 of 97 (14.43%) subjects in the treatment group at 35 and 90 days compared with 5 of 92 (5.44%) in the placebo group. Eleven of the 14 subjects who were negative for HP in the treatment group were negative on both test days, while only 2 of the 5 subjects in the placebo group were negative on both test days. The investigators concluded that subjects consuming cranberry juice had a better chance of becoming HP negative than those consuming placebo ($\chi^2 = 4.43$; $P = 0.04$) (Zhang *et al.*, 2005). Some subjects did respond to treatment, but overall response to treatment was poor. Cranberry may prove to be effective in treating HP, but in a more concentrated form. This study was however well-designed and contained many of the critical elements that define a good clinical trial. The sample size was much larger in this trial than in any of the previous ones, treatment duration was much longer, subjects were randomised, and both investigators and subjects were blinded.

Methodological issues

In-vitro methods

Susceptibility testing (minimum inhibitory concentration)

To compare results between studies standardisation of methodology is an absolute necessity. To help standardise in-vitro methodology it is recommended to use protocols set forth by the Clinical and Laboratory Standards Institute (CLSI), formerly known as the National Committee for Clinical Laboratory Standards (NCCLS). The agar dilution procedure outlined in this section has been used extensively in our laboratory and others when testing botanicals with good results. The standardised botanical extracts or pure compounds should be dissolved in a minimal volume of solvent. Common solvents used to dissolve the extracts or pure compounds consist of dimethyl sulphoxide (DMSO), methanol, or sterile distilled water. Final concentrations to be tested should range from 1–100 μg/mL (twofold dilutions) for each botanical extract or pure compound. When testing any botanical extract or pure compound, antibiotics used for standard treatment in patients with HP should also be tested to serve as controls; clarithromycin, metronidazole, and amoxicillin are recommended. The final concentration of the antibiotics should be as follows: clarithromycin, 0.001–0.25 μg/mL; amoxicillin, 0.001–0.25 μg/mL; metronidazole, 16–256 μg/mL. One millilitre of each concentration should be added to 19 mL of molten Mueller-Hinton agar (pH 7.3; 50°C) supplemented with 10% sterile defibrinated horse blood (Hartzen *et al.*, 1997; Meyer *et al.*, 1997). In the laminar flow hood, the botanical extract or pure compound and molten agar medium should be thoroughly mixed by gently inverting three times and pouring into sterile Petri dishes. Petri dishes should be left to cool in the laminar flow hood. Growth control plates consisting of 20 mL of agar medium should be included in each experiment. Petri plates incorporating minimal to maximum volumes of any solvents (i.e. DMSO, etc.)

used in dissolving the botanical extracts or pure compounds should be included as growth controls to ensure that the viability of the organisms is not affected by the solvents.

For susceptibility testing, HP should be inoculated on to 5% sheep blood agar plates and incubated at 37°C in a 10% CO_2 atmosphere for at least 3 days. The organisms should be subcultured once to ensure reliable growth. An inoculum of each HP isolate should be prepared by suspending the organism in 4.5 mL of sterile Mueller-Hinton broth and adjusting the turbidity to that of a 2.0 McFarland Standard using a spectrophotometer at 625 nm. This density produces a suspension of approximately 1×10^6 CFU/mL of HP. The isolates are inoculated on to agar plates, containing the botanical extracts, via a 32-prong inoculating device (Steers Replicator). This device delivers 8 μL per spot resulting in a final inoculum of approximately 1×10^4 CFU/spot. After the spots have dried, the plates are incubated at 37°C in 10% CO_2 and examine for growth at 72 h. It is recommended to perform all procedures in duplicate or triplicate. The MIC will be determined for each botanical extract or pure compound. The MIC is defined as the lowest concentration of a botanical extract or pure compound at which there is no visible growth (Mahady *et al.*, 2002, 2003a,b,c; NCCLS, 2005).

Combination studies

Antibiotic resistance against clarithromycin and metronidazole is now routinely observed for HP but can often be overcome with combination treatment. Additive or synergistic interactions between antibiotics can increase eradication rates and may prevent acquired resistance from occurring (Meyer *et al.*, 1997; Pendland *et al.*, 2000). Similarly, botanical extracts or pure compounds may also act synergistically with antibiotics, enhancing antimicrobial activity and reducing the emergence of resistant strains.

Combination effects of botanical extracts or pure compounds and antibiotics should be determined by the agar dilution checkerboard assay and evaluated using fractional inhibitory concentration (FIC) index as described (Kobayashi *et al.*, 1992; Pillai *et al.*, 2005; Botelho, 2000). The MIC protocol remains the same as in the section above with one exception; the agar plates are prepared with 1 mL of botanical extract or pure compound concentration, 1 mL of antibiotic concentration and 18 mL of molten Mueller-Hinton agar (pH 7.3; 50°C) supplemented with 10% sterile defibrinated horse blood (Pillai *et al.*, 2005). It is recommend that the concentrations tested range from five dilutions below the MIC to twice the MIC (MICs are determined by the susceptibility procedures outlined in the section above). Twofold dilutions should again be used. All possible combinations, including a control without any antibiotic, should be tested and performed in duplicate or triplicate. Synergy results should be quantified with the FIC index calculated from both the FIC values of the botanical extracts or pure compounds and antibiotics (Botelho, 2000; Pillai *et al.*, 2005). The FIC index should be used to determine if synergy, addition or antagonism occurs as a result of interactions between the botanical extracts or pure compounds and antibiotics. Using this method, the FIC index is interpreted as follows: $\leqslant$0.5, synergy; $>$0.5–1, additive; $>$1–4, indifference; $>$4, antagonism. Combinations that exert a synergistic effect should undergo further testing using the time-kill methodology. Statistical analyses should be performed using Student's *t* test and $P < 0.05$ is considered significant. In-vitro combination studies will indicate which combinations of botanical extracts or pure compounds and antibiotics would be applicable for in-vivo testing and at what dose.

Bactericidal activity (time-kill studies)

Combinations of botanical extracts or pure compounds and antibiotics that were found to be synergistic in the combination studies should be further tested for bactericidal activity. Time-kill methodology is performed using CLSI/NCCLS guidelines (NCCLS, 2005). HP strain ATCC 43504 is cultured in 10 mL of Brucella broth with 10% fetal bovine serum (FBS) and 0.1% β-cyclodextrin (Sigma) and incubated at 37°C with 10% CO_2 for 24 h (Dai *et al.*, 2005). To ensure optimal growth prior to drug exposure, HP should be subcultured three times into fresh broth and incubated for 24 h each time (NCCLS, 2005). Test tubes containing 10 mL Brucella broth with 10% fetal bovine serum, 0.1% β-cyclodextrin and predetermined concentrations of botanical extract or pure compound and antibiotic (as determined from combination studies described earlier) are inoculated with log-phase growth organisms to obtain a final inoculum of 10^6 CFU/mL. Control tubes should include botanical extract or pure compound, antibiotic, and agent-free broth. For concentrations greater than or equal to the MIC, drug carryover tests should be performed. The final inoculum is confirmed at time 0 and subsequent viable counts should be done at 2, 4, 6, 8, 10, 12 and 24 h. Sampling for viable colony counts is done by removing 0.5 mL samples of the broth at the specified times. The 0.5 mL samples should be serially diluted in test tubes containing 4.5 mL of sterile normal saline to produce tenfold dilutions. A 50 µL aliquot of the dilutions should be inoculated on to 5% sheep blood agar plates using a spiral plater or other plating technique. The plates are incubated at 37°C in 10% CO_2 and colony counts are performed after 3 days. All procedures should be performed in duplicate or triplicate. Killing rates are determined by plotting $\log_{10}$ colony counts (CFU/mL) against time. A bactericidal effect is determined by a $\geqslant 3 \log_{10}$ (99.9% killing) decrease in CFU at the specified time. Synergy is defined as a $\geqslant 2 \log_{10}$ decrease in CFU/mL between the combination and the most active constituent.

In-vivo methods

Animal protocols

To make comparisons between treatment options in HP research, methodologies should be standardised. The following are suggested research approaches which if followed would result in standardised research practices. Treatment with botanical extracts or pure compounds and antibiotics in combination or alone should be based on the data obtained from in-vitro studies. Specific pathogen-free (SPF) Mongolian gerbils, approximately 5–7 weeks old have been used in animal studies (Kataoka *et al.*, 2001; Iimuro *et al.*, 2002; Matsubara *et al.*, 2003). For the experimental inoculation of the gerbil, HP (strain dependent on the results of in-vitro studies), should be grown in Brucella broth supplemented with 2.5% heat-inactivated fetal bovine serum at 37°C for 2–3 days. The gerbils should be fasted for 24 h prior to oral inoculation with sterilised Brucella broth (control) or HP (5×10^6 CFU/mL) applied in a volume of 0.4 mL using an oral catheter. After inoculation, each animal should be fasted another 4 h then given a normal diet. Drinking water can be provided ad lib throughout the entire experiment. A daily dose of the botanical or a combination of antibiotics and botanicals should be administered intragastrically. It is recommended to monitor body weight weekly, diet intake twice weekly, and drink intake three times weekly. The animals should be monitored daily for their general health. Thus, the in-vivo study for each treatment should have a total of five arms per botanical or pure compound:

- negative control group (no HP challenge)
- positive control group (HP challenge but no treatment)
- one arm for antibiotic alone
- one group with botanical alone
- combination treatment group.

The animals should receive their treatments for a total of 2 weeks, starting the day of inoculation or six weeks after the challenge with HP. Both these treatment timelines are needed to assess outcomes of treatment starting immediately after inoculation as opposed to treatment six weeks after inoculation when the infection is well established. At the end of the treatment period, all animals are euthanised under CO_2 and their stomachs resected for histology.

Determination of gastric lesions

Each stomach should be opened along the greater curvature and washed with saline. The macroscopic gastric lesions (oedema and haemorrhage) should be recorded. The stomachs must be opened and pinned for the determination of gastric lesions, oedema and haemorrhage; it is recommended that this is done by two blinded investigators. The macroscopic score is graded as follows:

- 0 = normal
- 1 = mild oedema and haemorrhagic erosions but no gastric ulcers
- 2 = oedema, haemorrhage and gastric ulcers
- 3 = severe oedema, haemorrhage and multiple gastric ulcers.

If gastric lesions are apparent, then liver, spleen and kidney tissues should be assessed. After macroscopic examination of gastric lesions, the measurement of the wet weight of the whole stomach, including forestomach and glandular stomach should be done. Half of the glandular mucosa must be scraped for detection of colonising HP, and the residual part is formalin-fixed and embedded in paraffin for histological observation. Pathological diagnosis of gastritis is made according to the criteria described previously (Israel *et al.*, 2001; Brzozowski *et al.*, 2003).

Detection of H. pylori *colonisation in the gastric mucosa*

To detect HP colonisation in the gastric mucosa of treated and untreated animals, half of the stomach should be excised after examination and homogenised in 1 mL of phosphate-buffered saline using a homogeniser, followed by dilution with PBS. One hundred microlitres of diluted homogenate should be inoculated on to segregating agar plates for HP and incubated at 37°C under microaerobic conditions. After 5 days, colony counts should be performed to determine the level of HP colonisation of each stomach (Brzozowski *et al.*, 2003).

Determination of inflammatory parameters

Infections caused by HP stimulate an overproduction of pro-inflammatory cytokines causing inflammation. HP challenge is also associated with an over-expression of COX-2 in the gastric mucosal tissues (Aguilera *et al.*, 2001). Data indicate that HP-induced inflammation, acute and/or chronic, can be decreased by standardised botanical extracts. HP-induced inflammation is mediated by elevated pro-inflammatory cytokines (including IL-β, IL-6, IL-8 and TNF-α) and prostaglandin E2 (PGE2). The transcription factor NF-κB and the MAPK cascade appear to augment cytokine and prostaglandin production (Seo *et al.*, 2004). In-vitro data indicate that selected botanical extracts or pure compounds inhibit NF-κB transcriptional response, and release of IL-β, IL-6, IL-8 and TNF-α. Therefore, enzyme-linked immunoassay (ELISA) should be used to measure concentrations of IL-1, TNF-α and PGE2 in serum and tissue. The mRNA expression of IL-1, IL-6, IL-8, TNF-α and COX-2 should be measured in gastric tissues and liver, using reverse transcriptase PCR to assess how the botanical extracts affect HP-induced inflammation and the nuclear fraction of these tissues should be isolated with an electrophoretic mobility shift assay (EMSA), completed to measure NF-κB.

Prior to sacrifice, blood should be collected from the gerbils by cardiac puncture (8–10 mL) and microcentrifuged to separate the serum. The serum should be stored at −70 °C until needed for further analysis. To measure tissue cytokine and prostaglandin concentrations (IL, TNF, and PGE2) in the gastric and liver tissues, the tissue must be homogenised. The tissue sample (0.1 g) should be homogenised at 25 000 rpm in TRIS lysis buffer containing protease-inhibitor cocktail for 2 min. Samples should then be centrifuged for 10 min at 10 000 × *g* and tissue TNF, IL and PGE_2 concentrations will be determined using ELISA kits. Results should be expressed as milligrams of cytokine per gram of tissue.

The mRNA expression of IL, TNF-α and COX-2 in the gastric mucosa and liver are quantitated by RT-PCR normalised for the housekeeping gene GAPDH densitometry. mRNA should be isolated using TRIzol (Gibco Invitrogen Corp., Carlsbad, CA) according to manufacturer instructions. The amount and quality of the mRNA is confirmed by spectrophotometer analysis (optical density 1.8–2.0) and agarose gel electrophoresis. Each sample should then be reverse transcribed using the GeneAmp RNA PCR kit (Perkin Elmer, Foster City, CA). The RT reaction consists of cycling for 15 min at 42°C, followed by 95°C for 5 min and finished by 5°C for 5 min in a thermocycler. For the PCR analyses, each primer pair is tested to determine the annealing temperature and the linear reaction range. The PCR reaction includes heating to 95°C for 105 s to activate the Taq polymerase, then through approximately 25 cycles of heating and cooling from 99°C for 15 s to 60°C for 30 s. Holding at 72°C for 7 min completes the reaction. The linearity of the PCR reaction should be checked during various cycles. The PCR products are then separated by electrophoresis on a 1% agarose gel stained with ethidium bromide to quantify the intensity of the banding pattern. The gels should then be scanned into a densitometer for semi-quantitative analysis of the mRNA expression.

Nuclear protein extracts should be prepared from gastric and liver tissue using aliquots of frozen tissue mixed with liquid nitrogen and ground to powder using a mortar and pestle. Solution A (4 mL, 0.6% NP-40, 150 mmol/L NaCl, 10 mmol/L HEPES [pH 7.9], 1 mmol/L EDTA, 0.5 mmol/L PMSF) is added to the contents in the mortar and then all of the contents are placed in a tissue homogeniser. Five strokes of the pestle should lyse the cells. Transfer the contents to a 15-mL tube and centrifuge at 2000 rpm for 30 s to form a pellet. The supernatant containing intact nuclei should then be transferred to 50-mL Corex tubes, incubated on ice for 5 min, and centrifuged for 10 min at 5000 rpm. The nuclear pellets are then resuspended in solution B (300 L, 25% glycerol, 20 mmol/L HEPES [pH 7.9], 420 mmol/L NaCl, 1.2 mmol/L $MgCI_2$, 0.2 mmol/L EDTA, 0.5 mmol/L DTT, 0.5 mmol/L PMSF, 2 mmol/L benzamidine, 0.5 g/mL pepstatin, 0.5 g/mL leupeptin, 0.5 g/mL aprotinin) and incubated on ice for 30 min. The mixture is then transferred to micro-centrifuge tubes and the nuclei are pelleted by centrifugation at 14 000 rpm for 1 min. Supernatants containing nuclear proteins should then be aliquoted and stored at −70°C for further analysis.

EMSA is used to measure the presence of NF-κB in the nucleus (Novak *et al.*, 2002; Babcock *et al.*, 2003). For each sample, 5–10 μg of total nuclear protein should be incubated with the labelled double-stranded probe and 5 μg of poly(dI-dC) in binding buffer for 20 min at 25°C. Specific competition should be done by adding 100 ng of unlabelled NF-κB or AP-1 double-stranded binding probe to the reaction. The mixtures are then run on a 5% poly-acrylamide gel electrophoresis in ×1 Tris-glycine-EDTA buffer (NF-κB) or 0.25mult Tris-borate-EDTA buffer (AP-1). The gels should then be vacuum-dried and exposed to radiographic film.

Clinical studies

Once in-vitro and in-vivo studies have been completed and the tested compound has shown adequate anti-HP activity, controlled clinical trials in subjects infected with HP should be performed. The studies that are available in the literature are lacking, in that they are poorly designed (Martin and Ernst, 2003).

Prior to attempting human studies, standardised botanical extracts or pure compounds must be developed based on in-vitro and animal data. Clinical studies should have both a control group (no treatment or standard treatment) and the necessary treatment groups (active botanicals). Clinical trials should be double-blinded to eliminate investigator or study subject biases (Powers, 2005). Subjects should be randomised into control and treatment groups. Sample size is an important consideration too when developing a trial, the number of subjects enrolled should be large enough to detect differences between the treatment groups but small enough not to incur more expense. Type I error is usually set at less than 0.05 (also known as alpha), this means there is a 5% chance that the study results were coincidental.

Subjects enrolled into clinical trials should have documented infection by HP (Martin and Ernst, 2003). A diagnostic test, such as a urea breath test or endoscopy, should be done prior to the study beginning and repeated again at the end of treatment. Clinical symptoms of HP infection (dyspepsia, stomach ache, etc.) should be collected prior to treatment and again at the completion of treatment to access any improvements. Any side-effects reported by study subjects should be recorded. Treatment durations can vary depending on whether the botanical or pure compound is being used alone (longer durations of treatment required) or in combination with antibiotics (usually 7–14 days), but should be for an appropriate amount of time as deemed by the investigators. Diagnostic tests should be repeated 4–6 weeks after the completion of treatment along with a repeat assessment of clinical symptoms.

Conclusions

HP infection is of great concern worldwide because of its association with gastric cancer (Owen, 2003). Resistance to available antimicrobials is on the rise not only in the United States but in developing countries (Duck *et al.*, 2004). This increase in resistance has opened the door for research into herbal medicines. In recent years there have been numerous in-vitro studies published describing herbal medicine activity against HP. These studies have led to animal research and some clinical studies in humans. There is a great need for continued study in this area. Included in this chapter are some recommended standardised procedures for the study of herbal products against HP.

References

Aguilera A, Codoceo R, Bajo MA, *et al.* (2001). *Helicobacter pylori* infection: a new cause of anorexia in peritoneal dialysis patients. *Perit Dial Int* 21 (supp. 3): S152–S156.

Babcock TA, Kurland A, Helton WS, *et al.* (2003). Inhibition of activator protein-1 transcription factor activation by Omega-3 fatty acid modulated of mitogen-activated protein kinases signaling kinases. *J Parenter Enteral Nutr* 27: 176–180.

Bhamarapravati S, Pendland SL, Mahady GB (2003). Extracts of spice and food plants from Thai traditional medicine inhibit the growth of the human carcinogen *Helicobacter pylori*. *Vivo* 17: 541–544.

Botelho MG (2000). Fractional inhibitory concentration index of combinations of antibacterial agents against cariogenic organisms. *J Dent* 28: 565–570.

Brzozowski T, Konturek PC, Kwiecien S, *et al.* (2003). Tripe eradication therapy counteracts functional impairment associated with *Helicobacter pylori* infection in Mongolian gerbils. *J Physiol Pharmacol* 54: 33–51.

Cassel-Beraud AM, Le Jan J, Mouden JC, *et al.* (1991). Preliminary study of the prevalence of *Helicobacter pylori* in Tananarive, Madagascar and the antibacterial activity in vitro of 13 Malagasy medicinal plants on this germ. *Arch Inst Pasteur Madagascar* 59: 9–23.

Dai G, Cheng N, Dong L, *et al.* (2005). Bactericidal and morphological effects of NE-2001, a novel synthetic agent directed against *Helicobacter pylori*. *Antimicrob Agents Chemother* 49: 3468–3473.

Duck WM, Sobel J, Pruckler JM, *et al.* (2004). Antimicrobial resistance incidence and risk factors among *Helicobacter pylori*-infected persons, United States. *Emerg Infect Dis* 10 (6): 1088–1094.

Fabry W, Okemo P, Ansorg R (1996). Activity of East African medicinal plants against *Helicobacter pylori*. *Chemotherapy* 42: 315–317.

Frenck RW, Clemens J (2003). *Helicobacter* in the developing world. *Microbes Infect* 5: 705–713.

Frigo P, Lang C, Reisenberger K, *et al.* (1998). Hyperemesis gravidarum associated with *Helicobacter pylori* seropositivity. *Obstet Gynecol* 91: 615–617.

Goodwin CS (1997). *Helicobacter pylori* gastritis, peptic ulcer, and gastric cancer: clinical and molecular aspects. *Clin Infect Dis* 25: 1017–1019.

Graham DY (1989). Evolution of concepts regarding *Helicobacter pylori*: from a cause of gastritis to a public health problem. *Am J Gastroenterol* 89: 469–472.

Graham DY, Anderson SY, Lang T (1999). Garlic or jalapeno peppers for treatment of *Helicobacter pylori* infection. *Am J Gastroenterol* 94: 1200–1202.

Hamasaki N, Ishii E, Tominaga K, *et al.* (2000). Highly selective antibacterial activity of novel alkyl quinolone alkaloids from a Chinese herbal medicine, Gosyuyu (Wu-Chu-Yu), against *Helicobacter pylori in vitro*. *Microbiol Immunol* 44: 9–15.

Hartzen HS, Anderson LP, Bremmelgaard A (1997). Antimicrobial susceptibility testing of 230 *Helicobacter pylori* strains: importance of medium, inoculum, and incubation time. *Antimicrob Agents Chemother* 41: 2634–2639.

Hirayama F, Takagi S, Yokoyama Y, *et al.* (1996a). Establishment of gastric *Helicobacter pylori* infection in Mongolian gerbils. *J Gastroenterol* 31 (supp. 9): 24–28.

Hirayama F, Takagi S, Kusuhara H, *et al.* (1996b). Induction of gastric ulcer and intestinal metaplasia in Mongolian gerbils infected with *Helicobacter pylori*. *J Gastroenterol* 31: 755–757.

Hohenberger P, Gretschel S (2003). Gastric cancer. *Lancet* 362: 305–315.

IARC Working Group (1994). Schistosomes, liver flukes and *Helicobacter pylori*. IARC Working Group on the Evaluation of Carcinogenic Risks to Humans, Lyon, June 7–14. *IARC Monogr Eval Carcinog Risks Hum* 61: 1–241.

Iimuro M, Shibata H, Kawamori T, *et al.* (2002). Suppressive effects of garlic extract on *Helicobacter pylori*-induced gastritis in Mongolian gerbils. *Cancer Lett* 187: 61–68.

Ingolfsdottir K, Hjalmarsdottir MA, Sigurdsson A, *et al.* (1997). *In vitro* susceptibility of *Helicobacter pylori* to protolichesterinic acid from the lichen *Cetraria islandica*. *Antimicrob Agents Chemother* 41: 215–217.

Isenberg JI (1991). Acid-peptic disorders. In: Yamada T, Alpers D H, Owyang C, eds. *Textbook of Gastroenterology*. Philadelphia: JB Lippincott Co, 1231–1349.

Israel D, Salama N, Arnold C, *et al.* (2001). *Helicobacter pylori* strain-specific differences in genetic content, identified by microarray, influence host inflammatory responses. *J Clin Invest* 107: 611–620.

Jonkers D, van den Broek E, van Dooren I, *et al.* (1999). Antibacterial effect of garlic and omeprazole on *Helicobacter pylori*. *J Antimicrob Chemother* 43: 837–839.

Kadota S, Basnet P, Ishii E, *et al.* (1997). Antibacterial activity of trichorabdal A from *Rabdosia trichocarpa* against *Helicobacter pylori*. *Zentralbl Bakteriol* 286: 63–67.

Kataoka M, Hirata K, Kunikata T, *et al.* (2001). Antibacterial action of tryptanthrin and kaempferol, isolated from the indigo plant (*Polygonum tinctorium* Lour.), against *Helicobacter pylori*-infected Mongolian gerbils. *J Gastroenterol* 36: 5–9.

Kobayashi Y, Uchida H, Kawakami Y (1992). Synergy with aztreonam and arbekacin or tobramycin against *Pseudomonas aeruginosa* isolated from blood. *J Antimicrob Chemother* 30: 871–872.

Laine L, Fendrick AM (1998). *Helicobacter pylori* peptic ulcer disease. Bridging the gap between knowledge and treatment. *Postgrad Med* 103: 231–238.

Lindkvist P, Asrat D, Nilsson I, *et al.* (1996). Age acquisition of *Helicobacter pylori* infection: comparison of a high and a low prevalence country. *Scand J Infect Dis* 28: 181–184.

Lindsberg PJ, Grau AJ (2003). Inflammation and infections as risk factors for ischemic stroke. *Stroke* 4: 2518–2532.

Mahady GB, Pendland SL (1999). Garlic and *Helicobacter pylori*. *Am J Gastroenterol* 95: 309–310.

Mahady GB, Pendland SL (2000). Red wine and resveratrol inhibit the growth of *Helicobacter pylori in vitro*. *Am J Gastroenterol* 95: 1849.

Mahady GB, Pendland SL, Yun G, *et al.* (2002). Turmeric (*Curcuma longa*) and curcumin inhibit the growth of *Helicobacter pylori*, a group 1 carcinogen. *Anticancer Res* 22: 4179–4181.

Mahady GB, Pendland SL, Yun GS, *et al.* (2003a). Ginger (*Zingiber officinale* Roscoe) and the gingerols inhibit the growth of Cag A strains of *Helicobacter pylori*. *Anticancer Res* 23: 3699–3702.

Mahady GB, Pendland SL, Chadwick LR, (2003b). Resveratrol and red wine extracts inhibit the growth of *CagA* strains of *Helicobacter pylori in vitro*. *Am J Gastroenterol* 98: 1440–1441.

Mahady GB, Pendland SL, Stoia A, *et al.* (2003c). In vitro susceptibility of *Helicobacter pylori* to isoquinoline alkaloids from *Sanguinaria canadensis* and *Hydrastis canadensis*. *Phytother Res* 17: 217–221.

Mahady GB, Pendland SL, Stoia A, *et al.* (2005). In vitro susceptibility of *Helicobacter pylori* to botanical extracts used traditionally for the treatment of gastrointestinal disorders. *Phytother Res* 19: 988–991.

Martin K, Ernst E (2003). Herbal medicines for treatment of bacterial infections: a review of controlled clinical trials. *J Antimicrob Chemother* 51: 241–246.

Matsubara S, Shibata H, Ishikawa F, *et al.* (2003). Suppression of *Helicobacter pylori*-induced gastritis by green tea extract in Mongolian gerbils. *Biochem Biophys Res Commun* 310: 715–719.

Meyer JM, Ryu S, Pendland SL (1997). In vitro synergy testing of clarithromycin and 14-hydroxyclarithromycin with amoxicillin or bismuth subsalicylate against *Helicobacter pylori*. *Antimicrob Agents Chemother* 41: 1607–1608.

Moss SF, Sood S (2003). *Helicobacter pylori*. *Curr Opin Infect Dis* 16: 445–451.

National Committee for Clinical Laboratory Standards (NCCLS) (1999). *Methods for Determining Bactericidal Activity of Antimicrobial Agents; Approved Guideline*. NCCLS document M26-A. National Committee for Clinical Laboratory Standards, Wayne, PA.

National Committee for Clinical Laboratory Standards (2003). *Methods for Dilution Antimicrobial Susceptibility Tests for Bacteria that Grow Aerobically*, 6th ed. Approved standard M7-A6. National Committee for Clinical Laboratory Standards, Wayne, PA.

National Committee for Clinical Laboratory Standards. Clinical Laboratory Standards Institute/NCCLS (2005). *Performance Standards for Antimicrobial Susceptibility Testing*, 15th informational supplement. CLSI/NCCLS document M100-S15. Clinical and Laboratory Standards Institute, Wayne, PA.

Nir Y, Potasman I, Stermer E, *et al.* (2000). Controlled trial of the effect of cinnamon extract on *Helicobacter pylori*. *Helicobacter* 5: 94–97.

Novak TE, Babcock TA, Jho DH, *et al.* (2002). NF-κB inhibition by Omega-3 fatty acids modulates LPS-stimulated macrophages TNF-α transcription. *Am J Physiol Lung Cell Mol Physiol* 284 (1): L84–89.

O'Gara EA, Hill DJ, Maslin DJ (2000). Activities of garlic oil, garlic powder, and their diallyl constituents against *Helicobacter pylori*. *Appl Environ Microbiol* 66(5): 2269–2273.

Owen DA (2003). Gastritis and carditis. *Mod Pathol* 16: 325–341.

Pendland SL, Prause JL, Neuhauser MN, *et al.* (2000). In vitro activities of a new ketolide, ABT-773, alone and in combination with amoxicillin, metronidazole, or tetracycline against *Helicobacter pylori*. *Antimicrob Agents Chemother* 44: 2518–2520.

Pillai SK, Moellering RC, Eliopoulis GM (2005). Antimicrobial combinations. In: Lorian V, ed. *Antibiotics in laboratory medicine*, 5th ed. Philadelphia: Lippincott Williams & Wilkins, 365–440.

Powers JH (2005). Interpreting the results of clinical trials on antimicrobial agents. In: Mandell G L, Bennett J E, Dolin R, eds. *Mandell, Bennett, & Dolin: Principles and Practice of Infectious Diseases*, 6th ed. Philadelphia: Churchill Livingstone, 619–628.

Ramirez-Ramos A, Gilman RH, Leon-Barua R, *et al.* (1997). Rapid recurrence of *Helicobacter pylori* infection in Peruvian patients after successful eradication. *Clin Infect Dis* 25: 1027–1031.

Seo JH, Lim JW, Kim H, *et al.* (2004). *Helicobacter pylori* in a Korean isolate activates mitogen-activated protein kinases, AP-1, and NF-κB and induces chemokine expression in gastric epithelial AGS cells. *Lab Invest* 84: 49–62.

Shinchi K, Ishii H, Imanishi K, *et al.* (1997). Relationship of cigarette smoking, alcohol use, and dietary habits with *Helicobacter pylori* in Japanese men. *Scand J Gastroenterol* 32: 651–655.

Sivam GP, Lampe JW, Ulness B, *et al.* (1997). *Helicobacter pylori* – in vitro susceptibility to garlic (*Allium sativum*) extract. *Nutr Can* 27: 118–121.

Stamatis G, Kyriazopoulos P, Golegou S, *et al.* (2003). In vitro anti-*Helicobacter pylori* activity of Greek herbal medicines. *J Ethnopharmacol* 88: 175–179.

Tabak M, Armon R, Potasman I, *et al.* (1996). In vitro inhibition of *Helicobacter pylori* by extracts of thyme. *J Appl Bacteriol* 80: 667–672.

World Health Organization (2003). *World Health Report*. WHO, Geneva, Switzerland, 1–50.

Yesilada E, Gurbuz I, Shibata H (1999). Screening of Turkish antiulcerogenic folk remedies for anti-*Helicobacter pylori* activity. *J Ethnopharmacol* 66: 289–293.

Zhang L, Ma J, Pan K, *et al.* (2005). Efficacy of cranberry juice on *Helicobacter pylori* infection: a double-blind, randomized placebo-controlled trial. *Helicobacter* 10: 139–145.

12

Evaluation of the efficacy of herbal medicinal products used to treat cardiovascular diseases

Subir Kumar Maulik and Mohua Maulik

Introduction

Cardiovascular diseases (CVD) constitute one of the major causes of disability and death all over the world. Increased mechanisation, Westernisation of lifestyle and genetic factors, coupled with an increase in life expectancy owing to control of infectious diseases, have contributed to its rise in the developing world as well.

Despite remarkable advances in the identification of various risk factors and our enhanced knowledge regarding the aetiopathogenesis of CVD and molecular targeting for drug development, effective drug management of CVD still eludes medical researchers. There continues to be an unmet need for better and safer drugs to treat as well as to prevent CVD. In this regard, it is important to remember that many of the CVD are preventable, either by lifestyle modification and/or by drugs.

The past few decades have witnessed the introduction of a remarkable number of not only new drugs, but also new classes of drugs, for the treatment of CVD. These include calcium-channel blockers, angiotensin-converting enzyme inhibitors, angiotensin-receptor blockers, various hypolipidaemic agents, and various antiplatelet drugs. On the other hand, a few of the older drugs, such as digoxin, the first to be introduced to treat heart failure, have taken a back seat, not only because of their serious side-effect profile, as well as the discovery of safer and more effective drugs, but also as a consequence of improved understanding of CVD mechanisms.

Herbal medicine and CVD

Cardiovascular drugs include many whose origin can be traced to natural sources, e.g. digoxin (*Digitalis purpurea*), reserpine (*Rauwolfia serpentina*), aspirin (bark of willow *Salix* spp.) and taxol (*Taxus brevifolia*), the last one being used in drug-eluting stents to prevent restenosis following coronary angioplasty. All these examples demonstrate the vast potential of herbal products, their extracts and active principles in the management of CVD.

In many countries, there is a rich tradition of herbal medicine, and herbal preparations are available to patients, for which a prescription from a medical practitioner is not required. Moreover, many of these herbal preparations are prescribed legally by practitioners of some locally recognised alternative systems of medicine but, unfortunately, authentic information about the source and reliability of these herbal preparations is very often not available. Even in many developing countries, over-the-counter herbal preparations are widely used, but have hardly any regulatory control. In view of these issues, there is a global need for adopting guidelines for screening for efficacy, safety and quality (standardisation) of these preparations.

In this chapter, screening methods for herbal products for ischaemic heart disease, hypertension and heart failure are discussed. Cardiac arrhythmias and some cardiomyopathies are not dealt with here because of their more complex aetiopathogenesis and lower incidence, respectively.

Screening for efficacy of herbal preparations in CVD

There is a need to reconsider and reassess our traditional approach for identifying pharmacological activities with reference to our current knowledge and understanding of CVD. For instance, about a half-century ago, drugs with potential positive inotropic effect were thought to be useful candidates for use in heart failure, but today, beta-blockers, which are primarily cardiodepressants, are preferred over positive inotropic agents, even in advanced stages of heart failure! Therefore, understanding the pathological processes behind these diseases is essential before embarking on the task of screening for pharmacological effects. Hence, this chapter first familiarises the reader with the current understanding of different CVDs, to enable informed decision regarding the choice of model best suited to the plant under scrutiny and its particular potential properties.

Ischaemic heart disease

Ischaemic heart disease (IHD) develops largely because of the reduction in blood supply to the heart muscles, mostly caused by narrowing of the coronary arteries by atherosclerosis. Atherosclerosis is a chronic condition associated with accumulation of lipids in blood vessels, leading to the occlusion of blood flow and much focus has been on the role of low-density lipoprotein (LDL), and of oxidatively modified LDL, in the initiation and progression of this disease. LDL is in fact a metabolic end-product of the triglyceride-rich lipoproteins (i.e., very-low-density lipoproteins) but triglycerides are also implicated as contributors to atherosclerosis (Le and Walter, 2007).

Atherosclerosis starts very early in life, but the rapidity with which the disease advances may vary from individual to individual, depending on their genetic make up and other modifiable risk factors, such as diet, physical activity and dyslipidaemia. Therefore, lifestyle modifications, alone or in combination with drugs, are crucial in positively modulating this crucial factor of IHD (Genest, 2000).

Screening for hypolipidaemic activities

Dyslipidaemia and atherosclerosis are major initiating factors of IHD, and presently, even in normolipidaemic patients, certain hypolipidaemic drugs, such as statins, have been found to be useful in reducing acute events (Inoue and Node, 2007). Any indication regarding whether a plant extract can positively modulate the lipid levels, particularly the HDL-C levels, may be useful in obtaining important preliminary information about the therapeutic potential of a plant. Faecal concentrations of cholesterol and any effect on HMG-CoA reductase activity may be carried out (Visavadiya and Narasimhacharya, 2007).

Several models are available currently to detect hypolipidaemic activities (Yanni, 2000; Moghadasian *et al.*, 2001; Russell and Proctor, 2006) but most animal models involve cholesterol-enriched, diet-induced hyperlipidaemia. Either the plant extracts are administered along with cholesterol-enriched diet (pretreatment) or after hyperlipidaemia (post-treatment) has set in.

The pretreatment schedule helps to bring forward any potential preventive property regarding the development of dyslipidaemia, while the post-treatment protocol indicates the curative potential, if any. Both these protocols are valuable, but a practical difficulty associated with the diet-induced hyperlipidaemia model is that lipid levels tend to return to normal once the cholesterol-enriched diet is discontinued.

If any positive effect of a herbal product is observed on total-cholesterol, LDL-cholesterol, VLDL-cholesterol and HDL-cholesterol levels, it is worth carrying the investigation further. In addition, screening for effects on LpA and oxidised LDL are also useful as they play critical roles in the pathogenesis of CVD (Siess, 2006). Oxidised LDL is difficult to assess in animal models, as suitable immunoassay kits are not available from reliable sources. An ELISA method using anti-oxLDL monoclonal antibodies (mAb) has been described by Gidlund *et al.* (1996). As an alternative, in-vitro oxidisability of LDL fraction and the effect of the plant extract on it may be used (Yuan and Kitts, 2002; Hidiroglou *et al.*, 2004).

Rats are very resistant to development of hyperlipidaemia by cholesterol-enriched diet. This may be because the lipid metabolism of rats is primarily based on HDL, rather than on LDL (as in humans), which possibly offers resistance to the development of atherosclerosis. This is also true for mice. However, there are a few researchers who have reported success in this matter (Bennani-Kabchi *et al.*, 2000; El-Beshbishy *et al.*, 2006; Singab *et al.*, 2006).

Rabbits are more widely used for this purpose (Kolodgie *et al.*, 1996; Kaminura, 1999). Larger mammals, such as minipigs, have also been used (Theilmeier, 2002). A variety of genetic models of hyperlipidaemia, particularly in mice, have been used and are probably the most suitable (Zhang *et al.*, 1992; Schreyer *et al.*, 1998; Jiang *et al.*, 2003; Johansson *et al.*, 2005).

As atherosclerosis is the root cause of IHD, any plant extract having antiatherosclerotic property will be worth investigating. The different stages of atherosclerosis, from fatty streaks to full-blown lesions can be used for screening, and can underscore the usefulness of a plant product in preventing the progression of atherosclerosis. In addition to macroscopic and microscopic studies to assess the effects on atherosclerosis in large blood vessels, e.g. the aorta, estimation of certain biochemical markers in the aortic tissue is also helpful in further establishing the credentials of the plant product.

Levels of some major oxidative stress parameters, such as malondialdehyde, superoxide dismutase, catalase and glutathione, provide important information (Antonello *et al.*, 2007) about how the plant product may benefit the 'microenvironment' in the arterial wall in preventing the oxidation of the LDL particles. As mentioned above, this latter phenomenon is a major aetiopathological factor in the initiation and progression of atherosclerosis (Siess, 2006). Effects of the plant product on certain cell adhesion molecules are important, because in IHD, platelet clot formation is initiated by these compounds, released in large amounts from an unstable atherosclerotic plaque (Kraaijeveld *et al.*, 2007).

Screening for coronary vasodilator activity

Plant products having coronary vasodilator activity can be useful as 'add-on' therapy in established cases of IHD. The Langendorff method is widely used for this purpose and is probably the oldest method for screening usefulness of a drug candidate in IHD.

The Langendorff in-vitro coronary vasodilator activity measurement

Langendorff (1895) set up the first isolated mammalian heart and the goal of experiments using it is to provide the isolated heart with oxygen and metabolites via a single cannula inserted into the ascending aorta. Blood or an oxygenated perfusate is flushed down the aorta towards the heart using an external pump. As a consequence of the retrograde perfusion of the aorta, the aortic valve closes, forcing the fluid into the coronary arteries during the diastolic period as it does in the normal cardiac cycle. The perfusate flows through the coronary system finally exiting via the coronary sinus in the right atrium.

In the 1960s, Neely *et al.* (1967) adapted the method which has since been used extensively, with a number of modifications (Zimmer, 1998). As autonomic control is absent in the isolated heart, it helps in understanding whether any vasodilator activity acts directly on the coronary arteries or not. Mechanistic studies may reveal whether the vasodilator action is mediated through nitric oxide (NO) activity (by studies in the presence or absence of NO synthase inhibitors), calcium-channel blocking, and alpha-blocking activity or through other mechanism(s). Vasodilatory effects may be measured by traditional methods or by more sophisticated electromagnetic or Doppler flow probes.

Screening for anti-ischaemic effects

Langendorff's method may also be used to identify any anti-ischaemic effect (other than coronary vasodilator activity) (Gauthaman *et al.*, 2001; Rajlakshmi *et al.*, 2003; Devi *et al.*, 2005). In the isolated heart, both global and regional ischaemia can be produced by stopping the flow (global) or ligating any coronary artery, usually the left anterior descending coronary artery (regional). Ischaemia can be induced permanently or coronary circulation can be reinstituted after a defined period of ischaemia. The latter is a model for ischaemic-reperfusion injury of heart.

Ischaemic-reperfusion injury (IR injury) constitutes a major pathological process in IHD and occurs when coronary flow is re-established after a period of ischaemia, caused spontaneously or by drugs or by other interventions, e.g. angioplasty and coronary artery bypass surgery. IR injury is responsible for acute adverse outcomes (such as cardiac arrhythmias, sometimes leading to cardiac standstill) or chronic adverse effects, such as stunned myocardium (reduced cardiac contractility in the absence of any coronary flow deficit) and, if it occurs repeatedly, it may lead to left ventricular dysfunction (heart failure).

Plant products may be screened for their effect(s), if any, on various parameters of IR injury, using different protocols involving variations in duration of ischaemia (from 20 min to a few hours) (Maulik *et al.*, 2001; Kumari *et al.*, 2004). Various haemodynamic, biochemical and pathological parameters can be measured to assess the degree of IR injury and the effects of any interventions. Haemodynamic parameters include left ventricular pressure, left ventricular developed pressure, left ventricular dP/dt (the rate of rise of left ventricular pressure) (all indices of left ventricular systolic functions) and left ventricular end-diastolic pressure (LVEDP) and left ventricular–dP/dt (the rate of fall of left ventricular pressure) (all indices of left ventricular diastolic functions). Biochemical parameters, such as oxidative stress parameters (mentioned earlier), cell adhesion molecules, heat shock protein 72 (HSP72) and nuclear factor (NF)-κB, can provide mechanistic information.

Pathological parameters are useful for assessing cell viability. TTC stain is widely used in differentiating between viable and dead tissue (Khalil *et al.*, 2006).

Light microscope examinations are essential to identify gross morphological changes, while electron microscopic studies help in identifying the effects on smaller subcellular structures, such as mitochondria and sarcoplasmic reticulum and sarcolemmal integrity. Immunohistochemical studies are widely practised these days to localise the expression of pathological substances inside the cell (Banerjee *et al.*, 2002).

Screening for cardiac preconditioning effect

Cardiac preconditioning is a very recently discovered phenomenon and is helpful in offering protection against cardiac ischaemia. By virtue of this phenomenon, repeated episodes of short-term ischaemia offer protection against any subsequent more severe ischaemic episode. Cardiac preconditioning can help to reduce infarct size and cardiac arrhythmias, as well as preserving left ventricular function following acute myocardial infarction (Rezkalla and Kloner, 2005; Bolli, 2007).

Various cellular mechanisms responsible for cardiac preconditioning have been identified, which include removal of reactive oxygen species (ROS) or reduced mitochondrial ROS production (Halestrap *et al.*, 2007), reduced release of activated neutrophils, reduced apoptosis and better microcirculatory perfusion compared with non-preconditioned tissue (Pasupathy and Vanniasinkam, 2005), activation of nitric oxide synthase (Cohen *et al.*, 2006), K channel activation (Das and Sarkar, 2007), induction of heat shock protein (HSP72) (Miller, 2001; Gauthaman *et al.*, 2005) and augmentation of endogenous antioxidants (Dhalla *et al.*, 2000a).

Although cardiac preconditioning occurs spontaneously, many drugs have been shown to induce cardiac preconditioning in the normal heart and it represents one of the most powerful cardioprotective phenomena. Hence, 'preconditioning mimetic' drugs may have a promising future in simulating ischaemic preconditioning and thereby providing a powerful tool against myocardial damage.

However, despite the effectiveness of ischaemic preconditioning and 'preconditioning mimetics' for protecting ischaemic myocardium, there are no preconditioning-based therapies that are routinely used in clinical medicine at the current time (Kloner and Rezkalla, 2006). In this regard, medicinal plants may be the ideal source for such agents since they are relatively safe to consume and hence may be given on a long-term basis to IHD patients.

Many plants, such as *Allium sativum* (Banerjee *et al.*, 2002; 2003; Saravanan and Prakash, 2004;) *Emblica officinalis* (Bhattacharya *et al.*, 2002; Rajak *et al.*, 2004) and *Terminala arjuna* (Karthikeyan *et al.*, 2003; Gauthaman *et al.*, 2005) have been shown to have significant antioxidant properties. Chronic administration of these agents in animals (rats) offers protection against subsequent in-vitro and in-vivo ischaemic injury and ischaemic-reperfusion injury. These agents augment the level of endogenous antioxidants of the heart on chronic administration, which subsequently prevented oxidative stress induced by ischaemic-reperfusion injury (Banerjee *et al.*, 2003a; Narang *et al.*, 2005; Sood *et al.*, 2005).

Ischaemic preconditioning may be studied in animals, such as the rat or dog, by appropriate variation in the in-vitro and in-vivo models of ischaemic-reperfusion models.

Hypertension

Hypertension is a major cause of morbidity and mortality across the world and hence an important public health problem (Bakris, 2007; Israili *et al.*, 2007). Apart from CVD, hypertension is also the most important modifiable risk factor for cerebral stroke, end-stage kidney disease and peripheral vascular disease.

Over the past several decades, extensive clinical and basic research and aggressive patient education have led to some decrease in mortality and morbidity rates associated with hypertension, but there is still a great need for antihypertensive agents that go beyond the lowering of blood pressure to treat the underlying pathophysiologic conditions that contribute to CVD.

The Seventh Report of the Joint National Committee (JNC VII) of Prevention, Detection, Evaluation, and Treatment of High Blood Pressure (Chobanian *et al.*, 2003), classified blood pressure (expressed in mmHg) for adults aged 18 years or older as follows.

- *Normal:* systolic lower than 120 mmHg, diastolic lower than 80 mmHg
- *Prehypertension:* systolic 120–139 mmHg, diastolic 80–99 mmHg
- *Hypertensive stage 1:* systolic 140–159 mmHg, diastolic 90–99 mmHg
- *Hypertensive stage 2:* systolic equal to or more than 160 mmHg, diastolic equal to or more than 100 mmHg.

Knowledge about the normal control of blood pressure and pathophysiological factors operating in hypertension is essential for targeting drug development and designing animal models for screening putative drug candidates.

Regulation of blood pressure

Arterial blood pressure is a product of cardiac output and peripheral vascular resistance, so determinants of blood pressure include factors that affect both cardiac output and arteriolar vascular physiology.

Normal blood pressure is regulated by a complex process. The major variables, such as cardiac output and peripheral vascular resistance are influenced by a variety of other factors (Ackermann, 2004). These include sodium intake, renal function, and mineralocorticoids and an increase in heart rate and contractility. Peripheral vascular resistance is dependent upon the sympathetic nervous system, humoral factors and local autoregulation. The sympathetic nervous system exerts its effects via the vasoconstrictor alpha-receptor (α1) effect or the vasodilator beta-receptor (β2) effect. The humoral actions on peripheral resistance are also mediated by various mediators, such as angiotensin-II and catecholamines (vasoconstrictors) or prostaglandins and kinins (vasodilators) (Sharma, 2007).

Pathogenesis of hypertension

The pathogenesis of essential hypertension (without any identifiable cause) is multifactorial (Bakris and Mensah, 2002). Genetic predisposition, excess dietary salt intake, and more than normal adrenergic tone have been proposed to play important roles in the causation of hypertension. The exact molecular mechanism(s) of genetic factor(s) in the development of essential hypertension has not yet been clearly established (Puddu *et al.*, 2007).

Target organ damage in hypertension

Brain (stroke), kidneys (renal failure), heart (ischaemic heart disease and cardiac hypertrophy) and eyes (retinopathy) are the major organs that are adversely affected because of chronic, untreated or poorly treated hypertension.

Need for drug development in hypertension

Although at present there are a large number of drugs available for the treatment of hypertension, adequate blood pressure control remains a challenge in clinical medicine (Flaa and Kjeldsen, 2006). Use of multiple drugs is a common practice. Many drugs have a number of adverse effects which limit patient compliance, while others have contraindications which limit their use. Consequently, there is a strong need to develop newer drugs for hypertension and herbs could play a role in this respect.

Methods to induce experimental hypertension

Several models have been developed to assess antihypertensive potential of test compounds, some of which are described below. However, a general point of precaution for all such in-vivo experiments, indeed for any cardiovascular model, is that careful attention should be paid to choice of anaesthesia, which can depress or stimulate the cardiovascular system and play havoc with the experimental findings.

Acute renal hypertension in rats

Clamping of the left renal artery for 4 hours stimulates synthesis of renin, which, on release of the clamp, is released into the circulation and catalyses the formation of angiotensin II from angiotensin I causing acute hypertension.

This method was first described by Goldblatt (Goldblatt *et al.*, 1934). In anaesthetised male Sprague–Dawley rats, the left renal artery is occluded for 3.5–4 h. Blood pressure is measured via a cannula in the carotid artery and connected to a pressure transducer. Following a stable blood pressure state, ganglionic blockade is achieved with intravenous pentolinium and the renal arterial clip removed, causing a rise in blood pressure soon afterwards. The test substance is then administered by intravenous injection via the jugular vein at predetermined doses (Vogel *et al.*, 2002).

Chronic renal hypertension in rats

Various modifications of the Goldblatt model have been described for several animal species to produce chronic hypertension in animals. One of these modifications is the 1K1C (one-kidney, one-clip) method in rats (Vogel *et al.*, 2002). In anaesthetised male Sprague–Dawley rats the renal artery is dissected clean and a U-shaped silver clip is slipped around it near the aorta. The size of the clip is adjusted using Schaffenburg forceps (Schaffenburg, 1959) so that the internal gap ranges from 0.25–0.38 mm. The right kidney is removed through a flank incision after ligating the renal pedicle and skin incisions closed. About 4–5 weeks later, blood pressure is measured and rats with blood pressure values higher than 150 mmHg are selected for the experiments (Vogel *et al.*, 2002).

In another modification, right nephrectomy is performed on anaesthetised rats. After a 1-week recovery period, the nephrectomised rats are subjected to left renal artery constriction and systolic blood pressure measured twice a week with the tail-cuff method using a programmed electrosphygmomanometer. Acute unclipping experiments are carried out 4 weeks later (Huang and Tsai, 1998).

Another useful experimental model is that of the 2K1C (two-kidney, one-clip) Goldblatt model (Goldblatt, 1995) in which hypertension is induced by unilateral stenosis of the renal artery. The clip is not severe enough to cause ischaemia; but the reduced renal perfusion pressure stimulates increased renin synthesis and release from the clipped kidney.

Other modifications of the method

Many other modifications of the method of inducing renal hypertension have been made (Grollman, 1944; Stanton, 1971), e.g. the kidney is exposed through a lumbar incision, the renal capsule is removed by gentle traction, and a figure-of-eight ligature is applied being tight enough to deform the kidney but not tight enough to cut the tissue (Vogel *et al.*, 2002). Renal hypertension may also be induced in the rat by encapsulating both kidneys with latex rubber capsule moulds (Abrams and Sobin, 1947).

Chronic renal hypertension in larger animals

The principle is essentially the same as that originally described by Goldblatt. In this model, abdominal incision is made in anaesthetised dogs to expose one kidney (Vogel *et al.*, 2002). The kidney is wrapped in cellophane and then replaced. The contralateral kidney is removed after ligation of the artery, vein and ureter. After closure of the abdomen, the animals are allowed to recover. Six weeks following surgery, blood pressure is measured using a tail-cuff method. Only animals with a systolic blood pressure higher than 150 mmHg are considered to be hypertensive and are taken up for further studies on evaluating potential antihypertensive compounds. For the experiment, blood pressure is recorded either by the non-invasive tail-cuff method or by direct measurement via an implanted arterial cannula. Blood pressure recording is made at pre-determined time schedules, before and after the oral administration of the potential antihypertensive compound. Drug administration is repeated for 5 days.

Neurogenic hypertension in dogs

Blood pressure is finely regulated by the vasomotor centre which receives input from the baroreceptor areas of the carotid sinus and aortic arch. Stimulation of these afferent fibres exerts an inhibitory influence on the vasomotor centre, while sectioning leads to a persistent rise in blood pressure. The neurogenic hypertension model is based on this phenomenon (Vogel *et al.*, 2002).

In adult anaesthetised dogs, both the carotid sinus nerves are isolated, ligated and sectioned and a bilateral vagotomy is performed to produce neurogenic hypertension (mean arterial pressure more than 150 mmHg). The animal is allowed to equilibrate for around 30 min before testing of antihypertensive compounds is started. Heart rate, arterial pressure, left ventricular pressure, Pmax and dP/dt are recorded using appropriate pressure transducers connected to a polygraph (Vogel *et al.*, 2002).

The neurogenic hypertension model is useful for acute experiments. However, it is less useful for chronic experiments since the elevated blood pressure caused by buffer nerve section is more labile than that caused by renal ischaemia.

Neurogenic hypertension through baroreceptor denervation has also been described in rabbits (Angell-James, 1984) and in rats (Krieger, 1984).

Desoxycorticosterone acetate – salt-induced hypertension in rats

Mineralocorticoids induce hypertension by their sodium-retaining properties, leading to increase in plasma and extracellular volume. This hypertensive effect is enhanced by salt loading and unilateral nephrectomy in rats. In this model, the left kidney is removed from anaesthetised male Sprague–Dawley rats. The rats are injected twice weekly with subcutaneous desoxycorticosterone acetate for 4 weeks. Drinking water is replaced with a 1% NaCl solution. The blood pressure starts to rise after 1 week and reaches systolic values between 160 and 180 mmHg after 4 weeks (Vogel *et al.*, 2002).

Genetic hypertension in rats

Okamoto *et al.* (1963) developed a strain of spontaneously hypertensive rats from mating one Wistar male rat with spontaneously occurring high blood pressure with a female with slightly elevated blood pressure. By inbreeding over several generations, a high incidence of hypertension with blood pressure values of 200 mmHg or more was achieved. These strains were called spontaneously hypertensive rats. Hypertension in these rats is clearly hereditary and genetically determined, thus comparable with primary hypertension in humans. Cardiac hypertrophy (Sen *et al.*, 1974) has been observed in these rats.

Several substrains of spontaneous hypertensive rats were separated by the group of Okamoto *et al.* (1974) including the stroke-prone model. These rats have an increased sympathetic tone and show a high incidence of haemorrhagic lesions of the brain with motor disturbances followed by death (Yamori *et al.*, 1983).

Increase of blood pressure of spontaneously hypertensive rats is determined by multiple genetic loci (Deng and Rapp, 1992; Dubey *et al.*, 1993). With the newer technologies, not only can these loci be defined but also with the transgenic animals, new models in hypertension research and models to screen for antihypertensive agents can be established. The rat strain, TGR (mREN2)27, as a monogenetic model in hypertension research has been described by Peters *et al.* (1993). For review see Herrera and Ruiz-Opazo (2005).

Spontaneously hypertensive rats are widely used for the screening of potential antihypertensive compounds. Of the various models available, most work has been done on the Wistar-Kyoto strain and in the near future, transgenic rats with well-defined genomes are likely to be the preferred choice (Vogel *et al.*, 2002).

Endothelial dysfunction

Furchgott and Zawadzki (1980) first reported that the presence of the intact endothelial cells is essential for acetylcholine to induce relaxation in the underlying vascular smooth muscle, and the phenomenon where endothelial cells do not act in this way was named 'endothelial dysfunction'. Endothelial dysfunction is an early marker of atherosclerosis. It has been associated with a number of cardiovascular diseases, such as hypertension, atherosclerosis, but also with physiological and pathophysiological processes, including ageing, heart and renal failure, coronary syndrome, microalbuminuria, dialysis, thrombosis, intravascular coagulation, Type 1 and Type 2 diabetes, impaired glucose tolerance, insulin resistance, hyperglycaemia, obesity, hypercholesterolaemia, to name but a few (Félétou and Vanhoutte, 2006; Frick and Weidinger, 2007).

Endothelial dysfunction is characterised by a reduction in the bioavailability of vasodilators, particularly nitric oxide, and an increase in the activity of vasoconstrictors, including angiotensin II and ROS (Schulman *et al.*, 2005). ROS may importantly contribute to endothelial dysfunction through inactivation of endothelium-derived nitric oxide (Dhalla *et al.*, 2000b). Herbal preparations with potential antioxidant properties may be screened for their putative effects on endothelial dysfunction.

Screening for endothelial dysfunction

Endothelial dysfunction has been widely studied in vessels from hypertensive animals, such as the aorta of the spontaneously hypertensive rats. Several biological markers have been used as indicators of endothelial dysfunction. The soluble adhesion molecules, such as sICAM-1 and sVCAM-1, are increased in inflammatory processes. Both markers are increased in coronary artery disease. E-selectin is specific for the endothelium and is increased in coronary artery disease and diabetes mellitus. Other endothelium-specific markers are soluble thrombomodulin (Constans and Conri, 2006) and von Willebrand factor (Blann *et al.*, 2002).

Endothelial dysfunction may also be assessed noninvasively by determining brachial artery flow-mediated dilatation. Flow may be measured by Doppler and intravascular ultrasound in coronary circulation, laser Doppler in skin and by venous occlusion plethysmography in peripheral muscular arteries. Similar studies may be performed ex vivo using isolated resistance arteries obtained from fat subcutaneous biopsies (Joannides *et al.*, 2006).

Congestive heart failure

Considerable progress in our knowledge and management of congestive heart failure (CHF) has been made during the past few years. However, the incidence, prevalence, mortality and economic costs of heart failure are steadily increasing with decreasing mortality because of better management of various conditions, such as acute myocardial infarction and hypertension, that cause heart failure. Survival of patients with CHF depends on the duration and severity of the disease as well as on therapeutic strategies.

CHF is a complex clinical syndrome in which a number of factors, apart from mechanical failure of the heart muscle, such as ventricular remodelling, neurohumoral activation, cytokine overexpression, as well as vascular and endothelial dysfunction play critical contributory roles (Pacher, 2001).

The leading causes of CHF are IHD (Klein and Gheorghiade, 2004) and hypertension (Baker, 2002). Other causes of CHF include primary myocardial diseases, such as dilated cardiomyopathy and valvular heart disease (7–8%) (Kannel, 2000).

Regardless of the aetiology, activation of the neurohumoral and the cytokine system seems to play a critical role in CHF. There is activation of the neurohumoral system which results in increased noradrenaline release. There is also activation of both local and plasma renin-angiotensin systems in patients with symptomatic heart failure (Adams, 2004).

The importance of cytokines as mediators of disease progression has been recently highlighted. They are believed to cause endothelial dysfunction, oxidative stress, induction of anaemia, necrotic and/or apoptotic myocyte cell death, myocardial fibrosis, and depression of myocardial function (Candia *et al.*, 2007). Circulating levels of tumour necrosis factor-α (TNF-α) (Henriksen and Newby, 2003), brain natriuretic peptide (BNP) and interleukin-6 (Maeda *et al.*, 2000) are increased and positively related to the severity of heart failure. In addition, endothelin plays a significant role in the pathogenesis of CHF. Apart from being the most potent vasoconstrictor, endothelin mediates pathologic hypertrophy and fibrosis of both ventricular and vascular tissues, it potentiates the effects of other neurohormones and acts as a proarrhythmic agent (Teerlink, 2005).

Extracellular matrix and changes in collagen composition have been shown to occur in heart failure. Enhanced myocardial stress initiates structural remodelling of the heart. This involves cardiomyocyte hypertrophy and changes in the amount of collagen, collagen phenotype and collagen cross-linking resulting in a stiffer ventricle ultimately leading to diastolic and systolic dysfunction (Brower *et al.*, 2006).

The above discussion has been made with the purpose of highlighting the recent understanding of CHF pathophysiology and that pharmacotherapy of CHF has moved far beyond digitalis and diuretics, which provide just symptomatic relief, without having any effect on disease progression. Hence, herbal preparations, potentially useful in heart failure may be screened for properties in the light of these recent aetiopathological mechanisms of CHF.

Animal models of heart failure

The ideal animal model for heart failure should closely mimic heart failure in humans, i.e. it should exhibit:

- haemodynamic changes that include increased cardiac filling pressures and low cardiac output
- activation of the sympathetic nervous system and increased secretion of hormones, such as renin, angiotensin, aldosterone, vasopressin, atrial natriuretic factor and endothelin
- Evidence of clinical features such as cardiomegaly, lung and peripheral oedema and decreased exercise tolerance.

Moreover, the model should be reproducible, inexpensive and technically simple to establish and study (Arnolda *et al.*, 1999).

Clearly, there is no perfect animal model of heart failure that exhibits all the features mentioned above and the best way to circumvent the issue is to choose the model that is best suited to the purpose of the study.

A variety of animal models have been developed for studying heart failure and include pressure loading, volume loading, myocardial infarction, etc. Each model may be used to study a particular dysfunctional aspect of CHF, for instance ventricular hypertrophy, cellular derangements and vascular changes may be assessed through pressure-loading models. For studying the pathogenesis of hormone and electrolyte disturbances, volume-loading models may be more suited. Canine coronary artery microembolisation has been used to generate ischaemia-induced dilation and dysfunction in the left ventricle. Rapid ventricular pacing has been used in both dogs and pigs to reproduce the characteristics of dilated cardiomyopathy. Models of myocardial infarction or destruction are likely to be the most suitable for assessing novel therapy provided that peripheral reflexes are maintained. For a greater clinical relevance, studies should be conducted on conscious animals with intact reflexes (Smith and Nuttall, 1985; Yarbrough and Spinale, 2003).

The rat model of heart failure

Rats have been the most widely used animal in which heart failure has been induced by various methods. Rats are relatively inexpensive and are easier to handle, making them the models of choice for many investigators. However, the rat as a model for heart failure has a number of limitations, as there are significant differences from the human heart. The most obvious one is that of the resting heart rate, which is five times that of the human heart. Other differences include electrophysiological (rat heart exhibits a very short action potential and usually lacks a plateau phase) and excitation-contraction differences (Hasenfuss, 1998).

Rat coronary ligation model

Myocardial infarction following coronary artery ligation in rats is a commonly used model of heart failure (Goldman and Raya, 1995). In this model, the left coronary artery is partially ligated, leading to CHF as a consequence of chronic myocardial ischaemia. Total ligation of the artery also leads to CHF but high mortality rates limit use of this model.

Rat aortic-banding model

A large number of studies have shown that aortic banding (pressure-overload heart failure) in rats causes left ventricular hypertrophy and after several months, a subset of these aortic-banded animals develop heart failure. Cardiac hypertrophy is a compensatory process that leads to a heart better suited for the functional demands caused by cardiac muscle dysfunction or loss. Because cardiac myocytes are terminally differentiated, hypertrophied heart muscle cells demonstrate an increase in protein content rather than an increase in cell number (Hasenfuss, 1998).

Transgenic animals are very useful models to study the factors involved in the pathogenesis of cardiac hypertrophy. To achieve this goal, rodents lacking or overexpressing a specific gene are subjected to banding of the abdominal aorta, which leads to cardiac hypertrophy caused by pressure overload on the heart (Barbosa *et al.*, 2005).

Mouse model of chronic volume overload

Overt congestive heart failure associated with myocardial hypertrophy in the mouse may also be used as a model of CHF. In a model, in anaesthetised female C57/BL6 mice, the aorta is temporarily clamped proximal to the renal arteries. Thereafter a shunt is made between the aorta and inferior vena cava. Four weeks after shunt induction, mice show significant cardiac hypertrophy, increase in left ventricular end-diastolic pressure and left ventricular contractility. Plasma concentrations of atrial natriuretic peptide, as well as ventricular expression of atrial and brain natriuretic peptide mRNA, are also reported to be significantly increased in mice with shunt (Scheuermann-Freestone *et al.*, 2001).

Dahl salt-sensitive hypertensive rats

These rats develop systemic hypertension after receiving a high-salt diet (Rapp and Dene, 1985). Hypertension causes cardiac hypertrophy and there is a transition from compensated hypertrophy to failure in these rats. Concentric left ventricular hypertrophy develops at 8 weeks, followed by marked left ventricular dilatation and overt clinical heart failure at 15–20 weeks. High mortality rates are also observed in this model.

Spontaneously hypertensive heart failure rats

Development of heart failure occurs earlier (4–18 months) in some spontaneously hypertensive rats (Okamoto, 1969) that have a genetic abnormality. In these animals, plasma renin activity and aldosterone levels progressively increase with age (Hasenfuss, 1998). Spontaneously hypertensive heart failure, a genetic model predisposed to hypertension and heart failure, may also be used for screening purposes (McCune *et al.*, 1995).

Rabbits, guinea pigs and Syrian hamsters have also been used in developing heart failure models in a similar fashion.

Heart failure models in large animals

Left ventricular function and volumes in dog can be more accurately and conveniently studied than in rodents. Further, unlike the rat, excitation-contraction coupling processes in dog appear to be more similar to those of the human myocardium (Hasenfuss, 1998; Fuller *et al.*, 2007). However, dog models are more expensive, in addition to having ethical constraints.

Chronic rapid-pacing-induced heart failure

Chronic rapid pacing at above 200 beats per minute in healthy dogs produces congestive heart failure within a few weeks. Haemodynamic changes occur as soon as 24 h after rapid pacing, with continued deterioration in ventricular function for up to 3–5 weeks, resulting in end-stage heart failure. Within 48 h after termination of pacing, haemodynamic variables approach control levels, and left ventricular ejection fraction shows significant recovery with subsequent normalisation after 1–2 weeks (Shinbane *et al.*, 1997). Thus, in this model, heart failure is reversible when pacing is stopped. The exact pathogenesis in this model is still unclear.

Coronary artery ligation-induced congestive heart failure

Left coronary artery ligation has been used to produce myocardial infarction and CHF in dogs.

About 2–3 months after infarction, there are clinical signs of heart failure, including left ventricular dilatation, decreased left ventricular ejection fraction, and neurohumoral activation similar to that occurring in humans. The progression from left ventricular dysfunction to heart failure and the influence of pharmacological interventions can be studied.

The model has several disadvantages. Because of extensive collateral circulation, there are important differences in the pattern of infarction between the human and the dog. The model is time-consuming, technically demanding and expensive. The model is also associated with high mortality and with a high incidence of arrhythmias (Hasenfuss, 1998).

Volume overload

Arteriovenous fistula or destruction of the mitral valve in dogs cause volume overload and subsequently heart failure. Experimental mitral regurgitation is produced in closed-chest dogs by disruption of chordae tendinae or valve leaflets. This results in left ventricular hypertrophy and dilatation within 12 weeks, followed by heart failure. Neurohumoral activation and activation of the tissue renin-angiotensin system is observed (Villarreal *et al.*, 1987).

Conclusions

Herbs offer the promise of both prevention and cure for CVD. Many societies unquestioningly accept their safety and efficacy. While numerous investigators have scientifically studied the pharmacological activities of herbal medicinal plants, often most 'therapeutic' claims are based on rather far-fetched extrapolations. However, before they are globally accepted for use in the treatment of these diseases, there is an urgent need for a conserted effort to screen for their efficacy in a proper perspective and in the light of current knowledge of disease mechanisms using newer sophisticated methodologies. Further, there is also a need to subject them to a reasonable degree of safety studies and last, but not least, to ensure product standardisation.

In this chapter, several models that may be useful for the screening of potentially active herbal medicines in CVD have been briefly touched upon and the list is by no means complete. However, the primary purpose was to familiarise the reader with the issues involved in the screening of drugs of herbal origin and that each model is associated with it unique advantages and disadvantages. The trick is to have a very clear picture of what the goal of the screening is, i.e. what condition is the herb likely to cure and what the possible modes of action are, and then choose the model best suited to these objectives.

References

Abrams M, Sobin S (1947). Latex rubber capsule for producing hypertension in rats by perinephritis. *Proc Soc Exp Biol Med* 64: 412–416.

Ackermann U (2004). Regulation of arterial blood pressure. *Surgery (Oxf)* 5: 120a–120f. doi: 10.1383/surg.22.5.120a.33383.

Adams KF Jr (2004). Pathophysiologic role of the renin-angiotensin-aldosterone and sympathetic nervous systems in heart failure. *Am J Health Syst Pharm* 61 (supp. 2): S4–S13.

Angell-James JE (1984). Neurogenic hypertension in the rabbit. In: de Jong (ed) *Handbook of Hypertension, Vol. 4: Experimental and Genetic Models of Hypertension*. Elsevier Science Publ, pp. 364–397.

Antonello M, Montemurro D, Bolognesi M, *et al.* (2007). Prevention of hypertension, cardiovascular damage and endothelial dysfunction with green tea extracts. *Am J Hypertens* 20: 1321–1328.

Arnolda LF, Llewellyn-Smith IJ, Minson JB (1999). Animal models of heart failure. *Aust N Z J Med* 29: 403–409.

Baker DW (2002). Prevention of heart failure. *J Card Fail* 5: 333–346.

Bakris GL (2007). Current perspectives on hypertension and metabolic syndrome. *J Manag Care Pharm* 5 Suppl: S3–S5.

Bakris GL, Mensah GA (2002). Pathogenesis and clinical physiology of hypertension. *Cardiol Clin* 2: 195–206.

Banerjee SK, Dinda AK, Manchanda SC, Maulik SK (2002). Chronic garlic administration protects rat heart against oxidative stress induced by ischemic reperfusion injury. *BMC Pharmacol* 2: 16.

Banerjee SK, Mukherjee PK, Maulik SK (2003). Garlic as an antioxidant: the good, the bad and the ugly. *Phytother Res* 2: 97–106.

Banerjee SK, Sood S, Dinda AK, *et al.* (2003a). Chronic oral administration of raw garlic protects against isoproterenol-induced myocardial necrosis in rat. *Comp Biochem Physiol C Toxicol Pharmacol* 4: 377–386.

Barbosa ME, Alenina N, Bader M (2005). Induction and analysis of cardiac hypertrophy in transgenic animal models. *Methods Mol Med* 112: 339–352.

Bennani-Kabchi N, Kehel LE, Bouayadi F, *et al.* (2000). New model of atherosclerosis in insulin resistant rats: hypercholesterolemia combined with D2 vitamin. *Atherosclerosis* 1: 55–61.

Bhattacharya SK, Bhattacharya A, Sairam K, Ghosal S (2002). Effect of bioactive tannoid principles of *Emblica officinalis* on ischemia-reperfusion-induced oxidative stress in rat heart. *Phytomedicine* 2: 171–174.

Blann AD, McCollum CN, Lip GY (2002). Relationship between plasma markers of endothelial cell integrity and the Framingham cardiovascular disease risk-factor scores in apparently healthy individuals. *Blood Coagul Fibrinolysis* 13: 513–518.

Bolli R (2007). Preconditioning: a paradigm shift in the biology of myocardial ischemia. *Am J Physiol Heart Circ Physiol* 292: H19–H27.

Brower GL, Gardner JD, Forman MF, *et al.*(2006). The relationship between myocardial extracellular matrix remodeling and ventricular function. *Eur J Cardiothorac Surg* 4: 604–610.

Candia AM, Villacorta H Jr Mesquita ET (2007). Immune-inflammatory activation in heart failure. *Arq Bras Cardiol* 3: 183–190, 201–208.

Chobanian AV, Bakris GL, Black HR, *et al.* (2003). National Heart, Lung, and Blood Institute Joint National Committee on Prevention, Detection, Evaluation, and Treatment of High Blood Pressure; National High Blood Pressure Education Program Coordinating Committee. The Seventh Report of the Joint National Committee on Prevention, Detection, Evaluation, and Treatment of High Blood Pressure: the JNC 7 report. *JAMA* 289: 2560–2572.

Cohen MV, Yang XM, Downey JM (2006). Nitric oxide is a preconditioning mimetic and cardioprotectant and is the basis of many available infarct-sparing strategies. *Cardiovasc Res* 2: 231–239.

Constans J, Conri C (2006). Circulating markers of endothelial function in cardiovascular disease. *Clin Chim Acta* 368: 33–47.

Das B, Sarkar C (2007). Pharmacological preconditioning by levosimendan is mediated by inducible nitric oxide synthase and mitochondrial KATP channel activation in the in vivo anesthetized rabbit heart model. *Vascul Pharmacol* 4: 248–256.

Deng Y, Rapp JP (1992). Cosegregation of blood pressure with angiotensin converting enzyme and atrial natriuretic receptor genes using Dahl salt-sensitive rats. *Nature Genetics* 1: 267–272.

Devi R, Banerjee SK, Sood S, Dinda AK, Maulik SK (2005). Extract from *Clerodendron colebrookianum* Walp protects rat heart against oxidative stress induced by ischemic-reperfusion injury (IRI). *Life Sci* 77: 2999–3009.

Dhalla NS, Elmoselhi AB, Hata T, Makino N (2000a). Status of myocardial antioxidants in ischemia-reperfusion injury. *Cardiovasc Res* 47: 446–456.

Dhalla NS, Temsah RM, Netticadan T (2000b). Role of oxidative stress in cardiovascular diseases. *J Hypertens* 18: 655–673.

Dubey CH, Vincent M, Samani NJ, *et al.* (1993). Genetic determinants of diastolic and pulse pressure map to different loci in Lyon hypertensive rats. *Nature Genet* 3: 354–357.

El-Beshbishy HA, Singab AN, Sinkkonen J, Pihlaja K (2006). Hypolipidemic and antioxidant effects of *Morus alba* L. (Egyptian mulberry) root bark fractions supplementation in cholesterol-fed rats. *Life Sci* 23: 2724–2733.

Félétou M, Vanhoutte PM (2006). Endothelial dysfunction: a multifaceted disorder (The Wiggers Award Lecture). *Am J Physiol Heart Circ Physiol* 3: H985–H1002.

Flaa A, Kjeldsen SE (2006). Are all the hypertensives made equal? *Herz* 4: 323–330.

Frick M, Weidinger F (2007). Endothelial function: a surrogate endpoint in cardiovascular studies? *Curr Pharm Des* 17: 1741–1750.

Fuller GA, Bicer S, Hamlin RL, Yamaguchi M, *et al.* (2007). Increased myosin heavy chain-beta with atrial expression of ventricular light chain-2 in canine cardiomyopathy. *J Card Fail* 8: 680–686.

Furchgott RF, Zawadzki JV (1980). The obligatory role of the endothelial cells in the relaxation of arterial smooth muscle by acetylcholine. *Nature* 288: 373–376.

Gauthaman K, Maulik M, Kumari R *et al.* (2001). Effect of chronic treatment with bark of *Terminalia arjuna*: a study on the isolated ischemic-reperfused rat heart. *J Ethnopharmacol* 75: 197–201.

Gauthaman K, Banerjee SK, Dinda AK, *et al.* (2005). *Terminalia arjuna* (Roxb.) protects rabbit heart against ischemic-reperfusion injury: role of antioxidant enzymes and heat shock protein. *J Ethnopharmacol* 3: 403–409.

Genest JG Jr. (2000). Dyslipidemia and coronary artery disease. *Can J Cardiol* 16 Suppl A: 3A–4A.

Gidlund M, Damasceno NRT, Lindoso JAL, *et al.* (1996). Monoclonal antibodies against low density lipoprotein with various degrees of oxidative modification. *Braz J Med Biol Res* 29: 1625–1628.

Goldblatt H, Lynch J, Hanzal RF, Summerville WW (1934). Studies on experimental hypertension: I. The production of persistent elevation of systolic blood pressure by means of renal ischemia. *J Exp Med* 59: 347–379.

Goldblatt, PJ (1995). The Goldblatt experiment: a conceptual paradigm. In: *Hypertension: pathophysiology, diagnosis and management*. J. H. Laragh and B. M. Brenner, Eds. New York: Raven p. 23–35.

Goldman S, Raya TE (1995). Rat infarct model of myocardial infarction and heart failure. *J Card Fail* 2: 169–177.

Grollman A (1944). A simplified procedure for inducing chronic renal hypertension in the mammal. *Proc Soc Exp Biol Med* 57: 102–104.

Guidance for Industry (2007). Botanical drug products draft guidance. Available at: http://www.fda.gov/cder/guidance (accessed 9 Dec 2007).

Hansson GK (2005). Inflammation, atherosclerosis, and coronary artery disease. *N Engl J Med* 352: 1685–1695.

Halestrap AP, Clarke SJ, Khaliulin I (2007). The role of mitochondria in protection of the heart by preconditioning. *Biochim Biophys Acta* 8: 1007–1031.

Hasenfuss G (1998). Animal models of human cardiovascular disease, heart failure and hypertrophy. *Cardiovasc Res* 1: 60–76.

Herrera VL, Ruiz-Opazo N (2005). Genetic studies in rat models: insights into cardiovascular disease. *Curr Opin Lipidol* 2: 179–191.

Henriksen, PA, Newby DE (2003). Therapeutic inhibition of tumour necrosis factor alpha in patients with heart failure: cooling an inflamed heart. *Heart* 1: 14–18.

Hidiroglou N, Gilani GS, Long L, *et al.* (2004). The influence of dietary vitamin E, fat, and methionine on blood cholesterol profile, homocysteine levels, and oxidizability of low density lipoprotein in the gerbil *J Nutr Biochem* 12: 730–740.

Huang WC, Tsai RY (1998). Nitric oxide synthesis inhibition retards surgical reversal of one-kidney Goldblatt hypertension in rats. *Hypertension* 3: 534–540.

Inoue T, Node K (2007). Statin therapy for vascular failure. *Cardiovasc Drugs Ther* 4: 281–295.

Israili ZH, Hernández-Hernández R, Valasco M (2007). The future of antihypertensive treatment. *Am J Ther* 2: 121–134.

Joannides R, Bellien J, Thuillez C (2006). Clinical methods for the evaluation of endothelial function – a focus on resistance arteries. *Fundam Clin Pharmacol* 3: 311–320.

Johansson ME, Hagg U, Wikstrfm J, *et al.* (2005). Haemodynamically significant plaque formation and regional endothelial dysfunction in cholesterol-fed apoE-/- mice. *Clin Sci* 108: 531– 538.

Jiang F, Jones GT, Husband AJ, Dusting GJ (2003). Cardiovascular protective effects of synthetic isoflavone derivatives in apolipoprotein E-deficient mice. *J Vasc Res* 40: 276–284.

Kaminura R, Suzuki S, Sakamoto H, *et al.* (1999). Development of atherosclerotic lesions in cholesterol-loaded rabbits. *Exp Anim* 48: 1–7.

Kannel WB (2000). Incidence and epidemiology of heart failure. *Heart Fail Rev* 2: 167–173.

Karthikeyan K, Bai BR, Gauthaman K, *et al.* (2003). Cardioprotective effect of the alcoholic extract of *Terminalia arjuna* bark in an in vivo model of myocardial ischemic reperfusion injury. *Life Sci* 21: 2727–2739.

Khalil PN, Siebeck M, Huss R *et al.* (2006). Histochemical assessment of early myocardial infarction using 2, 3, 5-triphenyltetrazolium chloride in blood-perfused porcine hearts. *J Pharmacol Toxicol Methods* 3: 307–312.

Klein L, Gheorghiade M (2004). Coronary artery disease and prevention of heart failure. *Med Clin North Am* 5: 1209–1235.

Kloner RA, Rezkalla SH (2006). Preconditioning, postconditioning and their application to clinical cardiology. *Cardiovasc Res* 2: 297–307.

Kolodgie FD, Katocs AS, Largis EE, *et al.* (1996). Hypercholesterolemia in the rabbit induced by feeding graded amounts of low-level cholesterol. *Atheroscler Thromb Vasc Biol* 16: 1454– 1464.

Kraaijeveld AO, de Jager SC, van Berkel TJ, *et al.* (2007). Chemokines and atherosclerotic plaque progression: towards therapeutic targeting? *Curr Pharm Des* 13: 1039–1052.

Krieger EM (1984). Neurogenic hypertension in the rat. In: de Jong (ed.) *Handbook of Hypertension, Vol. 4: Experimental and Genetic Models of Hypertension.* Elsevier Science Publ, pp. 350–363.

Kuei-Meng W, Farrelly J, Birnkrant D, *et al.* (2004). Regulatory toxicology perspectives on the development of botanical drug products in the United States. *Am J Ther* 11: 213–217.

Kumari R, Manchanda SC, Maulik SK (2004). Effect of pre- and posttreatment of losartan in feline model of myocardial ischemic-reperfusion injury. *Methods Find Exp Clin Pharmacol* 1: 39–45.

Langendorff O (1895). Untersuchungen am überlebenden Säugethierherzen. *Pflügers Arch ges Physiol* 61: 291.

Le NA, Walter MF (2007). The role of hypertriglyceridemia in atherosclerosis. *Curr Atheroscler Rep* 2: 110–115.

Maeda K, Tsutamoto T, Wada A, *et al.* (2000). High levels of plasma brain natriuretic peptide and interleukin-6 after optimized treatment for heart failure are independent risk factors for morbidity and mortality in patients with congestive heart failure. *J Am Coll Cardiol* 365: 1587–1593.

Maulik SK, Kumari R, Maulik M, *et al.* (2001). Captopril and its time of administration in myocardial ischaemic-reperfusion injury. *Pharmacol Res* 2: 123–128.

McCune SA, Park S, Radin MJ, Jurin RR (1995). The SHHF/Mcc-fa^{cp} rat model: a genetic model of congestive heart failure. In: Singal PK, Dixon IMC, Beamish RE, Dhalla NS, eds. *Mechanisms of Heart Failure.* Boston, Mass: Kluwer Academic Publishers pp. 91–106.

Miller MJ (2001). Preconditioning for cardioprotection against ischemia reperfusion injury: the roles of nitric oxide, reactive oxygen species, heat shock proteins, reactive hyperemia and antioxidants–a mini review. *Can J Cardiol* 10: 1075–1082.

Moghadasian MH, Frohlich JJ, McManus BM (2001). Advances in experimental dyslipidemia and atherosclerosis. *Lab Invest* 819: 1173–1183.

Narang D, Sood S, Thomas M, *et al.* (2005). Dietary palm olein oil augments cardiac antioxidant enzymes and protects against isoproterenol-induced myocardial necrosis in rats. *J Pharm Pharmacol* 11: 1445–1451.

Neely JR, Liebermeister H, Battersby EJ, Morgan HE (1967). Effect of pressure development on oxygen consumption by isolated rat heart. *Am J Physiol* 212: 804–814.

Okamoto K, Aoki K (1963). Development of a strain of spontaneously hypertensive rats. *Jap Circulat J* 27: 282–293.

Okamoto K (1969). Spontaneous hypertension in rats. *Int Rev Exp Patho* 7: 227–270.

Okamoto K, Yamori Y, Nagaoka A (1974). Establishment of the stroke prone spontaneously hypertensive rat (SHR). *Circ Res* Suppl 34/35: 1143–1153.

Pacher R (2001). Pathogenesis of heart failure. *Semin Nephrol* 3: 273–277.

Pasupathy S, Homer-Vanniasinkam S (2005). Ischaemic preconditioning protects against ischaemia/reperfusion injury: emerging concepts. *Eur J Vasc Endovasc Surg* 2: 106–115.

Peters J, Munter K, Bader M, *et al.* (1993). Increased adrenal rennin in transgenic hypertensive rats, TGR (mREN2)27, and its regulation by cAMP, angiotensin II, and calcium. *J Clin Invest* 91: 742–747.

Puddu P, Puddu GM, Cravero E, *et al.* (2007). The genetic basis of essential hypertension. *Acta Cardiol* 3: 281–293.

Rajak S, Banerjee SK, Sood S, *et al.* (2004). *Emblica officinalis* causes myocardial adaptation and protects against oxidative stress in ischemic-reperfusion injury in rats. *Phytother Res* 1: 54–60.

Rapp JP, Dene H (1985). Development and characteristics of inbred strains of Dahl salt-sensitive and salt-resistant rats. *Hypertension* 3 Pt 1: 340–349.

Rajlakshmi D, Banerjee SK, Sood S, Maulik SK (2003). In-vitro and in-vivo antioxidant activity of different extracts of the leaves of *Clerodendron colebrookianum* Walp in the rat. *J Pharm Pharmacol* 12: 1681–1686.

Rezkalla SH, Kloner RA (2005). Preconditioning and the human heart. *Panminerva Med* 2: 69–73.

Russell JC, Proctor SD (2006). Small animal models of cardiovascular disease: tools for the study of the roles of metabolic syndrome, dyslipidemia, and atherosclerosis. *Cardiovasc Pathol* 6: 318–330.

Saravanan G, Prakash J (2004). Effect of garlic (*Allium sativum*) on lipid peroxidation in experimental myocardial infarction in rats. *J Ethnopharmacol* 1: 155–158.

Schaffenburg CA (1959). Device to control constriction of main renal artery for production of hypertension in small animals. *Proc Soc Exp Biol Med* 101: 676–677.

Sen S, Tarazi RC, Kharallah, PA, Bumpus FM (1974). Cardiac hypertrophy in spontaneously hypertensive rats. *Circ Res* 35: 775–781.

Scheuermann-Freestone M, Freestone NS, *et al.* (2001). A new model of congestive heart failure in the mouse due to chronic volume overload. *Eur J Heart Fail* 5: 535–543.

Schreyer SA, Wilson DL, LeBoeuf RC (1998). C57BL/6 mice fed high fat diets as models for diabetes-accelerated atherosclerosis. *Atherosclerosis* 136: 17–124.

Schulman IH, Zachariah M, Raij L (2005). Calcium channel blockers, endothelial dysfunction, and combination therapy. *Aging Clin Exp Res* 4 (supp.): 40–45.

Sharma S (2007). Hypertension. http://www.emedicine.com/med/TOPIC1106.HTM (accessed 2 Dec 2007).

Shinbane JS, Wood MA, Jensen DN, *et al.* (1997). Tachycardia-induced cardiomyopathy: a review of animal models and clinical studies. *J Am Coll Cardiol* 4: 709–715.

Siess W (2006). Platelet interaction with bioactive lipids formed by mild oxidation of low-density lipoprotein. *Pathophysiol Haemost Thromb* 35: 292–304.

Singab AN, Sinkkonen J, Pihlaja K (2006). Hypolipidemic and antioxidant effects of *Morus alba* L. (Egyptian mulberry) root bark fractions supplementation in cholesterol-fed rats. *Life Sci* 23: 2724–2733.

Smith HJ, Nuttall A (1985). Experimental models of heart failure. *Cardiovasc Res* 4: 181–186.

Sood S, Narang D, Dinda AK, Maulik SK (2005). Chronic oral administration of *Ocimum sanctum* Linn. augments cardiac endogenous antioxidants and prevents isoproterenol-induced myocardial necrosis in rats. *J Pharm Pharmacol* 1: 127–133.

Stanton HC (1971). Experimental hypertension. In: Schwartz A (ed) *Methods in Pharmacology*, Appleton-Century-Crofts, Meredith Corporation. New York, Vol 1, pp. 125–150.

Teerlink JR (2005). Endothelins: pathophysiology and treatment implications in chronic heart failure. *Curr Heart Fail Rep* 4: 191–197.

Theilmeier G, Verhamme P, Dymarkowski S, *et al.* (2002). Hypercholesterolemia in minipigs impairs left ventricular response to stress. *Circ* 106: 1140– 1146.

Villarreal D, Freeman RH, Davis JO, *et al.* (1987). Atrial natriuretic factor secretion in dogs with experimental high-output heart failure. *Am J Physiol* 4 Pt 2: H692–H696.

Visavadiya NP, Narasimhacharya AV (2007). Ameliorative effect of *Chlorophytum borivilianum* root on lipid metabolism in hyperlipaemic rats. *Clin Exp Pharmacol Physiol* 34: 244–249.

Vogel HG, Vogel HW, Scholken AB *et al.* (Eds) (2002). *Drug Discovery and Evaluation: pharmacological assays,* 2nd edn. Berlin Heidelberg, Germany: Springer-Verlag, pp. 172–179.

Wu K-M, DeGeorge J, Atrakchi A, *et al.* (2000). A special update from the United States Food and Drug Administration: preclinical issues and status of investigation of botanical drug products in the United States. *Toxicol Lett* 111: 199–202.

Yamori Y, Horie R, Nara Y, Kihara M (1983). Pathogenesis, prediction and prevention of stroke in stroke-prone SHR. In: Stefanovich V (ed.) *Stroke: animal models.* Pergamon Press, Oxford, New York, Paris, Kronberg pp. 99–113.

Yanni AE (2000). The laboratory rabbit: an animal model of atherosclerosis research. *Lab Anim* 3: 246–256.

Yarbrough WM, Spinale FG (2003). Large animal models of congestive heart failure: a critical step in translating basic observations into clinical applications. *J Nucl Cardiol* 1: 77–86.

Yuan YV, Kitts DD (2002). Dietary fat source and cholesterol interactions alter plasma lipids and tissue susceptibility to oxidation in spontaneously hypertensive (SHR) and normotensive Wistar Kyoto (WKY) rats. *Mol Cell Biochem* 232: 33–47.

Zhang SH, Reddick RL, Piedrahita JA *et al.* (1992). Spontaneous hypercholesterolemia and arterial lesions in mice lacking apolipoprotein *E*. *Science* 258: 468–471.

Zimmer HG (1998). The isolated perfused heart and its pioneers. *News Physiol Sci* 13: 203–210.

13

Herbal medicinal products as antiangiogenic agents: perspectives and evaluation

Royce Mohan

Introduction

Angiogenesis is the morphogenic process by which new blood vessels develop from a pre-existing vasculature. This process occurs during embryonic development and feeds the oxygen and nutrient requirements of growing tissues and organs (Battegay, 1995). Blood vessels are lined internally by vascular endothelial cells, of mesenchymal origin. These endothelial cells are tightly compacted as a monolayer and display a cobblestone-like appearance. The endothelial cells also fulfil a role in maintenance of blood–brain and blood–retinal barrier and restrict the passage of blood components to inner tissues. However, when the vasculature is inflamed or injured such as in an oedema, substances from the blood can leak out; and the ability of the endothelial cell to re-populate the damaged tissue and re-establish cell–cell contact is critical for vascular homeostasis. In adults, the vasculature is usually dormant, except in certain instances, such as, during ovulation and menstruation in the female, and upon injury when tissue repair is required.

The vascular endothelium is thus an important beacon of humoral homeostasis and continues to guide the clinical diagnosis of underlying stress and disease (Meyers and Gokce, 2007). In fact, the silent and debilitating disease diabetes is at times diagnosed during a visit to the ophthalmologist for poor vision, which results from diabetic retinal capillaries leaking and causing vision impairment (Ryan, 2007).

Pathological angiogenesis is an underlying disease process in tumour growth where it supports the expansion of the tumour mass in size and also acts as a means to aid tumour cells to metastasise to distal organs (Folkman, 1995; Carmeliet *et al.* 1996). In fact, it is known that tumour masses can only grow to sizes where oxygen can diffuse through tissue (approximately 200 μm), hence, without establishment of new blood vessels, tumour cells are limited in their microscopic volume (Folkman, 1972b; Neeman *et al.*, 1997; Evans and Koch, 2003). The revolutionary paradigm that blocking new blood vessel growth (antiangiogenesis) could be a therapeutic means to 'starve' a tumour and thus arrest tumour development was at first strongly opposed by the oncology research community, who believed that directly killing the tumour cells with potent cytotoxins was the most effective means to cure cancers (Folkman, 1971).

However, targeted strategies to cause interference with blood vessel formation have begun to open up antiangiogenesis as a new modality in therapeutic discovery (Figg *et al.*, 2002; Ferrara and Kerbel, 2005). Today this idea has changed the treatment of cancers, with the clinical success of the neutralising antibody drug Avastin (bevacizumab), an anti-angiogenic agent which binds to vascular endothelial growth factor (VEGF), a critical survival and growth-stimulatory protein for new blood vessel growth (Ruegg and Mutter, 2007). Because it is believed that existing blood vessels are not affected by angiogenesis inhibitors, the quest to find new treatment options that do not possess the undesirable side-effects of currently used anticancer cytotoxic drugs has turned patient awareness to this new class of anticancer drugs. In this respect, researchers and clinicians have also begun looking seriously to the wealth of herbal medicines (Paper, 1998; Fan *et al.*, 2006; Yance and Sagar, 2006), many of which tout efficacy without the side-effects of radiation and chemotherapy.

Although much of our knowledge about the basic mechanisms of angiogenesis and clinical practice in the field of antiangiogenesis has come about from work done in the oncology field, it should be pointed out that there is a wide range of non-oncological diseases of no less importance as burdens to society that are angiogenic-dependent (Folkman, 1972a, 1995; Healy *et al.*, 1998). Furthermore, the list of angiogenic diseases awakens us to how critical blood vessel homeostasis is to organ functions, and it is also important to note that the promotion of angiogenesis is necessary in other clinical conditions that result from a lack of adequate vascularisation, such as ischaemic heart disease and diabetic ulcers (Shireman, 2007; Velazquez, 2007).

From ground-breaking work done by Folkman, a whole range of diseases can now be classified as having excessive angiogenesis or insufficient vascularisation (Table 13.1). He raised the hypothesis that tumour angiogenesis results when the net levels of stimulators of new blood vessel growth exceed that of inhibitors and devoted his laboratory in Boston, USA, to identifying the body's endogenous activators (and inhibitors) of tumour angiogenesis (Folkman *et al.*, 1971). Thirty-five years later, there are over 20 such protein effectors, which have been identified and shown to possess angiomodulatory activity (Carmeliet and Jain, 2000). By demonstrating validation in a wide range of cell culture, organ and animal models of angiogenesis (Norrby, 2006; Ucuzian and Greisler, 2007), it is possible to provide therapeutic doses of angio-inhibitory molecules to block angiogenesis, and contrarily, pro-angiogenic molecules to stimulate new blood vessel growth. The ability to discover new angiomodulatory agents and assess their effectiveness in controlling angiogenesis was enabled by the development of a number of in-vitro and in-vivo angiogenesis assays (Table 13.2) (Auerbach *et al.*, 2003).

Tests to examine effects of plant extracts on angiogenesis

Growth of blood vessels within a matrix

In-vitro vessel formation is assessed by measuring the total length of new blood vessels formed in a matrix over a period of time. Typically, endothelial cells are cultured within a matrix of fibroblasts in the absence or presence of the test compound. The matrix is supplied with fresh medium every third day and, after 11 days, the cells are washed and fixed. A staining reagent is applied to show the blood vessels formed from the endothelial cells and then quantified using a scanner attached to a computer which is able to process the images captured (Newman *et al.*, 2004).

Use of genetically modified zebra fish

The embryos of the zebra fish (*Danio rerio*) have been used extensively in recent studies for several

Table 13.1 Angiogenesis in human diseases

Organ	Disease manifestation	Comments
Blood vessels	Vascular malformations caused by abnormal remodelling, haemangioma and atherosclerosis from increased vascularisation	Localised lesions due to vascular malformation; congestive heart failure resulting from atherosclerosis
Eye	Diabetic retinopathy and wet age-related macular degeneration from increased vascularisation	Blindness due to leaky vessels in diabetic retina; blindness from proliferating choroidal blood vessels
Skin	Psoriasis from increased vascularisation that becomes tortuous and enlarged; decubitus (stasis) ulcers from insufficient vascularisation; Kaposi's sarcoma, allergic oedema, and neoplasms from increased vascularisation	Psoriasis appears as scaly, raised red lesions as a common form of this disease; stasis ulcers are open surface wounds that fail to heal
Bone and joints	Increased vascularisation of synovial joints in arthritis and of bone tissue in cancers	Inflammation of synovium in rheumatoid arthritis leads to joint destruction; destruction of cartilage in osteoarthritis causes pain and impaired mobility
Heart, skeletal muscle	Increased vascularisation of heart due to work overload; ischaemic heart and limb disease from insufficient vascularisation	Contractile dysfunction of heart tissue leads to heart failure; coronary heart disease manifests as a result of occlusion of blood vessels and poor oxygen supply
Adipose tissue	Increased vascularisation of fat tissue	Fat cells accumulate around new blood vessels causing obesity
Uterus, ovary	Increased vascularisation of uterine tissue, endometrium, ovary	Uterine tissue becomes dysfunctional from excessive bleeding; endometriosis can cause ectopic pregnancy, miscarriage and also infertility
Brain	Increased vascularisation in brain tumours; insufficient vascularisation of brain can lead to strokes	Gliomas and glioblastomas are incurable diseases of brain; stroke can incapacitate the cognitive and functional aspects of the brain

Adapted from Carmeliet and Jain, 2000.

types of biological activity. Transgenic lines are used which express the green fluorescent protein GCFP to visualise vasculogenesis in the tail region. The extent of vascularisation can be quantified by computer-aided image analysis and is taken as a model of angiogenesis (Friedrich *et al.*, 2004).

Three-dimensional endothelial cell sprouting assay

Sprouting of endothelial cells is an early event in angiogenesis, which follows vasodilation and degradation of matrix (Kurz, 2000) and it represents a valuable target for therapies because it takes place so early in the angiogenic process. The degradation of matrix is accomplished by the family of matrix metalloproteinases (MMPs) (Caserman and Lah, 2004). The mechanisms by which sprouts progress to form a lumen and ultimately become competent to support blood flow are largely unknown. Therefore, the study of the early steps of vessel sprouting can point to new therapeutic directions once key targets in these pathways have been identified.

The most promising in-vitro assays for elucidating relevant molecules and pathways necessary for endothelial cell morphogenesis are those using three-dimensional extracellular matrices, because endothelial cells experience a richer, more complex physical environment than cells cultured on two-dimensional surfaces (Ucuzian and Greisler, 2007). The collagen I and fibrin matrices represent the major matrix environments where angiogenic events

Table 13.2 In vitro and in in vivo angiogenesis assays

Assay	Measurement	Comments
Cell proliferation	Inhibition of cell doubling opposing stimulatory effect of a defined angiogenic factor	Cytostatic activity blocks cell proliferation without causing cell death
Cell migration	Inhibition of cell migration opposing stimulatory effect of a defined angiogenic factor such as VEGF or bFGF	The extension of endothelial cell processes allows cells to migrate over a substratum
Invasion	Inhibition of cell invasion opposing stimulatory effect of a defined angiogenic factor	The growth of endothelial cells through a porous membrane or matrix in response to a chemotactic factor
Sprouting	Inhibition of migration, invasion and tube formation in a 3D matrix of collagen I or fibrin opposing stimulatory effect of a defined angiogenic factor	An integrated assay which couples vascular invasion, tube formation and maturation in 3D matrix
Matrigel cord assay	Inhibition of cord assembly by endothelial cells on complex matrix derived from tumour stroma opposing stimulatory effect of a defined angiogenic factor	Endothelial cells assemble into cords over the matrix
CAM in vivo	Inhibition of blood vessel growth in the CAM of a fertilised developing chicken egg	The developing vasculature of the CAM is highly sensitive inhibitors of angiogenesis
Corneal angiogenesis in vivo	Inhibition of de novo capillary growth in cornea opposing stimulatory effect of a defined angiogenic factor	Blood vessels from surrounding scleral vessel supply invade the avascular cornea in response to slow-release growth factor implanted in cornea
Matrigel in vivo	Inhibition of blood vessel growth into a Matrigel plug implanted in abdominal region of mouse	Blood vessels invade the Matrigel plug in response to stimulus from growth factor impregnated plug

CAM = chorioallantoic membrane.

take place (Ryan and Barnhill, 1983). For example, during endothelial sprouting there is the induced expression of endogenous growth factors, transcription factors and signalling molecules, endothelial cell differentiation markers and adhesion molecules and a marked down-regulation of positive regulators of the cell cycle and ubiquitin-proteasome genes (Bell *et al.*, 2001). In stark comparison, the angiogenesis-screening assay using the basement-membrane matrix Matrigel, which measures the ability of endothelial cells to form a meshwork of cords on a tumour cell-derived matrix is markedly independent of transcriptional events (Zimrin *et al.*, 1995), and protein synthesis (Laterra and Goldstein, 1991). These and other drawbacks with the Matrigel gel assay (Vernon *et al.*, 1992) limit its scope for screening purposes. In the endothelial cell sprouting assay (3D-ECSA) (Korff and Augustin, 1998), endothelial cells are induced over a period of 24 h to form spheroids by aggregating. The spheroids are next seeded in suspension in a collagen I matrix by gelling at 37°C. Exogenous growth factors, such as VEGF, when added to the three-dimenional culture, stimulate the growth of vessel-like structures that grow out from the spheroid. Extracts and drugs being tested for angiogenesis inhibition are added along with VEGF. The sprouting extent and its inhibition are observed after a period of 18–24 h, which allows one to readily identify agents that block vessel development. The assay has been used by our laboratory to identify several classes of angiogenesis inhibitors, one of which is withaferin A from the medicinal plant *Withania somnifera* (Mohan *et al.*, 2004).

The angiogenic balance: a paradigm for herbal medicine

Several traditional medicine systems, such as those used in China and India (Ayurveda, Siddha and Unani) explain disease as the imbalances in the body's humoral and local effectors of normal physiology. In contrast, Western medicine identifies targets and designs therapeutic agents to affect particular diseased proteins/factors. Traditional or ethnomedicines lay emphasis on multiple modalities, focusing, on the one hand, on reducing the disease burden with the use of complex mixtures of principal active agents, while, on the other hand, also laying equal emphasis on reducing the undesired effects of these principal active agents with secondary substances to alleviate drug-induced toxicities (Pal, 1997; Garodia *et al.*, 2007). Considering this complex paradigm, two important aspects regarding herbal products need to be considered. One is focused on understanding the molecular factors that contribute to the pathobiology of disease and the other to the toxicology of drug activity. Using modern tools of analytical chemistry, biochemistry and molecular biology, molecular descriptors (genomics, proteomics, metabolomics), the activity of plant extracts and their principal active components on cellular and animal models can be understood mechanistically and are providing a wealth of information that serve hypotheses on which targets are tractable and how best to affect their functions to reverse disease (Wen and Han, 2004; Ventura, 2005; Wang *et al.*, 2005; Ma *et al.*, 2006; Ulrich-Merzenich *et al.*, 2007).

Herbal products with angiogenesis-inhibitory activity

Angiogenesis modulators are present in a wide range of plant products, some of which are also consumed on a daily basis through diets in certain ethnic populations. In addition, herbal products derived from specific medicinal plants known for their curative properties on chronic angiogenesis-dependent conditions are also gaining recognition for their principal active agents.

Curcuma longa (turmeric)

The staple in India's armoury of wound-healing plants is the common spice plant *C. longa*, used for injuries, burns, and as an all-purpose, topical anti-inflammatory (Singh, 2007). The principal active substance is curcumin. The use of curcumin as an inhibitor of angiogenesis has only recently been appreciated, despite great interest in this natural product for cancer chemoprevention (Singh and Khar, 2006). We showed that local delivery of curcuminoid pellets (2 mg), implanted in the cornea of rabbits, blocked angiogenesis induced by fibroblast growth factor 2, and even oral delivery of curcuminoids to mice blocked angiogenesis induced by the same growth factor in the mouse corneal model of neovascularisation (Mohan *et al.*, 2000).

The anti-angiogenic activity of this class of inhibitor was demonstrated as acting through the targeting of gene expression of MMP-9, a critical proteolytic enzyme that cleaves gelatinous substrates of the vascular basement membrane. This gene expression blockade of MMP-9 was found to occur through the inhibition of AP-1 and NF-κB transcription factors, two critically important activators of proliferative and inflammatory cytokine genes (Mohan *et al.*, 2000; Bhandarkar and Arbiser, 2007). The use of turmeric in promoting growth of blood vessels to heal wounds has also been remarkable. Contrary to the anti-angiogenic activity of curcumin, its wound-healing properties are mediated through promotion of angiogenesis (Maheshwari *et al.*, 2006; Thangapazham *et al.*, 2007).

The mechanism of this natural product is believed to be dependent on disease contexts. For instance, it was shown that one of curcumin's targets is the kinase that is responsible for activating the multipurpose signalling complex, the COP9 signalosome (Henke *et al.*, 1999). This complex lies at the interface of a number of divergent stress signalling cascades, acting as a central modulator of stress response. The COP9 signalosome activates the expression of VEGF in tumour cells providing the cells with survival advantage by stimulating blood vessels. In this manner, curcumin's anti-angiogenic activity causes the inhibition of VEGF expression. On the other hand, cyclo-oxygenase (COX)-2 is also shown to associate with COP9 signalosome, where this enzyme is targeted for proteosomal degradation (Neuss *et al.*, 2007).

Yet another interesting finding is that curcumin regulates the expression of the Id proteins through their association with the COP9 signalosome (Berse *et al.*, 2004). Thus, complex, broad and effective activities of curcumin (Thangapazham *et al.*, 2006) fall into a category of compounds that would best be described as 'homeostatins', which would be agents that act on stressors of dis-homeostasis but do not perturb cellular balances under homeostasis. The non-pungent flavour of turmeric has also made this spice broadly appealing for oral ingestion, albeit the compound is not readily bioavailable to target organs at doses that would be necessary for severe conditions. A Phase 1 study of oral daily dose of 8 g curcumin consumed for 4 months showed no toxic effects, other than nausea and diarrhoea, but higher doses were not acceptable to patients because of the bulk substance (Hsu and Cheng, 2007). Since a daily oral dose of 3.6 g of curcumin in the clinical setting is found to be detectable in colorectal tissues, the proposed protective effect of curcumin is largely limited to organ tissues which are exposed to the drug. Thus, the rather poor pharmacokinetic and dynamic characteristics resulting possibly from sulphation and glucuronidation of curcumin has precluded this otherwise highly effective agent to be developed for other cancers. However, novel advances in nanoparticle formulation have succeeded in making this natural product more bioavailable (Singh, 2007). It remains to be seen whether the clinical benefits of such formulations of curcumin will advance to angiogenic-dependent disease which could benefit from the therapeutic action of this homeostatin.

Panax ginseng (ginseng)

The roots of *P. ginseng* are highly revered in the Far East for their medical properties (Gillis, 1997). The main active principles that target blood vessels are the ginsenosides. Unlike turmeric, whose dual actions of angiomodulatory activity can be shown to result from a single compound (curcumin), the activity of ginseng is attributed to different subclasses of ginsenosides such as Rb1 and Rg1 (Yue *et al.*, 2007). At doses of 1 nmol/L to 1 μmol/l, 20(R)-Rg_3 showed dose-dependent inhibition of endothelial cell proliferation and inhibition of VEGF-induced chemoinvasion and tube formation. Additionally, in the Matrigel plug assay in mice, 600 nmol/L of Rg_3 reduced blood vessel growth by fivefold compared with controls (Yue *et al.*, 2006). Rg_3 also reduces the expression of MMP-2 and MMP-9, metalloproteinases that are involved in tube formation and invasion. Like Rg_3, the ginsenoside Rb_1 also demonstrates anti-angiogenic activity.

Notwithstanding the important anti-angiogenic activities of ginseng, it is shown that when Rb_1 is combined with Rg_1 in differing amounts these mixed ginsenosides can either induce or restrict blood vessel growth based on their compositional ratios (Sengupta *et al.*, 2004). This is because the panaxatriols represented by Rg_1 and Rb_1 have proangiogenic activity. The proangiogenic mechanism of Rg_1, which induces endothelial cell proliferation, is related to stimulation genes involved in cytoskeletal dynamics, cell–cell adhesion and migration (Yue *et al.*, 2005). It would appear that the cognitive supportive activity of ginseng derives from promotion of angiogenesis, or at least the stabilisation of blood vessels that are diseased in ageing brains of humans, while that of its use in the treatment of cancer would result from the anti-angiogenic activity of Rb_1 or Rg_3. *Panax ginseng,* which is rich in Rb_1, is reported to exert preventative activity in diverse cancer models, whereas Sanqi ginseng, which is rich in Rg_1 ginsenoside, has been employed in treatment of trauma injuries that require the promotion of capillary growth (Sengupta *et al.*, 2004; Yue *et al.*, 2007). Given these very interesting findings on the mechanism of ginseng varieties, it is imperative that the individual bioactive agents and their abundance be characterised in formulation of ginseng extracts.

Withania somniferia (ashwagandha)

This herb plant has invigorating and tonic uses in Ayurvedic medicine (Mishra *et al.*, 2000; Upton, 2000). Some of the popular uses of the roots of this plant are for the treatment of arthritic conditions and for bleeding disorders that result from menstrual dysfunction (Begum and Sadique, 1988). Hypothesising that an underlying angiogenic mechanism is targeted by the extracts of *W. somnifera*, we investigated the extracts of this plant for the presence of angiogenesis inhibitors by exploiting the 3D-ECSA (Mohan *et al.*, 2004). The combination of bioactivity testing in the 3D-ECSA along with assessment in the Matrigel model of angiogenesis revealed that the angiogenic inhibitory activity present in the methanolic extracts was enriched about fivefold upon further fractionation into chloroform-soluble substances. In assessing the molecular mechanism targeted by the chloroform-enriched fraction, it was found that the DNA binding activity of transcription factor NF-κB was specifically and potently inhibited by the chloroform extract (IC_{50} 10 μg/mL) (Mohan *et al.*, 2004). Further fractionation of the chloroform extract using HPLC afforded isolation of discrete peaks, which were individually tested for inhibitory activity in the 3D-ECSA. We characterised two of these compounds as withaferin A (Mohan *et al.*, 2004) and withanolide D (Bargagna-Mohan *et al.*, 2005). The anti-angiogenic activity of withaferin A and withanolide D result from potent targeting of NF-κB activity (IC_{50} = 0.5 μM) via a mechanism linked to upstream interference with the critical protein quality control complex, the ubiquitin proteasome pathway (UPP), a therapeutic target for a range of angio-inflammatory diseases (Mitsiades *et al.*, 2005).

The UPP is a cytoplasmic proteolytic complex that regulates protein expression during signal transduction by causing the destruction of critical factors, which are involved in the cell cycle, apoptosis, differentiation and inflammatory response (Crews, 2003). Withaferin A exerts its cytostatic effect on endothelial cells at substantially lower doses, causing blockade of the cell cycle (IC_{50} 12 nmol/L) via UPP-dependent down-regulation of the critical cell cycle regulator, cyclin D1 (Mohan *et al.*, 2004) (Figure 13.1). Based on these findings, it could be further

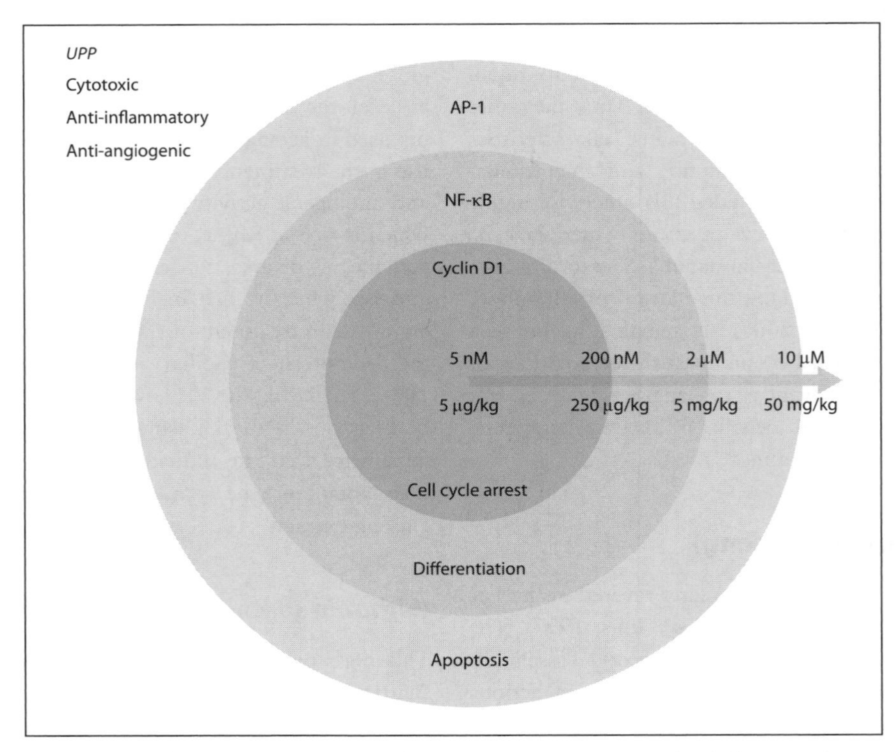

Figure 13.1 The dose-related ubiquitin proteasome pathway (UPP)-targeting activities of withaferin A. In human umbilical vein endothelial cells, the IC_{50} for inhibition of proliferation and sprouting (differentiation and NF-κB) is 12 nmol/L and 500 nmol/L, respectively (Mohan *et al.*, 2004). At concentrations above 2 μmol/L, withaferin A induces apoptosis. The corresponding doses in mg/kg of withaferin A shown below the arrow are our estimates for use in mice based on our investigations (Mohan *et al.*, 2004; Bargagna-Mohan *et al.*, 2007).

demonstrated that the in-vivo inhibition of angiogenesis by withaferin A was also significantly lower in the basic-fibroblast growth factor stimulated Matrigel plug model, being highly effective between 7 and 200 μg/kg/day (Mohan *et al.*, 2004). On the other hand, assessment of withaferin A in the corneal inflammatory model of neovascularisation revealed that doses between 500 μg/kg/day and 2 mg/kg/day reduced corneal angiogenesis by 50 and 80%, respectively (Mohan, unpublished data). In testing other genetic backgrounds of mice (129 SVEV) compared with previously used C57BL6 lines in the corneal inflammatory model of neovascularisation, we found that withaferin A at 2 mg/kg/day was highly effective, resulting in inhibition of 73% (Bargagna-Mohan *et al.*, 2007). Taken together, our strategy for isolation and investigation of anti-angiogenic natural products from medicinal plants has proven to be successful with discovery of withaferin A's angiogenesis inhibitory activity (Mohan *et al.*, 2004; Bargagna-Mohan *et al.*, 2005; Bargagna-Mohan *et al.*, 2007).

Perturbation of the UPP is responsible for various diseases states. For example, tumour cells possess a highly active proteasome which results in over stimulation of cell proliferation. In addition, proteasome inhibition also results in blockade of angiogenesis by causing apoptosis of vascular endothelial cells and inhibition of VEGF expression (Hamner *et al.*, 2007). Intriguingly, unlike proteasome inhibitors which directly target the enzymatic site of the 20S proteosome, withaferin A interferes with the UPP by an indirect mechanism. This UPP-targeting mechanism was recently shown to be due to binding by withaferin A to the type III intermediate filament protein vimentin (Bargagna-Mohan *et al.*, 2007). The anti-angiogenic response to 2 mg/kg/day withaferin A treatment in the corneal inflammatory model of neovascularisation is found to be 3-fold-lower in vimentin-deficient mice than corresponding wild-type mice (Bargagna-Mohan *et al.*, 2007).

The multiple dose-related activities of withaferin A, and structurally related withanolides that possess anti-angiogenic activity, can be distinguished (see Figure 13.1). At low nanomolar concentrations withaferin A's anti-angiogenic activity is related to cytostatic blockade of the cell cycle in G1 phase (Mohan *et al.*, 2004), whereas at sub-to-low micromolar concentrations, withaferin A targets cell differentiation associated with tubule formation and inflammatory activation of NF-κB (Mohan *et al.*, 2004). At doses higher than 2 micromolar, withaferin A induces apoptosis via a mechanism linked to cleavage of vimentin and F-actin aggregation (Bargagna-Mohan *et al.*, 2007). Given such differences in the mechanisms of withaferin A with respect to its dose, one has to be careful in how extracts from this plant are prepared and of the exact amounts and proportions of the bioactive withanolides present. Studies have shown that extracts obtained from different cultivars of *W. somnifera* (Negi *et al.*, 2000), or from different geographical locations (Sangwan *et al.*, 2007) have a wide range in amounts of withanolides. Thus it is imperative not only that there be standardising criteria to provide exact concentrations of the major chemical substances present in withania extracts but that these extracts also be biologically tested for efficacy for their intended use. Due to the heavy demand for *W. somnifera*, scientific attempts to produce these desirable compounds under defined laboratory conditions are being attempted (Sangwan *et al.*, 2007). It may soon be possible to then use such techniques to produce metabolites under highly controlled environments. In addition, the application of genetic engineering approaches to modify biosynthetic pathways in plants and plant cells so that desired metabolites are preferentially generated is another modern technology now being used to solve some of the issues of seasonal influences on natural product biosynthesis (Bandyopadhyay *et al.*, 2007).

Hypericum perforatum (St John's wort)

The widely used herb for depression, St John's wort, is also the source of anti-angiogenic agents, hypericin and hyperforin. Attention to the angiogenesis-inhibitory activity of hyperforin has attracted attention not only to the broader uses of this plant in human diseases, but also to the potential side-effects (Mandavilli, 2003), especially so in patients who may have other vascular complications where an anti-angiogenic agent would have contradiction. The mode of action of hyperforin is due to inhibition of MMP-9 expression (Quiney *et al.*, 2006), an enzyme that is responsible for basement membrane degradation during blood vessel growth. In addition, hyperforin inhibits microtubules which prevent endothelial cells from forming capillary tubes (Quiney *et al.*, 2006). Also, in other models hyperforin was shown to target component(s) within G-protein signalling cascades that regulate Ca^{2+} homeostasis, and inhibit neutrophil invasion and block inflammatory activation, suggesting that the target of this natural product is present on both vascular and inflammatory components that act in synergy during many angiogenic diseases. Interestingly, a dose of *Hypericum* extract 900 mg/day used as an antidepressant (which supplies 0.4 μmol/L of hyperforin) was shown to down-regulate production of the angiogenic cytokine interferon-gamma in activated T-cells with concomitant inhibition of MMP-9 expression (Cabrelle *et al.*, 2008). On the other hand, hypericin is also a potent angiogenesis inhibitor that targets activity of a related proteinase, MT1-MMP and is also responsible for inhibiting signalling events that trigger MAP kinase (Lavie *et al.*, 2005). Hypericin administered at 2 mg/kg intraperiteoneally, blocks activating phosphorylation of ERK1/2, which is required for the transactivation of hypoxia-inducible factor 1 alpha (HIF-1α) and in VEGF-induced blood vessel growth in models employing photodynamic therapy (Yee *et al.*, 2005; Bhuvaneswari *et al.*, 2007). Additionally, hypericin 3–50 μmol/L inhibits the activity of the proteasome complex in a dose-dependent manner (Pajonk *et al.*, 2005). This upstream activity is shown to block activation of transcription factor NF-κB at doses of between 6 and 50 μmol/L. It is noteworthy to point out some of the adverse effects of this plant, which include sensitivity to sunlight and drug interactions with selective serotonin reuptake and protease inhibitors, as well as intermenstrual bleeding or altered menstrual bleeding in users of oral contraceptives (De Smet, 2002), which may result from inherent proteasome inhibitory activity of hypericin-containing extracts of St John's wort.

Camellia sinensis (green tea)

Epidemiological evidence has raised the interest in green tea consumption for prevention of cancers and cardiovascular diseases, and invigorated scientific research to identify the biologically active substances of tea extracts (Yance and Sagar, 2006). One of the major ingredients of green tea, (−)epigallocatechin gallate (EGCG), a flavonoid, was shown to inhibit angiogenesis and have chemopreventive activity (Garbisa *et al.*, 2001; Cao *et al.*, 2002). Using data derived from rodent studies (Fassina *et al.*, 2004), a Phase 1 study of green tea extract was performed. Cohorts of adults with cancer were administered oral GTE with water with doses provided one or three times daily for 4 weeks (Pisters *et al.*, 2001). The maximum-tolerated dose was 4.2 g/m^2 once daily or 1.0 g/m^2 three times daily. Thus, a dose for anti-angiogenic activity in humans was calculated to be 1 g/m^2 three times per day (equivalent to 120 mL or 7–8 Japanese cups) for human consumption (Sagar *et al.*, 2006a). As much as 200–500 mg of green tea consisting of 50% (−)EGCG is believed to be the pharmacological dose for angiogenesis prevention (Sagar *et al.*, 2006b). Dose-limiting adverse effects of (−)EGCG are gastrointestinal and neurological, for which the coadministered presence of caffeine in green tea extracts is thought to be responsible for these side-effects (Pisters *et al.*, 2001). (−)EGCG has also been shown to inhibit COX-2 activity (Surh *et al.*, 2001), an enzyme that is well known to be a target for anti-angiogenesis. The angiopreventive activity of (−)EGCG is also believed to result from inhibition of MMP-2 and MMP-9 activities (Tosetti *et al.*, 2002). Furthermore, unlike other bioactive flavonoids that show inhibition of NF-κB activation, (−)EGCG is found to inhibit the DNA binding activity of inflammatory cytokine interleukin-1α-induced NF-κB, whereas flavonoids such as genistein do not produce this effect (Muraoka *et al.*, 2002). It is likely that angio-inflammatory pathways that up-regulate IL-1β may be targets of this class of natural product, differentiating EGCG products from other flavonoids. Thus, this class of flavonoid may be more suitable for use in inflammatory angiogenic diseases.

Vitis vinifera (red grapes)

Red wine consumption is believed to be protective of the cardiovascular system (Brouillard *et al.*, 1997), as evidenced in the prevention of the progression of atherosclerosis even in people who consume high amounts of red meat and cholesterol-containing foods (Zern and Fernandez, 2005). This was thought to be due to the major cardioprotective polyphenolic compounds found in skins and seeds of red grapes. One of these red wine polyphenolic compounds

(RWPC), is the natural product resveratrol. The anti-angiogenic mechanisms of resveratrol are known to be complex; since it inhibits proliferation of endothelial cells at 25 μmol/L, with inhibitory effects on cell migration and vessel tube formation occurring at 25 to 50 μmol/L (Hu *et al.*, 2007).

Interestingly, the inhibitory activity of resveratrol on metalloproteinases MMP-9 was observed at 6.25 μmol/L, whereas on MMP-2 activity was at 25 μmol/L. Resveratrol inhibits VEGF-induced angiogenesis by interfering with reactive oxygen species-dependent Src kinase activation, and down-regulates the expression of angiogenic cytokines, including interleukin-8 and VEGF (Lin *et al.*, 2003). It is interesting that RWPCs also show dose-dependent opposite effects on angiogenesis. In rats, 0.2 mg/kg/day of RWPCs caused a pro-angiogenic effect while higher daily doses of 2 mg/kg of RWPC (equivalents found in seven glasses of red wine) showed anti-angiogenic activity in the post-ischaemic model of hind limb neovascularisation (Baron-Menguy *et al.*, 2007). It was found that the low-dose (1/10 glass) angiogenic effect occurs through overexpression of PI3 kinase-AKT-NOS pathway leading to increased VEGF production without affecting MMP production. Intriguingly, in the non-ischaemic leg, neither the low nor high dose of RWPC affected angiogenesis or blood flow (Baron-Menguy *et al.*, 2007). Thus, it appears that a prior disease condition needs to manifest, to observe these pharmacological effects of RWPC. Since normal tissues did not appear to be responsive to either high or low dose effects of RWPCs, it cannot be inferred that these extracts are safe. For instance, others have shown that RWPCs at high doses can induce hypotension, decreased cardiac reactivity in rats (Ralay Ranaivo *et al.*, 2004). Interest in pharmacological activity of RWPCs has led to isolation of other principal active agents. Delphinidin, an abundant anthocyanin from RWPCs at high dose has been shown to inhibit vascularisation and blood flow at 0.6 m/kg per day, suggesting that the anti-angiogenic activity of RWPCs is derived, in part, from delphinidin (Baron-Menguy *et al.*, 2007).

Conclusions

The field of antiangiogenesis has greatly benefitted from discoveries of targets for therapeutic development from which angiogenesis-inhibitory drugs such as Avastin have emerged for treatment of colon cancer (Rugo, 2004). However, the literature is also beginning to see the emergence of undesirable side-effects of angiogenesis inhibitors. While it was once believed that adult tissues do not remodel their vasculature, it is now known that the microvasculature of the trachea and digestive system is not in a state of quiescence. Indeed, in mice, Avastin has been observed to cause normal mucosal capillaries in the trachea to regress. However, this drug-induced side-effect is ameliorated by cessation of Avastin treatment, indicative of the plasticity of the microvasculature to drug effects, and that developing safer treatments should involve careful examination of these preclinical and clinical results. As witnessed with natural product drugs emerging from traditional medicines (Corson and Crews, 2007), the guide to finding and developing highly effective and safe treatments for angiogenic diseases will need to integrate traditional knowledge with modern analytical methods of assessment and molecular pathobiology.

As the population ages, we are beginning to see many more diseases that result from vessel diseases which could benefit from angiomodulation. In these cases, one has to also remember that the physical constitution of older patients to drug activity is poorer because of weaker metabolism, reduced blood flow and general cellular ageing processes. More and more, the older patient groups will move towards more palatable medicines as older people are increasingly becoming dependent on multiple medications to support their different chronic conditions. In this context, it is critical to know contradictions to anti-angiogenesis drugs. Other clinical adverse effects of anti-angiogenic drugs include gastrointestinal perforations of the bowels, arterial blood clots, and hypertension (Yang *et al.*, 2003). The clinical manifestation of drug resistance to anti-angiogenic agents draws attention to yet another facet of cumulative toxic effects (Yu *et al.*, 2002). That is, while the endothelial cell which is genetically stable does not become resistant to drug action, the genetic alterations that decrease the vascular dependence of tumour cells can influence the therapeutic response of tumours to angiogenesis inhibitors.

Herbal products that strive to restore the angiogenic balance must demonstrate standardisation in material quality, biological/pharmacological efficacy, and safety principles because many of the active principles have opposite effects on blood vessel growth when their concentrations or compositions are altered.

References

Auerbach R, Lewis R, Shinners B, Kubai L, Akhtar N (2003). Angiogenesis assays: a critical overview. *Clin Chem* 49: 32–40.

Bandyopadhyay M, Jha S, Tepfer D (2007). Changes in morphological phenotypes and withanolide composition of Ri-transformed roots of *Withania somnifera*. *Plant Cell Rep* 26: 599–609.

Bargagna-Mohan P, Gambaro R, Mohan R (2005). *Withanolides: A new class of angiogenesis inhibitors*. Paper presented at 229th American Chemical Society National Meeting (San Diego, CA, American Chemical Society).

Bargagna-Mohan P, Hamza A, Kim YE *et al.* (2007). The tumor inhibitor and antiangiogenic agent withaferin A targets the intermediate filament protein vimentin. *Chem Biol* 14: 623–634.

Baron-Menguy C, Bocquet A, Guihot AL *et al.* (2007). Effects of red wine polyphenols on postischemic neovascularization model in rats: low doses are proangiogenic, high doses anti-angiogenic. *Faseb J* 21: 3511–3521.

Battegay EJ (1995). Angiogenesis: mechanistic insights, neovascular diseases, and therapeutic prospects. *J Mol Med* 73: 333–346.

Begum VH, Sadique J (1988). Long term effect of herbal drug *Withania somnifera* on adjuvant induced arthritis in rats. *Indian J Exp Biol* 26: 877–882.

Bell SE, Mavila A, Salazar R, Bayless KJ *et al.* (2001). Differential gene expression during capillary morphogenesis in 3D collagen matrices: regulated expression of genes involved in basement membrane matrix assembly, cell cycle progression, cellular differentiation and G-protein signaling. *J Cell Sci* 114: 2755–2773.

Berse M, Bounpheng M, Huang *et al.* (2004). Ubiquitin-dependent degradation of Id1 and Id3 is mediated by the COP9 signalosome. *J Mol Biol* 343: 361–370.

Bhandarkar SS, Arbiser JL (2007). Curcumin as an inhibitor of angiogenesis. *Adv Exp Med Biol* 595: 185–195.

Bhuvaneswari R, Gan YY, Yee KK *et al.* (2007). Effect of hypericin-mediated photodynamic therapy on the expression of vascular endothelial growth factor in human nasopharyngeal carcinoma. *Int J Mol Med* 20: 421–428.

Brouillard R, George F, Fougerousse A (1997). Polyphenols produced during red wine ageing. *Biofactors* 6: 403–410.

Cabrelle A, Dell'aica I, Melchiori L *et al.* (2008). Hyperforin down-regulates effector function of activated T lymphocytes and shows efficacy against Th1-triggered CNS inflammatory-demyelinating disease. *J Leukoc Biol* 83: 212–219.

Cao Y, Cao R, Brakenhielm E (2002). Antiangiogenic mechanisms of diet-derived polyphenols. *J Nutr Biochem* 13: 380–390.

Carmeliet P, Ferreira V, Breier G *et al.* (1996). Abnormal blood vessel development and lethality in embryos lacking a single VEGF allele. *Nature* 380: 435–439.

Carmeliet P, Jain RK (2000). Angiogenesis in cancer and other diseases. *Nature* 407: 249–257.

Caserman S, Lah TT (2004). Comparison of expression of cathepsins B and L and MMP2 in endothelial cells and in capillary sprouting in collagen gel. *Int J Biol Markers* 19: 120–129.

Corson TW, Crews CM (2007). Molecular understanding and modern application of traditional medicines: triumphs and trials. *Cell* 130: 769–774.

Crews CM (2003). Feeding the machine: mechanisms of proteasome-catalyzed degradation of ubiquitinated proteins. *Curr Opin Chem Biol* 7: 534–539.

De Smet PA (2002). Herbal remedies. *N Engl J Med* 347: 2046–2056.

Evans SM, Koch CJ (2003). Prognostic significance of tumor oxygenation in humans. *Cancer Lett* 195: 1–16.

Fan TP, Yeh JC, Leung KW *et al.* (2006). Angiogenesis: from plants to blood vessels. *Trends Pharmacol Sci* 27: 297–309.

Fassina G, Vene R, Morini M *et al.* (2004). Mechanisms of inhibition of tumor angiogenesis and vascular tumor growth by epigallocatechin-3-gallate. *Clin Cancer Res* 10: 4865–4873.

Ferrara N, Kerbel RS (2005). Angiogenesis as a therapeutic target. *Nature* 438: 967–974.

Figg WD, Kruger EA, Price DK *et al.* (2002). Inhibition of angiogenesis: treatment options for patients with metastatic prostate cancer. *Invest New Drugs* 20: 183–194.

Folkman J (1971). Tumor angiogenesis: therapeutic implications. *N Engl J Med* 285: 1182–1186.

Folkman J (1972a). Angiogenesis in psoriasis: therapeutic implications. *J Invest Dermatol* 59: 40–43.

Folkman J (1972b). Anti-angiogenesis: new concept for therapy of solid tumors. *Ann Surg* 175: 409–416.

Folkman J (1995). Angiogenesis in cancer, vascular, rheumatoid and other disease. *Nat Med* 1: 27–31.

Folkman J, Merler E, Abernathy C, Williams G (1971). Isolation of a tumor factor responsible for angiogenesis. *J Exp Med* 133: 275–288.

Friedrich EB, Liu E, Sinha S *et al.* (2004). Integrin-linked kinase regulates endothelial cell survival and vascular development. *Mol Cell Biol* 24: 8134–8144.

Garbisa S, Sartor L, Biggin S *et al.* (2001). Tumor gelatinases and invasion inhibited by the green tea flavanol epigallocatechin-3-gallate. *Cancer* 91: 822–832.

Garodia P, Ichikawa H, Malani N *et al.* (2007). From ancient medicine to modern medicine: ayurvedic concepts of health and their role in inflammation and cancer. *J Soc Integr Oncol* 5: 25–37.

Gillis CN (1997). *Panax ginseng* pharmacology: a nitric oxide link? *Biochem Pharmacol* 54: 1–8.

Hamner JB, Dickson PV, Sims TL *et al.* (2007). Bortezomib inhibits angiogenesis and reduces tumor burden in a murine model of neuroblastoma. *Surgery* 142: 185–191.

Healy DL, Rogers PA, Hii L, Wingfield M (1998). Angiogenesis: a new theory for endometriosis. *Hum Reprod Update* 4: 736–740.

Henke W, Ferrell K, Bech-Otschir D *et al.* (1999). Comparison of human COP9 signalsome and 26S proteasome lid. *Mol Biol Rep* 26: 29–34.

Hsu CH, Cheng AL (2007). Clinical studies with curcumin. *Adv Exp Med Biol* 595: 471–480.

Hu Y, Sun CY, Huang J *et al.* (2007). Antimyeloma effects of resveratrol through inhibition of angiogenesis. *Chin Med J (Engl)* 120: 1672–1677.

Korff T, Augustin HG (1998). Integration of endothelial cells in multicellular spheroids prevents apoptosis and induces differentiation. *J Cell Biol* 143: 1341–1352.

Kurz H (2000). Physiology of angiogenesis. *J Neurooncol* 50: 17–35.

Laterra J, Goldstein GW (1991). Astroglial-induced in vitro angiogenesis: requirements for RNA and protein synthesis. *J Neurochem* 57: 1231–1239.

Lavie G, Mandel M, Hazan S *et al.* (2005). Anti-angiogenic activities of hypericin in vivo: potential for ophthalmologic applications. *Angiogenesis* 8: 35–42.

Lin MT, Yen ML, Lin CY *et al.* (2003). Inhibition of vascular endothelial growth factor-induced angiogenesis by resveratrol through interruption of Src-dependent vascular endothelial cadherin tyrosine phosphorylation. *Mol Pharmacol* 64: 1029–1036.

Ma ZC, Gao Y, Wang YG *et al.* (2006). Ginsenoside Rg1 inhibits proliferation of vascular smooth muscle cells stimulated by tumor necrosis factor-alpha. *Acta Pharmacol Sin* 27: 1000–1006.

Maheshwari RK, Singh AK, Gaddipati J *et al.* (2006). Multiple biological activities of curcumin: a short review. *Life Sci* 78: 2081–2087.

Mandavilli A (2003). Natural-born killers. *Nat Med* 9: 634–635.

Meyers MR, Gokce N (2007). Endothelial dysfunction in obesity: etiological role in atherosclerosis. *Curr Opin Endocrinol Diabetes Obes* 14: 365–369.

Mishra LC, Singh BB, Dagenais S (2000). Scientific basis for the therapeutic use of *Withania somnifera* (ashwagandha): a review. *Altern Med Rev* 5: 334–346.

Mitsiades CS, Mitsiades N, Hideshima T, Richardson PG, Anderson KC (2005). Proteasome inhibitors as therapeutics. *Essays Biochem* 41: 205–218.

Mohan R, Hammers HJ, Bargagna-Mohan P *et al.* (2004). Withaferin A is a potent inhibitor of angiogenesis. *Angiogenesis* 7: 115–122.

Mohan R, Sivak J, Ashton P *et al.* (2000). Curcuminoids inhibit the angiogenic response stimulated by fibroblast growth factor-2, including expression of matrix metalloproteinase gelatinase B. *J Biol Chem* 275: 10405–10412.

Muraoka K, Shimizu K, Sun *et al.* (2002). Flavonoids exert diverse inhibitory effects on the activation of NF-κ. *Transplant Proc* 34: 1335–1340.

Neeman M, Abramovitch R, Schiffenbauer YS *et al.* (1997). Regulation of angiogenesis by hypoxic stress: from solid tumours to the ovarian follicle. *Int J Exp Pathol* 78: 57–70.

Negi MS, Singh A, Lakshmikumaran M (2000). Genetic variation and relationship among and within *Withania* species as revealed by AFLP markers. *Genome* 43: 975–980.

Newman SP, Leese MP, Purohit A *et al.* (2004). Inhibition of in vitro angiogenesis by 2-methoxy- and 2-ethyl-estrogensulfamates. *Int J Cancer* 109: 533–540.

Neuss H, Huang X, Hetfeld BK *et al.* (2007). The ubiquitin- and proteasome-dependent degradation of COX-2 is regulated by the COP9 signalosome and differentially influenced by coxibs. *J Mol Med* 85: 961–970.

Norrby K (2006). In vivo models of angiogenesis. *J Cell Mol Med* 10: 588–612.

Pajonk F, Scholber J, Fiebich B (2005). Hypericin – an inhibitor of proteasome function. *Cancer Chemother Pharmacol* 55: 439–446.

Pal MN (1997). Philosophy of medicine according to Ayurveda. *Bull Indian Inst Hist Med Hyderabad* 27: 103–118.

Paper D (1998). Natural products as angiogenesis inhibitors. *Planta Med* 64: 686–695.

Pisters KM, Newman RA, Coldman B *et al.* (2001). Phase I trial of oral green tea extract in adult patients with solid tumors. *J Clin Oncol* 19: 1830–1838.

Quiney C, Billard C, Mirshahi P *et al.* (2006). Hyperforin inhibits MMP-9 secretion by B-CLL cells and microtubule formation by endothelial cells. *Leukemia* 20: 583–589.

Ralay Ranaivo H, Diebolt M, Andriantsitohaina R (2004). Wine polyphenols induce hypotension, and decrease cardiac reactivity and infarct size in rats: involvement of nitric oxide. *Br J Pharmacol* 142: 671–678.

Ruegg C, Mutter N (2007). Anti-angiogenic therapies in cancer: achievements and open questions. *Bull Cancer* 94: 753–762.

Rugo HS (2004). Bevacizumab in the treatment of breast cancer: rationale and current data. *Oncologist* 9 Suppl 1: 43–49.

Ryan GJ (2007). New pharmacologic approaches to treating diabetic retinopathy. *Am J Health Syst Pharm* 64: S15–21.

Ryan TJ, Barnhill RL (1983). Physical factors and angiogenesis. *Ciba Found Symp* 100: 80–94.

Sagar SM, Yance D, Wong RK (2006a). Natural health products that inhibit angiogenesis: a potential source for investigational new agents to treat cancer – Part 1. *Curr Oncol* 13: 14–26.

Sagar SM, Yance D, Wong RK (2006b). Natural health products that inhibit angiogenesis: a potential source for investigational new agents to treat cancer – Part 2. *Curr Oncol* 13: 99–107.

Sangwan RS, Chaurasiya ND *et al.* (2007). Withanolide A biogeneration in in vitro shoot cultures of ashwagandha (*Withania somnifera* Dunal), a main medicinal plant in Ayurveda. *Chem Pharm Bull* (Tokyo) 55: 1371–1375.

Sengupta S, Toh SA, Sellers LA *et al.* (2004). Modulating angiogenesis: the yin and the yang in ginseng. *Circulation* 110: 1219–1225.

Shireman PK (2007). The chemokine system in arterio-genesis and hind limb ischemia. *J Vasc Surg* 45 (Suppl A): A48–56.

Singh S (2007). From exotic spice to modern drug? *Cell* 130: 765–768.

Singh S, Khar A (2006). Biological effects of curcumin and its role in cancer chemoprevention and therapy. *Anticancer Agents Med Chem* 6: 259–270.

Surh YJ, Chun KS, Cha HH *et al.* (2001). Molecular mechanisms underlying chemopreventive activities of anti-inflammatory phytochemicals: down-regulation of COX-2 and iNOS through suppression of NF-κB activation. *Mutat Res Sep* 1: 243–268, 480–481.

Thangapazham RL, Sharma A, Maheshwari RK (2006). Multiple molecular targets in cancer chemoprevention by curcumin. *AAPS J* 8: E443–449.

Thangapazham RL, Sharma A, Maheshwari RK (2007). Beneficial role of curcumin in skin diseases. *Adv Exp Med Biol* 595: 343–357.

Tosetti F, Ferrari N, De Flora S, Albini A (2002). Angioprevention: angiogenesis is a common and key target for cancer chemopreventive agents. *Faseb J* 16: 2–14.

Ucuzian AA, Greisler HP (2007). In vitro models of angiogenesis. *World J Surg* 31: 654–663.

Ulrich-Merzenich G, Zeitler H, Jobst D *et al.* (2007). Application of the '-Omic-' technologies in phytomedicine. *Phytomedicine* 14: 70–82.

Upton R (2000). 'Ashwagandha' Root in *American Herbal Pharmacopoeia* (Santa Cruz, CA), pp. 1–25.

Velazquez OC (2007). Angiogenesis and vasculogenesis: inducing the growth of new blood vessels and wound healing by stimulation of bone marrow-derived progenitor cell mobilization and homing. *J Vasc Surg* 45 Suppl A, A39–47.

Ventura C (2005). CAM and cell fate targeting: molecular and energetic insights into cell growth and differentiation. *Evid Based Complement Alternat Med* 2: 277–283.

Vernon RB, Angello JC, Iruela-Arispe ML *et al.* (1992). Reorganization of basement membrane matrices by cellular traction promotes the formation of cellular networks in vitro. *Lab Invest* 66: 536–547.

Wang M, Lamers RJ, Korthout HA *et al.* (2005). Metabolomics in the context of systems biology: bridging traditional Chinese medicine and molecular pharmacology. *Phytother Res* 19: 173–182.

Wen JK, Han M (2004). Application of genomics and proteomics in study of traditional Chinese medicine. *Zhong Xi Yi Jie He Xue Bao* 2: 323–325.

Yance DR, Jr, Sagar SM (2006). Targeting angiogenesis with integrative cancer therapies. *Integr Cancer Ther* 5: 9–29.

Yang JC, Haworth L, Sherry RM *et al.* (2003). A randomized trial of bevacizumab, an anti-vascular endothelial growth factor antibody, for metastatic renal cancer. *N Engl J Med* 349: 427–434.

Yee KK, Soo KC, Olivo M (2005). Anti-angiogenic effects of Hypericin-photodynamic therapy in combination with Celebrex in the treatment of human nasopharyngeal carcinoma. *Int J Mol Med* 16: 993–1002.

Yu JL, Rak JW, Coomber BL *et al.* (2002). Effect of p53 status on tumor response to antiangiogenic therapy. *Science* 295: 1526–1528.

Yue PY, Mak NK, Cheng YK *et al.* (2007). Pharmacogenomics and the Yin/Yang actions of ginseng: anti-tumor, angiomodulating and steroid-like activities of ginsenosides. *Chin Med* 2: 6.

Yue PY, Wong DY, Ha WY *et al.* (2005). Elucidation of the mechanisms underlying the angiogenic effects of ginsenoside Rg(1) in vivo and in vitro. *Angiogenesis* 8: 205–216.

Yue PY, Wong DY, Wu PK *et al.* (2006). The angiosuppressive effects of 20(R)- ginsenoside Rg3. *Biochem Pharmacol* 72: 437–445.

Zern TL, Fernandez ML (2005). Cardioprotective effects of dietary polyphenols. *J Nutr* 135: 2291–2294.

Zimrin AB, Villeponteau B, Maciag T (1995). Models of in vitro angiogenesis: endothelial cell differentiation on fibrin but not matrigel is transcriptionally dependent. *Biochem Biophys Res Commun* 213: 630–638.

14

Herbs affecting the central nervous system

David O Kennedy

Introduction

Herbal medicines have been utilised for their psychoactive and psychotropic properties throughout recorded history. However, in comparatively recent times we have become accustomed to the generally accepted notion that synthetic medicines will be more efficacious than natural products, although this view tends to overlook the fact that many medicinal products derived from nature. However, psychotropic agents comprised only 3 out of 84 new drugs of natural origin (Newman and Cragg, 2007).

One of these three is galantamine, originally derived from the Caucasian snowdrop (*Galanthus woronowii* Losinsk.) and now synthesised. Galantamine is interesting in that, having been initially identified on the basis of traditional ethnic use, it both validates the principles of an ethnopharmacological route to drug discovery (Heinrich and Teoh, 2004), and it also underlines the difficulty in translating most herbal medicines into 'mainstream' medicines. The reason for the latter is that although galantamine represents a potential improvement over the other cholinesterase-inhibiting treatments for Alzheimer's disease, in that it has demonstrated efficacy and is both a competitive inhibitor of acetylcholinesterase and allosteric modulator at nicotinic cholinergic receptor sites (Loy and Schneider, 2006), it also represents a single, isolated alkaloid.

In contrast to this, although the mechanisms of action of most established herbal medicines in this domain are far from clear, they could all be described as having multiple potentially active constituents and manifold potential mechanisms of action. It is unlikely that any will provide us with the next 'galantamine'. However, it is notable that a number of 'single action' synthetic psychotropic medications represent a poor cost–benefit profile in terms of efficacy and side-effects (e.g. the cholinesterase inhibitors for Alzheimer's disease) and the complexity of the central nervous system (CNS) does suggest that the polypharmacology offered by, for instance, *Ginkgo biloba*, *Salvia* species, *Hypericum perforatum* (St John's wort) or *Melissa officinalis*, may well provide more efficacious, better-tolerated, alternative treatments for disorders affecting the CNS.

The range of candidate herbal products with CNS effects is substantial. Zhang (2003) reviews the evidence pertaining to traditional medicinal herbal extracts that have undergone screening in animal models pertinent to psychiatric conditions and identifies more than 80 herbal extracts with evidence of potential efficacy. This contrasts with the current evidence base in humans, which is agglomerating around the handful of candidate extracts reviewed below.

The following therefore represents a brief summary of the putative bioactive components and mechanisms, and behavioural effects of the CNS active herbal products that have been subjected to significant research and/or demonstrated some potential efficacy in humans. For brevity it does not include combinations of herbs, or those that have not yet been tested in humans, nor does it include several herbal extracts that have a single, small, human study, and therefore resist any assessment as yet.

The herbal extracts are grouped into those that have predominantly been investigated for their effects on 'mood', 'sleep' and 'cognitive performance'. This chapter deals more on the results shown by scientific testing than on methods used, which can be found in the original papers referenced in the chapter.

Mood

Crocus sativus L. (saffron)

The stigmas of *Crocus sativus* L. contain a number of potentially bioactive compounds including a number of carotenoids (crocins), monoterpenes and flavonoids, including quercetin and kaempferol (Tarantilis *et al.*, 1995). Rodent behaviour models have demonstrated that *C. sativus* extracts can ameliorate scopolamine-induced memory performance (Pitsikas and Sakellaridis, 2006) and that crocins can enhance memory performance and attenuate scopolamine-induced memory deficits (Pitsikas *et al.*, 2007).

In humans, four double-blind, controlled trials, each with relatively small samples of 40 patients with mild-to-moderate depression, have demonstrated that 6–8 weeks of administration of dried ethanol extracts of *C. sativus* stigmas (15 mg) and petals (30 mg) are more effective than placebo (Akhondzadeh *et al.*, 2005; Moshiri *et al.*, 2006) and as effective as fluoxetine (but with no placebo control) (Noorbala *et al.*, 2005; Basti *et al.*, 2007) in ameliorating the symptoms of depression, as assessed by the Hamilton Depression Rating Scale. While *C. sativus* has been included on the basis that these studies show some promise, the evidence base requires research conducted in larger cohorts.

Hypericum perforatum L. (St John's wort)

Hypericum perforatum L. has been in recorded medicinal use from the time of the ancient Greeks (Di Carlo *et al.*, 2001). *Hypericum* extracts contain a number of groups of potentially bioactive constituents including flavonoids, phenolic acids, naphthodianthrones and phloroglucinols (Tatsis *et al.*, 2007).

The bioactive properties of St John's wort include inhibition of the neuronal re-uptake of serotonin, dopamine, noradrenaline, γ-aminobutyric acid (GABA) and L-glutamate, and increased neurotransmitter sensitivity and receptor binding (Butterweck, 2003; Mennini and Gobbi, 2004). These effects have been variously attributed over time to the naphthodianthrones, e.g. hypericin, pseudohypericin, protohypericin and protopseudohypericin, (Meruelo *et al.*, 1988), the phloroglucinol hyperforin (Zanoli, 2004) and the range of flavonoid constituents (Butterweck *et al.*, 2000).

Given their ability to modulate a wide range of neurotransmitter systems, it is not surprising that extracts and constituents have been shown to exert a plethora of effects relevant to behaviour in animal models. These include neuroprotective effects, an attenuation of cognitive impairment and improved cognitive performance (Kumar, 2006).

In humans the vast majority of research has focused on the antidepressant effects of *H. perforatum* extracts. In this domain a number of reviews and meta-analyses summarising the evidence have been published in the past 8 or 9 years. The two most recent reviews adequately encompass the considerable body of work in this area. In the first of these meta-analyses, Roder *et al.*, (2004) assessed the evidence from randomised, controlled trials for the efficacy of standardised extracts (dosage: 300–1200 mg/day) in the treatment of mild-to-moderate depression. They concluded that these extracts had a significant effect on symptoms in comparison with placebo, and performed as well as synthetic antidepressants.

A subsequent Cochrane review by Linde *et al.* (2005) included a total of 37 trials judged to be methodologically adequate that had assessed St John's wort in comparison with either placebo or standard antidepressants. In common with Roder *et al.* (2004), the authors conclude that the extracts seems to be more effective than placebo and as effective as standard antidepressants for treating mild-to-moderate depressive symptoms. However, beneficial effects for treating major depression appear minimal, although this latter conclusion may reflect a simple lack of research addressing this question. A subsequent review of reviews and meta-analyses (Pilkington *et al.*, 2006) also confirmed the general consensus that St John's wort is effective in the treatment of depression.

Given evidence of similar levels of efficacy as synthetic antidepressants, a further advantage of *H. perforatum* extracts is that they are generally found to be better tolerated. However, they can affect the metabolism of several medications resulting in reduced plasma concentrations (Ernst, 2004).

Melissa officinalis L. (lemon balm)

Melissa officinalis is a perennial, lemon-scented herb, used medicinally for over 2000 years, particularly for improved memory and mental function. Its contemporary usage includes as a mild sedative, in disturbed sleep, and in the attenuation of the symptoms of nervous disorders, including the reduction of excitability, anxiety, and stress (Kennedy and Scholey, 2006).

Potentially active constituents include a number of monoterpenoid aldehydes (including citronellal, neral and geranial), flavonoids and polyphenolic compounds (most notably rosmarinic acid) (Carnat *et al.*, 1998; Hohmann *et al.*, 1999) and monoterpene glycosides (Mulkens *et al.*, 1985).

Extracts have been shown to have both nicotinic and muscarinic cholinergic receptor-binding properties in human brain homogenates (Perry *et al.*, 1996; Wake *et al.*, 2000; Kennedy *et al.*, 2003) and essential oils have appreciable acetylcholinesterase-inhibitory properties (Perry *et al.*, 1996; Ferreira *et al.*, 2006). Extracts also have antioxidant properties (Lamaison *et al.*, 1991; Tagashira and Ohtake, 1998; Mantle *et al.*, 2000; Ferreira *et al.*, 2006) which are putatively attributable to their flavonoid content (Hohmann *et al.*, 1999).

In behavioural terms, a number of studies involving rodents suggest specific 'calming' or sedative effects following both essential oil (Wagner and Sprinkmeyer, 1973) and an hydroalchoholic extract of *M. officinalis* (Soulimani *et al.*, 1991).

A series of randomised, double-blind, placebo-controlled, balanced-crossover trials have also assessed the cognitive and mood effects of single doses of *M. officinalis* in humans. Two of these studies assessed the effects of a commercial lemon-balm methanolic, which lacked in-vitro nicotinic and muscarinic receptor-binding properties. In the first (Kennedy *et al.*, 2002a), three separate, single doses of *M. officinalis* extract (300 mg, 600 mg, and 900 mg) were compared with placebo, with 20 participants undergoing weekly assessments. The results demonstrated a dose-dependent impairment of memory function, with concomitant reductions in ratings of 'alertness' restricted to the highest dose and increased 'calmness' following the lowest dose.

In the second study (Kennedy *et al.*, 2004a), the two lower doses (300 mg, 600 mg) were investigated using a multitasking laboratory stressor paradigm, with the highest dose again leading to reduced ratings of alertness and increased ratings of calmness during the stressor battery. The pattern of results from these two studies is broadly in line with the traditional mildly sedative and calming properties of these extracts.

To assess the effects of *M. officinalis* with cholinergic receptor-binding properties, a further experiment (Kennedy *et al.*, 2003a) was conducted in two distinct phases. In the first phase, cholinergic receptor-binding properties were established across a number of samples, with the dried leaf with the highest nicotinic and muscarinic receptor-binding properties being administered in a placebo-controlled, double-blind, balanced crossover study assessing the cognitive performance and mood effects of several single doses (600, 1000, 1600 mg dried leaf). In this case, while the lowest of the three doses evinced similar memory decrements as those seen in the previous study, the highest dose both increased 'calmness' and improved memory performance. The results from these three studies suggest that lemon balm owes its mildly sedative properties to something other than cholinergic receptor binding.

Two recent double-blind, placebo-controlled studies have also assessed the effects of *M. officinalis* in patients with dementia. Ballard *et al.* (2003) examined the effect of essential oil aromatherapy (in comparison with vegetable oil) on ratings of agitation and quality of life of 71 patients with severe dementia. After 4 weeks' treatment, patients in the active treatment group were rated, in comparison with the placebo group, as being less agitated, less socially withdrawn, and as engaging in more time spent in constructive activities. Akhondzadeh *et al.* (2003) also assessed the effects of 60 drops/day of a tincture in 35 patients with mild-to-moderate dementia (20 verum, 15 placebo) who completed their 16-week trial. At the study endpoint, the results showed a clear cognitive advantage (ADAS-cog and Clinical Dementia Rating) and reduced agitation for the group taking the tincture.

Piper methysticum L.f. (kava)

Drinks and extracts made from the rhizome and roots of kava have been used for millennia in the South Pacific both recreationally and medicinally to reduce fatigue and induce relaxation and sleep (Lebot, 1992).

The major bioactive constituents of kava are styryl α-pyrones generally referred to as kavapyrones or, more commonly, kavalactones. Contemporary commercial Kava extracts are generally standardised to contain approximately 30–70% of kavalactones. It should be noted that leaves and stem contain potentially hepatotoxic alkaloids (Folmer *et al.*, 2006) but these are not generally considered to be responsible for the severe liver toxicity in a few individuals reported in recent years, which has led to severe curtailment of its use in many countries.

The exact mechanism underlying the central nervous system effects of kavalactones is poorly delineated to date. Kavalactones have been shown, at the most fundamental level, to modulate neuronal excitability via voltage-dependent calcium channels. They also modulate activity in the serotonergic, glutamatergic and dopaminergic neurotransmitter systems (Cairney *et al.*, 2002). In addition, kava's anxyolitic properties have been attributed to interactions with *N*-methyl-D-aspartic acid (Bilia *et al.*, 2002) and GABA receptors (Davies *et al.*, 1992; Jussofie *et al.*, 1994), although the evidence regarding the latter is inconsistent (Garrett *et al.*, 2003). Modulation of β-adrenergic activity may also play a role in their behavioural effects (Singh and Singh, 2002).

With regards to kava's anxiolytic effects, Pittler and Ernst's (2003) Cochrane review meta-analysed the randomised, controlled trials extant at that time. Twelve studies met their inclusion criteria and they concluded that, in comparison with placebo, kava extracts (administered for between 1 day and 24 weeks and containing between 105 and 280 mg of kavalactones) were associated with a significant reduction in anxiety on the Hamilton Anxiety (HAM-A) scale. Witte *et al.* (2005) went on to meta-analyse the six studies included in the latter analysis that had administered the standardised acetonic extract WS1490, and again found a significant treatment-related anxiolytic effect in comparison with placebo. With regards to behaviour, Cairney *et al.* (2002) note that a number of small studies have assessed the cognitive effects of kava. However, because of the methodology employed in these studies, the question is largely unresolved.

The focus of recent research has shifted away from efficacy and firmly towards putative negative side-effects and potential drug interactions of kava, since the publication of several case reports of treatment-related liver failure. These reports led to the withdrawal of kava by many national authorities, although the strength of the evidence on which these decisions were based is contested by many (Schulz *et al.*, 2003). Similary, it has been suggested that kava is capable of a host of theoretical drug interactions, for which hard evidence of specific cases is lacking (Ankea and Ramzan, 2004).

Sleep

Valeriana officinalis L. (valerian)

Extracts from the roots and rhizomes of *Valeriana officinalis* L. have a long, cross-cultural tradition of medicinal usage, mainly as mild sedatives and anxiolytics (Houghton, 1988), but they also demonstrate spasmolytic properties (Circosta *et al.*, 2007). The effects of valerian may be attributable to a number of potentially active constituents, including monoterpenes and sesquiterpenes, including the genus-specific valepotriates and valerenic acid. Root extracts also contain appreciable levels of GABA (Houghton, 1999), constituents which bind to a variety of neurotransmitter receptors (Marder *et al.*, 2003) including $GABA_A$ (Wasowski *et al.*, 2000), where they perform as an allosteric modulator of subunit specific $GABA_A$ channels (Khom *et al.*, 2007), adenosine A_1 receptors where they also exert a range of allosteric effects (Lacher *et al.*, 2007), and act on the $5HT_{1A}$ (Bodesheim and Holzl, 1997) and the $5\text{-}HT_{5A}$ receptors (Dietz *et al.*, 2005), which are implicated in circadian rhythms and anxiety.

Research in humans has tended to concentrate on the role of valerian in attenuating sleep disturbance. Stevinson and Ernst (2000) reviewed the 19 randomised, controlled trials that assessed its effects on sleep and insomnia, and concluded from the nine that reached their inclusion criteria, that the efficacy of valerian in this respect was 'promising but not fully conclusive'.

Similarly, a systematic review of randomised, controlled trials of valerian (Bent *et al.*, 2006) for improving sleep quality included 16 eligible studies. However, it was noted that the majority of studies had some methodological problems. Allowing for the possibility of a publication bias, the authors concluded that the evidence to date only 'suggested' that valerian improved sleep quality.

Valerian has also been reported to have a similar effect to benzodiazepines, with similar positive effects from 6 weeks' administration of 600 mg/day of valerian extract to those produced by 10 mg/day of oxazepam on sleep quality and waking symptoms in 202 non-organic insomnia outpatients (Ziegler *et al.*, 2002). Additionally a number of studies have reported a benefit to sleep following a valerian/hops combination (e.g. Schmitz and Jackel, 1998; Fussel *et al.*, 2000).

It is also interesting to note that, whereas no effect of valerian on psychomotor performance, alertness or concentration has been reported the morning after administration (Gerhard *et al.*, 1996; Kuhlmann *et al.*,1999), acute doses of valerian led to a significant deterioration in performance in vigilance and information-processing tasks 1–2 h after acute daytime administration (Gerhard *et al.*, 1996). Valerian is also often indicated for anxiety, but a recent Cochrane review (Miyasaka *et al.*, 2006) concluded that there was insufficient evidence of efficacy in this since only one pilot study (Andreatini *et al.*, 2002) was found to be eligible for inclusion according to their criteria. Taibi *et al.* (2007) interpret the literature as failing to show any convincing pattern of behavioural effects but *V. officinalis* extracts are associated with markedly less negative side-effects than benzodiazepines, with levels similar to placebo across clinical trials.

Cognitive performance

Bacopa monniera Wettst. (water hyssop)

Bacopa monniera has been used in Ayurvedic medicine for some 3000 years. Its traditional and contemporary indications include anxiety and cognitive performance and the active constituents are thought to be triterpenoid saponins, of which the most prevalent are known as bacoside A and B (Russo and Borelli, 2005).

Potential CNS-relevant mechanisms include an enhancement of protein kinase activity in the hippocampus (Singh and Dhawan, 1997), interactions with the cholinergic (Bhattacharya *et al.*, 1999; Das *et al.*, 2002) and monoaminergic (Singh and Dhawan, 1997; Sheikh *et al.*, 2007) neurotransmitter systems, and antioxidant properties (Bhattacharya *et al.*, 2000; Anbarasi *et al.*, 2006).

B. monniera extracts have been shown in animal models to protect cognitive function in the face of a number of challenges (Bhattacharya *et al.*, 1999; Das *et al.*, 2002) and exert anxiolytic effects in stress paradigms (Bhattacharya *et al.*, 2000; Shanker and Singh, 2000).

In humans the behavioural effects have received little methodical attention. However, several double-blind, placebo-controlled studies have assessed the cognitive and mood effects of *B. monniera* extracts. In the first of these Stough *et al.* (2001a) investigated the effects of 5 and 12 weeks' administration of 300 mg of a standardised (55% bacosides) extract in 46 healthy adult participants. By the 12-week endpoint, self-ratings of 'anxiety state', and cognitive tasks assessing speed of early information processing, verbal learning rate and memory consolidation were beneficially modulated in the group taking extract.

A second study using the same extract (Roodenrys *et al.*, 2002), involving 76 middle-aged participants, demonstrated a lack of any cognitive or mood effect following 3 months' administration of 300 or 450 mg extract (depending on body weight). However, an assessment 6 weeks after the end of the trial showed that the group taking extract had outperformed placebo on a single task, a 'delayed recall of word pairs' task. The authors tentatively interpret this as a possible attenuation of 'forgetting', but allow for the effect being a statistical anomaly. Given the lack of a clear effect from these two studies, *B. monniera* requires further research.

Ginkgo biloba L. (gingko)

Ginkgo biloba extract contains a number of species-specific flavonoids and the terpenoids: bilobalide and ginkgolides A, B, C and J (Kleijnen and Knipschild, 1992). Potential CNS-relevant mechanisms of action include:

- a potential antagonism of platelet activating factor (e.g. Akiba *et al.*, 1998; Krane *et al.*, 2003)
- enhanced nitric oxide bioavailability (Koltermann *et al.*, 2007)
- scavenging and inhibition of free radicals (Droy-Lefaix, 1997; Ramassamy, 2006)
- modulation of a number of neurotransmitter systems (Ahlemeyer and Krieglstein, 2003; Shah *et al.*, 2003; Defeudis and Drieu, 2004; Lee *et al.*, 2004; Ahmad *et al.*, 2005)
- beneficial effects on blood viscosity and circulation (Ahlemeyer and Krieglstein, 2003; Santos *et al.*, 2003 Galduroz *et al.*, 2007)
- both in-vitro and in-vivo protection against hypoxic challenges (Oberpichler *et al.*, 1988; Klein *et al.*, 1997; Jannsens *et al.*, 1999)
- in-vivo neuro-protective properties (Tadano *et al.*, 1998; Lee *et al.*, 2002; Ahlemeyer and Krieglstein, 2003)
- increased cerebral perfusion in humans (Santos *et al.*, 2003).

There is also some evidence of cognitive enhancement in both younger (Stough *et al.*, 2001b) and older (Mix and Crews, 2000, 2002) 'cognitively intact' populations administered 120 mg or 180 mg of gingko extract for 7 days or longer, although evidence in this respect is not unequivocal (Moulton *et al.*, 2001; Solomon *et al.*, 2002).

Several placebo-controlled, balanced crossover experiments, with relatively small sample sizes have also demonstrated improved cognitive performance in young adults following single doses of GBE (Hindmarch, 1986; Warot *et al.*, 1991; Rigney *et al.*, 1999; Kennedy *et al.*, 2000). In the last of these studies, Kennedy *et al.* (2000) demonstrated linear, dose-dependent speeding of attention task performance for the two highest doses under investigation (240 mg, 360 mg gingko extract), and improved memory following the lowest dose (120 mg) in 20 participants. A later re-analysis of the data for the lowest dose not only confirmed this memory enhancement effect but also suggested modest but significant slowing on attention tasks following this typical daily dose (Kennedy *et al.*, 2007b).

A large number of studies have assessed the efficacy of chronic administration of *Ginkgo biloba* in the amelioration of the cognitive declines associated with ageing and dementia. In this respect a comprehensive Cochrane review (Birks *et al.*, 2002) meta-analysed the 33 extant studies involving cohorts with dementia or age-related cognitive impairment that met their inclusion criteria. The authors concluded that 'Overall there is promising evidence of improvement in cognition and function associated with Ginkgo'. However, in a recent update and re-analysis, Birks and Grimley-Evans (2007) added a further three studies and deleted two studies and, in terms of cognitive function, fractionated their analyses by the length of treatment and the instrument employed. While there was evidence of improvement either following some treatment durations or dependent on the cognitive assessment instrument utilised, their revised overall conclusion was that the evidence with regards overall efficacy in dementia or cognitive impairment is 'inconsistent and unconvincing'.

Two potentially interesting randomised, controlled trials have also been published recently. Napryeyenko and Borzenko (2007) investigated the effects of ginkgo in 400 patients with mild-to-moderate dementia who also had concomitant neuropsychiatric symptoms (who would be expected to show more rapid decline than average) and demonstrated significant improvements in cognitive functioning and neuropsychiatric symptoms following 6 months' treatment with the extract Egb 761. A single trial (Woelk *et al.*, 2007) has also assessed the effects of two doses of Egb 761 in people with anxiety disorders. Results showed a significant dose-related improvement in Hamilton Rating Scale for Anxiety and a number of clinical measures. With regards safety, Birks and Evans (2007) conclude that *Ginkgo biloba* appears to be safe and comparable with placebo in terms of negative side-effects across studies.

Panax ginseng C.A. Mey. (ginseng)

'Ginseng' is generally taken to refer to the dried root of several species in the plant genus *Panax* (Araliaceae family). The most widely used family member is *P. ginseng,* which has a medicinal history stretching back more than 5000 years (Yun, 2001).

The major active constituents of the *Panax* genus are thought to be the species-specific saponins, also known as ginsenosides, of which over 30 have been identified (Tachikawa *et al.*, 1999).

Ginsenosides have a number of effects relevant to general health, including bolstering of the immune system, anti-inflammatory, antihepatotoxic and anticarcinogenic effects (Radad *et al.*, 2006). With regards to brain function, ginseng exerts a number of central and peripheral physiological effects that are potentially relevant. These include a host of neuroprotective properties, cardiovascular effects, modulation of the hypothalamic–pituitary–adrenal axis, neurotransmission (Kennedy and Scholey, 2003; Radad *et al.*, 2006), and glucoregulation (Reay *et al.*, 2005, 2006, 2007). While ginsenosides are known to exert a plethora of effects at a cellular level, a number of authors have suggested that the modulation of nitric oxide synthesis contributes to many of their wider effects (Gillis, 1997; Achike and Kwan, 2003; Kennedy and Scholey, 2003) including those within the CNS.

Animal behaviour models suggest that ginsenosides have antistress and anxiolytic effects (e.g. Park *et al.*, 2005; Carr *et al.*, 2006; Lee *et al.*, 2006), moderate fatigue (Min *et al.*, 2003; Voces *et al.*, 2004), improve memory in impaired rodents (Nishijo *et al.*, 2004) and improve learning and memory in several hippocampal/amygdala-dependent behavioural tasks in intact rodents (Kurimoto *et al.*, 2004). Potential mechanisms of the latter include the ability to foster neurogenesis (Qiao *et al.*, 2005) and modulate long-term potentiation in the hippocampus (Zhang and Zhang, 2000; Wang and Zhang, 2001).

In humans there is no clear evidence from controlled studies of ergogenic or antifatigue effects. Similarly, while a number of studies have demonstrated improvements in subjective 'wellbeing' or 'quality of life' attributable to ginseng monotherapy (Sotaniemi *et al.*, 1995; Marasco *et al.*, 1996; Wiklund *et al.*, 1999; Ellis and Reddy, 2002), a number of other studies have failed to find this effect (Hallstrom *et al.*, 1982; Ussher *et al.*, 1995; Thommessen and Laake, 1996; Cardinal and Engels, 2001). However, it should be noted that the lack of clear efficacy in these domains may reflect methodological shortcomings (Kennedy and Scholey, 2003).

A number of randomised, double-blind, placebo-controlled, balanced-crossover studies investigating single doses of *P. ginseng* have identified positive cognitive effects in healthy young adults. The most consistent finding is of improved secondary memory performance following standardised ginseng extract G115 alone (Kennedy *et al.*, 2001a, 2002b, 2004), and in combination with both *Ginkgo biloba* (Kennedy *et al.*, 2001b, 2002b) and guarana (*Paullinia cupana*) (Kennedy *et al.*, 2004). Improvements have also been noted in the speed of performing attention tasks (Kennedy *et al.*, 2004b; Sünram-Lea *et al.*, 2004) and significantly shortened latency of the P300 component of auditory evoked potentials measured by EEG, along with overall topographical modulation of electrical activity (Kennedy *et al.*, 2003b).

Two studies have also concomitantly measured glucoregulatory effects and cognitive performance during 'glucose sensitive', mentally demanding task performance. In the first of these, Reay *et al.* (2005) demonstrated significantly reduced fasted blood glucose levels and concomitant improvements in performance and reductions in self-ratings of mental fatigue in healthy young participants following 200 mg or 400 mg of G115. In the second study, Reay *et al.* (2006) used the same methodology and the most effective dose from the previous study (200 mg) but added a further factor: presence or absence of glucose 75 g. The results directly replicated the cognitive improvements, attenuation of mental fatigue and reduced blood glucose levels seen following ginseng alone in the previous study, but showed that these effects were largely abolished by coadministration with glucose.

The cognitive effects of longer-term dosage with ginseng has not been investigated to a great extent. In two early, double-blind, placebo-controlled studies, D' Angelo *et al.* (1986) and Sorensen and Sonne (1996) demonstrated improvements restricted to one or two task outcomes from within a large selection of tasks following ginseng 200 mg and 400 mg/day. Similarly, a recent double-blind, placebo-controlled pilot study (n = 16) using a balanced crossover design in an investigation of 8 weeks' treatment with 200 mg Korean *Panax ginseng* demonstrated improvements that were limited to two working memory tasks from within a larger battery, and one (social relations) of four scales from within the World Health Organization – Quality of Life scale (Kennedy *et al.*, 2007a).

P. ginseng monopreparations are rarely associated with adverse events or drug interactions (Coon and Ernst, 2002).

Salvia officinalis L. and *Salvia lavandulifolia* Vahl (sage)

The most commonly consumed species of the large genus *Salvia* are *S. officinalis* (garden sage) and *S. lavandulaefolia* (Spanish sage). Indications have traditionally included beneficial central nervous system effects, principally with regards mood and memory (Perry *et al.*, 1999).

It has been suggested that the monoterpenoid constituents of sage, e.g. 1,8-cineole, contribute to the physiological activity of the whole herb (Perry *et al.*, 2001). Extracts also contain a number of polyphenolic compounds, most notably rosmarinic acid and methyl carnosate (Hohmann *et al.*, 1999). Concentration-dependent inhibition of acetylcholinesterase in postmortem human brain homogenates was demonstrated by essential oils of both herbs and alcoholic extracts of both fresh and dried *S. officinalis* leaf (Perry *et al.*, 1999) and dose-dependent inhibition of human acetylcholinesterase by Spanish sage essential oil has also been shown (Perry *et al.*, 2000; Savelev *et al.*, 2004) and in vivo in the striatum and hippocampus of aged rats following oral administration (Perry *et al.*, 2002).

Acetylcholinesterase inhibition has been shown to involve synergistic interactions and antagonisms (Savelev *et al.*, 2003). Two studies have also demonstrated inhibition of butyrylcholinesterase in human erythrocytes (Savelev *et al.*, 2004; Kennedy *et al.*, 2006) and others have shown the antioxidant and free-radical scavenging properties of both sages (Lamaison *et al.*, 1991; Hohmann *et al.*, 1999; Mantle *et al.*, 2000; Perry *et al.*, 2001). This latter study also demonstrated anti-inflammatory actions by the extract and its geraniol and α-pinene monoterpenoid constituents.

Several other potentially CNS-relevant properties have also been demonstrated including an oestrogenic activity of Spanish sage and the monoterpenoid component geraniol (Perry *et al.*, 2001) and benzodiazepine receptor binding by fractions of a methanol extract of *S. officinalis* (Kavvadias *et al.*, 2003).

Five double-blind, placebo-controlled, randomised, balanced-crossover studies in healthy humans have assessed the behavioural effects of single doses of sage with in-vitro cholinesterase-inhibiting properties (the number of participants was 20, 24, 20, 30, 36 respectively). Tildesley *et al.* (2003) assessed the effects of three doses of *S. lavandulaefolia* essential oil and showed significant memory improvements in 20 healthy young participants following the two lowest doses (50 μL, 100 μL). In a subsequent study, Tildesley *et al.* (2005) examined the effects of 25 and 50 μL of the same oil in 24 participants and demonstrated that improved memory performance was most marked for the lowest dose of 25μL. Both doses also resulted in significantly increased ratings of 'contentedness' and 'calmness'.

The memory-enhancing effects in a healthy young population have also been confirmed in a recent study (Kennedy *et al.*, 2007a) into the effects of 50 μL *S. officinalis* essential oil. This study also demonstrated improved mood (alertness) and reduced ratings of mental fatigue during an extended period of cognitive demand. A further study (Scholey *et al.*, 2008) assessed the effects of four separate single doses of an ethanolic extract of *S. officinalis* in an elderly cohort. Once again the results showed clear improvements in memory performance, with this most marked for the lower two doses.

In one further study, Kennedy *et al.* (2006) also assessed the effects of two doses (300, 600 mg) of dried *S. officinalis* leaf with both acetylcholinesterase and butyrylcholinesterase-inhibitory properties on mood and performance of a psychological stressor multitasking battery. The results showed that the lower dose reduced anxiety and the higher dose increased ratings of 'alertness', 'calmness' and 'contentedness'. Task performance was also improved for the higher dose at both post-dose sessions, but reduced for the lower dose at the later testing session.

A single, double-blind, placebo-controlled trial has also assessed the effects of 16 weeks' administration of an *S. officinalis* alcoholic tincture in 30 patients with Alzheimer's disease (Akhonzadeh *et al.*, 2003b). Those in the verum group were shown to have significantly improved scores on the Alzheimer's Disease Clinical Assessment Scale cognitive subscale (ADAS-cog) at the study endpoint at 16 weeks. Clinical dementia rating scores were also significantly improved at the end of the study.

Why do herbal extracts have an effect on the central nervous system?

One common theme within this brief review of CNS-active herbs is the multiplicity of potential mechanisms of action. Interestingly, while the literature on the in-vitro, in-vivo, animal and human behavioural effects of herbal extracts is enormous, and growing exponentially (Zhang, 2003), the simple question of why bioactives from plants have CNS effects in mammals is largely overlooked. Herbal extracts owe their bioactive effects to a vast array of 'secondary metabolites' that are not directly involved, either in the plant's metabolism or indeed in its immediate ability to survive. Instead, these chemical compounds have developed via evolutionary and ecological pressure to serve a variety of functions that enhance the plant's longer-term survivability, e.g. the provision of colour, a host of localised protective roles (e.g. antioxidant, free-radical scavenging, ultraviolet absorption, antiproliferative, antiviral, etc.), roles in interplant relationships (e.g. allelopathic defence against competitors), interactions with a range of heterotrophs, including defence against fungi and bacteria, deterrence and attraction of insects and herbivores, and even symbiotic hormonal and central nervous system interactions with higher life forms, most notably insects (Harborne, 1993; Tahara, 2007).

It seems axiomatic that the physiological effects of consuming secondary metabolites within mammals can therefore be seen as being as a result of the similarity in biological processes across the eukaryotes, in this case the plant and animal kingdoms. The effects within humans may be merely a coincidental consequence of this similarity, but they may also take the form of a similar action as that exerted by the plant over other external organisms (e.g. insects), or alternatively a similar action to that which occurs within the plant itself. As an example of the former, acetylcholine is the major excitatory CNS neurotransmitter in insects (Gundelfinger and Schulz, 2000), and a range of extracts that have beneficial properties within the acetylcholine neurotransmitter system at low doses in humans may owe these properties to compounds functioning as toxic, predation deterrents within plant–insect relationships.

With regard to secondary metabolites exerting similar effects in their source plant and mammals, examples may include similarities in the protective effects conferred on the end-consumer. These include not only CNS-relevant antioxidant effects but also the more general antifungal/viral, antiproliferative, anti-ultraviolet light, etc. effects of consuming many secondary metabolites in mammals. In this respect, and inextricably linked to several of these general protective effects, it is interesting to note that the ubiquitous signalling molecule, nitric oxide, acts in plants in a similar manner as it does in animals (Arasimowicz and Floryszak-Wieczorek, 2007). In plants it plays a key role in several processes including protection during physical stress, disease and ageing (Crawford and Guo, 2005). In mammals this distinction is also clearly seen in the three isoforms of nitric oxide synthase, the enzyme responsible for nitric oxide synthesis. Two of these produce nitric oxide at a comparatively slow rate and contribute to a host of homeostatic physiological processes important to health. The third isoform, inducible nitric oxide synthase, on the other hand, produces nitric oxide at a rapid rate during immune and inflammatory responses to stressors and, when overactivated or activated for prolonged periods, is implicated in a range of pathological conditions (Achike and Kwan, 2003).

What is particularly intriguing is that the expression of potentially bioactive secondary metabolites during plant stress, for example, hypericin produced in the cells of *Hypericum perforatum* L., is related to nitric oxide production (Xu *et al.*, 2005), and that the secondary metabolite components of a number of herbal medicines play a role in the regulation of nitric oxide homeostasis in mammalian tissue models. As an example, a number of authors have suggested that the ginsenoside constituents of *Panax ginseng* may owe their efficacy in various domains to their ability to enhance constitutive nitric oxide synthesis throughout the tissues of the body, including the brain (Kennedy and Scholey, 2003). Similarly, the active components of *Ginkgo biloba* L. and a wide range of polyphenols from a number of sources have beneficial effects both in increasing constitutive nitric oxide synthase activity, thereby potentially improving, for instance, vascular tone and cerebral tissue perfusion, while also reducing the potentially damaging overproduction of inducible nitric oxide synthase (Achike and Kwan, 2003).

Given that neuronal nitric oxide synthase is also present throughout the brain, that levels are related to mood disorders (Karolewicz *et al.*, 2004) and that nitric oxide functions as a neurotransmitter in its own right (Jurado *et al.*, 2004), and is involved in synaptic plasticity and hippocampal long-term potentiation (LTP) (Blackshaw *et al.*, 2003) and general memory processes (Prast and Philippu, 2001), it becomes tempting to suggest that some of the CNS effects of herbal extracts are via the commonalities with regards to this signalling molecule.

Conclusions

From the hundreds of medicinal herbs that have demonstrated potential CNS-relevant properties in-vitro, and the 80 that have been assessed in animal models (Zhang, 2003), the above describes only nine that have been subjected to more than cursory, methodologically adequate investigation in humans. For two of them (*Bacopa monniera* and *Crocus sativus*), the research base is currently weak but may improve with time. Only four have generated enough research to be subjected to the meta-analyses favoured by the medical establishment.

One commonality between them is that they all possess multiple, potentially bioactive constituents, and may exert a multiplicity of CNS-relevant physiological effects. There are good arguments to be made for offering a polypharmacological treatment for complex CNS conditions. However, the very complexity of these potential treatments will hinder their application in a wider medical setting.

Overall, a great deal of more focused research is required to reach a full understanding of the bioactive constituents of plants (including the issues of standardisation and replication of extracts), their effects in mammalian physiological systems and their efficacy.

References

Achike FI, Kwan C (2003). Nitric oxide, human diseases and the herbals that affect the nitric oxide signaling. *Clin Exp Pharmacol Physiol* 30: 605–615.

Ahlemeyer B, Krieglstein J (2003). Neuroprotective effects of *Ginkgo biloba* extract. *Cell Mol Life Sci* 60: 1779–1792.

Ahmad M, Saleem S, Ahmad AS *et al.* (2005). *Ginkgo biloba* affords dose-dependent protection against 6-hydroxydopamine-induced parkinsonism in rats: Neurobehavioural, neurochemical and immunohistochemical evidences. *J Neurochem* 93 (1): 94–104.

Akhondzadeh S, Noroozian M, Mohammadi M *et al.* (2003). *Melissa officinalis* extract in the treatment of patients with mild to moderate Alzheimer's disease: a double blind, randomised, placebo controlled trial. *J Neurol Neurosurg Psychiatry* 74: 863–866.

Akhondzadeh S, Tahmacebi-Pour N, Noorbala AA *et al.* (2005). *Crocus sativus* L. in the treatment of mild to moderate depression: a double-blind, randomized and placebo-controlled trial. *Phytother Res* 19: 148–151.

Akiba S, Kawauchi T, Oka T *et al.* (1998). Inhibitory effect of the leaf extract of *Ginkgo biloba* L. on oxidative stress-induced platelet aggregation. *Biochem Mol Biol Int* 46: 1243–1248.

Anbarasi K, Vani G, Balakrishna K *et al.* (2006). Effect of bacoside A on brain antioxidant status in cigarette smoke exposed rats. *Life Sci* 78: 1378–1384.

Andreatini R, Sartori VA, Seabra MLV *et al.* (2002). Effect of valepotriates (valerian extract) in Generalised Anxiety Disorder: a randomized placebo-controlled pilot study. *Phytother Res* 16: 650–654.

Ankea J, Ramzan I (2004). Pharmacokinetic and pharmacodynamic drug interactions with Kava (*Piper methysticum* Forst. f.). *J Ethnopharmacol* 93: 153–160.

Arasimowicz M, Floryszak-Wieczorek J (2007). Nitric oxide as a bioactive signalling molecule in plant stress responses. *Plant Sci* 172: 876–887.

Ballard CG, O'Brien JT, Reichelt K *et al.* (2003). Aromatherapy as a safe and effective treatment for the management of agitation in severe dementia: the results of a double-blind, placebo-controlled trial with Melissa. *J Clin Psychiatr* 63: 553–558.

Basti AA, Moshiri E, Noorbala A *et al.* (2007). Comparison of petal of *Crocus sativus* L. and fluoxetine in the treatment of depressed outpatients: A pilot double-blind randomized trial. *Prog Neuro-Psychopharmacol Biol Psychiatr* 31: 439–442.

Bent S, Padula A, Moore D *et al.* (2006). Valerian for sleep: a systematic review and meta-analysis. *Am J Med* 119: 1005–1012.

Bhattacharya SK, Bhattacharya A, Kumar A *et al.* (2000). Antioxidant activity of *Bacopa monniera* in rat frontal cortex, striatum and hippocampus. *Phytother Res* 14: 174–179.

Bhattacharya SK, Kumar A, Ghosal S (1999). Effect of *Bacopa monniera* on animal models of Alzheimer's disease and perturbed central cholinergic markers of cognition in rats. In: *Molecular Aspects of Asian Medicines*. Ed D.V. Siva Sankar. PJD Publications, New York.

Bilia RA, Gallori S, Vincieri FF (2002). Kava-kava and anxiety: Growing knowledge about the efficacy and safety. *Life Sci* 70: 2581–2597.

Birks J, Grimley Evans J (2007). Ginkgo biloba for cognitive impairment and dementia. *Cochrane Database of Systematic Reviews* Issue 2: CD003120. DOI: 10.1002/14651858.CD003120.pub2.

Birks J, Grimley EV, Van Dongen M (2002). *Ginkgo biloba* for cognitive impairment and dementia. *Cochrane Database of Systematic Reviews* Issue 4: CD003120.

Blackshaw S, Eliasson MJ, Sawa A *et al.* (2003). Species, strain and developmental variations in hippocampal neuronal and endothelial nitric oxide synthase clarify discrepancies in nitric oxide-dependent synaptic plasticity. *Neuroscience* 119: 979–990.

Bodesheim U, Holzl J (1997). Isolierung, Strukturaufklärung und Radioreceptor-assays von Alkaloiden und Lignan aus Valeriana officinalis L. *Pharmazie* 52: 386–391.

Butterweck V (2003). Mechanism of action of St John's wort in depression: what is known? *CNS Drugs* 17: 539–562.

Butterweck V, Jurgemlienk G, Nahrstedt A *et al.* (2000). Flavonoid from *Hypericum perforatum* show antidepressant activity in the forced swimming test. *Planta Med* 66: 3–6.

Cairney S, Maruff P, Clough AR (2002). The neurobehavioural effects of kava. *Aust NZ J Psychiatr* 36: 657–662.

Cardinal BJ, Engles HJ (2001). Ginseng does not enhance psychological well-being in healthy young adults: results of a double blind, placebo controlled randomized clinical trail. *J Am Diet Assoc* 101: 655–660.

Carnat AP, Carnat A, Fraisse D *et al.* (1998). The aromatic and polyphenolic composition of lemon balm (*Melissa Officinalis* L. subsp. *Officinalis*) tea. *Pharm Acta Helv* 72: 301–305.

Carr MN, Bekku N, Yoshimura H (2006). Identification of anxiolytic ingredients in ginseng root using the elevated plus-maze test in mice. *Eur J Pharmacol* 531: 160–165.

Circosta C, De Pasqualea R, Samperia S *et al.* (2007). Biological and analytical characterization of two extracts from *Valeriana officinalis*. *J Ethnopharmacol* 112: 361–367.

Coon JT, Ernst E (2002). *Panax ginseng* – A systematic review of adverse effects and drug interactions. *Drug Saf* 25: 323–344.

Crawford NM, Guo F (2005). New insights into nitric oxide metabolism and regulatory functions. *Trends Plant Sci* 10: 195–200.

D'Angelo L, Grimaldi R, Caravaggi M *et al.* (1986). A double-blind, placebo-controlled clinical study on the effect of a standardized ginseng extract on psychomotor performance in healthy volunteers. *J Ethnopharmacol* 16: 15–22.

Das A, Shanker G, Nath C *et al.* (2002). A comparative study in rodents of standardized extracts of *Bacopa monniera* and *Ginkgo biloba*. *Pharmacol Biochem Behav* 73: 893–900.

Davies LP, Drew CA, Duffield P *et al.* (1992). Kava pyrones and resin: studies on GABAA, GABAB and benzodiazepine binding sites in rodent brain. *Pharmacol Toxicol* 71: 120–126.

DeFeudis FV, Drieu K (2004). "Stress-alleviating" and "vigilance-enhancing" actions of *Ginkgo biloba* extract (EGb 761). *Drug Dev Res* 62 (1): 1–25.

Di Carlo G, Borrelli F, Ernst E *et al.* (2001). St. John's wort: Prozac from the plant kingdom. *Trends Pharmacol Sci* 22: 292–297.

Dietz BM, Mahady GB, Pauli GF *et al.* (2005). Valerian extract and valerenic acid are partial agonists of the 5-HT5a receptor in vitro. *Mol Brain Res* 138: 191–197.

Droy-Lefaix MT (1997). Effect of the antioxidant action of *Ginkgo biloba* extract (Egb 761) on aging and oxidative stress. *Age* 20: 141–149.

Ellis JM, Reddy P (2002). Effects of *Panax ginseng* on quality of life. *Ann Pharmacother* 36: 375–279.

Ferreira A, Proenc C, Serralheiro MLM *et al.* (2006). The in vitro screening for acetylcholinesterase inhibition and antioxidant activity of medicinal plants from Portugal. *J Ethnopharmacol* 108: 31–37.

Folmer F, Blasius R, Morceau F (2006). Inhibition of TNFα-induced activation of nuclear factor κB by kava (*Piper methysticum*) derivatives. *Biochem Pharmacol* 71: 1206–1218.

Fussel A, Wolf A, Brattstrom A (2000). Effect of a fixed valerian-Hop extract combination (Ze 91019) on sleep polygraphy in patients with non-organic insomnia: a pilot study. *Eur J Med Res* 18: 5: 385–390.

Galduróz JCF, Antunes HK, Santos RF (2007). Gender- and age-related variations in blood viscosity in normal volunteers: A study of the effects of extract of *Allium sativum* and *Ginkgo biloba*. *Phytomedicine* 14: 447–451.

Garrett KM, Basmadjian G, Khan IA *et al.* (2003). Extracts of kava (*Piper methysticum*) induce acute anxiolytic-like behavioral changes in mice. *Psychopharmacology* 170: 33–41.

Gerhard U, Linnenbrink N, Georghiadou C *et al.* (1996). Vigilanzmindernde Effekte zweier pflanzlicher Schlafmittel [Vigilance-decreasing effects of two plant-derived sedatives]. *Rev Suisse Med Prax* 85: 473–481.

Gillis CN (1997). *Panax ginseng* pharmacology: a nitric oxide link? *Biochem Pharmacol* 4: 1–8.

Gundelfinger E, Schulz R (2000). Insect nicotinic acetylcholine receptors: genes, structure, physiological and pharmacological properties, In: *Handbook of experimental pharmacology*, Eds. F. Clementi, D. Fornasari, and C. Gotti. Berlin: Springer-Verlag. pp. 497–521.

Hallstrom C, Fulder S, Carruthers M (1982). Effects of ginseng on the performance of nurses on night duty. *Comparat Med East West* 6: 277–282.

Harborne JB (1993). *Introduction to Ecological Biochemistry*, 4th edn. London Elsevier.

Heinrich M, Teoh HL (2004). Galanthamine from snowdrop – the development of a modern drug against Alzheimer's disease from local Caucasian knowledge. *J Ethnopharmacol* 92: 147–162.

Hindmarch I (1986). Activity of *Ginkgo biloba* extract on short-term memory. *Presse Med* 15: 1592–1594.

Hohmann J, Zupko I, Redei D *et al.* (1999). Protective effects of the aerial parts of *Salvia Officinalis*, *Melissa Officinalis* and *Lavandula angustifolia* and their constituents against enzyme-dependent and enzyme-independent lipid peroxidation. *Planta Med* 65: 576–578.

Houghton PJ (1988). The biological activity of Valerian and related plants. *J Ethnopharmacol* 22: 121–142.

Houghton PJ (1999). The scientific basis for the reputed activity of Valerian. *J Pharm Pharmacol* 51: 505–512.

Janssens D, Remacle J, Drieu K *et al.* (1995). Protection of mitochondrial respiration activity by bilobalide. *Biochem Pharmacol* 58: 109–119.

Jurado S, Sanchez-Prieto J, Torres M (2004). Elements of the nitric oxide/cGMP pathway expressed in cerebellar granule cells: biochemical and functional characterisation. *Neurochem Int* 45: 833–843.

Jussofie A, Schmiz A, Hiemke C (1994). Kavapyrone enriched extract from *Piper methysticum* as modulator of the GABA binding site in different regions of rat brain. *Psychopharmacology* 116: 469–474.

Karolewicz B, Szebeni K, Stockmeier CA *et al.* (2004). Low nNOS protein in the locus coeruleus in major depression. *J Neurochem* 91 (5): 1057–1066.

Kavvadias D, Monschein V, Sand P *et al.* (2003). Constituents of sage (*Salvia officinalis*) with in vitro affinity to human brain benzodiazepine receptor. *Planta Med* 69: 113–117.

Kennedy DO, Scholey AB, Wesnes KA (2001a). Differential, dose-dependent changes in cognitive performance and mood following acute administration of *Ginseng* to healthy young volunteers. *Nutri Neurosci* 4: 295–310.

Kennedy DO, Haskell CF, Wesnes KA *et al.* (2004b). Improved cognitive performance in humans volunteers following administration of guarana (*Paulinia cupana*) extract: comparison and interaction with *Panax ginseng*. *Pharmacol Biochem Behav* 79: 401–411.

Kennedy DO, Jackson PA, Haskell CF *et al.* (2007a). Modulation of cognitive performance following single doses of 120mg *Ginkgo biloba* extract administered to healthy young volunteers. *Hum Psychopharmacol Clin Exp* 22: 559–556.

Kennedy DO, Little W, Scholey AB (2004a). Attenuation of laboratory induced stress in humans following acute administration of *Melissa officinalis* (Lemon Balm). *Psychosom Med* 66: 607–613.

Kennedy DO, Pace S, Haskell C *et al.* (2006). Effects of cholinesterase inhibiting sage (*Salvia officinalis*) on mood, anxiety and performance on a psychological stressor battery. *Neuropsychopharmacology* 31: 845–852.

Kennedy DO, Reay JL, Scholey AB (2007b). Effects of 8 weeks administration of Korean *Panax ginseng* extract on the mood and cognitive performance of healthy individuals. *J Ginseng Res* 1: 34–43.

Kennedy DO, Scholey AB (2003). Ginseng: potential for the enhancement of cognitive performance and mood. *Pharmacol Biochem Behav* 75: 687–700.

Kennedy DO, Scholey AB (2006). The psychopharmacology of European herbs with cognition enhancing properties. *Curr Pharm Des* 12: 4613–4623.

Kennedy DO, Scholey AB, Drewery L *et al.* (2003b). Topographic EEG effects of single doses of *Panax ginseng* and *Ginkgo biloba*. *Pharmacol Biochem Behav* 75: 701–709.

Kennedy DO, Scholey AB, Tildesley NTJ *et al.* (2002a). Modulation of mood and cognitive performance following acute administration of single doses of *Melissa officinalis* (Lemon Balm). *Pharmacol Biochem Behav* 72: 953–964.

Kennedy DO, Scholey AB, Wesnes K (2001b). Differential, dose dependent changes in cognitive performance following acute administration of a *Ginkgo biloba/Panax ginseng* combination to healthy young volunteers. *Nutrit Neurosci* 4: 399–412.

Kennedy DO, Scholey AB, Wesnes KA (2002b). Modulation of cognition and mood following administration of single doses of *Ginkgo biloba*, *Ginseng* and a *Ginkgo/Ginseng* combination to healthy young adults. *Physiol and Behav* 75: 1–13.

Kennedy DO, Wake G, Savelev S *et al.* (2003a). Modulation of mood and cognitive performance following administration of single doses of *Melissa officinalis* (Lemon balm) with human CNS nicotinic and muscarinic receptor binding properties. *Neuropsychopharmacology* 28: 1871–1881.

Khom S, Baburin I, Timin E *et al.* (2007). Valerenic acid potentiates and inhibits GABAA receptors: Molecular mechanism and subunit specificity. *Neuropharmacology* 53: 178–187.

Kleijnen J, Knipschild P (1992). *Ginkgo biloba*. *Lancet* 12: 340 (8833): 1474.

Klein J, Chatterjee SS, Loffelholz K (1997). Phospholipid breakdown and choline release under hypoxic conditions: inhibition by bilobalide, a constituent of *Ginkgo biloba*. *Brain Res* 755: 347–350.

Koltermann A, Hartkorn A, Koch E *et al.* (2007). *Ginkgo biloba* extract EGb 761 increases endothelial nitric oxide production in vitro and in vivo. *Cell Mol Life Sci* 64: 1715–1722.

Krane S, Kim SR, Abrell LM *et al.* (2003). Microphysiometric measurement of PAF receptor responses to ginkgolides. *Helv Chim Acta* 86: 3776–3786.

Kuhlmann J, Berger W, Podzuweit H *et al.* (1999). The influence of valerian treatment on 'reaction time, alertness and concentration' in volunteers. *Pharmacopsychiatry* 32: 235–241.

Kumar V (2006). Potential medicinal plants for CNS disorders: an overview. *Phytother Res* 20: 1023–1035.

Kurimoto H, Nishijo H, Uwano T *et al.* (2004). Effects of nonsaponin fraction of red ginseng on learning deficits in aged rats. *Physiol Behav* 82: 345–355.

Lacher SK, Mayera R, Sichardt K *et al.* (2007). Interaction of valerian extracts of different polarity with adenosine receptors: Identification of isovaltrate as an inverse agonist at A1 receptors. *Biochem Pharmacol* 73: 248–258.

Lamaison JL, Petitjean-Freytet C, Carnat A (1991). Medicinal Lamiaceae with antioxidant properties, a potential source of rosmarinic acid. *Pharm Acta Helv* 66: 185–188.

Lebot V, Merlin M, Lindstrom L (1992). *Kava, the Pacific Drug*. New Haven, Yale University Press.

Lee EJ, Chen HY, Wu TS *et al.* (2002). Acute administration of *Ginkgo biloba* extract (EGb 761) affords neuroprotection against permanent and transient focal cerebral ischemia in Sprague-Dawley rats. *J Neurosci Res* 68: 636–645.

Lee SH, Jung BH, Kim SY *et al.* (2006). The anti-stress effect of ginseng total saponin ginsenoside Rg3 and Rb1 evaluated by brain polyamine level under immobilization stress. *Pharmacol Res* 54 (1): 46–49.

Lee TF, Chen CF, Wang LCH (2004). Effect of ginkgolides on beta-amyloid-suppressed acetylocholine release from rat hippocampal slices. *Phytother Res* 18 (7): 556–560.

Linde K, Mulrow CD, Berner M *et al.* (2005). St John's Wort for depression. *The Cochrane Database of Systematic Reviews* Issue 3: CD000448. doi: 10.1002/14651858.CD000448.pub2.

Loy C, Schneider L (2006). Galantamine for Alzheimer's disease and mild cognitive impairment. *Cochrane Database of Systematic Reviews* Issue 1: CD001747. DOI: 10.1002/14651858.CD001747.pub3.

Mantle D, Eddeb F, Pickering A (2000). Comparison of relative antioxidant activities of British medicinal plant species in vitro. *J Ethnopharmacol* 72: 47–51.

Marasco A, Vargas Ruiz R, Salas Villagomez A *et al.* (1996). Double-blind study of a multivitamin complex supplemented with ginseng extract. *Drugs Exp Clin Res* 22: 323–329.

Marder M, Viola H, Wasowski C *et al.* (2003). 6-methylapigenin and hesperidin: new Valeriana flavonoids with activity on the CNS. *Pharmacol Biochem Behav* 75: 537–545.

Mennini T, Gobbi M (2004). The antidepressant mechanism of *Hypericum perforatum*. *Life Sci* 75: 1021–1027.

Meruelo D, Lavie G, Lavie D (1988). Therapeutic agents with dramatic antiretroviral activity and little toxicity at effective doses: aromatic polycyclic diones hypericin and pseudohypericin. *Proc Natl Acad Sci USA* 85: 5230–5234.

Min YK, Chung SH, Lee JS *et al.* (2003). Red ginseng inhibits exercise-induced increase in 5-hydroxytryptamine synthesis and tryptophan hydroxylase expression in dorsal raphe of rats. *J Pharmacol Sci* 93: 218–221.

Mix JA, Crews WD (2000). An examination of the efficacy of *Ginkgo biloba* extract EGb761 on the neuropsychologic functioning of cognitively intact older adults. *J Altern Complement Med* 6: 219–229.

Mix JA, Crews WD (2002). A double-blind, placebo-controlled, randomized trial of *Ginkgo biloba* extract EGb 761 (R) in a sample of cognitively intact older adults: neuropsychological findings. *Hum Psychopharmacol Clin Exp* 17: 267–277.

Miyasaka LS, Atallah AN, Soares BGO (2006). Valerian for anxiety disorders. *Cochrane Database of Systematic Reviews* Issue 4: CD004515. DOI: 10.1002/14651858.CD004515.pub2.

Moshiri E, Basti AA, Noorbala A *et al.* (2006). *Crocus sativus* L. (petal) in the treatment of mild-to-moderate depression: A double-blind, randomized and placebo-controlled trial. *Phytomedicine* 13: 607–611.

Moulton PL, Boyko LN, Fitzpatrick JL *et al.* (2001). The effect of *Ginkgo biloba* on memory in healthy male volunteers. *Physiol Behav* 73: 659–665.

Mulkens A, Stephanou E, Kapetenadis I (1985). Heterosides a genines volatiles dans les feuilles de *Melissa Officinalis* L. (Lamiaceae). *Pharm Acta Helv* 60: 276–278.

Napryeyenko O, Borzenko I (2007). *Ginkgo biloba* special extract in dementia with europsychiatric features: A randomised, placebo-controlled, double-blind clinical trial. *Arzneimittelforschung* 57: 4–11.

Newman DJ, Cragg GM (2007). Natural products as

sources of new drugs over the last 25 years. *J Nat Prod* 70: 461–477.
Nishijo H, Uwano T, Zhong YM *et al.* (2004). Proof of the mysterious efficacy of ginseng: Basic and clinical trails: Effects of red ginseng on learning and memory deficits in an animal model of amnesia. *J Pharmacol Sci* 95: 145–152.
Noorbala AA, Akhondzadeh S, Tahmacebi-Pour N *et al.* (2005). Hydro-alcoholic extract of *Crocus sativus* L. versus fluoxetine in the treatment of mild to moderate depression: a double-blind, randomized pilot trial. *J Ethnopharmacol* 97: 281–284.
Oberpichler H, Beck T, Abdel-Rahman MM *et al.* (1988). Effects of *Ginkgo biloba* constituents related to protection against brain damage caused by hypoxia. *Pharmacol Res Commun* 20: 349–368.
Park JH, Cha HY, Seo JJ *et al.* (2005). Anxiolytic-like effects of ginseng in the elevated plus-maze model: Comparison of red ginseng and sun ginseng. *Prog Neuro-Psychopharmacol Biol Psychiatr* 29: 895–900.
Perry EK, Pickering AT, Wang WW *et al.* (1999). Medicinal plants and Alzheimer's disease: from ethnobotany to phytotherapy. *J Pharm Pharmacol* 51: 527–534.
Perry N, Court G, Bidet N *et al.* (1996). European herbs with cholinergic activities: potential in dementia therapy. *Int J Geriatr Psychiatr* 11: 1063–1069.
Perry NSL, Houghton PJ, Jenner P *et al.* (2002). *Salvia lavandulaefolia* essential oil inhibits cholinesterase in vivo. *Phytomedicine* 9: 48–51.
Perry NSL, Houghton PJ, Sampson J *et al.* (2001). In-vitro activities of *S. lavandulaefolia* (Spanish Sage) relevant to treatment of Alzheimer's disease. *J Pharm Pharmacol* 53: 1347–1356.
Perry NSL, Houghton PJ, Theobald A *et al.* (2000). In-vitro inhibition of human erythrocyte acetylcholinesterase by *Salvia lavandulaefolia* essential oil and constituent terpenes. *J Pharm Pharmacol* 52: 895–902.
Pilkington K, Boshnakova A, Richardson J (2006). St John's wort for depression: Time for a different perspective? *Complement Ther Med* 14: 268–281.
Pitsikas N, Sakellaridis N (2006). *Crocus sativus* L. extracts antagonize memory impairments in different behavioural tasks in the rat. *Behav Brain Res* 173: 112–115.
Pitsikas N, Zisopoulou S, Tarantilis PA *et al.* (2007). Effects of the active constituents of *Crocus sativus* L., crocins on recognition and spatial rats' memory. *Behav Brain Res* 183: 141–146.
Pittler MH, Ernst E (2003). Kava extract versus placebo for treating anxiety. *Cochrane Database of Systematic Reviews* Issue 1: CD003383. DOI: 10.1002/14651858. CD003383.
Prast H, Philippu A (2001). Nitric oxide as modulator of neuronal function. *Prog Neurobiol* 64: 51–68.
Qiao CX, Den R, Kudo K *et al.* (2005). Ginseng enhances contextual fear conditioning and near genesis in rats. *Neurosci Res* 51: 31–38.
Radad K, Gille G, Liu L *et al.* (2006). Use of ginseng in medicine with emphasis on neurodegenerative disorders. *J Pharmacol Sci* 100: 175–186.
Ramassamy C (2006). Emerging role of polyphenolic compounds in the treatment of neurodegenerative diseases: A review of their intracellular targets. *Eur J Pharmacol* 545: 51–64.
Reay JL, Kennedy DO, Scholey AB (2005). Single doses of *panax ginseng* (G115) reduce blood glucose levels and improve cognitive performance during sustained mental activity. *J Psychopharmacol* 4: 357–365.
Reay JL, Kennedy DO, Scholey AB (2006). The glycaemic effect of single doses of panax ginseng (G115) in young healthy volunteers. *Br J Nutr* 96: 639 – 642.
Reay JL, Kennedy DO, Scholey AB (2007). Effects of *Panax ginseng*, consumed with and without glucose, on blood glucose levels and cognitive performance during sustained 'mentally demanding' tasks. *J Psychopharmacol* 20: 771–781.
Rigney U, Kimber S, Hindmarch I (1999). The effects of acute doses of standardised *Ginkgo biloba* extract on memory and psychomotor performance in volunteers. *Phytother Res* 13: 408–415.
Roder C, Schaefer M, Leucht S (2004). Meta-analysis of effectiveness and tolerability of treatment of mild to moderate depression with St John's wort. *Fortschr Neurol Psychiatr* 72: 330–343.
Roodenrys S, Booth D, Bulzoni S *et al.* (2002). Chronic effects of Brahami (*Bacopa monnieri*) on human memory. *Neuropsychopharmacology* 27: 279–281.
Russo A, Borelli F (2005). *Bacopa monniera*, a reputed nootropic plant: an overview. *Phytomedicine* 12: 305–317.
Santos RF, Galduroz JCF, Barbieri A *et al.* (2003). Cognitive performance, SPECT, and blood viscosity in elderly non-demented people using *Ginkgo biloba*. *Pharmacopsychiatry* 36: 127–133.
Savelev S, Okello E, Perry NSL *et al.* (2003). Synergistic and antagonistic interactions of anticholinesterase terpenoids in *Salvia lavandulaefolia* essential oil. *Pharmacol Biochem Behav* 75: 661–668.
Savelev SU, Okello EJ, Perry EK (2004). Butyryl and acetylcholinesterase inhibitory activities in essential oils of *Salvia* species and their constituents. *Phytother Res* 18: 315–324.
Schmitz M, Jackel M (1998). Comparative study for assessing quality of life of patients with exogenous sleep disorders (temporary sleep onset and sleep interruption disorders) treated with a hops-valerian preparation and a benzodiazepine drug. *Wien Med Wochenschr* 148: 291–298.
Scholey AB, Tildesley NTJ, Perry EK *et al.* (2008). Modulation of cognitive performance following acute administration of *Salvia officinalis* (sage) in healthy older volunteers: A randomised double blind, placebo controlled study. *Psychopharmacology* 198: 127–139.
Shah ZA, Sharma P, Vohora SB (2003). *Ginkgo biloba* normalises stress-elevated alterations in brain catecholamines, serotonin and plasma corticosterone levels. *Eur Neuropsychopharmacol* 13: 321–325.
Shanker G, Singh HK (2000). Anxiolytic profile of standardized Brahmi extract. *Indian J Pharmacol* 32: 152.

Sheikh N, Ahmad A, Siripurapua KB *et al.* (2007). Effect of *Bacopa monniera* on stress induced changes in plasma corticosterone and brain monoamines in rats. *J Ethnopharmacol* 111: 671–676.

Singh HK, Dhawan BN (1997). Neuropsychopharmacological effects of the Ayurvedic nootropic *Bacopa monniera* Linn (Brahmi). *Indian J Pharmacol* 29: S359–S365.

Singh YN, Singh NN (2002). Therapeutic potential of kava in the treatment of anxiety disorders. *CNS Drugs* 16: 731–743.

Solomon PR, Adams F, Silver A *et al.* (2002). Ginkgo for memory enhancement – A randomized controlled trial. *JAMA* 288: 835–840.

Sorensen H, Sonne J (1996). A double masked study of the effects of ginseng on cognitive functios. *Curr Ther Res* 57: 959–968.

Sotaniemi EA, Haapakoski E, Rautio A (1995). Ginseng therapy in non-insulin diabetic patients. *Diabetes Care* 18: 1373–1375.

Soulimani R, Fleurentin J, Mortier F *et al.* (1991). Neurotropic action of the hydroalcoholic extract of *Melissa officinalis* in the mouse. *Planta Med* 57: 105–109.

Stevinson C, Ernst E (2000). Valerian for insomnia: a systematic review of randomized clinical trials. *Sleep Med* 1: 91–99.

Stough C, Lloyd J, Clarke J *et al.* (2001a). The chronic effects of an extract of *Bacopa monniera* (Brahmi) on cognitive function in healthy human subjects. *Psychopharmacology* 156: 481–484.

Stough C, Clarke J, Lloyd J *et al.* (2001b). Neuropsychological changes after 30-day *Ginkgo biloba* administration in healthy participants. *Int J Neuropsychopharmacol* 4: 131–134.

Sünram-Lea SI, Birchall RJ, Wesnes KA *et al.* (2004). The effect of acute administration of 400mg of *Panax ginseng* on cognitive performance and mood in healthy young volunteers. *Curr Topics Nutr Res* 3: 65–74.

Tachikawa E, Kudo K, Harada K *et al.* (1999). Effects of ginseng saponins on reponses induced by various receptor stimuli. *Eur J Pharmacol* 369: 23–32.

Tadano T, Nakagawasai O, Tan-no K *et al.* (1998). Effects of *ginkgo biloba* extract on impairment of learning induced by cerebral ischemia in mice. *Am J Chin Med* 26: 127–132.

Tagashira M, Ohtake Y (1998). A new antioxidative 1, 3-benzodioxole from *Melissa officinalis*. *Planta Med* 64: 555–558.

Tahara S (2007). A journey of twenty-five years through the ecological biochemistry of flavonoids. *Biosci Biotechnol Biochem* 71: 1387–1404.

Tarantilis PA, Tsoupras G, Polissiou M (1995). Determination of saffron (*Crocus sativus* L.) components in crude plant extract using high-performance liquid chromatography-UV/visible photodiode-array detection-mass spectrometry. *J Chromatogr* 699: 107–118.

Tatsis EC, Boeren S, Exarchou V, Troganis AN, Vervoort J, Gerothanassis IP (2007). Identification of the major constituents of *Hypericum perforatum* by LC/SPE/NMR and/or LC/MS. *Phytochemistry* 68: 383–393.

Thommessen B, Laake K (1996). No identifiable effect of ginseng (Gericomplex) as an adjuvant in the treatment of geriatric patients. *Aging* 8: 417–420.

Tildesley NTJ, Kennedy DO, Perry EK *et al.* (2003). *Salvia lavandulaefolia* (Spanish Sage) enhances memory in healthy young volunteers. *Pharmacol Biochem Behav* 75: 669–674.

Tildesley NTJ, Kennedy DO, Perry EK *et al.* (2005). Cognitive and mood effects of acute administration of *Salvia lavandulaefolia* (Spanish Sage) to healthy young volunteers. *Physiol Behav* 83: 699–709.

Ussher JM, Dewberry C, Malson H, Noakes J (1995). The relationship between health related quality of life and dietary supplementation in British middle managers: A double blind placebo controlled study. *Psychol Health* 10: 97–111.

Voces J, Cabral de Oliveira AC, Preito JG *et al.* (2004). Ginseng administration protects skeletal muscle from oxidative stress induced by acute exercise in rats. *Brazil J Med Biol Res* 37: 1863–1871.

Wagner H, Sprinkmeyer L (1973). Über die pharmakologische Wirkung von Melissengeist *Dtsch Apoth Ztg* 113: 1159–1166.

Wake G, Court J, Pickering A *et al.* (2000). CNS acetylcholine receptor activity in European medicinal plants traditionally used to improve failing memory. *J Ethnopharmacol* 69: 105–114.

Wang XY, Zhang JT (2001). NO mediates ginsenoside Rg1-induced long-term potentiation in anesthetized rats. *Acta Pharmacol Sin* 22: 657–662.

Warot D, Lacomblez L, Danjou P *et al.* (1991). Comparative effects of *ginkgo biloba* extracts on psychomotor performances and memory in healthy subjects. *Therapie* 46: 33–36.

Wasowski C, Marder M, Viola H *et al.* (2002). Isolation and identification of 6-methylapigenin, a competitive ligand for the brain GABAA receptors, from *Valeriana wallichii* D.C. *Planta Med* 68: 934–936.

Wiklund IK, Mattsson K, Lingren R *et al.* (1999). Effects of a standardized ginseng extract on quality of life and physiological parameters in symptomatic postmenopausal women: a double blind placebo controlled trial, *Int J Clin Pharmacol Res* 19: 89–99.

Witte S, Loew D, Gaus W (2005). Meta-analysis of the efficacy of the acetonic kava-kava extract WS®1490 in patients with non-psychotic anxiety disorders. *Phytother Res* 19: 183–188.

Woelk H, Arnoldt KH, Kieser M, Hoerr R (2007). *Ginkgo biloba* special extract EGb. *J Psychiatr Res* 761: 49–55.

Zanoli P (2004). Role of hyperforin in the pharmacological activities of St John's wort. *CNS Drug Rev* 10: 203–218.

Zhang Z (2003). Therapeutic effects of herbal extracts and constituents in animal models of psychiatric disorders. *Life Sci* 75: 1659–1699.

Zhang DS, Zhang JT (2000). Effect of total ginsenoside on synaptic transmission in dentate gyrus in rats. *Acta Pharm Sin* 35: 185–188.

Ziegler G, Ploch M, Miettinen-Baumann A *et al.* (2002). Efficacy and tolerability of valerian extract LI 156 compared with oxazepam in the treatment of non-organic insomnia – a randomized, double-blind, comparative clinical study. *Eur J Med Res* 7: 480–486.

15

Herbs used to treat respiratory conditions other than infections

Anwarul Hassan Gilani and Arif-ullah Khan

Introduction

Physiology of the respiratory system and asthma

The respiratory system is composed of the lungs and the air passages, the muscles of the thorax, of pleural sacs and nerves. The air passage consists of the paired nasal cavities, pharynx, larynx, trachea and bronchial tree (Catcott, 1964). The trachea bifurcates to form the primary bronchi which further divide into secondary bronchi leading to smaller respiratory bronchioles terminating in alveoli, through which oxygen passes from air into blood and carbon dioxide passes from blood into air (Singh, 1997).

On the lungs and air passages, receptors such as adrenoceptor, histamine and muscarinic are present, which are responsible for regulation of different physiological functions. Stimulation of β-adrenergic receptors decreases smooth tone of the airways and inhibits the release of inflammatory mediators from mast cells (Carstains *et al.*, 1985). Muscarinic receptors in airways belong to M_3 subtypes, which occur almost exclusively in proximal airways (Barnes, 1987), and mediate contractile responses and increase the mucous secretion. Histamine receptors of H_1-type are present on bronchial muscle, causing contraction of smooth muscles, but have little physiological role; thus antihistaminic drugs have limited therapeutic contribution.

The hyperactivity of respiratory smooth muscles results in airway constriction leading to asthma (Reed, 1974; Barnes, 1986). Most of the disorders of the respiratory system, other than infectious diseases, results from the hyperactivity of airways. Asthma is a major congestive respiratory disorder, characterised by episodic wheezing, cough and chest tightness associated with airflow obstruction (Howarth, 1997). The worldwide prevalence of asthma has been increasing, particularly in children (Croner and Kjellman, 1992; Lenfant, 1995). According to the World Health Organization (WHO), it affects about 5–10% of adults (Lowhagen, 1999) and 10% of children globally (Lazaro *et al.*, 1999; Malhotra, 2000). The mortality rates from asthma have been increasing steadily over recent decades (Ulrik and Frederiksen, 1995). According to the National Center for Health Statistics, the death rate from asthma in the United States increased from 0.8 per 100 000 in 1971 to 2 per 100 000 in 1991 (Sly, 1994).

The pathogenesis of asthma is multifactorial and multicellular since macrophages, mast cells, eosinophils, neutrophils and platelets are involved in its pathogenesis (Joseph *et al.*, 1983). The cells produce an arsenal of mediators such as bradykinin, histamine, leukotrienes, platelet-activating factor, prostaglandins and thromboxane which interact in a complex way to produce numerous pathological effects. These include constriction of airway smooth muscle, increased microvascular leakage, mucus secretion and recruitment of inflammatory cells into airways (Sasaki *et al.*, 1993; Cookson, 1999). Histopathological studies of patients with asthma have shown inflammation in the airways with infiltration of inflammatory cells, particularly eosinophils, disruption of airway epithelium and mucus hypersecretion, thus indicating that airway inflammation may underlie bronchial hyperresponsiveness (Dunnill, 1960).

Asthma is classified into extrinsic and intrinsic types. The extrinsic type generally appears in early stages of life in individuals with a family history of either asthma or various allergies including hay fever, eczema and dermatitis. The intrinsic type, on the other hand, develops at around 40 years of age and occurs because of non-specific factors (common cold, exercise or emotion) that may trigger the asthmatic attack. Many stimuli including viral infection, environmental allergens, animal dander, stress, air pollutants, emotion (fear, anger, frustration), cold air and changes in weather enhance symptoms of asthma and alter airway physiology (Wilson, 1992; Khan and Hazir, 1995).

In many instances asthma has been found to run in families and multiple genes are involved in its expression (Postma, 1999). In the traditional Greco-Arab Unani system of medicine, the human race is divided genetically into four classes based on their susceptibility to develop different diseases, i.e, choleric, sanguine, phlegmatic and melancholic. Those who have the tendency to develop asthmatic disorders belong to the phlegmatic category (Tobyn, 1997). It has been observed that such individuals with sensitive airways respond adversely and develop bronchoconstriction and/or cough when taking allopathic medicines, such as angiotensin-converting enzyme inhibitors.

Drugs used to treat asthma

The common classes of drugs with proven efficacy in asthma are bronchodilators such as β_2-agonists, anticholinergics, phosphodiesterase inhibitors, while glucocorticosteroids, mass cell stabilisers and leukotriene modifiers are used usually as preventive therapy in chronic cases (Rang *et al.*, 1999). More recently, Ca^{2+} antagonists and potassium channel openers have been added to the list of potential bronchodilators (Rang *et al.*, 1999; Undem, 2006). All bronchodilators currently in use are known to manifest cardiac stimulation as a serious side-effect, particularly when given orally (Undem, 2006). Inhalers are used to avoid cardiac side-effects, but are very expensive and beyond the reach of a large part of the population in developing countries, so alternate measures are being explored for safe and cost-effective treatment.

Herbs in this regard have potential not only as a source of new clinical drugs but are also gaining popularity in the form of crude herbal products or botanicals (Harrison, 1998; Gilani and Rahman, 2005). Interestingly, a constituent of *Aspalathus linearis* (a popular herbal tea in South Africa, commonly known as rooibos) is chrysoeriol, a flavonoid, and was found to exhibit high selectivity for airways compared with other smooth muscles, so placing itself amongst the candidates to be developed for congestive airways disorders (Khan and Gilani, 2006).

Pathology of coughing

Cough is a spasmodic contraction of the thoracic cavity that results in abrupt release of air from the lungs. It is usually very sudden in onset and very often repetitive. The cough reflex is complex, involving the central and peripheral nervous system as well as the smooth muscle of the bronchial tree. It has been suggested that irritation of the bronchial mucosa causes bronchoconstriction, which in turn stimulates cough receptors (which probably represent a specialised type of stretch receptor) located in tracheobronchial passages. The cough reflex probably includes several mechanisms or centres that are distinct from the mechanisms involved in the regulation of respiration (Irwin and Madison, 2000). Excessive cough is one of the most common symptoms for which the patient seeks medical care and may represent up to one-third of a pulmonologist's outpatient referrals. Persistent severe cough, seen in interstitial lung disease or bronchiectasis, may impair respiration as well as disrupt sleep and social functioning. Bronchospasm, syncope, rib fractures and urinary incontinence are all potential complications (Irwin and Madison, 2002). On the basis of duration, cough has been divided into acute (less than 3 weeks' duration), subacute (3–8 weeks) and chronic (more than 8 weeks) types.

The causes of acute cough are viral or bacterial infection, pneumonia, pulmonary embolism and pulmonary oedema. The most common causes of subacute and chronic cough are asthma, weather changes, smoking, inflammation of larynx or pharynx and allergies.

The drugs that directly or indirectly can affect the cough are diverse. Cough may be the first, or the only, symptom of asthma or allergy and in such cases bronchodilators and antihistaminergics have been shown to reduce cough without having significant central effects. The drugs acting primarily on central or peripheral nervous system components of the cough reflex are opioid agents, i.e. codeine and dextromethorphan, which are structurally related to morphine and act on the cough centre of the medulla, increasing the cough threshold and thus depressing the cough (Irwin and Madison, 2000).

Medicinal plants used to treat respiratory disorders

According to the WHO, about three-quarters of the world population relies on traditional remedies (mainly herbs) to fulfil their healthcare needs (WHO, 2003). In developing countries, remedies prepared by traditional healers from plants of the local flora are the only drugs available for a large number of people. It is not uncommon that a single plant possesses a wide range of medicinal applications. Several scientific studies, in parallel to this, have also shown the presence of synergistic and/or side-effect-neutralising combinations in plants, which is the result of the presence of multiple constituents in a single plant (Gilani and Rahman, 2005). Herbs have always played an important role in the treatment of respiratory diseases and *Atropa belladonna* is one such example, with folkloric repute to treat asthma. This species is the source of atropine, a prototype antimuscarinic drug, which has a wide range of clinical applications including asthma (Rang *et al.*, 1999).

Chinese traditional medicine has also claimed to treat many diseases, especially bronchial asthma (Hsieh, 1996). The number of plants considered useful for respiratory disorders is surprisingly large. Some of the species, which have been shown to be effective in the disorders of airway hyperactivity in experimental animals or clinical trials, confirming their traditional use in respiratory disorders, are listed in Table 15.1.

Plants mentioned for their effect against potassium-induced contraction are considered to be calcium-channel blockers (CCBs) as high K^+ (>30 mmol/L) is known to cause smooth-muscle contraction via Ca^{2+} influx through voltage-dependent calcium channels (Bolton, 1979). Interestingly, we found some novel combinations and observed that CCB-like constituents are abundantly present in plants and usually coexist with other active constituents, such as phosphodiesterase inhibitors and anticholinergics (Gilani and Rahman, 2005).

The drugs used in conventional medicine as bronchodilators in asthmatic conditions belong to the catagories of β_2-adrenoceptor stimulants (salbutamol), phosphodiesterase inhibitors (theophylline) and anticholinergics (ipratropium), all of which cause cardiac stimulation as a side-effect (Rang *et al.*, 1999). Calcium antagonists (which are devoid of cardiac stimulant effect) have been shown to possess therapeutic usefulness in asthma in recent years (Ahmed, 1992). These have an inhibitory effect, opposite to what is seen with currently used anti-asthmatic drugs. Hence, it is logical to combine Ca^{2+} antagonists with any of the above mentioned bronchodilators to achieve an enhanced bronchodilator effect with neutralisation of cardiac side-effects.

Based on the assumption that medicinal plants do contain such combinations of activities, a few plants with folkloric use in asthma were screened. Interestingly, two popular plants, commonly used in asthma

Table 15.1 Studies on medicinal plants useful in respiratory disorders

Plant	Model of study	Effect	Reference
Aegle marmelos	Histamine-induced constriction of guinea pig isolated trachea	Bronchodilation	Arul *et al.*, 2004
Allium sativum	Histamine and acetylcholine-induced constriction of guinea pig isolated trachea and a clinical study in patients with asthma	Bronchodilation anti-asthmatic	Aqel *et al.*, 1991; Clement *et al.*, 2005
Aloe vera	Patients with asthma	Anti-asthmatic	Clement *et al.*, 2005
Alstonia scholaris	Carbachol-mediated bronchoconstriction in anaesthetised rats	Bronchodilation	Channa *et al.*, 2005
Anchietia salutaris	Guinea pig lung parenchymal strips contracted with prostaglandin and U46619	Bronchodilation	Gambero and Gomes, 1998
Artemisia caerulescens	Histamine and acetylcholine-induced bronchoconstriction in anaesthetised guinea pigs and their isolated trachea	Bronchodilation	Moran *et al.*, 1989
Artemisia capillaris	Patients with asthma	Improved expiratory flow volume	Fu, 1989
Aspalathus linearis	Low K^+-contracted guinea pig isolated trachea	Bronchodilation	Khan and Gilani, 2006
Bacopa monniera	Carbachol-induced bronchoconstriction in anaesthetised rats	Bronchodilation	Dar and Channa, 1997
Borago officinalis	K^+ and carbachol-induced contraction of isolated rabbit trachea	Bronchodilation	Gilani *et al.*, 2007
Capparis spinosa	Antigen and histamine-induced bronchoconstriction in anaesthetised guinea pigs	Bronchodilation	Trombetta *et al.*, 2005
Carum copticum	Carbachol, histamine and K^+-induced constriction of isolated guinea pig trachea	Bronchodilation	Boskabady *et al.*, 1998; Boskabady and Shaikhi, 2000; Gilani *et al.*, 2005a
Cecropia glaziovi	Histamine-induced bronchospasm in guinea pigs	Bronchodilation	Jr *et al.*, 2007
Cinnamomum massoiae	IgE-dependent histamine release from the RBL-2H3 mast cells	Mast cell stabiliser	Ikawati *et al.*, 2001
Cordia curassavica	Patients with asthma	Anti-asthmatic	Clement *et al.*, 2005
Crocus sativus	Methacholine and K^+ induced guinea pig isolated tracheal contraction	Bronchodilation	Boskabady and Aslani, 2006
Crossopteryx febrifuga	Citric acid-induced cough and antigen-induced bronchospasm in guinea pig	Antitussive, bronchodilation	Occhiuto *et al.*, 1999
Curcuma longa	Carbachol and K^+-induced constriction of isolated guinea pig trachea	Bronchodilation	Gilani *et al.*, 2005b
Cymbopogon citratus	Patients with asthma	Anti-asthmatic	Clement *et al.*, 2005
Datura stramonium	Patients with asthma	Decreased the airway resistance	Charpin *et al.*, 1979

Table 15.1 *(continued)*

Plant	Model of study	Effect	Reference
Drymis winteri	Guinea pig isolated trachea precontracted with bradykinin, prostaglandin, capsacin, substance P, neurokinin A-(4–10), U 46619, ovalbumin and compound 48/80	Bronchodilation	Sayah *et al.*, 1997
Echinacea purpurea	Patients with asthma	Anti-asthmatic	Clement *et al.*, 2005
Entada africana	Citric acid-evoked cough and histamine-induced bronchoconstriction in guinea pig	Antitussive, bronchodilation	Occhiuto *et al.*, 1999
Eryngium foetidium	Patients with asthma	Anti-asthmatic	Clement *et al.*, 2005
Eucalyptus globulus	IgE-dependent histamine release from the RBL-2H3 mast cells	Mast cell stabiliser	Ikawati *et al.*, 2001
Eucommia ulmoides	Patients with asthma	Improved expiratory flow volume	Fu, 1989
Hibiscus sabdariffa	Guinea pig isolated trachea	Bronchodilation	Ali *et al.*, 1991
Hydrastis canadensis	Carbachol-induced constriction of guinea pig isolated trachea and a clinical study in patients with asthma	Bronchodilation anti-asthmatic	Abdel-Haq *et al.*, 2000; Clement *et al.*, 2005
Hymenocallis tubiflora	Patients with asthma	Anti-asthmatic	Clement *et al.*, 2005
Hyoscyamus niger	Carbachol and K^+ precontracted guinea pig isolated trachea	Bronchodilation	Gilani *et al.*, 2008a
Hypericum perforatum	Carbachol and K^+ precontracted guinea pig trachea	Bronchodilation	Gilani *et al.*, 2005c
Leonotis nepetifolia	Patients with asthma	Anti-asthmatic	Clement *et al.*, 2005
Liriope platyphylla	Airway inflammation and hyperresponsiveness in murine model of asthma	Anti-asthmatic	Lee *et al.*, 2005
Lycium chinense	Patients with asthma	Improved expiratory flow volume	Fu, 1989
Mangifera indica	Acetycholine and histamine precontracted rat isolated trachea	Bronchodilation	Agbonon *et al.*, 2005
Matricaria chamomilla	Patients with asthma	Anti-asthmatic	Clement *et al.*, 2005
Myristica fragrans	Patients with asthma	Anti-asthmatic	Clement *et al.*, 2005
Nigella sativa	Carbachol, histamine and K^+-mediated tracheal constriction and measurement of respiratory rate and intratracheal pressure in guinea pigs	Bronchodilation	El-Tahir *et al.*, 1993; Gilani *et al.*, 2001
Ocimum gratissimum	Patients with asthma	Anti-asthmatic	Clement *et al.*, 2005
Phyllanthus urinaria	Carbachol-induced constriction of guinea pigs isolated trachea	Bronchodilation	Paulino *et al.*, 1996
Phymatodes scolopendria	Carbachol, histamine, K^+-induced constrictions of isolated trachea and histamine inhalation to guinea pig	Bronchodilation	Ramanitrahasimbola *et al.*, 2005

(*continued overleaf*)

Table 15.1 *(continued)*

Plant	Model of study	Effect	Reference
Pimpinella anisum	Methacholine-induced constriction of guinea pig isolated trachea	Bronchodilation	Boskabady and Ramazani-Assari, 2001
Plantago major	IgE-dependent histamine release from the RBL-2H3 mast cells	Mast cell stabiliser	Ikawati *et al.*, 2001
Pluchea ovalis	Acetycholine precontracted rat isolated trachea	Bronchodilation	Agbonon *et al.*, 2002
Pogostemon cablin	Patients with asthma	Improved expiratory flow volume	Fu, 1989
Portulaca oleracea	Measurement of forced expiratory volume, peak expiratory flow, maximal mid-expiratory flow and specific airway conductance in patients with asthma	Improved the pulmonary functions	Malek *et al.*, 2004
Psoralea corylifolia	Patients with asthma	Improved expiratory flow volume	Fu, 1989
Pteleopsis suberosa	Citric acid-induced cough in guinea pig	Antitussive	Occhiuto *et al.*, 1999
Rauwolfia ligustrina	Guinea pig isolated trachea precontracted with carbachol	Bronchodilation	Medeiros and Calixto, 1996
Rosa damascena	Methacholine and K^+-induced guinea pig isolated tracheal contraction	Bronchodilation	Boskabady *et al.*, 2006a
Rosmarinus officinalis	Acetylcholine and K^+-induced constriction of rabbit isolated tracheal smooth muscle	Bronchodilation	Aqel, 1991
Sarcococca saligna	Carbachol and K^+-induced constriction of guinea pig and rabbit trachea	Bronchodilation	Ghayur and Gilani, 2006a
Solanum trilobatum	Measurement of forced expiratory volume, peak expiratory flow, maximal mid-expiratory flow and specific airway conductance in patients with asthma	Improved the pulmonary functions	Govindan *et al.*, 1999
Solanum xanthocarpum	Measurement of forced expiratory volume, peak expiratory flow, maximal mid-expiratory in patients with asthma	Improved the pulmonary functions	Govindan *et al.*, 1999
Stemona tuberosa	Carbachol, histamine and K^+ precontracted guinea pig isolated trachea	Bronchodilation	Liao *et al.*, 1997
Terminalia bellerica	Carbachol and K^+ precontracted guinea pig isolated trachea	Bronchodilation	Gilani *et al.*, 2008b
Thymus vulgaris	Methacholine and K^+-induced contraction of guinea pig isolated trachea	Bronchodilation	Boskabady *et al.*, 2006b
Tussilago farfara	Patients with asthma	Improved expiratory flow volume	Fu, 1989
Viscum coloratum	Patients with asthma	Improved expiratory flow volume	Fu, 1989

Ganguly T, Badheka LP, Sainis KB (2001). Immunomodulatory effects of *Tylophora indica* in conA induced lymphoproliferation. *Phytomedicine* 8: 249.

Ganguly T, Sainis KB (2001). Inhibition of cellular immune responses by *Tylophora indica* in experimental models. *Phytomedicine* 8: 242.

Ganju L, Karan D, Chanda S *et al.* (2003). Immunomodulatory effects of agents of plant origin. *Biomed Pharmacother* 57: 296–300.

Gautam M, Diwanay S, Gairola S *et al.* (2004). Immunoadjuvant potential of *Asparagus racemosus* aqueous extract in experimental system. *J Ethnopharmacol* 91: 251–255.

Geetha S, Sai Ram M, Singh V *et al.* (2002). Anti-oxidant and immunomodulatory properties of seabuckthorn (*Hippophae rhamnoides*) – an in vitro study. *J Ethnopharmacol* 79: 373–378.

Germain RN (1994). MHC dependent antigen processing and peptide presentation. *Cell* 76: 287–289.

Ghule BV, Murugananthan G, Nakhat PD, Yeole PG (2006). Immunostimulant effects of *Capparis zeylanica* Linn. leaves. *J Ethnopharmacol* 108: 311–315.

Godhwani S, Godhwani J, Vyas DS (1988). *Ocimum sanctum* – a preliminary study evaluating its immunoregulatory profile in albino rats. *J Ethnopharmacol* 24: 193–198.

Gokhale AB, Damre AS, Saraf MN (2003). Investigations into the immunomodulatory activity of *Argyreia speciosa*. *J Ethnopharmacol* 84: 109–111.

Gottlieb AA, Gottlieb MS, Scholes VE (1987). Reconstitution of immune functions in AIDS/ARC. *Concepts Immunopathol* 4: 261–274.

Govindarajan R, Vijayakumar M, Pushpangadan P (2005). Antioxidant approach to disease management and the role of 'Rasayana' herbs of Ayurveda. *J Ethnopharmacol* 99: 165–178.

Gupta A, Khajuria A, Singh J *et al.* (2006). Immunomodulatory activity of biopolymeric fraction RLJ-NE-205 from *Picrorhiza kurroa*. *Int Immunopharmacol* 6: 1543–1549.

Hadden JW (1993). Immunostimulants. *Trends Pharmacol Sci* 14: 169.

Hafeez BB, Haque R, Parvez S *et al.* (2003). Immunomodulatory effects of fenugreek (*Trigonella foenum graecum* L.) extract in mice. *Int Immunopharmacol* 3: 257–265.

Haq A, Lobo PI, Al-Tufail M *et al.* (1999). Immunomodulatory effect of *Nigella sativa* proteins fractionated by ion exchange chromatography. *Int J Immunopharmacol* 21: 283–295.

Havsteen BH (2002). The biochemistry and medical significance of the flavonoids. *Pharmacol Ther* 96: 67–202.

Hu S, Concha C, Lin F, Persson WK (2003). Adjuvant effect of Ginseng extracts on the immune response to immunization against *Staphylococcus aureus* in dairy cattle. *Vet Immunol Immunopathol* 91: 29–37.

Huisman MMH, Fransen CTM, Kamerling JP *et al.* (2001). The CDTA-soluble pectic substances from soybean meal are composed of rhamnogalacturonan and xylogalacturonan but not homogalacturonan. *Biopolymers* 58: 279–294.

Janeway CA, Medzhitov R (2002). Innate immune recognition. *Ann Rev Immunol* 20: 197–216.

Jayaram S, Walwaikar PP, Rajadhyaksha SS (1993). Evaluation of efficacy of a preparation containing a combination of Indian medicinal plants in patients of generalized weakness. *Indian Drugs* 30: 498–500.

Jayathirtha MG, Mishra SH (2004). Preliminary immunomodulatory activities of methanol extracts of *Eclipta alba* and *Centella asiatica*. *Phytomedicine* 11: 361–365.

Kapil A, Sharma S (1997). Immunopotentiating compounds from
T. cordifolia. *J Ethnopharmacol* 58: 89–95.

Klimp AH, de Vries EG, Scherphof GL, Daemen T (2002). A potential role of macrophage activation in the treatment of cancer. *Crit Rev Oncol Hematol* 44: 143–161.

Kumar P, Kuttan RV, Kuttan GG (1994). Chemoprotective action of 'Rasayana' against cyclophosphamide toxicity. *Tumori* 80: 306–308.

Lakshmi V, Pandey K, Puri A, Saxena RP, Saxena KC (2003). Immunostimulant principles from *Curculigo orchioides*. *J Ethnopharmacol* 89: 181–184.

Makare N, Bodhankar S, Rangari V (2001). Immunomodulatory activity of alcoholic extract of *Mangifera indica* L. in mice. *J Ethnopharmacol* 78: 133–137.

Manjrekar PN, Jolly,. CI, Narayanan S (2000). Comparative studies of the immunomodulatory activity of *Tinospora cordifolia* and *Tinospora sinensis*. *Fitoterapia* 71: 254–257.

Marcinkiewicz J (1997). Neutrophil chloramines: missing links between innate and acquired immunity. *Immunol Today* 18: 577–579.

Mathew S, Kuttan G (1999). Immunomodulatory and antitumour activities of *Tinospora cordifolia*. *Fitoterapia* 70: 35–43.

Mediratta PK, Sharma KK, Singh S (2002). Evaluation of immunomodulatory potential of *Ocimum sanctum* seed oil and its possible mechanism of action. *J Ethnopharmacol* 80: 15–20.

Mehrotra S, Mishra KP, Maurya R *et al.* (2002). Immunomodulation by ethanolic extract of *Boerhaavia diffusa* roots. *Int Immunopharmacol* 2: 987–996.

Mehrotra S, Mishra KP, Maurya R *et al.* (2003). Anticellular and immunosuppressive properties of ethanolic extract of *Acorus calamus* rhizome. *Int Immunopharmacol* 3: 53–61.

Mukherjee R, Dash PK, Ram GC (2005). Immunotherapeutic potential of *Ocimum sanctum* (L) in bovine subclinical mastitis. *Res Vet Sci* 79: 37–43.

Mungantiwar AA, Nair AM, Shinde UA *et al.* (1999). Studies on the immunomodulatory effects of *Boerhaavia diffusa* alkaloidal fraction. *J Ethnopharmacol* 65: 125–131.

Oberholzer A, Oberholzer C, Moldawer LL (2000). Cytokine signaling – regulation of the immune response in normal and critically ill states. *Crit Care Med* 28: N3–12.

Pandey R, Maurya R, Singh G *et al.* (2005). Immunosuppressive properties of flavonoids isolated from Boerhaavia diffusa Linn. *Int Immunopharmacol* 5: 541–543.

Panossian A, Davtyan T, Gukassyan N *et al.* (2002). Effect

of Andrographolide and Kan Jang – fixed combination of extract SHA-10 and extract SHE-3 – on proliferation of human lymphocytes, production of cytokines and immune activation markers in the whole blood cells culture. *Phytomedicine* 9: 598–605.

Patwardhan B, Kalbag D, Patki PS *et al.* (1990). Search of immunomodulatory agents: a review. *Indian Drugs* 28: 348–358.

Patwardhan B, Vaidya ADB, Chorghade M (2004). Ayurveda and natural products. *Drug Discov Curr Sci* 86: 789–799.

Pulhmann J, Knaus U, Tubaro L, Schaefer W, Wagner H (1992). Immunologically active metallic ion containing polysaccharides from *Achyrocline satureioides*. *Phytochemistry* 31: 2617.

Puri A, Sahai R, Singh KL *et al.* (2000). Immunostimulant activity of dry fruits and plant materials used in Indian traditional medical system for mothers after child birth and invalids. *J Ethnopharmacol* 71: 89–92.

Puri A, Saxena RP, Guru PY *et al.* (1992). Immunostimulant activity of picroliv, the iridoid glycoside fraction of *Picrorhiza kurroa*, and its protective action against *Leishmania donovani* infection in hamsters 1. *Planta Med* 58: 528–532.

Puri A, Saxena R, Saxena RP *et al.* (1994). Immunostimulant activity of *Nyctanthes arbor tristis* L. *J Ethnopharmacol* 42: 31–37.

Puri HS (2003). *'Rasayana' – Ayurvedic herbs for longevity and rejuvenation.* Taylor and Francis, London.

Pushpangadan P, Govindarajan R (2005). Need for developing protocol for collection/cultivation and quality parameters of medicinal plants for effective regulatory quality control of herbal drugs. In: *Proceedings International Conference Of Botanicals*, Kolkata, India.

Rasool M, Varalakshmi P (2006). Immunomodulatory role of *Withania somnifera* root powder on experimental induced inflammation: An in vivo and in vitro study. *Vasc Pharmacol* 44: 406–410.

Rivera E, Daggfeldt A, Hu S (2003). Ginseng extract in aluminum hydroxide adjuvanted vaccines improves the antibody response of pigs to porcine parvovirus and *Erysipelothrix rhusiopathiae*. *Vet Immunol Immunopathol* 91: 19–27.

SaiRam M, Sharma SK, Ilavazhagan G, *et al.* (1997). Immunomodulatory effects of NIM-76, a volatile fraction form Neem oil. *J Ethnopharmacol* 55: 133–139.

Sendl A, Mulinaci N, Vincieri FF, Wagner H (1993). Anti-inflammatory and immunologically active polysaccharides from *Sedum telephium*. *Phytochemistry* 4: 1357.

Sharma ML, Raob CS, Duda PL (1994). Immunostimulatory activity of *Picrorhiza kurroa* leaf extract? *J Ethnopharmacol* 41: 185–192.

Sharma ML, Khajuria A, Kaul A *et al.* (1988). Effect of Salai guggal ex *Boswellia serrata* on cellular and humoral immune responses and leucocyte migration. *Agents Actions* 24: 161–164.

Sharma ML, Kaul A, Khajuria A *et al.* (1996). Immunomodulatory activity of boswellic acids (pentacyclic triterpene acids) from *Boswellia serrata*. *Phytother Res* 10: 107–112.

Shekhani MS, Shah PM, Yasmin A *et al.* (1990). An immunostimulant sesquiterpene glycoside from *Sphaeranthus indicus*. *Phytochemistry* 29: 2573–2576.

Singh D, Aggarwal A, Mathias A, Naik S (2006). Immunomodulatory activity of *Semecarpus anacardium* extract in mononuclear cells of normal individuals and rheumatoid arthritis patients. *J Ethnopharmacol* 108: 398–406.

Sohni YR, Bhatt RM (1996). Activity of a crude extract formulation in experimental hepatic amoebiasis and in immunomodulation studies. *J Ethnopharmacol* 54: 119–124.

Sunila ES, Kuttan G (2004). Immunomodulatory and antitumor activity of *Piper longum* Linn. and piperine. *J Ethnopharmacol* 90: 339–346.

Suresh K, Vasudevan DM (1994). Augmentation dependent cellular of murine natural killer cell and antibody cytotoxicity activities by *Phyllanthus emblica* a new immunomodulator. *J Ethnophartnacol* 44: 55–60.

Thakur RS, Puri HS, Hussain A (1989). *Major Medicinal Plants of India*. Central Institute of Medicinal and Aromatic Plants, Lucknow, India.

Thatte UM, Dahanukar SA (1986). Ayurveda and contemporary scientific thought. *Trends Pharmacol Sci* 7: 247.

Thatte UM, Chhabria SN, Karandikar SM *et al.* (1987). Protective effects of Indian medicinal plants against cyclophosphamide neutropenia. *J Postgrad Med* 33: 185–188.

Tiwari U, Rastogi B, Singh P *et al.* (2004). Immunomodulatory effects of aqueous extract of *Tridax procumbens* in experimental animals. *J Ethnopharmacol* 92: 113–119.

Tzianabos AO (2000). Polysaccharide immunomodulators as therapeutic agents: structural aspects and biological function. *Clin Microbiol Rev* 13: 523–533.

Upadhyaya SN (1997). Natural products with immunomodulatory activity. In: *Immunomodulation* Eds. CK Katiyar, NB Brindavanam, P Tiwari, DBA Narayana. Narosa Publishing House, New Delhi, pp. 163–187.

Uthaisangsook S, Day NK, Bahna SL *et al.* (2002). Innate immunity and its role against infections. *Ann Allergy Asthma Immunol* 88: 253–264.

Vincken JP, Schols HA, Oomen RJFJ *et al.* (2003). If homogalacturonan were a side chain of rhamnogalacturonan I. Implications for cell wall architecture. *Plant Physiol* 132: 1781–1789.

Wagner H (1990). Search for plant derived natural products with immunostimulatory activity. *Pure Appl Chem* 62: 1217.

Wagner H (1994). *Therapy and Prevention With Immunomodulatory and Adaptogenic Plant Drugs. Update – Ayurveda.* Ayurveda Press, Bombay, pp. 24–26.

Wagner H (1999). Ayurvedic herbs and the immune system. In: *Immunomodulatory agents from plants.* Eds. SA Dhanukar, UM Thatte and NM Rege, Verlag, Basel, Switzerland, pp. 289–323.

Wagner H, Stuppner H, Schafer W, Zenk M (1988). Immunologically active polysaccharides of *Echinacea purpurea* cell cultures. *Phytochemistry* 27: 119.

Waksman BH (1980). Adjuvants and immunoregulation by lymphoid cells. In: *Immunostimulation*, Eds. L Chedid, PA Meicher and HJ Meuller-Eberhard, Springer-Verlag, Berlin, pp. 5.

Wang XS, Liu L, Fang JN (2005). Immunological activities and structure of pectin from *Centella asiatica*. *Carbohydrate Pol* 60: 95–101.

Willats WGT, McCartney L, Mackie W *et al.* (2001). Pectin: cell biology and prospects for functional analysis. *Plant Mol Biol*. 47: 9–27.

Wybran J (1988). Immunomodulation. *Curr Opin Immunol* 1: 251–252.

Yamada H, Kiyohara H (1999). Complement-activating polysaccharides from medicinal herbs. In: *Immunomodulatory Agents from Plants*. Ed. H Wagner, Birkhâuser Verlag, Basel, pp. 161–202.

Zhou H, Deng YM, Xie Q (2006). The modulatory effects of the volatile oil of ginger on the cellular immune response in vitro and in vivo in mice. *J Ethnopharmacol* 105: 301–305.

Ziauddin M, Phansalkar N, Patki, P *et al.* (1996). Studies on the immunomodulatory effects of Ashwagandha. *J Ethnopharmacol* 50: 69–76.

17

Tests on Indian and Peruvian medicinal plants used for wound healing

Tuhin Kanti Biswas, Srikanta Pandit and Shrabana Chakrabarti

Introduction

Healing of wounds is a natural phenomenon but it may lack quality, promptness and aesthetics (Ramesh, 1993). Research on wound healing has only recently received much attention in modern biomedical research. Extracts and new molecules from natural sources are being investigated for the management of various types of wound, with particular attention being paid to agents used in different traditional systems of medicine.

An insight on the global ancient historical roots revealed that the earliest medical writings deal extensively with wound care. Seven of the 48 case reports included in the Smith Papyrus (1700 BC) describe wounds and their management and the ancient physicians of Egypt, Greece, India and Europe developed methods of treatment for wounds, including the removal of foreign bodies, suturing, covering wounds with clean materials and protecting injured tissues from corrosive agents.

A 'wound' can be defined as a bodily injury caused by physical means with disruption of the normal continuity of the structure (Saraf and Pandey, 1996). Wounds can be classified into three types:

- non-specific
- specific
- malignant.

A non-specific wound can again be classified as:

- traumatic
- inflammatory
- nutritional or trophic.

A specific wound is mainly caused by some specific infection and/or a specific internal cause. Clinically, healing of wounds occurs in two ways: healing by first intention (primary healing) and healing by second intention (secondary healing or healing by granulation).

Wound healing involves a complex series of interactions between different cell types, cytokine mediators, and the extracellular matrix. The phases of normal wound healing include haemostasis, inflammation, proliferation, and remodelling. Different phases of wound healing are recognised, although the wound healing process is continuous, with each phase overlapping the next.

Because successful wound healing requires adequate blood and nutrients to be supplied to the site of damage, the overall health and nutritional status of the patient influences the outcome of the damaged tissue.

The objective in wound management is to heal the wound in the shortest time possible, with minimal pain and discomfort to, and scarring of, the patient. At the site of wound closure, a flexible and fine scar with high-tensile strength is desired. Research into the complex dynamics of tissue repair has identified several nutritional cofactors involved in tissue regeneration, including vitamins A, C, and E, zinc, arginine, glutamine and glucosamine (Mackay and Miller, 2003).

There is no drug in clinical use that can directly act as a wound-healing drug although antibiotics, steroids and non-steroidal anti-inflammatory drugs are used for the treatment of wounds, but they have many drawbacks.

Natural products of diverse origin from medicinal plants, animal products, metals and minerals are reported to have potential wound-healing activity, with medicinal plants being the main materials used. This chapter elaborates on some medicinal plants traditionally used for wound healing, with special reference to pharmacognosy, phytochemistry, pharmacology and clinical effects.

Research in the field of wound healing has increased greatly since the discovery of growth factors. Brown *et al.* (1989), probably first described the use of growth factors, especially epidermal growth factor (EGF), for the healing of wounds in rat. However, this agent is not only expensive but may result in cytotoxic effects.

Selection criteria of medicinal plants

Traditional leads

Ayurvedic system of medicine

Many wound-healing medicinal plants are mentioned in Ayurveda, one of the Indian traditional systems of medicine, designated with the term *Vranaropaka*. About 164 medicinal plants are mentioned in various Ayurvedic classic texts – such as *Charaka Samhita, Sushruta Samhita, Astanga Hridaya* and *Bhabaprakash Nighantu* – for their wound-healing properties. Some of the important medicinal plants are shown in Table 17.1 as well as scientifically evaluated to some extent (Biswas and Mukherjee, 2003).

Unani system of medicine

Unani medicine originated in Greece and, as a result of Islamic influence, was later established in India. Description of wounds occurs in the Unani system of medicine in a scattered manner but, in general, the term *Ghao* is described for wounds (Singh, 1985), but there is also a description of corneal ulcer under the term *Kuru-hul-en*. Many important formulations are found in Unani texts such as *Dakhili, Tamrikh Janghar, Marham Ajib, Marham Safedaw Kakuri, Marham Sartan* and *Marham Syaha* (Singh, 1979). In almost all Unani formulations, the drugs are prepared in an ointment base (*Marham*). Very few of the medicinal plants mentioned in Unani have been scientifically tested for their wound-healing activity but there are reports on *Cordia dichotoma* (Kuppast and Nayak, 2006) and henna leaves (*Lawsonia inermis*) in animal experimental models (Sakarkar *et al.*, 2004).

South Indian traditional folklore

India has a rich ethnic diversity and other 'tribal' medical systems exist. An ethnobotanical survey has been made in the Kanchipuram district, Tamil Nadu, India which includes information on plants used for wound healing by the local traditional healers (Table 17.2) (Muthu *et al.*, 2006). Santals are the tribal people of the eastern part of India, living in the area known as Santal Parganas. They maintain their health and cure diseases using only natural remedies.

Table 17.1 List of important botanicals used in Ayurveda for wound healing activity

Sl. No.	Botanical name	Common name	Family	Parts used	Indications in Ayurveda
1	*Aegle marmelos* Corr.	Bilwa	Rutaceae	Leaves	Diabetic wounds
2	*Albizzia lebbeck* Benth.	Shirish	Leguminoceae	Stem bark	Septic wounds
3	*Azadirachta indica* A. Juss	Nim	Meliaceae	Leaves	Wounds
4	*Berberis aristata* DC.	Daruharidra	Berberidaceae	Wood	Septic wounds
5	*Calotropis gigantea* Linn.	Rajarka	Asclepiadaceae	Latex	Wounds
6	*Calotropis procera* Ait.	Akanda	Asclepiadaceae	Latex	Fistula-in-ano
7	*Cedrus deodara* Roxb.	Devdaru	Anonaceae	Leaves	Syphilitic ulcers
8	*Centella asiatica* Linn.	Mandukaparni	Umbelliferae	Whole plant	Wounds
9	*Curcuma longa* Linn.	Haridra	Zingiberaceae	Tuber	Wounds
10	*Cynodon dactylon* L.	Durva	Gramineae	Whole plant	Wounds
11	*Embelia ribes* Burm.	Bidanga	Myrsinaceae	Fruits	Wounds
12	*Euphorbia nerifolia* L.	Snuhi	Euphorbiaceae	Latex	Wounds
13	*Ficus benghalensis* L.	Vad	Moraceae	Stem bark	Wounds, abscess, syphilitic wounds
14	*Ficus racemosa* Linn.	Jagyadumur	Moraceae	Leaves	Wounds
15	*Glycyrrhiza glabra* L.	Jasthimadhu	Leguminoseae	Root	Wounds
16	*Jasminum auriculatum* Vahl.	Juthika	Oleaceae	Flower	Wounds
17	*Moringa oleifera* Lam. Syn.	Sajina	Moringaceae	Root	Wounds, abscess
18	*Papaver somnifera* L.	Ahiphena	Papaveraceae	Seeds	Wounds
19	*Pterocarpus santalinus* Linn.	Raktachandan	Papilionaceae	Heart wood	Wounds, syphilitic wounds
20	*Rubea cordifolia* L.	Manjistha	Rubiaceae	Root	Septic wounds
21	*Shorea robusta* Gaertn. f.	Shala	Dipterocarpaceae	Resin	Wounds
22	*Symplocos racemosa* Roxb.	Lodhraka	Symplocaceae	Stem bark	Wounds, diabetic wounds, abcess
23	*Tinospora cordifolia* Linn.	Gulancha	Menispermaceae	Leaves	Wounds
24	*Vateria indica* Linn.	Sarja	Dipterocarpaceae	Resin	Wounds
25	*Withania somnifera* Dunal	Aswagandha	Solanaceae	Root	Wounds

The experts in medical management amongst the Santals are known as *Ojha*.

Many plants are reported for managing various types of wounds under the traditional language, e.g. *Kadar nari rehef (Asparagus racemosus)* for *Jari phutauk* (wounds in the tongue), *Nim* (*Azadirachta indica*) for *Ghao* (open sores), *Loa lore* (*Ficus glomerata*) for *Gand Ghao* (adenitis), *Akona rehef* (*Calotropis gigantea*) for *Goda ghao* (sores on the leg), *Lal Chandan* (*Pterocarpus santalinus*) for *Pachiari Ghao* (burns).

Very little scientific study has so far been carried out on these plants for wound-healing activity, complicated by the difficulty of understanding the

Table 17.2 Medicinal plants used by traditional healers from the Kancheepuram district of Tamil Nadu

Family	Plant	Medicinal uses
Acanthaceae	*Asystasia gangetica* (L.) T. Anderson	Leaf powder is mixed with coconut oil and applied topically for wound healing (burn wound)
Amaranthaceae	*Achyranthes aspera* L. *Aerva lanata* (L.) Juss. Ex Schult.	Leaf paste is applied topically to treat cuts and wounds Wounds can be treated by oral ingestion of juice of the whole plant
Asteraceae	*Tridax procumbens* L.	Leaf paste is applied topically on cuts and wounds
Capparaceae	*Cleome viscose*	Leaf paste is used topically to heal wounds
Fabaceae	*Pongamia pinnata*	Juice of root is mixed with equal amount of coconut milk, boiled and applied topically to cure wound
Lythraceae	*Lawsonia inermis* L.	Leaf powder is mixed with coconut oil and applied topically to treat cuts and wounds
Menispermaceae	*Tinospora cordifolia* Miers.	Leaf paste is applied topically to treat wounds
Mimosaceae	*Acacia leucophloea* (Roxb.) Willd. *Mimosa pudica* L.	Paste of fresh stem bark is applied topically to treat cuts and wounds Pinch of leaf paste is applied topically to treat cuts and wounds
Rhamnaceae	*Zizyphus mauritiana* Lam.	Dried bark powder is applied topically to treat wounds
Rutaceae	*Aegle marmelos* Corr.ex.Roxb	Leaf paste is applied topically to heal wounds
Verbenaceae	*Lippia nodiflora* Mich.	Paste of leaves is applied topically to treat swellings and wounds

language of the Santals. Bodding (1986) is the only researcher who has studied in detail the rituals and medicines used by Santals, producing a useful text that can act as a base for ethnopharmacological studies.

Traditional leads of Peru

In Latin America, the use of traditional remedies is still very strong and the World Health Organization (WHO) estimates that it comprises about 40% of all healthcare in the region. Peru is a good example and has a high biodiversity; 21 462 species of plants and animals being reported, 5855 of them endemic (Instituto Nacional de Estadística e Informática, 2005).

There is a long history of many plant species being used in traditional medicine and Peru's National Program in Complementary Medicine and the Pan American Health Organization recently compared complementary medicine to allopathic medicine in clinics and hospitals within the Peruvian social security system. This survey included a wound-healing study and revealed that general inflammation of the body was mentioned in 63 applications (2.5%), and 59 plant species (11.5%) were used for such conditions. In addition, throat and tonsil infections were treated with seven species (1.4%). Wound infections and bleeding resulting from accidents are very common in the northern Peruvian work environment, and are a major concern, especially in rural areas. A total of 8.4% of all plants (43 species) were used for the treatment of wounds and an additional 12 species (2.3%) were used in applications which involved the treatment of bleeding and haemorrhages (Bussman and Sharon, 2006).

Phytochemical leads

Numerous bioactive plant compounds have been tested for their wound-healing potential in clinical application. Among the most frequently studied are resveratrol, a polyphenol present in red wine and grape seed, epigallocatechin-3-gallate from green tea and curcumin from *Curcuma longa* (Dulak, 2005). Embelin, a quinone from the leaves of *Embelia ribes,* has been found to increase cross-linking of collagen fibres with an absence of monocytes (Kumara Swamy *et al.*, 2007). Three fractions from a hydroalcohol extract of the bark of *Terminalia arjuna* have been assessed for the healing of rat dermal wounds using in-vivo models. Fraction I, consisting mainly of tannins, showed a maximum increase in the tensile strength of incision wounds and also displayed antimicrobial activity against tested microorganisms such as *Pseudomonas aeruginosa, Escherichia coli, Staphylococcus aureus* and *Streptococcus pyogenes* (Chaudhari and Mengi, 2006).

The wound-healing effect of *Opuntia ficus-indica* was reported to be due to the presence of polysaccharides (molecular weight ranging from 10^4–10^6 Da) (Trombetta *et al.*, 2006). Several species of *Croton* (Euphorbiaceae) are used by Indian and Mestizo populations of Peru and Ecuador for the purpose of acceleration of wound healing. The alkaloid taspine was isolated from *Croton lechleri* of the Amazon rainforest and was tested in vivo using an incision wound model in rats, as well as in the in-vitro fibroblast proliferation assay. The in-vivo study with taspine revealed that there was a significant ($P < 0.001$) gain of tensile strength (>600 g/mm^2) with taspine at a dose of 250 μg after 12 days of treatment, and in vitro there was a significant ($P < 0.05$) increase in proliferation of fibroblast cells (6×10^4) with taspine at a dose of 100 μg (Porras-Reyes *et al.*, 1993).

Evaluation of wound-healing medicinal plants

Botanical and phytochemical evaluation

The necessity of correct botanical identification and the use of phytochemical constituents is discussed in Chapter 27.

Phytochemical profile

It is essential to define a phytochemical profile before any pharmacological or clinical studies are carried out. Chromatography is the most important technique for doing this but simple tests for phytochemical groups are sometimes used.

Preparation of plant extracts and dosage form

There are many techniques for preparation of a standardised plant extract. Most polar components of medicinal plants can be obtained by conventional aqueous or 80% ethanol extract, by soaking the coarse powder of the plant in the required amount of solvent (distilled water or 80% ethanol) for about 24 h. Extraction without applying heat will avoid decomposition of many components present. Most of the research on wound-healing plant drugs has been performed with these two types of extracts. They are mostly applied topically as 5–10% w/w in ointment base but sometimes by the oral or intraperitoneal route.

Investigations into toxicity

Dermal toxicity studies should be performed for topical applications of plant extracts respectively. Acute dermal toxicity/irritation can be induced by topical application of the solution prepared from the plant product and compared with known dermal toxic chemicals such as 0.1% dinitrochlorobenzene (DNCB) in dimethyl sulphoxide (DMSO). The erythema produced within 24 h should be noted and compared with known agents on the basis of the erythema and its severity as assessed by an arbitrary scoring system (http://www.rosecityarchery.com).

Pharmacological approach

Wound healing is the process of repair and regeneration that follows injury to the skin and other soft tissues. Initially there is an inflammatory response and the cells below the dermis begin to increase collagen production. Finally the gap is filled up with the regeneration of epithelial tissue. There are three stages to the process of wound healing:

- inflammation
- proliferation
- remodelling.

The need to verify traditional claims and to understand the detail underlying the mechanisms of wound healing by various plants has prompted researchers to develop specific wound models in animals and also in-vitro tests.

Selection of animals for wound-healing research

Wound-healing research has traditionally been categorised as either basic experimental animal work or clinical human research, although there are models that are applicable to both categories. Clinical research studies are normally based on results from experimental research, so the successful treatment of a patient's problem wound is therefore based on knowledge from both experimental and clinical research. Animal models provide invaluable information for the human wound-healing response but problems may arise with the extrapolation, interpretation and implementation of the results to clinical situations. A good example is the use of growth factors, which have shown beneficial effects on healing in animals but until now have shown much less of an effect clinically.

The most important relevant animal model which can be considered for wound-healing research is the rat, as shown by Sourla *et al.* (2000) who observed that there are many similarities between the physiological nature of the skin of rats and human beings. One problem is that no animal models of chronic wounds such as venous leg ulcers, diabetic ulcers or pressure ulcers are presently available. For these reasons the use of human models, despite the ethical and methodological problems, is preferable in wound-healing research (Gottrup, 2001).

Animal wound models

Prior to infliction of wounds, preferably over the dorsal area of the animal (rat), the region needs to be depilated and cleaned well with 70% ethanol. Permissible anaesthetic agents such as ketamine in a scheduled dose are injected before the artificial production of a wound. It is also important that all experiments should be approved by an ethical committee and carried out in accordance with international guidelines for humane use of animals in research.

Excision wound model

The excision wound model can be used in Sprague–Dawley rats following the method of Morton and Malon (1972). It is the most relevant model to human wounds because of the wide margin of wounds with full thickness usually performed with punch biopsy instruments of specific diameter. This model is the best because the assessment of physical and biochemical characters can be done clearly and it enables measurement of the wound contraction size (mm^2), healing period, tensile strength (g), estimation of tissue DNA, RNA, protein or hydroxyproline as well as histopathological examination.

Detailed scientific pharmacological evaluation was reported by Rasik *et al.* (1996) with the Indian medicinal plant *Euphorbia nerifolia* L. in guinea pigs, and work was performed using *Butea monosperma* on full-thickness, excised wounds (Sumitra *et al.*, 2005). Most of the work on excised wounds is performed by cutting a section of a particular area on the back of the animal with simple scissors and a scalpel (Diwan *et al.*, 1982; Hegde *et al.*, 2005). Interesting and promising results have been obtained with *Tridax procumbens, Cassia alata, Eleusine coracan* and *Paspalum scorbiculatum*.

This method has some drawbacks because it could hamper the maintenance of the wound edge as well as the measurement of the wound-contraction area. The best way to inflict the excision wound is with standard punch biopsy instruments such as Acupunch (Acu derm Inc., Florida, USA).

Incision-wound model

The method of Ehrlich *et al.* (1968) is commonly used where an incision-wound model is inflicted. This model is performed initially only to assess the wound-healing activity of unknown medicinal plants prior to detailed study. The incision model is the best for understanding the breaking strength of the wound following application of the plant extract. Several medicinal plants from a variety of geographical areas were all tested in this model to evaluate their wound-healing effect, particularly by measuring tensile strength and all gave significant results for improvement. Active plants included *Ocimum sanctum* (Shetty *et al.*, 2006), the Mexican medicinal plant *Hylocereus undatus* (Perez *et al.*, 2005) and the Peruvian medicinal plant *Anredera diffusa* (Moura-Letts *et al.*, 2006).

Dead-space wound model

This is a special technique for the infliction of wounds in animal models and applicable especially for the assessment of the capability of the formation of granulation tissue, which is responsible for the formation of the wound bed, as well as remodelling of wounds. Dead-space wounds can be produced in animals under light anaesthesia by inserting a sterilised cylindrical glass pith (2.5 cm × 0.3 cm) on either side of the dorsal paravertebral surface of the rat (Turner, 1965). After a certain time, granulation tissue deposits over the pith and is collected, dried and finally weighed. The greater the mass of deposited tissue, the better is the indication for healing capability.

Several medicinal plants were found to have potent activity by this technique, e.g. the Indian medicinal plant *Vernonia arborea* HK given orally at a dose of 30 mg/mL and simultaneously by local application in ointment form at a concentration of 5% (w/w) was found to generate a significant amount of granulation tissue (Manjunathan *et al.*, 2005).

In another study, the fresh juice of the leaves of *Tridax procumbens,* at a daily dose of 1 mL/kg by intraperitoneal route for 8 days, was administered to rats with a dead-space wound, along with a separate study on incised and excised wounds. The result showed decreased levels of granuloma (32.00 ± 3.00) compared with the control group (57.00 ± 4.50) indicating that the plant could prevent post-healing keloid formation (Diwan *et al.,* 1982). Therefore, the dead-space wound model reflects the therapeutic efficacy of a drug as well as its potentiality in prevention of post-healing hazards.

Diabetic wound model

The diabetic wound model is important in evaluating any medicinal plant for its activity in chronic and complicated wounds. Usually this is performed in streptozotocin-induced (65 mg/kg body weight in citrate buffer at pH 4.2) adult, diabetic rats. Excised wounds are produced in the conventional way as described earlier and efficacy of plants can be assessed following the conventional physical, biochemical, histological and molecular parameters. The advantage of this model is that the plants that exhibit activity in this model can be considered to be ideal candidates for the repair of normal secondary wounds as well as diabetic wounds in clinical practice. The medicinal plants thus far showing activity in diabetic wound models are *Aloe vera* (Chithra *et al.*, 1998), *Pterocarpus santalinus* (Biswas *et al.*, 2004) and *Hylocereus undata* (Perez *et al.*, 2005).

Observation criteria

Physical parameters

Wound-contraction size

Measurement of wound-contraction size is an important physical marker of healing. This can be done by tracing around the wound during the period of treatment. From these traces, areas can be determined and expressed in square millimetres. Biswas *et al.* evaluated the effect of *P. santalinus* on wound-contraction size in punch, burn and diabetic wound models using the same method (Biswas, 2004). It was observed from this study that the plant extract was able to contract the wounds significantly ($P < 0.05$) in all three models. The ethanol extract of *Catharanthus roseus* flower gave highly significant ($P < 0.001$) contraction of wound size (mm^2) in the excised wound model from days 1–20 post-wounding (Nayak and Pereira, 2006). Similarly wound-contraction size was used as a physical parameter while studying the wound-healing effect of *Hylocereus undatus* on diabetic rats (Perez *et al.*, 2005). The ethanol extract of leaves of *Embelia ribes* also showed a high rate of wound contraction in excision, incision and dead-space wound models using Swiss Albino rats.

Tensile strength

Tensile strength is another parameter for the assessment of healing of wounds. It gives direct evidence of genesis of collagen fibres, essential for formation of a wound bed. In collagen fibre formation, three basic protein components – glycine, proline and hydroxyproline – are drawn together to give maximum strength, which is reflected as an increase in tensile strength (Freifelder, 1987). Almost all the medicinal plants that have been investigated for wound-healing activity have been tested for their effect on tensile strength of the wound. Tensile strength can be measured by a tensilometer (Bostford, 1941) and the value is expressed in grams. Good examples of tensile-strength generation in wounds have been observed with 0.5% and 1% aqueous extract of the latex of *Euphorbia nerifolia* in excised wounds (Rasik *et al.,* 1996). Biswas *et al.* (2004) observed that there were significant increases ($P < 0.05$) in tensile strength in all three models with the plant *Pterocarpus santalinus*.

Period of healing

Measurement of the healing period also reflects the two physical parameters: wound contraction size and tensile strength. A shorter healing time indicates the capability of a plant extract to improve wound healing. *Centella asiatica* applied to excised wounds required a maximum of 24 days for epithelialisation (Rao *et al.*, 1996) but *Allamanda cathartica* L. and *Laurus nobilis* L. required only 15 days for healing of excised wounds (Nayak *et al.*, 2005). *Pterocarpus santalinus*, on the other hand was found to be more promising and required only 9 days in the punch-wound model and a maximum of 18 days in the burn-wound model (Biswas *et al.*, 2004), indicating that it is a useful plant for improving the healing process.

Biochemical parameters

Several compounds that directly regulate the healing process are useful as biochemical markers. The most important biochemical factors which reflect the healing potentiality are total protein, DNA, RNA and hydroxyproline. All these biochemical factors can be estimated at the end of the healing of varieties of wounds.

Role of total protein

There are several proteins that are involved in the extracellular formation of collagen fibrils and maturation of collagen, e.g. chondroitin, its sulphates and dermatan sulphate. The protein elastin is a major component of connective tissue and is responsible for cross-linking of collagen (Irvin, 1981). Total protein can be estimated from healed wound tissue according to the methods of Lowry *et al.* (1951). The alcoholic extract of bark of *Butea monosperma* (Sumitra *et al.*, 2005), wholegrain flour of finger millet and kodo millet (Hegde *et al.*, 2005) generated sufficient amounts of total protein to indicate that the plant extract was responsible for collagen cross-linking of collagen, as well as helping collagen fibre formation. The total protein content from the healed wound tissue was also measured in the case of *Vanda roxburghii*, an epiphytic orchid, giving a moderately significant increase in protein content in granulation tissue when the plant extract was used compared with control (Nayak *et al.*, 2005).

Role of tissue DNA

During the process of wound healing, the proliferation of cells for epithelialisation and collagenesis occurs through mitosis. In the early phase of nuclear repair (karyogenesis) there is repair of nucleic acids such as DNA. DNA synthesis has an important role in the healing process by means of chromosome replication (Watson *et al.*, 1987). DNA of healed wound tissue can be estimated by the thymidine incorporation assay method but the commonest method that can be adopted for this purpose is that of Burton (1956) using diphenylamine reagent. The medicinal plant that is able to generate DNA at a promising rate can be considered as an ideal wound healer. *Euphorbia nerifolia* was able to generate 6.13 mg/g of DNA with 0.5% aqueous extract and 12.41 mg/g of DNA with 1% extract after 7 days of treatment while *Pterocarpus santalinus* generated 2.45 mg/g on the 9th day in the excised model, backing up results obtained by other measurements.

Role of tissue RNA

Messenger RNA (mRNA) is synthesised within the nucleus of fibroblasts during the healing process. mRNA can be estimated from tissue by the orcinol reagent technique (Stroev and Makarova, 1989) from wound tissue and was used in the demonstration of the activity of *Hylocereus undatus* and *Pterocarpus santalinus*.

Estimation of tissue hydroxyproline

Hydroxyproline formation reflects direct evidence of collagen fibre formation since it is one of the important members of triple helix collagen. Estimation of hydroxyproline can be performed with the technique of Woessner (1961). Evidence of hydroxyproline generation in the wound area has been demonstrated for several medicinal plant extracts, e.g. *Vernonia arborea* (Manjunathan *et al.*, 2005). The hydroxyproline-generation capability of *Allamanda cathartica* and *Laurus nobilis* was 67.1 and 49.50 mg/g, respectively (Nayak *et al.*, 2005). *Catharanthus roseus* flower extract generated 63 mg/g of tissue hydroxyproline, indicating its high proficiency in the mechanism of wound repair (Nayak and Pereira, 2006) and the 0.5% aqueous extract of *Euphorbia nerifolia* latex synthesised 52 mg/g hydroxyproline in tissue and interestingly this did not increase with higher doses.

Histological investigations

Histological examination is useful to give a detailed picture of the healing process at different time intervals. A common method that can be followed for assessment of histological examination of treated wound tissue is staining with haematoxylin and eosin, which gives a general view of the formation of tissues such as collagen fibres and epithelialisation. For more specific information about the infiltration of collagen, elastin and reticulin, the most important protein for healing of wounds, it is better to use the Van-Gieson stain (Singh and Sulochana, 1997), Eigert Resorcin-Fuschin (Mallory, 1961) or Gridley modification of the silver impregnation method of staining (Gridley, 1951). The paste of the rhizome of the Indian medicinal plant *Curcuma longa* was tested in excised wounds on rabbits and evidence was recorded by histological examination using these stains that there was a well-characterised genesis of collagen, elastin and reticulin (Kundu *et al.*, 2005).

Molecular biological investigations

There are many ways to determine the mechanisms of action of medicinal plants for wound-healing activity. Matrix metalloproteinase (MMP) expression is an important parameter but the simplest method is a SDS-polyacrylamide gel electrophoresis (SDS-PAGE) study with the wound tissue of different days treatment. The technique was followed for evaluation of *Pterocarpus santalinus* wound-healing activity in the punch model. Results of this study showed that *P. santalinus* could generate protein of gradually higher molecular weights from day 3 to day 5 and finally up to day 7. All the larger proteins are responsible for the formation of ground substance in the wound area (Biswas *et al.*, 2004).

Clinical evidence for wound-healing medicinal plants

Objectives

The main object of a clinical trial is to test the effect of a drug in humans. Topical application of several synthetic agents, e.g. antibiotics (especially neomycin), preservatives (parabenes) and other substances used in topical applications to the skin may cause allergic contact dermatitis (Anon., 1995) and may result in a delay in the healing process (Demling, 1985). In these situations, products of plant origin may be useful alternatives, although only a few medicinal plants have so far been tested and reported to have wound-healing activity. The parameters for observation of efficacy of wound-healing medicinal plants in the human model tends to be more dependent on physical examination rather than using biochemical parameters. Pre-clinical studies should be performed before any humans are exposed to extracts, particularly with open complicated wounds and/or toxic and impure medicinal plants.

During clinical research with any plant drugs, careful attention must be paid to the dressing of the wound. Most studies on traditional medicines rarely maintain the aseptic condition of the wounds and this may cause unwanted infection, leading to non-healing of wounds or other complications such as serious infections. It is desirable to use agents such as 70% ethanol or 6% hydrogen peroxide for debridement of wounds and these usually do not interfere with the wound-healing property of the plant extracts. It is not recommended that wound dressings be changed daily since this might cause delay in healing owing to delay in granulation tissue formation. The wound areas should also be kept aerated so that sufficient oxygen can enter in the wound area, essential for early healing.

Physical parameters for observation

Wound-contraction size

Assessment of wound-healing potentiality can be achieved through measuring the wound-contraction area (mm^2). The plant that shows rapid reduction of the wound area is considered to be a good agent. The wound size can be recorded by area-measuring scales. During measurement of the wound-contraction area, it is mandatory to measure it from all aspects and all directions. If there are multiple numbers of wounds, measurement is to be taken for all and it should be done by addition of all the data. In a study with turmeric powder (*Curcuma longa*) on patients with common surgical wounds, reductions of wound area were found to be very significant, indicating its proficiency as an ideal wound healer of natural origin (Surh, 2002).

Granulation

Granulation can be observed by eye and is characterised by the formation of red, brittle tissues observed during the post-wounding period. Granulation is the early phase of scar formation before epithelialisation, caused by the extruding nature of fibrous tissue in the wound area. Granulation tissue is essential to wound repair and is a highly vascular and cellular tissue in which the collagen and ground substance of connective tissues are synthesised. The size of the final fibrous scar is proportional to the amount of granulation tissue formed (Irvin, 1981).

The quality of granulation is considered to be an important parameter for observation. A study with the ointment prepared from the Indian medicinal plant *Pterocarpus santalinus* revealed that the granulation in five patients with lower-extremity wounds appeared at an early stage with evidence of proper maintenance of quality. The study was conducted in chronic and complicated non-healing wounds, infected wounds and accidental injury; all of which were in a serious condition before the treatment and repaired with good aesthetic quality and with proper features of granulation. It was observed that granulation tissue could be generated within a very short period, almost half that given by conventional therapeutic measurements (Biswas *et al.*, 2004).

Cicatrisation, epithelialisation and angiogenesis

These three parameters for assessment of wound-healing activity are mainly concerned with final closure of the wound by development of new epithelial tissue (Gabbiani *et al.*, 1971). Fibrosis is characterised by formation of whitish scar formation over the wound area, neoangiogenesis is characterised by bleeding on removal of granulation and/or fibrous tissue and epithelialisation is characterised by remodelling of the wound area. Early occurrence of these features in clinical models indicates quality formation of extracellular matrix, formation of matrix metalloproteinases by means of collagenesis and prevention of apoptosis or keloid formation (Ehrlich *et al.* 1994).

Aloe vera, Chamaemelum nobile (commonly known as chamomile) and *Centella asiatica* are good examples of plant drugs that showed early genesis of cicatrisation, epithelialisation and neoangiogenesis in wound-healing models. The gel of *Aloe vera* is a common remedy for wound healing and is claimed to increase epithelialisation and reduce inflammation, but clinical studies are equivocal as to its effectiveness. However, a study was conducted with a glycoprotein fraction, isolated and named G1G1M1DI2, and showed that it produced significant [^{3}H] thymidine uptake in squamous carcinoma cells. The effect of G1G1M1DI2 on cell migration was confirmed by accelerated wound healing on a monolayer of human keratinocytes in vitro (Choi *et al.*, 2001). This indicates that the gel might accelerate the cicatrisation and epithelialisation in human wounds in a clinical setting.

A similar study with the 6% aqueous extract of *Buddleja globosa* exhibited proliferation of keratinocytes as well as slowing down the contraction of the lattice when tested at concentrations of 50 and 100 μg/mL (Houghton *et al.*, 2005). Both the in-vitro studies of *Aloe vera* and *Buddleja globosa* indicate that these two plants have a definite role in promoting wound healing by means of cicatrisation and epithelialisation owing to their keratinocyte-proliferating activities. However, direct clinical evidence is needed to establish their mechanism of action.

Asiaticoside, a triterpene compound from *Centella asiatica* (Apiaceae) is reported to hasten the fibroblast cell formation in human collagen-I which is mainly responsible for cicatrisation. Gota kola (*Centella asiatica*) increases blood supply to connective tissue. It promotes rapid wound healing by accelerating tissue growth. It also exhibits an antimicrobial action by dissolving the covering of certain viruses and bacteria (http://www.docharrison.com/webedit). In a study on human fibroblast cell culture with the triterpenoid fraction of C. *asiatica,* rapid formation of fibroblast cells was observed with the formation of new blood vessels as well as epithelial tissue (Tennai *et al.,* 1986).

In a double-blind clinical trial, the therapeutic efficacy of chamomile extract was tested on 14 patients. The drying effect of this plant causes early epithelialisation and the decrease in the weeping wound area, as well as the drying tendency, was statistically significant (Glowania *et al.* 1987).

The plant extract *Calendula officinalis* was evaluated in 34 patients with chronic venous leg ulcers on the basis of the epithelialisation as observed by wound-contraction size. There was a 14.52% decrease in wound size in chronic venous leg ulcers with this plant after 3 weeks of treatment (Duran *et al.*, 2005).

Haematological observation

Inflammation in the early stage of wounds is characterised by the involvement of a number of haematological factors. During the early phase of inflammation, polymorphonuclear neutrophils account for the major part of the initiation of repair mechanism. Erythrocytes undergo rouleux formation, with a resulting increase in the erythrocyte sedimentation rate, and lymphocytes undergo proliferation for the genesis of new blood vessels. Therefore, the assessment of the healing mechanism in human subjects can be identified by estimation of these various haematological parameters. The most important haematological parameters that are helpful in the evaluation of medicinal plants for their wound-healing potentiality in human subjects are described below.

Differential count of leucocytes

Neutrophils are considered to be chemotaxic agents of inflammation, which prepare the environment for beginning the repair mechanism. At the early phase of wounding the number of neutrophils is increased and, as the healing process progresses, the number of neutrophils gradually decreases. Eosinophils migrate at the later stage of the healing process and heparin and histamines are produced by basophils, which are responsible for the destruction of unwanted materials at the wound site. Monocytes, by their phagocytic property, engulf the microorganisms so that the healing can be achieved. Lymphocytes are the most important variety of leucocytes that are responsible for either the generation of fibroblast or collagen cells or are directly converted to fibroblast cells (Rubin and Farber, 1996).

The present authors evaluated the ointment prepared from three Indian medicinal plants, i.e. *Pterocarpus santalinus, Ficus benghalensis* and *Cynodon dactylon*, for their wound-healing properties in human models, with a variety of wounds such as surgical wounds, burns and complicated wounds of the lower extremity. Besides conventional physical parameters, haematological parameters were also added as objectives, and included the estimation of differential leucocyte counts at different times in the therapy. Results revealed that there were tendencies to a decrease in neutrophil count as healing progressed, while there was a remarkable increase in lymphocytes, indicating the process of genesis of fibrosis, and a decrease in both the eosinophils as well as monocytes, owing to the inflammatory processes being overcome. *Pterocarpus santalinus* gave better results than other two plants used, i.e. *Ficus benghalensis* and *Cynodon dactylon.* The results of *P. santalinus* were found to be similar to the standard topical antibiotic framycetin (P = 0.05–0.001).

Erythrocyte sedimentation rate

Erythrocyte sedimentation rate (ESR) indicates the degree of inflammation and if it is greater than 20 mm (unless known to be pre-existent), this indicates that the healing process is hampered (Weber *et al.*, 2005). The Peterborough Healthcare Wound Management Committee, June 2004, also recommended estimation of ESR for the assessment of wound healing. In an experimental study with *Terminalia chebula*, it was observed that, besides several biochemical parameters such as estimation of DNA, ESR has been used for the assessment of the wound repair mechanism (Suguna *et al.*, 2002).

A comparative clinical study with the ointment prepared from *Pterocarpus santalinus, Ficus benghalensis* and *Cynodon dactylon* on 54 patients of varieties of wounds showed that there were remarkable reductions in ESR with the progress of the healing process (Table 17.3) when compared with the standard topical antibiotic framycetin. Therefore, these three medicinal plants might be able to control

Table 17.3 Effect of ointments prepared from *Pterocarpus santalinus*, *Ficus benghalensis* and *Cynodon dactylon* on human models of wounds on the basis of different haematological parameters in comparison with framycetin

Treatment groups	Differential counts of WBC (%) N		L		E		M		ESR (mm/h)	
	BT	AT	BT	AT	BT	AT	BT	AT	BT	AT
P. santalinus (n = 0)	70.93 ± 4.13	64.96 ± 3.72**	24.73 ± 2.22	28.93 ± 2.43**	3.93 ± 0.18	2.71 ± 0.17*	2.14 ± 0.16	1.53 ± 0.12*	25.96 ± 2.01	14.75 ± 1.79**
F. benghalensis (n = 12)	64.83 ± 3.99	64.67 ± 3.98	28.00 ± 2.76	29.97 ± 2.82*	5.00 ± 0.65	4.17 ± 0.54	2.33 ± 0.18	1.87 ± 0.14*	38.67 ± 2.32	35.17 ± 2.30
C. dactylon (n = 12)	67.33 ± 4.01	67.00 ± 4.00	28.50 ± 2.34	29.33 ± 2.29*	3.33 ± 0.15	2.67 ± 0.13*	0.83 ± 0.09	1.00 ± 0.10	37.67 ± 2.29	35.33 ± 2.23
Framycetin (n = 10)	70.67 ± 4.12	65.50 ± 3.70**	24.67 ± 2.21	31.00 ± 2.91**	3.16 ± 0.17	3.00 ± 0.16*	1.50 ± 0.13	1.00 ± 0.10*	25.83 ± 1.99	12.50 ± 1.01**

Data are represented as mean ± SEM.
WBC = white blood count; ESR = erythrocyte sedimentation rate; N = neutrophil; L = lymphocytes; E = eosinophil; M = monocytes; BT = before treatment; AT = 30 days after treatment.
*$P<0.05$; **$P<0.001$ (unpublished).

the inflammatory process followed by healing of wounds.

Other assessment criteria

Besides the two parameters noted above for clinical evaluation of medicinal plants for their wound-healing activity, other measurements to evaluate the oxygen supply in the wound area can be used, especially for chronic venous leg ulcers or diabetic foot. Another important parameter is the estimation of antioxidants and superoxide levels from serum, as these directly reflect the potential of that particular medicinal plant for wound healing. However, a review of the literature reveals that no clinical study has so far been carried out with any medicinal plants, probably because of the lack of facilities or no relevant clinical research with medicinal plants for wound-healing activity.

Conclusions

Much attention is being paid in the field of biomedical research to wound healing at all levels. Major problems lie in wound infection and loss of body immunity and the main objective of wound-healing research is to exclude all these problems by maintaining the hygienic condition of wounds, prompt healing of the wound area and maintenance of its cosmetic aspects. In modern medicine, there are rarely any drugs or prescriptions that can fulfil all of these aspects. Modern techniques such as vacuum-assisted closure therapy (Steenvoorde *et al.*, 2004) are being introduced but this therapy is very expensive, and not affordable for many in the world, especially in developing countries.

Because of such economic restrictions, many people in such countries depend on traditional medicines, especially from plant sources, for maintaining their health and for disease cures. It has been observed in this chapter that most of the wound-healing research on medicinal plants is limited to a certain extent and has rarely been done to the full extent of clinical research. The exception is *Pterocarpus santalinus* which can be categorised as a wound-healing medicinal plant of level 3, which has been examined in detail both in experimental and clinical models.

The level 2 medicinal plants for wound-healing activity comprise those that have given good results at an experimental pharmacological level. Examples are *Euphorbia nerifolia, Aspillia africana, Curcuma longa* and *Aloe vera*. There are some medicinal plants that show good effects at the initial levels of pharmacological screening, especially in the incision model, which can be designated level 1 wound-healing medicinal plants, e.g. *Aegle marmelos* and *Cassia alata*. It is, therefore, necessary to perform level 2 and level 3 research for the level 1 group of wound-healing plants, and level 3 for level 2 group of medicinal plants, to bring them to a position where they can be considered to be viable medicinal agents.

Acknowledgement

The authors thankfully acknowledge Prof. Biswapati Mukherjee for his guidance, enormous inspiration and valuable suggestions.

References

Anon. (1995). *Treatment of venous leg ulcers: recommendations*. Workshop on Treatment of Venous Leg Ulcers, Statens Legemiddelkontroll, Upsala, Sweden, 1995, 5: 9–37.

Biswas TK, Muherjee B (2003). Plant medicine of Indian origin for wound healing activity. *Int J Lower Ext Wounds* 2: 25–39.

Biswas TK, Maity LN, Mukherjee B (2004). Wound healing potential of *Pterocarpus santalinus* Linn.: a pharmacological evaluation. *Int J Lower Ext Wounds* 3: 143–150.

Bodding PO (1986). List of Santal Prscriptions. In: *Studies in Santal Medicine and Connected Folklore*, Parts I–III. Calcutta, The Asiatic Society, pp. 161–393.

Bostford TW (1941). The tensile strength of sutured skin wounds during healing. *Surg Gynaecol Obst* 62: 690–697.

Brown G, Nanney LB, Grifen J *et al.* (1989). Enhancement of wound healing by topical treatment with epidermal growth factor. *New Engl J Med* 321: 76–79.

Burton K (1956). A study of the condition and mechanism of the diphenylamine reaction for the colorimetric estimation of deoxyribonucleic acid. *Biochem J* 62: 315–321.

Bussmann WR, Sharon D (2006). Traditional medicinal plant use in Northern Peru: tracking two thousand years of healing culture. *J Ethnobiol Ethnomed* 2: 47: 1–18.

Craig MA, Karchesy JJ, Blythe LL *et al.* Toxicity studies on western juniper oil (*Juniperus occidentalis*) and Port-Orford-cedar oil (*Chamaecyparis lawsoniana*) extracts utilizing local lymph node and acute dermal irritation assays. Rose City Archery, Oregon State University, Corvallis. http://www.rosecityarchery.com.

Chithra P, Sajithalal GB, Chandrakasan G (1998). Influence of *aloe vera* on the healing of dermal wounds in diabetic rats. *J Ethnopharmacol* 59: 195–201.

Choi SW, Son BW, Son YS *et al.* (2001). The wound-healing effect of a glycoprotein fraction isolated from *Aloe vera. Br J Dermatol* 145 (4): 535.

Demling RH (1985). Medical Progress: Burn. *New Engl J Med* 313 (22): 1389–1398.

Dulak J (2005). Nutraceuticals as anti-angiogenic agents: hopes and reality. *J Physiol Pharmacol* 56: 51–69.

Duran V, Matic M, Jovanovc M *et al.* (2005). Results of the clinical examination of an ointment with marigold (*Calendula officinalis)* extract. I The treatment of venous leg ulcers. *Int J Tissue React* 27: 101–106.

Ehrlich HP, Hunt TK (1968). Effect of cortisone and vitamin A on wound healing. *Ann Surg* 167: 324–328.

Ehrlich HP, Desmouliere A, Diegelman RF *et al.* (1994). Morphological and immunochemical differences between keloid and hypertrophic scar. *Am J Pathol* 56: 173–181.

Freifelder D (1987). Collagen – a multiprotein assembly. 2nd edn. In: *Molecular Biology*. Narosa Publishing House, Calcutta.

Gabbiani G, Ryan G, Majno G (1971). Presence of modified fibroblasts in granulation tissue and their possible role in wound contraction. *Experientia* 27: 549–550.

Glowania HJ, Raulin C, Swoboda M (1987). Effect of chamomile on wound healing – a clinical double-blind study. *Z Hautkr* 62: 1267–1271.

Gottrup F (2001). Experimental wound healing research, The use of models. *Eur Wound Manag Assoc J* 1(2): 5–7.

Gridley MF (1951). A modification of the silver impregnation method of staining reticular fibre. *Am J Clin Path* 21: 897–899.

Hegde PS, Anitha B, Chandra TS (2005). In vivo effect of whole grain flour of finger millet (*Eleusine coracana*) and kodo millet (*Paspalum scorbiculatum*). *Indian J Exp Biol* 43: 254–258.

Houghton PJ, Hylands PJ, Mensah AJ *et al.* (2005). In vitro tests and ethnopharmacological investigations: wound healing as an example. *J Ethnopharmacol* 100: 100–107.

Irvin TT (1981). The healing wound. In: *Wound Healing Principles and Practice*. London: Chapman & Hall, 1–34.

Instituto Nacional de Estadi-acutestica e Informa-acutetica (2005). *Perú: Compendio Estadístico 2005*, p. 50.

Kumara Swamy HM, Krishna V, Shankarmurthy K *et al.* (2007). Wound healing activity of embelin isolated from the ethanol extract of leaves of *Embelia ribes. Burm J Ethnopharmacol* 109: 205–213.

Kuppast IJ, Nayak PV (2006). Wound healing activity of *Cordia dichotoma* Forst. f. fruits. *Nat Prod Radiance* 5: 99–102.

Lowry OH, Rosebrough NJ, Farr A l *et al.* (1951). Protein measurement with folin – phenol reagent. *J Biol Chem* 193: 265–275.

MacKay D, Miller AL (2003). Nutritional support for wound healing. *Wound Healing, Altern Med Rev 8* (4): 359–377.

Mallory FB (1961). *Pathological Techniques*. New York, Hafner, 154–155.

Manjunathan BK, Vidya SM, Rashmi KV *et al* (2005). Evaluation of wound healing potency of *Vernonia arborea* HK. *Indian J Pharmacol* 37(4): 223–226.

Morton JJP, Malone MH (1972). Evaluation of vulneray activity by an open wound procedure in rats. *Arch Int Pharmacodyn* 196: 117–126.

Moura-Letts G, Villegas LF, Marcalo A *et al.* (2006). In vivo wound healing activity of oleanolic acid derived from the acid hydrolysis of *Anredera diffusa. J Nat Prod* 69: 978–979.

Muthu C, Ayyanar M, Raja N *et al.* (2006). Medicinal plants used by traditional healers in Kancheepuram District of Tamil Nadu, India. *J Ethnobiol Ethnomed* 2: 43: 1–10.

Nayak BS, Pereira LMP (2006). *Catharanthus roseus* flower extract has wound-healing activity in Sprague Dawley rats. *BMC Complement Altern Med* 6: 41–46.

Nayak BS, Suresh R, Rao AVC *et al* (2005). Evaluation of wound healing activity of *Vanda roxburghii* R.Br (Orchidacea): A preclinical study in a rat model. *Int J Lower Ext Wounds* 4: 200–204.

Perez GRM, Vargas SR, Ortiz HYD (2005). Wound healing properties of *Hylocereus undatus* on diabetic rats. *Phytother Res* 19: 665–668.

Porras-Reyes BH, Lewis WH, Roman J *et al.* (1993). Enhancement of wound healing by the alkaloid taspine defining mechanism of action. *J Physiol Soc Exp Biol Med* 203: 18–25.

Ramesh KV (1993). Wound repair: drug research and therapeutics. In: Tripathi S, Ed. *Update in Clinical Pharmacology*. Indian Pharmacological Society, Calcutta, India.

Rao GV, Shivakumar HG, Parthasarathi G. (1996). Influence of aqueous extract of *Centella asiatica* (Bramhi) on experimental wounds in albino rats. *Indian J Pharmacol* 28: 249–253.

Rasik AM, Shukla A, Patnaik GK *et al.* (1996). Wound healing activity of latex of *Euphorbia nerifolia* Linn. *Indian J Pharmacol* 28: 107–109.

Rubin E, Farber JL (1996). Repair, regeneration and fibrosis. In: *Pathology*, 2nd edn. Philadelphia. J. B. Lippincott and Company.

Sakarkar DM, Sakarkar UM, Shrikhande VN, *et al.* (2004). *Nat Prod Radiance* 3: 406–412.

Saraf S, Pandey SS (1996). *An overview on wound healing*. First National Conference on Wound Care, Varansi, India, Sept 28–29.

Shetty S, Udupa S, Udupa L *et al.* (2006). Wound healing activity of *Ocimum sanctum* Linn with supportive role of antioxidant enzymes. *Indian J Physiol Pharmacol* 50: 163–168.

Singh D (1979). *Unani Siddhayoga Samgraha*, 4th edn [in Hindi]. Calcutta: Shree Baidyanath Ayurveda Bhavan Ltd.

Singh D (1985). *Unani Treatments*, 3rd edn [in Hindi]. Calcutta: Shree Baidyanath Ayurveda Bhavan Ltd.

Singh UB, Sulochana S (1997). Special stain. In: *Handbook of Histological and Histochemiocal Techniques*, 2nd edn. Hyderabad, India, Premier, 42–43.

Sourla A, Richard V, Labrie F *et al.* (2000). Exclusive androgenic effect of dehydroepiandrosterone in sebaceous glands of rat skin. *J Endocrinol* 166: 455–462.

Steenvoorde P, Slotema E, Adhin S *et al* (2004). Deep infection after ilioinguinal node dissection: vacuum-assisted closure therapy? *Int J Lower Ext Wounds* 3: 223–226.

Stroev EA, Makarova VG (1989). Photocolorimetric methods for quantitating analysis of nucleic acids. In: *Laboratory Manual of Biochemistry*. Moscow: Mir Publishers.

Suguna L, Singh S, Sivakumar P *et al.* (2002). Influence of *Terminalia chebula* on dermal wound healing in rats. *Phytother Res* 16: 227–231.

Sumitra M, Manikandan P, Suguna L (2005). Efficacy of *Butea monosperma* on dermal wound healing in rats. *Int J Biochem Cell Biol* 37: 566–573.

Surh YJ (2002). Anti-tumor promoting potential of selected spices ingredients with anti-oxidative and anti-inflammatory activitie: a short review. *Food Chem Toxicol* 40: 1091–1097.

Tennai R, Zanaboni G, De Agostini M *et al.* (1986). Effect of titerpenoid fraction of *Centella asiatica* on macromolecules of the connective tissue matrix in human skin fibroblast cultures. *Int J Biochem* 37: 69–77.

Trombetta D, Puglia C, Perri D *et al* (2006). Effect of polysaccharides from *Opuntia ficus-indica* (L.) cladodes on the healing of dermal wounds in the rat. *Phytomedicine* 13: 352–358.

Turner RA (1965). *Screening Methods in Pharmacology*. New York, Academic Press, 168.

Watson JD, Hopkins NH, Roberts RW *et al.* (1987). The control of cell proliferation. In: *Molecular Biology of the Gene*. California: The Benjamin Cummings Publishing Co. Inc.

Weber EWG, Slappendel R, Prins MH *et al.* (2005). Blood transfusions and delayed wound healing after hip replacement surgery: effects on duration of hospitalization. *Anesth Analg* 100: 1416–1421.

18

Evidence of the efficacy of herbal medicinal products used for conditions associated with inflammation

Eva M Vigo, Samuel Seoane, Cristobal Fraga and Roman Perez-Fernandez

Introduction

Inflammation is a defence mechanism of living tissue in response to mechanical injury, tissue ischaemia, autoimmune processes or infectious agents. Clinically it is characterised by swelling, redness, heat, and often pain and loss of function.

This host defence is a highly regulated mechanism, to restrict its action to the time and place where it is necessary. Often, inflammation elicits a generalised sequence of events known as the acute phase response. This includes production of acute phase proteins by the liver, activation of the sympathetic nervous system, changes in cardiovascular function, altered neuroendocrine status, behavioural changes that lead to energy conservation, and the most common feature of infection, fever, which can limit bacterial proliferation.

These local and generalised inflammatory responses have clear benefits in infectious states when they are activated in a regulated manner for a defined period of time. An excessive or inadequate activation of the system, or failure in mechanisms of inactivation, can therefore have serious effects, leading to a number of diseases, including rheumatoid arthritis, chronic inflammatory bowel diseases, neurodegenerative disorders and asthma (Monaco *et al.*, 2004). Thus, inflammation is a major component of the damage caused by autoimmune diseases, but it is also a fundamental contributor to disorders such as diabetes, cancer and cardiovascular disease (Schwartsburd, 2003).

Numerous mediators are involved in inflammation processes, including mediators related to the arachidonic acid pathway (e.g. cyclo-oxygenase, lipoxygenase, and phospholipase A_2), and arachidonic acid-independent mediators (e.g. nitric oxide synthase, NF-κB, peroxisome proliferator-activated receptors, nonsteroidal anti-inflammatory drug-activated gene-1 and cytokines) (Figure 18.1) (Heller *et al.*, 1997; Kracht and Saklatvala, 2002).

Salicylate-containing plants have been used for relieving the signs of inflammation in several cultures

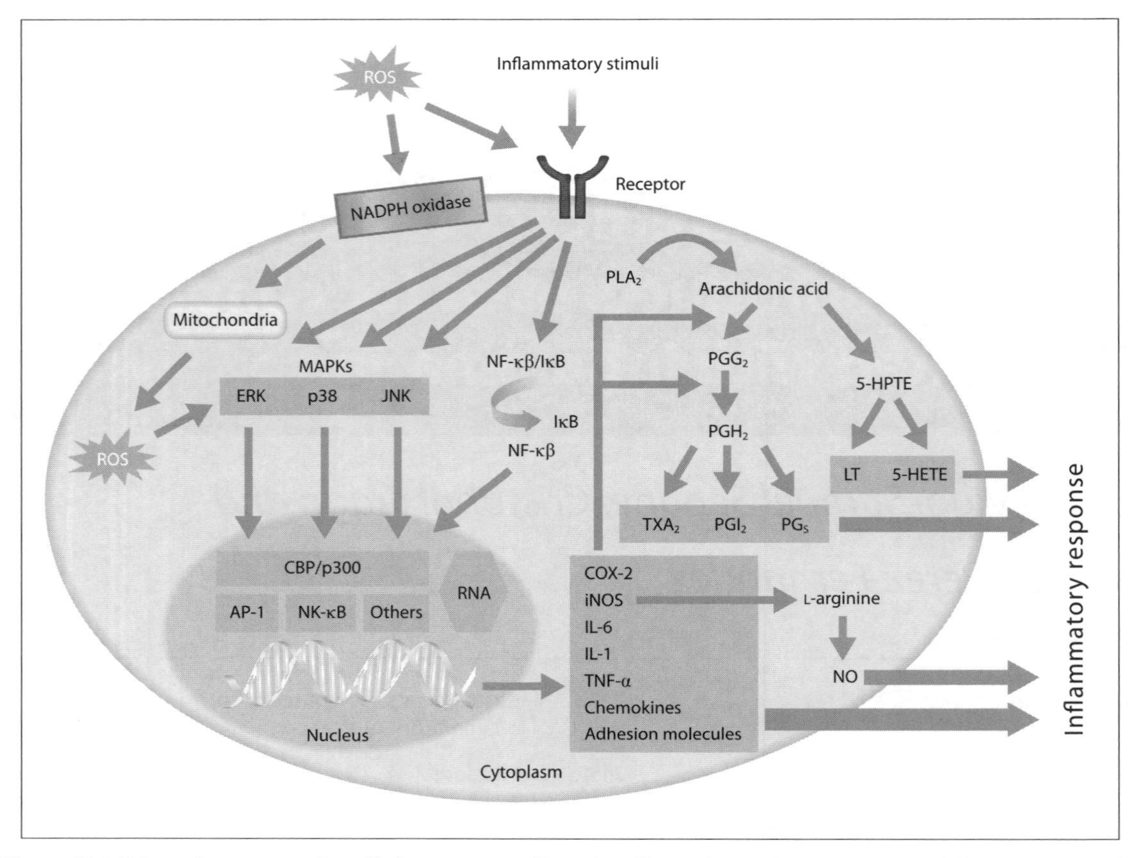

Figure 18.1 Schematic representation of inflammatory mediator signalling pathways. In response to pro-inflammatory stimuli (e.g. TNF-α, LPS, IFN-γ), specific cells induce receptor aggregation and activation of the mitogen-activated protein kinases (MAPKs) or the IκB, and thus activation of nuclear NF-κB and AP-1 proteins. Binding of these proteins and other transcription factors, coactivators, and RNA polymerase to specific regions of gene promoters results in activation of the transcription of specific genes, leading to the production of inflammatory mediators. Some of these newly synthesised proteins (e.g. iNOS and COX-2) may act on specific substrates (e.g. L-arginine and arachidonic acid, respectively) to induce new inflammatory mediators, such as nitric oxide and PGE2. Reactive oxygen species (ROS) oxidise several proteins, altering their conformation and up-regulating several signalling cascades, such as MAPK-dependent signalling pathways, leading to the activation of several redox-regulated transcription factors (e.g. AP-1 and NF-κB).

for centuries. A significant advance in the study of drugs with anti-inflammatory activity came in the early 1970s. During this decade, it was demonstrated that aspirin and other non-steroidal anti-inflammatory drugs inhibit cyclo-oxygenase and therefore synthesis of prostaglandins, key components in the inflammatory process. Since then, numerous investigators have addressed their research to developing drugs with the capacity to specifically inhibit inflammatory mediators. Steroidal and non-steroidal anti-inflammatory drugs (SAIDs and NSAIDs, respectively) are currently the most widely used drugs in the treatment of acute inflammatory disorders, despite their renal and gastric negative secondary effects, but have not been very successful in the treatment of chronic inflammatory diseases. Thus numerous research groups are focusing on the search for new and safe anti-inflammatory agents, and medicinal plants may represent a useful source of molecules for the development of drugs especially designed for the control of chronic inflammatory states (Sautebin, 2000; Calixto *et al.*, 2003, 2004; Kim *et al.*, 2004a; Yoon and Baek, 2005).

Newly developed molecular techniques with high selectivity and sensitivity are currently being widely used to study the mechanisms of action of herbal products on inflammation processes, whether through effects on gene transcription or on signal transduction.

Compared with chemically defined individual substances, the application of these tests to herbal preparations is laborious because they comprise mixtures of substances; in many cases the active ingredient(s) are unknown; and the composition and characteristics of what is nominally a single phyto-preparation may vary widely, depending on its origin and manufacturing procedure. Despite these difficulties, an increasing number of reports indicate that compounds derived from higher plants, extracts or extract fractions have medically useful effects on the pathophysiological processes involved in inflammation.

Inflammation mediators

Phospholipase A2, cyclo-oxygenases and lipoxygenases

Phospholipase A_2 (PLA_2) is the enzyme that governs the release of arachidonic acid from membrane lipids in cells. Several isoforms of PLA_2 have been discovered, and these isoforms are classified into three categories:

- secretory PLA_2 ($sPLA_2$)
- cytosolic PLA_2 ($cPLA_2$)
- calcium-independent PLA_2 ($iPLA_2$).

These PLA_2s are distributed in numerous tissues and cells. Once activated, PLA_2 releases arachidonic acid, which is subsequently metabolised by either of two enzymes, a prostaglandin endoperoxide H synthase (also called cyclo-oxygenase, COX) or a lipoxygenase (LOX). COX converts arachidonic acid into prostaglandins and thromboxanes, catalysing the stepwise conversion of arachidonic acid into the intermediates prostaglandin G_2 and prostaglandin H_2; the latter is subsequently transformed into prostacyclin I_2, thromboxane A_2, and prostaglandins D_2, E_2 and $F_{2\alpha}$ by specific synthases depending on the kind of tissue.

There are two different isoforms of cyclo-oxygenases (COX-1 and COX-2) and one variant (COX-3). COX-1 is a ubiquitous constitutive isoform that is expressed at constant levels throughout the cell cycle, and that is postulated to have housekeeping functions. This enzyme generates the prostaglandins responsible for physiological functions, including gastric mucosal integrity and regulation of renal blood flow. COX-2 was discovered separately (Kujubu *et al.*, 1991; Xie *et al.*, 1991): it is an inducible protein, induced by Src and tumour-promoting phorbol esters, showing 60% amino-acid sequence homology with the previously known COX-1. COX-2 is undetectable in many mammalian tissues, but its production is rapidly induced in cells involved in the inflammatory response, such as macrophages and mast cells, when these cells are stimulated by proinflammatory cytokines and/or bacterial lipopolysaccharide (LPS); this leads to production of much larger amounts of prostanoids than by COX-1 (Smith *et al.*, 1996).

In fact, COX-2 is thought to be the primary generator of the prostanoids that contribute to inflammation, acting in both the inflammation initiation and resolution phases. In view of this, it has been proposed that specific inhibition of COX-2 may be a better way of limiting inflammatory processes without affecting the synthesis of the prostaglandins required for normal physiological function. However, the relative contributions of COX-1 and COX-2 to inflammatory responses remain incompletely understood, and several studies have shown that prostanoids formed via COX-1 are also involved in inflammation processes (Vane *et al.*, 1998; Smith and Langenbach, 2002). The identification of the new variant COX-3, which is weakly inhibited by the NSAID acetaminophen, may contribute to the elucidation of the inflammatory process (Chandrasekharan *et al.*, 2002).

Lipoxygenases (LOXs) are enzymes involved in the generation of hydroxyeicosatetraenoic acid (HETE) and leukotriene compounds from arachidonic acid. Three LOX isoforms have been described in different cells and tissues: 15-LOX synthesises anti-inflammatory 15-hydroxyeicosatetraenoic acid (15-HETE), 12-LOX synthesises 12-HETE, which aggregates platelets and induces the inflammatory response, and 5-LOX synthesises 5-HETE and leukotrienes. Inhibition of the biosynthesis of inflammatory HETE mediators by blocking the activities of 5- and 12-LOXs is considered a possible way of treating inflammatory diseases (Parente and Perretti, 2003; Schneider and Bucar, 2005). When only COX enzymes are blocked, the LOX pathway leads to accelerated formation of leukotrienes, which suggests that dual inhibition of LOX and COX enzymes by specific drugs may be a sensible goal for research.

Nitric oxide (NO)

Nitric oxide (NO) is synthesised from the amino acid L-arginine by the NO synthase (NOS) enzymes in numerous mammalian cells and tissues. NO has diverse biological activities, including those involved in physiological regulation and activities contributing to pathological processes. The physiological actions of NO involve low concentrations (about 10^{-12} mol/L), with NO acting as a labile intracellular messenger in, for example, the regulation of vascular tone, neurotransmission in the brain or peripheral nerves. NO production is mediated by two enzymes, jointly termed constitutive nitric oxide synthases (cNOS), and originally detected in endothelial cells (eNOS) and in neurones (nNOS). The actions of this 'physiological' NO are mediated by a Ca^{2+}/calmodulin-dependent pathway. However, when NO is synthesised in large quantities (10^{-9} mol/L) by activated inflammatory cells, it shows cytotoxic properties and may be involved in the pathogenesis of acute or chronic inflammatory conditions (Moilanen *et al.*, 1999).

This NO production is mediated by an enzyme termed inducible nitric oxide synthase (iNOS), which is induced by several stimuli, including bacterial lipopolysaccharide and interferon-γ (IFN-γ). iNOS is present in macrophages and hepatocytes. Thus, during inflammation associated with different pathologies, NO production increases significantly (Kharitonov *et al.*, 1994) and may become cytotoxic. Moreover, the free-radical nature of NO and its high reactivity with oxygen to produce peroxynitrite ($ONOO^-$) makes NO a potent pro-oxidant molecule able to induce oxidative damage and become potentially harmful towards cellular targets (Epe *et al.*, 1996).

NO production induced by iNOS may thus reflect the degree of inflammation, and provides a useful way of assessing the effect of drugs on the inflammatory process. Conversely, inhibition of NO accumulation induced by inflammatory stimuli could be a useful strategy for treatment of inflammatory diseases (Hobbs *et al.*, 1999; Sautebin, 2000).

Nuclear transcription factor-κ

Considerable evidence indicates that the primary pathway involved in the initiation and amplification of inflammatory responses is the one that leads to activation of nuclear factor (NF)-κB transcription factors (Karin, 2005). NF-κB is a widely distributed protein located in the cytoplasm as an inactive heterodimer composed of a family of five subunits (Baeuerle and Baltimore, 1996). These protein complexes are retained in the cytoplasm by inhibitory (κB) proteins, hindering the translocation of NF-κB to the nucleus. NF-κB is activated by free radicals, inflammatory stimuli, endotoxins, ultraviolet light, carcinogens and tumour promoters. Once activated, specific protein kinases phosphorylate the κB proteins, inducing dissociation of NF-κB from κB. The phosphorylated IκaB is subsequently degraded by the proteasome, and NFκB is transported to the nucleus, where it induces transcription of numerous genes (Kracht and Saklatvala, 2002; Magne *et al.*, 2006). NF-κB regulates the transcription of various inflammatory cytokines, so agents that can suppress NF-κB are important candidate targets for drugs to prevent, delay the onset of, or treat many inflammatory diseases (Barnes and Karin, 1997; Ghosh and Karin, 2002).

Cytokines, chemokines and adhesion molecules

Cytokines are a group of molecules that are involved in many steps of the inflammatory response of which more than 100 have been identified (Haddad, 2002; Hopkins, 2003). Cytokines are generally classified as pro- or anti-inflammatory, depending on their role in the inflammatory process. In general, pro-inflammatory cytokines (i.e. interleukins IL-1β, IL-6, IL-8, IL-12 and tumour necrosis factor (TNF)-α) are involved in the initiation and amplification of the inflammatory response, whereas anti-inflammatory cytokines negatively modulate these events (i.e. IL-4, IL-10 and transforming growth factor (TGF)-β). Cytokines produced by cells such as macrophages, neutrophils and mast cells can act locally or systemically. They can induce their own production or even the secondary generation of other cytokines. Moreover, most cytokine actions involve the activation of transcription factors (e.g. NF-κB, AP-1) and protein kinases (e.g. mitogen-activated protein kinase), which subsequently regulate the expression of genes involved in the maintenance of the inflammatory situation (Haddad, 2002; Kracht and Saklatvala, 2002). In addition, cytokines are responsible for the induction of numerous enzymes such as iNOS and COX-2, as well as receptors (e.g. platelet-activating factor receptor, IL-2 receptor) and adhesion molecules (E-selectin, α and β-integrins) (Barnes and Karin, 1997; Donaldson *et al.*, 1997; Haddad, 2002).

Chemokines (e.g. IL-8 and eotaxin) are a group of cytokines that chemoattract and stimulate leucocytes at the site of inflammation. The chemokine system is extensive, with an estimated 50 chemokine ligands and 20 receptors. The effects of these molecules are mediated through G protein-coupled receptors. Once activated, chemokines enable leucocytes to migrate to the target tissues, a process also requiring activation of integrins. Numerous studies indicate that cytokines are implicated in the pathophysiology of various inflammatory diseases so the cytokine system constitutes an interesting target for the development of anti-inflammatory drugs (Tarrant and Patel, 2006).

Peroxisome proliferator-activated receptors and liver receptors

The peroxisome proliferator-activated receptors (PPARs) and the liver receptors (LXRs) are members of the nuclear hormone receptor superfamily that are mainly, or exclusively, regulated by ligands produced in a paracrine or autocrine manner. They transduce a wide variety of signals, including environmental, nutritional and inflammatory signals, into a defined and ordered set of cellular responses at the level of gene transcription (Daynes and Jones, 2002; Glass and Ogawa, 2006). Three PPAR (PPARα, PPARβ/δ and PPARγ) and two LXR (LXRα and LXRβ) isoforms have been identified and cloned.

Although the endogenous ligands that function to regulate PPAR activity in vivo remain poorly characterised, various types of fatty acid can bind to and activate PPARs. In addition, some of the eicosanoids that are derived from the metabolism of arachidonic acid, can also be effective ligand agonists for specific PPAR isoforms. PPARs also function as sensors and regulators of inflammatory responses through their ability to be activated by locally generated eicosanoids and can inhibit inflammatory gene expression by several mechanisms (Delerive *et al.*, 1999, 2003; Kelly *et al.*, 2004). It is probable that at least some of these mechanisms operate in a cell type-specific manner and recent studies (Pascual *et al.*, 2005) have given some explanation for how PPARγ represses inflammatory-response genes in a promoter-specific manner.

LXRs have recently been characterised as regulators of macrophage inflammatory pathways. Mice lacking LXRs show an exaggerated response to LPS, and synthetic LXR agonists inhibit the macrophage response to bacterial pathogens and antagonise the induction of a number of proinflammatory genes (Joseph *et al.*, 2003). LXR-sensitive genes overlap with genes that are sensitive to glucocorticoid receptor and/or PPARγ-mediated repression. Some of these are preferentially sensitive to LXR, indicating LXR-specific effects on the evolution of inflammatory responses, probably linked to inhibition of NF-κB activity (Joseph *et al.*, 2003).

The findings that nuclear receptors can modulate inflammatory immune responses in a gene- and signal-specific manner have a number of implications for the development and application of nuclear-receptor ligands in human disease. For example, in addition to atherosclerosis, PPARγ ligands have been suggested to ameliorate inflammation in animal models of inflammatory bowel disease, experimental autoimmune encephalomyelitis, arthritis and psoriasis. Indeed, several clinical trials have shown that PPARγ ligands reduce the severity of inflammation in patients with mild-to-moderate cases of ulcerative colitis (Glass and Ogawa, 2006).

Mitogen-activated protein kinase

Inflammatory mediators are produced in response to inflammatory stimuli that activate macrophages, and, subsequently, activation of intracellular signalling pathways. Primary inflammatory stimuli (microbial products) act through receptors of the Toll-like receptor family, and cytokines (e.g. IL-1β and TNF-α) through receptors of the IL-1 receptor (IL-1R) or TNF receptor families. Activation of receptors triggers major intracellular signalling pathways, namely mitogen-activated protein kinase (MAPK) pathways (Lee *et al.*, 1994; Lee and Young, 1996; Kyriakis and Avruch, 2001; Aggarwal, 2003) and the pathway leading to activation of the transcription factor NF-κB (Tak and Firestein, 2001; Aggarwal, 2003). TNF-α is a potent activator of NF-κB, which in turn is a potent inducer of TNF-α.

This positive feedback is a key feature in chronic inflammation. Lipopolysaccharide, a component of bacterial wall and commonly used inducer of the monocyte/macrophage cell lineage, acting via Toll-like receptor 4 (TLR4), also stimulates mitogen-activated protein (MAP) kinase cascades and the pathway leading to activation of NF-κB. Upon activation of the MAP kinases, transcription factors present in the cytoplasm or nucleus are phosphorylated and activated, leading to expression of target genes, resulting in a biological response. It has been demonstrated that MAP kinases have overlapping substrate specificities and phosphorylation of regulatory sites is shared among multiple protein kinases. These multiple interactions integrate the responses and activate separate sets of genes (Kyriakis and Avruch, 2001; Pearson *et al.*, 2001). A classic MAPK cascade is composed of

- an MAPK
- the kinase that activates the MAPK through phosphorylation of serine and tyrosine residues (called MAPK kinase, MKK, MEK, MAPKK, or MAP2K)
- the kinase that activates the MAP2K (called MKK kinase, MKKK, MEKK, MAPKKK, or MAP3K).

The MAP3Ks are activated through a variety of mechanisms, most of which are not entirely clear, in response to engagement of cell-surface receptors. Several distinct MAPK cascades have been identified, the three most common being the extracellular signal-regulated kinase, the Jun-N terminal kinase, and the p38 MAPK cascades. Each of the MAPK cascades has a distinct function, although a given stimulus, for example, TNF-α or IL-1, can activate all three MAPK cascades to a variable extent. The response specificity (i.e. the type of stimulus that activates any given cascade) is determined by the MAP3K (Karin, 2005).

The p38 MAPK cascade shares many features with the other MAPK cascades, and is associated with inflammation, cell growth, cell differentiation and cell death (Kyriakis and Avruch, 2001). Extracellular stimuli of the p38 MAP kinase pathway include a variety of cytokines (Pearson *et al.*, 2001) and a number of pathogenic stimuli activate p38 through various Toll-like receptors (Armant and Fenton, 2002). In most inflammatory cells, the main biological response of p38 is to initiate leucocyte recruitment and activation (Lee *et al.*, 1994; Lee and Young, 1996).

Free radicals

The term free-radical species refers to a variety of highly reactive molecules that can be divided into various categories, including reactive oxygen species (ROS), reactive nitrogen species (RNS), and reactive chlorine species (RCS). Important free-radical species include superoxide (O_2^-), the hydroxyl radical (OH^-), and the peroxyl radical (ROO^-) in the ROS group, and nitric oxide (NO) in the RNS group (Pop-Busui, 2006).

ROS and RNS occur as a result of several different processes:

- generated during irradiation by ultraviolet light, by X-rays or by gamma-rays
- products of metal-catalysed reactions
- present as pollutants in the atmosphere
- produced by neutrophils and macrophages during inflammation
- byproducts of mitochondria-catalysed electron transport reactions and other biochemical processes (Cadenas, 1989).

ROS and RNS play a dual role, being either beneficial or harmful to living systems. Beneficial effects of ROS involve physiological roles in cell responses to noxious stimuli such as in defence against infectious agents and in a number of cellular signalling systems. One further beneficial example of ROS at low concentrations is the induction of mitogenic responses.

In contrast, at high concentrations ROS can be important mediators of damage to cell structures, including lipids and membranes, proteins and nucleic acids (Poli *et al.*, 2004). ROS and metal ions primarily inhibit phosphatases, most probably by interacting with sulphydryl groups on their cystein residues, which are oxidised to form either intramolecular or intermolecular disulphide bonds. These structural changes alter protein conformations, leading to the up-regulation of several signalling cascades, most importantly those dependent on growth factor kinase, Src/Abl kinase, MAPK and PI-kinase. These cascades lead to the activation of several redox-regulated transcription factors.

Despite the actions of the cell's antioxidant defence system to counteract oxidative damage from ROS, such damage accumulates over the life cycle, and indeed, radical-related damage to DNA, to proteins and to lipids has been proposed to play a key role in the development of age-dependent diseases such as cancer, arteriosclerosis, arthritis, neurodegenerative disorders and other conditions (Valko *et al.*, 2006).

The term *oxidative stress* in essence refers to a serious imbalance between free-radical production and antioxidant defence mechanisms, potentially leading to tissue damage. Antioxidants have been defined as substances that are able, at relatively low concentrations, to compete with other oxidisable substrates, and thus to significantly delay or inhibit the oxidation of these substrates. This definition includes the enzymes superoxide dismutase, glutathione peroxidase, and catalase, as well as non-enzymatic compounds such as α-tocopherol (vitamin E), β-carotene, ascorbate (vitamin C) and glutathione. Currently the development of procedures to reduce adverse ROS production is one of the central issues in research on oxidative stress-related diseases. Swamping the system with antioxidants or overexpressing antioxidative enzymes may be just as detrimental as excessive exposure to free radicals and it is clear that a precisely balanced intermediate level of free radicals and radical-derived ROS is necessary.

Medicinal plants as a source of anti-inflammatory substances

Evaluation of therapeutic actions of herbal products

Research on anti-inflammatory substances has generally focused on nitric oxide production and arachidonic acid metabolism, signal transduction mechanisms in activated inflammatory cells, inflammatory cell functions (i.e. generation of free-radical species), and synthesis and actions of cytokines and related peptides involved in the inflammatory process. Any plant product that may interfere in any or all these systems can be considered as a potential candidate for anti-inflammatory therapy (Duwiejua and Zeitlin, 1993). It has been demonstrated in various inflammatory models, both in vivo (e.g. inflammation (erythema and oedema) of rodent ear, rat (or mouse) paw oedema test, adjuvant arthritis in rat or mouse and in vitro (e.g. inhibition of specific mediators involved in the inflammatory process in primary cell cultures or transformed cell lines) that various plant extracts and plant-derived bioactive compounds, are involved in reducing or suppressing inflammatory processes. Some of the tests that are commonly used to evaluate the anti-inflammatory activity from plant-derived compounds are now briefly reviewed.

In-vivo models of inflammation

Collagen-induced arthritis

An in-vivo murine model of arthritis was first described by Trentham *et al.* (1977). The collagen-induced arthritis is normally induced in mice or rats by immunisation with autologous or heterologous type II collagen in adjuvant. As in rheumatoid arthritis, pro-inflammatory cytokines, such as TNF-α, and IL-1β, are abundantly expressed in the arthritic joints of mice, and blockade of these molecules results in a reduction of disease severity (Williams, 2004).

Adjuvant-induced arthritis

A useful in-vivo rat model was originally described by Pearson *et al.* (1956). Adjuvant-induced arthritis is developed after injection of complete Freund's adjuvant in the footpad of Wistar rats (Mizushima *et al.*, 1972). It is a systemic disease that resembles rheumatoid arthritis, and is characterised by chronic evolution with recurrent inflammatory bouts resulting in periarticular, articular and bone lesions (Rotelli *et al.*, 2003).

Carrageenan-induced paw oedema

Carrageenan-induced paw oedema, originally described by Winter *et al.* (1962), is a good model of non-immune acute inflammatory reaction with which to assess the contribution of mediators involved in vascular changes associated with acute inflammation and to evaluate potential treatments. Mice or rats are injected with carrageenan in the paw to produce acute inflammation, involving an initial release of histamine and serotonin, a second phase mediated by kinins, and a third phase mediated by prostaglandins (Di Rosa *et al.*, 1971). This methodology has recently been used to evaluate the anti-inflammatory activity of several flavonoids (Rotelli *et al.*, 2003).

In-vitro models of inflammation

As commented above, mediators related (or unrelated) to the arachidonic acid pathway are involved in inflammatory diseases, and therefore assays of some of these compounds may be useful to evaluate biological properties of potential drug compounds (Calixto *et al.*, 2003, 2004). A number of primary and immortalised cell lines (e.g. RAW 264.7 and J774A.1, both mice monocyte macrophage cell lines) stimulated with endotoxin (e.g. LPS) and/or cytokine (e.g. IFN-γ), in the presence or absence of test compound, are currently used for the evaluation of their effects on inflammation mediator production, signal transduction pathway activation, transcription factor activity or gene expression.

Medicinal plant extracts and isolated plant compounds in the inflammatory process

Phytotherapy may be defined as the prevention and treatment of human diseases using plants, parts of plants or plant preparations. For most purposes, extracts are used (Gaedcke and Steinhoff, 2003). Herbal extracts range from simple infusions (herbal tea) to a purified single chemical entity. It is not always possible to isolate a single active principle, e.g. if it is very unstable, or unknown, or if a range of compounds are responsible for the biological activity. In this case bioassays can be performed using a suitable purified extract (Williamson *et al.*, 1996).

In this section, we review the mechanisms of action of some plant extracts and specific secondary metabolites (classified according to main chemical family, i.e. terpenes, phenolic compounds, and alkaloids) on the inflammatory process.

Plant extracts

Crude extracts from numerous species show some sort of anti-inflammatory activity (Duwiejua and Zeitlin, 1993). Here we review the most recent data related to the effects of plant extracts on inflammatory process mediators, in both in-vivo and in-vitro models. We focus on extracts with potent and specific effects that have been characterised in detail.

It has been reported that administration of *Uncaria tomentosa* (UT) inhibits LPS-induced iNOS expression and NO production in the RAW 264.7 cell line, through inactivation of NF-κB transcription factor (Sandoval-Chacon *et al.*, 1998). It also protects mice against ozone-induced lung inflammation, probably through antioxidant effects (Sandoval-Chacon *et al.*, 1998; Cisneros *et al.*, 2005).

Harpagophytum procumbens (HP, commonly known as Devil's claw) has been used in traditional southern African medical therapies for arthritis and low back pain (Stewart and Cole, 2005). The validity of HP as an effective anti-inflammatory and analgesic preparation, particularly in the relief of arthritic symptoms, has been investigated in numerous animal, clinical and in-vitro studies (Grant *et al.*, 2007). In studies of the mouse fibroblast cell line L929, it has been demonstrated that administration of aqueous extract of HP to LPS-induced L929 cells suppresses prostaglandin E_2 (PGE_2) synthesis and NO production by inhibiting COX-2 and iNOS expression (Jang *et al.*, 2003). These effects may be mediated by inhibition of NF-κB activation and/or of AP-1 activation (Kundu *et al.*, 2005; Huang *et al.*, 2006).

In a randomised double-blind pilot study, Chrubasik *et al.* (2003) evaluated the administration of an extract of HP versus administration of non-steroidal anti-inflammatory drugs to patients with acutely exacerbated low back pain. There were no intergroup differences, but the authors suggest that studies with larger numbers of patients will be needed to show equivalence.

It has also recently been demonstrated that oral administration of HP (960 mg of dry extract per day, during 8 consecutive weeks), to a sample of 259 patients with arthritis and other rheumatic conditions, significantly improved global pain, stiffness and function, as well as increases quality of life, reduces or stops concomitant pain medication, and is associated with few gastrointestinal side-effects, suggesting that HP is suitable for medium-term use as a potential treatment option for mild-to-moderate degenerative disorders (Warnock *et al.*, 2007). A recent review concluded that HP should not be neglected as a possible treatment for painful osteoarthritis and chronic low back pain before use of NSAIDs (Chrubasik *et al.*, 2007).

The mechanisms of action of *Eucalyptus globulus*, *Thymus vulgaris*, *Pinus sylvestris*, and *Plantago lanceolata* on inflammatory processes have been evaluated in vitro, in the murine macrophage cell line J774A.1 (Vigo *et al.*, 2004, 2005). All of these extracts showed a significant capacity to scavenge NO radicals released by an NO donor, PAPA-NONOate, and significantly inhibited iNOS expression, suggesting that their anti-inflammatory properties may reflect decreased NO production, whether caused by inhibitory effects on iNOS gene expression or to NO-scavenging activity.

The effects of cannabinoids on inflammatory processes have been reviewed recently (Walter and Stella, 2004; Klein, 2005). Synthetic and plant-derived Δ^9–tetrahydrocannabinol (THC) inhibits NO production in LPS/IFN-γ-stimulated mouse macrophages and in LPS-stimulated RAW 264.7 macrophages, but endogenous cannabinoids induce NO production. THC induces arachidonic acid release from RAW 264.7 macrophages, which implies a proinflammatory influence. With regard to cytokine production, THC inhibits the production of IFN-γ and the proinflammatory IL-12, as well as the expression of IL-12 receptors, and increases the expression of the anti-inflammatory IL-4.

Anandamide, an endogenous cannabinoid, inhibits pro-inflammatory TNF-α production, soluble cytokine receptors, and inhibits IL-6 and IL-8 in LPS-stimulated monocytes. Although these results indicate an anti-inflammatory effect of cannabinoids, there are other results suggesting that cannabinoids may in some cases be proinflammatory. Indeed, THC has been shown to increase release of IL-1β from macrophages. In addition, a synthetic cannabinoid, CP55940, but not anandamide or THC, induces pro-inflammatory IL-8 and monocyte chemotactic protein 1 (MCP-1) gene expression in unstimulated HL60 human leukaemia cells. These data suggest that the therapeutic use of these drugs in chronic inflammatory diseases needs to be reassessed.

Several extracts from plants used in traditional Chinese medicine to treat inflammatory conditions were evaluated by Li *et al.* (2003). The most potent for COX-1, COX-2, PLA_2, and 5-LOX inhibition was *Tripterygium wilfordii*, a plant containing triptolide, a diterpene that has been demonstrated to inhibit NF-κB activation (Kim *et al.*, 2004a). Extracts of *Alchornea cordifolia*, *Ulmus davidiana*, and *Pfaffia glomerata* have been evaluated for their anti-inflammatory effects in vivo in animal models and showed beneficial properties in the management of inflammatory states (Osadebe and Okoye, 2003; Kim *et al.*, 2005; Neto *et al.*, 2005). *Zingiber officinale* extract inhibits the induction of several genes involved in the inflammatory response (Grzanna *et al.*, 2005; Kim *et al.*, 2005; Zhou *et al.*, 2006). Finally, a hexane extract from the rhizome of *Curcuma comosa*, a plant traditionally used as an anti-inflammatory agent in Thailand, significantly suppressed NO/iNOS synthesis and IL-6 in immortalised microglia HAPI cells (Jantaratnotai *et al.*, 2006).

Terpenes

Terpenes are comprised of multiple C_5 units, and can be classified as monoterpenes (C_{10}), sesquiterpenes (C_{15}), diterpenes (C_{20}), triterpenes (C_{30}), and polyterpenes $(C_5)n$ where n is very large. Several terpenes have been shown to have anti-inflammatory activity, although triterpenes and sesquiterpenes are probably the most interesting.

Monoterpenes

Essential oils are composed mainly of monoterpenes, although essential oils are always mixtures of many compounds. One of the most widely studied monoterpenes is eucalyptol (1.8-cineole), which is present at a high concentration in eucalyptus oil. This compound is used in cough drops, and is believed to be responsible for the expectorant and cough-suppressing activities of eucalyptus extracts. 1.8-cineole significantly inhibits metabolites of arachidonic acid (leukotriene B_4 and PGE_2), as well as several cytokines (Juergens *et al.*, 1998a,b), suggesting that it may be of value for long-term treatment of airway inflammation in bronchial asthma. 1,8-Cineole also can prevent colitis induced by trinitrobenzene sulphonic acid, at least in part, by an antioxidant mechanism which may involve glutathione, one of the most abundant intracellular antioxidants (Santos *et al.*, 2004). With regard to the antioxidant capacity of monoterpenes, the essential oil of *Melaleuca alternifolia* (tea tree oil) significantly suppresses superoxide-induced production in human monocytes; mainly because of the effects of α-terpineol, a water-soluble component of this oil (Brand *et al.*, 2001).

Sesquiterpenes

In an interesting study, Siedle *et al.* (2004) performed a preliminary evaluation of the structure–activity relationships of 103 different serquiterpene lactones, and demonstrated that strong NF-κB inhibitory activity is correlated with the number of alkylate centres. Helenalin and parthenolide are probably the most extensively studied lactones. Lyss *et al.* (1998) were the first to demonstrate that helenalin (a sesquiterpene present in *Arnica montana* and *Arnica chamissonis* ssp. *foliosa*) inhibits the binding of transcription factor NF-κB to DNA, and thus substantially attenuates the inflammatory process. Since then, numerous studies have been performed using this compound as a selective NF-κB inhibitor, although it also inhibits both 5-lipoxygenase and leukotriene C_4 synthase (Tornhamre *et al.*, 2001), which seems to indicate that helenalin acts on both NF-κB and leukotriene pathways.

Parthenolide, the principal active component in medicinal plants such as *Tanacetum parthenium* (feverfew), *Magnolia grandiflora*, and *Smallanthus uvedalius*, is reported to have anti-inflammatory activity. In vitro, it inhibits IL-1 and TNF-α-mediated NF-κB activation (Bork *et al.*, 1997; Hehner *et al.*, 1999). and also inhibits the expression of inducible COX-2, pro-inflammatory cytokines and inducible nitric oxide synthase (Hwang *et al.*, 1996; Fukuda *et al.*, 2000). A recent study (Smolinski and Pestka, 2005) in vivo in animal models, found that only one gene, IL-6, was suppressed by parthenolide, and that the suppression was only moderate; this seems to indicate that further studies using animals as models should be performed.

Diterpenes

In view of the clinically effective antineoplastic activity, taxol (paclitaxel), originally isolated from *Taxus brevifolia*, is probably the best-known diterpene. This compound generates an LPS-like signal, increasing the production of several cytokines and nitric oxide (Kirikae *et al.*, 1996; Moos and Fitzpatrick, 1998). Kahweol and cafestol, two coffee diterpenes, suppress PGE_2, COX-2 and iNOS in LPS-activated RAW 264.7 macrophages (Kim *et al.*, 2004b,c). Triptolide, a diterpene extracted from *Trypterygium wilfordii*, inhibits NO production and iNOS expression through blockade of NF-κB and c-Jun NH2-terminal kinase activation (Kim *et al.*, 2004a). A recently discovered diterpene isolated from *Euphorbia peplus*, named pepluanone, inhibits both in vivo the carrageenin-induced rat paw oedema and in-vitro production of nitric oxide, PGE_2, and TNF-α by reducing iNOS, COX-2 and TNF-α mRNA levels through the down-regulation of NF-κB binding activity (Corea *et al.*, 2005).

Triterpenes

Triterpenes of oleane-, ursane- and lupane-types extracted from *Eriobotrya japonica* have been reported to have anti-inflammatory activity by reducing inflammatory effects on TPA-induced inflammation in mice (Banno *et al.*, 2005). Celastrol, a triterpene extracted from *Trypterigium wilfordii*, inhibits IL-1β, -6, -8, and TNF-α production by LPS-activated human mononuclear cells, and in activated whole blood and inflammatory human colonic biopsies, by reducing LPS-induced NF-κB translocation (Pinna *et al.*, 2004).

Ursolic acid, a pentacyclic triterpene carboxylic acid found in various plants, attenuates the expression of inducible nitric oxide synthase and COX-2 by repression of NF-κB in LPS- or IFN-γ-activated mouse macrophages (Suh *et al.*, 1998), but also triggers the release of intracellular macrophage migration inhibitory factor, a protein linked to pro-inflammatory events in resting macrophages (Ikeda *et al.*, 2005), which seems to suggest a dual action of ursolic acid depending on the biological status of macrophages. Saponins are triterpeneglycosides and many possess anti-inflammatory activity. Glycyrrhizin, a triterpene glycoside extracted from liquorice root (*Glycyrrhiza glabra*, has a variety of activities, including those related to inflammation (Duwiejua and Zeitlin, 1993).

Recently, it has been reported that glycyrrhizin induces production of several cytokines, and inhibition of IL-8 and eotaxin 1 chemokines (Dai *et al.*, 2001; Abe *et al.*, 2003; Matsui *et al.*, 2004). Other saponins isolated from *Platycodon grandiflorum* (Platycodi Radix) or from *Panax ginseng* inhibit the expression of LPS-induced iNOS and COX-2 mRNA and protein in RAW 264.7 macrophages without appreciable cytotoxic effects, through the blocking of NF-κB activation, and also suppress the pro-inflammatory cytokine PGE_2 (Ahn *et al.*, 2005; Park *et al.*, 2005).

Tetraterpenes

In addition to their better-known antioxidant effects, it has recently been demonstrated that carotenoids possess anti-inflammatory activity by inhibiting NO and PGE_2 production and iNOS, COX-2, TNF-α and IL-1β expression in both LPS-stimulated RAW 264.7 cells and primary cultures of mice macrophages, via suppression of IκB degradation and subsequent NF-κB activation by scavenging of intracellular ROS (Bai *et al.*, 2005). Using both in-vivo and in-vitro models, Shiratori *et al.* reported that fucoxanthin, a carotenoid found in common edible seaweed, suppresses the development of endotoxin-induced uveitis in rats and reduces PGE2, NO and TNF-α concentrations in the aqueous humour, with an anti-inflammatory effect on the eye comparable with the effect of prednisolone (Shiratori *et al.*, 2005).

Phenolic compounds

This group includes flavonoids, tannins, coumarins and phenolic acids, all of which show some degree of anti-inflammatory activity (Yoon and Baek, 2005).

Flavonoids

Flavonoids act as powerful antioxidants, providing high levels of protection against oxidative and free-radical damage, and the anti-inflammatory activities of flavonoids have been extensively reviewed (Kim *et al.*, 2004a; Yoon and Baek, 2005).

Apigenin, genistein, and kaempferol inhibit both COX-2 and iNOS in a dose-dependent manner in LPS-activated RAW 264.7 macrophages, and these effects may be mainly mediated through inhibition of IkB kinase activity (Liang *et al.*, 1999). In addition, administration of two of these compounds, apigenin and kaempferol, or another flavone, chrysin, to RAW 264.7 macrophages induced activation of PPAR-γ, which seems to indicate that inhibition of COX-2 and iNOS may be also mediated by PPAR-γ activation (Liang *et al.*, 2001). In these cells, quercetin and (−)-epigallocatechin-e-gallate also inhibit iNOS activity, but slightly enhance COX-2 activity (Liang *et al.*, 1999).

Apigenin, chrysin, or luteolin administration to LPS-stimulated human peripheral blood mononuclear cells inhibits TNF-α, IL-1β and IL-6 production, and increases apoptosis of monocytes (Hougee *et al.*, 2005). Luteolin also inhibits the activity of IL-5, a modulator of the chemotactic responses of eosinophils, which plays an important role in eosinophilia-associated allergic inflammation (Park *et al.*, 1999).

Using human endothelial cells as in-vitro models, it has been demonstrated that apigenin-inhibited IL-1α-induced prostaglandin synthesis and TNF-α-induced IL-6 and IL-8 production, suggesting that apigenin may act as a general inhibitor of cytokine-induced gene expression (Gerritsen *et al.*, 1995). In addition, apigenin blocks cytokine-induced intracellular adhesion molecule-1 (ICAM-1), which is associated with a variety of inflammatory diseases and modulation of ICAM-1 expression is an important therapeutic target.

This inhibitory effect of apigenin and other flavonoids on ICAM-1 is mediated by attenuation of mitogen-activated protein kinase (MAPK) activities (Chen *et al.*, 2004). Myricetin-3-OβD-glucuronide, isolated from *Epilobium angustifolium*, is a potent inhibitor, not only of COX-1 and COX-2 but also of 5-LOX (Porath *et al.*, 2005). A fraction of a blackberry extract with high anthocyanin content showed inhibitory effects on NO biosynthesis in the LPS-stimulated murine J774A.1 macrophage cell line, through inhibition of IκB degradation and thus blocking of NF-κB activation (Pergola *et al.*, 2006).

Several pioneer studies have demonstrated that chalcones inhibit inflammatory mediator generation (Ballesteros *et al.*, 1995). Suppression of iNOS and COX-2 induction by several chalcones has been reported (Herencia *et al.*, 1999; Hsieh *et al.*, 2000), and some of these compounds show potent scavenging of superoxide (Herencia *et al.*, 1998), but they also inhibit TNF-α- and LPS-induced NF-κB activation, and PPARγ ligand-binding activity (Alcaraz *et al.*, 2004; Jung *et al.*, 2006).

Tannins and phenolic acids

It has been reported that some caffetannins and related compounds inhibit 5-HETE and 5-LOX production, whereas others, such as caffeic acid and caffeoylmalic acid have been reported to enhance PGE_2 formation in a concentration-dependent fashion (Kimura *et al.*, 1987). In-vivo studies on proanthocyanidins from grape seeds and from blackcurrant (*Ribes nigrum*) showed reduction in carrageenan-induced paw oedema in rats, and inhibition of NOS activity and NO, IL-1β, TNF-α and PGE_2 levels in exudate (Li *et al.*, 2001; Garbacki *et al.*, 2004), but no effect on IL-6 and IL-10 levels (Garbacki *et al.*, 2004).

Contradictory results have been described with regard to the effect of gallotannin (GT) on poly(ADP-ribose) (PAR), an emerging key regulator of chromatin superstructure and transcription activation. Pharmacological inhibition of PAR formation impairs the expression of several genes, including those of the inflammatory response. It has been reported that in the RAW 264.7 macrophage cell line, GT inhibits PAR glycohydrolase (PARG), the sole depoly(ADP-ribosyl)ating enzyme, triggering nuclear accumulation of PAR and concomitant PAR-dependent expression of iNOS and COX-2, but not of IL-1β and TNF-α. Neither NF-κB nor AP-1 transcription factor were increased (Rapizzi *et al.*, 2004).

By contrast, a study of A549 type-II lung epithelial cells did not detect either a GT-dependent PAR increase or a PARG inhibition, but did detect potent inhibitory effects of GT on cytokine and chemokine expression, probably due to the antioxidant effect of GT, which inhibits NF-κB/AP-1 activation (Erdelyi *et al.*, 2005). It has previously been demonstrated that tannins (e.g. those isolated from *Terminalia catappa*) show potent antioxidant activity (Lin *et al.*, 2001).

Coumarins

Several coumarins have been reported that possess anti-inflammatory activity. Aesculetin and scopolin isolated from *Santolina oblongifolia* show marked activity as inhibitors of release of eicosanoids from ionophore-stimulated mouse peritoneal macrophages (Silvan *et al.*, 1996). Treatment of LPS-activated RAW 264.7 macrophage cells with any of several furanocoumarins isolated from *Ledebouriella seseloids* led to inhibition of NO production by decreasing iNOS expression (Wang *et al.*, 2000), while cloricromene, a coumarin derivative, protects agains collagen-induced arthritis in rats by reducing levels of iNOS, COX-2, nitrotyrosine and poly(ADP-ribose) synthetase (PARS) (Cuzzocrea *et al.*, 2000). Blocking of IL-1β-induced PGE_2 release by coumarins has been evaluated by several groups, finding that coumarins inhibit COX-2 expression and that this effect might be mediated, at least in part, through suppression of NF-κB activity (Lin *et al.*, 2002; Yang *et al.*, 2002).

Alkaloids

Phenanthroindolizidine alkaloids extracted from the stems of *Ficus septica* (Damu *et al.*, 2005) have been evaluated for their anti-inflammatory activity. Tylophorine and ficuseptine-A potently suppressed NO production and did not show significant cytotoxicity in LPS/IFN-γ-stimulated RAW 264.7 cells. Tylophorine also reduced TNF-α, iNOS and COX-2 protein levels, probably through inhibition of AP-1 activation (Yang *et al.*, 2006) and its analogue DCB 3503 had similar effects (You *et al.*, 2006).

Berberine, a benzodioxoloquinolizine alkaloid reduces carrageenan- and zymosan-induced paw oedema (Ivanovska and Philipov, 1996; Kuo *et al.*, 2004), probably by inhibition of iNOS, NO, COX-2 and PGE_2 production and increased IL-12 levels through activation of p38 MAPK (Kang *et al.*, 2002; Lee *et al.*, 2003).

Capsaicin has been shown to inhibit the in-vitro production of superoxide anions, hydrogen peroxide and nitrite radicals by macrophages (Joe and Lokesh, 1994). In LPS/IFN-γ-stimulated RAW 264.7

macrophages, capsaicin inhibits COX-2 and iNOS expression, and subsequently NO and PGE_2 production (Chen *et al.*, 2003). These effects seem to be mediated by inhibition by capsaicin of NF-κB and AP-1 activation (Han *et al.*, 2001; Chen *et al.*, 2003).

Sanguinarine shows antioxidant activity against spontaneous oxidation (Firatli *et al.*, 1994), and is a potent inhibitor of NF-κB activation (Chaturvedi *et al.*, 1997). Tetrandrine and fangchinoline, the major alkaloids of the tuberous root of the creeper *Stephania tetrandrae*, show anti-inflammatory effects in acute paw oedema assay, in adjuvant-induced arthritis, and in rat subcutaneous air pouch models of inflammation (Wong *et al.*, 1992; Whitehouse *et al.*, 1994). However, in-vitro studies showed varying results for these related alkaloids, suggesting different biochemical mechanisms of action (Choi *et al.*, 2000).

Oxymatrine, from *Sophora flavescens*, decreased TNF-α levels by inhibition of p38 MAPK in an in-vivo mouse model of oleic-acid-induced acute lung injury (Xu *et al.*, 2005). Brucine, an alkaloid extracted from the seeds of *Strychnos nux-vomica*, significantly reduced PGE_2 and 6-keto-$PGF_{1\alpha}$ levels in carrageenan-induced paw oedema and in Freund's complete adjuvant-induced arthritis in rat (Yin *et al.*, 2003).

Using in-vitro models, it has been demonstrated that stylopine (a major component of the leaf of *Chelidonium majus*) and rutaecarpine (isolated from the fruits of *Evodia rutaecarpa*) inhibit both COX-2 activity and PGE2 production (Moon *et al.*, 1999; Jang *et al.*, 2004), while stylopine also reduces levels of iNOS and NO, as well as of TNF-α (Jang *et al.*, 2004).

Finally, evodiamine, an alkaloid extracted from the fruit of *Evodia*, abolishes constitutive and inducible NF-κB activation by inhibiting IκBα kinase activation in several cell types (Takada *et al.*, 2005).

Conclusions

Inflammation is a complex physiopathological process in which an inflammatory stimulus produces a cascade of intracellular signalling leading to the synthesis of specific mediators that in turn induce the inflammatory response. Thus, evaluation of herbal substances that can either reduce levels/activity of pro-inflammatory mediators, or increase levels/activity of anti-inflammatory mediators, may be a useful strategy for studying their efficacy for the treatment of inflammatory disease. In this chapter, we analysed the mechanisms of action of stimuli that induce mediators involved in the inflammatory process, and reviewed the most recent studies, in both in-vivo and in-vitro models, about the ways in which certain plant extracts and/or isolated plant compounds may act on inflammatory signalling pathways to reduce inflammatory processes.

References

Abe M, Akbar F, Hasebe A *et al.* (2003). Glycyrrhizin enhances interleukin-10 production by liver dendritic cells in mice with hepatitis. *J Gastroenterol* 38: 962–967.

Aggarwal BB (2003). Signalling pathways of the TNF superfamily: a double-edged sword. *Nature Rev Immunol* 3: 745–756.

Ahn K-S, Noh E-J, Zhao H-L *et al.* (2005). Inhibition of inducible nitric oxide synthase and cyclooxygenase II by *Platycodon grandiflorum* saponins via suppression of nuclear factor-κB activation in RAW 264.7 cells. *Life Sci* 76: 2315–2328.

Alcaraz MJ, Vicente AM, Araico A, Domínguez *et al.* (2004). Role of nuclear factor-kappaB and heme oxygenase-1 in the mechanism of action of an anti-inflammatory chalcone derivative in RAW 264.7 cells. *Br J Pharmacol* 142: 1191–1199.

Armant MA, Fenton MJ (2002). Toll-like receptors: a family of pattern-recognition receptors in mammals. *Genome Biol* 3: 3011.1–3011.6.

Baeuerle PA, Baltimore D (1996). NF-κB: ten years after. *Cell* 87: 13–20.

Bai S-K, Lee S-J, Na H-J *et al.* (2005). β-Carotene inhibits inflammatory gene expression in lipopolysaccharide-stimulated macrophages by suppressing redox-based NF-κB activation. *Exp Mol Med* 37: 323–334.

Ballesteros JF, Sanz MJ, Ubeda A *et al.* (1995). Synthesis and pharmacological evaluation of 2′-hydroxychalcones and flavones as inhibitors of inflammatory mediator generation. *J Med Chem* 38: 2794–2797.

Banno N, Akihisa T, Tokuda H *et al.* (2005). Anti-inflammatory and antitumor-promoting effects of the triterpene acids from the leaves of *Eriobotrya japonica*. *Biol Pharm Bull* 28: 1995–1999.

Barnes PJ, Karin M (1997). Nuclear factor-κB: a pivotal transcription factor in chronic inflammatory diseases. *N Engl J Med* 336: 1066–1071.

Bork PM, Schmitz ML, Kuhnt M *et al.* (1997). Sesquiterpene lactone containing Mexican Indian medicinal plants and pure sesquiterpene lactones as potent inhibitors of transcription factor NF-κB. *FEBS Lett* 402: 85–90.

Brand C, Ferrante A, Prager RH *et al.* (2001). The water-soluble components of the essential oil of *Melaleuca alternifolia* (tea tree oil) suppress the production of superoxide by human monocytes, but not neutrophils, activated in vitro. *Inflamm Res* 50: 213–219.

Cadenas E (1989). Biochemistry of oxygen toxicity. *Annu Rev Biochem* 58: 79–110.

Calixto J, Otuki M, Santos A (2003). Anti-inflammatory compounds of plant origin. Part I. Action on arachidonic acid pathway, nitric oxide and nuclear factor κB (NF-κB). *Planta Med* 69: 973–983.

Calixto J, Campos M, Otuki M, Santos A (2004). Anti-inflammatory compounds of plant origin. Part II. Modulation of pro-inflammatory cytokines, chemokines and adhesion molecules. *Planta Med* 70: 93–103.

Chandrasekharan NV, Dai H, Roos KL *et al.* (2002). COX-3, a cyclooxygenase-l variant inhibited by acetaminophen and other analgesic/antipyretic drugs: cloning, structure, and expression. *Proc Natl Acad Sci* 99: 13926–13931.

Chaturvedi MM, Kumar A, Darnay BG *et al.* (1997). Sanguinarine (pseudochelerythrine) is a potent inhibitor of NF-kappaB activation, IkappaBalpha phosphorylation, and degradation. *J Biol Chem* 272: 30129–30134.

Chen C-C, Chow M-P, Huang W-C *et al.* (2004). Flavonoids inhibit tumor necrosis factor-α-induced up-regulation of intercellular adhesion molecule-1 (ICAM-1) in respiratory epithelial cells through activator protein-1 and nuclear factor-κB: structure-activity relationships. *Mol Pharmacol* 66: 683–693.

Chen C-W, Lee S-T, Wu W-T *et al.* (2003). Signal transduction for inhibition of inducible nitric oxide synthase and cyclooxygenase-2 induction by capsaicin and related analogs in macrophages. *Br J Pharmacol* 140: 1077–1087.

Choi H-S, Kim H-S, Min KR *et al.* (2000). Anti-inflammatory effects of fangchinoline and tetrandrine. *J Ethnopharmacol* 69: 173–179.

Chrubasik S, Model A, Black A, Pollak S (2003). A randomized double-blind pilot study comparing Doloteffin and Vioxx in the treatment of low back pain. *Rheumatology* 42: 141–148.

Chrubasik E, Roufogalis BD, Chrubasik S (2007). Evidence of effectiveness of herbal antiinflammatory drugs in the treatment of painful osteoarthritis and chronic low back pain. *Phytother Res* 21: 675–683.

Cisneros FJ, Jayo M, Niedziela L (2005). An *Uncaria tomentosa* (cat's claw) extract protects mice against ozone-induced lung inflammation. *J Ethnopharmacol* 96: 355–364.

Corea G, Fattorusso E, Lanzotti V *et al.* (2005). Discovery and biological evaluation of the novel naturally occurring diterpene pepluanone as antiinflammatory agent. *J Med Chem* 48: 7055–7062.

Cuzzocrea S, Mazzon E, Bevilaqua C *et al.* (2000). Cloricromene, a coumarine derivative, protects against collagen-induced arthritis in Lewis rats. *B J Pharmacol* 131: 1399–1407.

Dai J-H, Iwatani Y, Ishida T *et al.* (2001). Glycyrrhizin enhances interleukin-12 production in peritoneal macrophages. *Immunology* 103: 235–243.

Damu A-G, Kuo P-C, Shi L-S *et al.* (2005). Phenanthroindolizidine alkaloids from the stems of *Ficus septica*. *J Nat Prod* 68: 1071–1075.

Daynes RA, Jones DC (2002). Emerging roles of PPARs in inflammation and immunity. *Nat Rev Immunol* 2: 748–759.

Delerive P, De Bosscher K, Besnard S *et al.* (1999). Peroxisome proliferator-activated receptor α negatively regulates the vascular inflammatory gene response by negative cross-talk with transcription factors NF-κB and AP-1. *J Biol Chem* 274: 32048–32054.

Di Rosa M, Giround JP, Willougbby DA (1971). Studies of the mediators of the acute inflammatory response induced in rats in different sites by carrageenan and turpentine. *J Pathol* 104: 15–29.

Donaldson LF, Hanley MR, Villablanca AC (1997). Inducible receptors. *Trends Pharmacol Sci* 18: 171–181.

Duwiejua M, Zeitlin IJ (2003). Plants as a source of anti-inflammatory substances. In: *Drugs from Natural Products*, Eds. Harvey, A.L. Ellis Horwood, Chichester, UK, pp. 152–167.

Epe B, Ballmaier D, Roussyn I *et al.* (1996). DNA damage by peroxynitrite characterized with DNA repair enzymes. *Nucl Acids Res* 24: 4105–4110.

Erdelyi K, Kiss A, Bakondi E *et al.* (2005). Gallotannin inhibits the expression of chemokines and inflammatory cytokines in A549 cells. *Mol Pharmacol* 68: 895–904.

Firatli E, Unal T, Onan U *et al.* (1994). Antioxidative activities of some chemotherapeutics. A possible mechanism in reducing gingival inflammation. *J Clin Periodontol* 21: 680–683.

Fukuda K, Hibiya Y, Mutoh M *et al.* (2000). Inhibition by parthenolide of phorbol ester-induced transcriptional activation of inducible nitric oxide synthase gene in a human monocyte cell line THP-1. *Biochem Pharmacol* 60: 595–600.

Gaedcke F, Steinhoff B (2003). *Herbal Medicinal Products*. Medpharm Scientific: Stuttgart, pp. 1–28.

Garbacki N, Tits M, Angenot L *et al.* (2004). Inhibitory effects of proanthocyanidins from *Ribes nigrum* leaves on carrageenin acute inflammatory reactions induced in rats. *BMC Pharmacol* 4: 25.

Gerritsen ME, Carley WW, Ranges GE *et al.* (1995). Flavonids inhibit cytokine-induced endothelial cell adhesion protein gene expression. *Am J Pathol* 147: 235–237.

Ghosh S, Karin M (2002). Missing pieces in the NF-κB puzzle. *Cell* 109: S81–S96.

Glass CK, Ogawa S (2006). Combinatorial roles of nuclear receptors in inflammation and immunity. *Nat Rev Immunol* 6: 44–55.

Grant L, McBean DE, Fyfe L *et al.* (2007). A review of the biological and potential therapeutic actions of *Harpagophytum procumbens*. *Phytother Res* 21: 199–209.

Grzanna R, Lindmark L, Frondoza CG (2005). Ginger–an herbal medicinal product with broad anti-inflammatory actions. *J Med Food* 8: 125–132.

Haddad JJ (2002). Cytokines and related receptor-mediated signalling pathways. *Biochem Biophys Res Commun* 297: 700–713.

Han SS, Keum Y-S, Seo H-J *et al.* (2001). Capsaicin suppresses phorbol ester-induced activation of NF-κB/Rel and AP-1 transcription factors in mouse epidermis. *Cancer Lett* 164: 119–126.

Hehner SP, Hofmann TG, Dröge W *et al.* (1999). The anti-inflammatory sesquiterpene lactone parthenolide inhibits NF-kappa B by targeting the IκB kinase complex. *J Immunol* 163: 5617–5623.

Heller RA, Schena M, Chai A *et al.* (1997). Discovery and analysis of inflammatory disease-related genes using cDNA microarrays. *Proc Nat Acad Sci USA* 94: 2150–2155.

Herencia F, Ferrándiz ML, Ubeda A *et al.* (1998). Synthesis and anti-inflammatory activity of chalcone derivates. *Bioorg Med Chem Lett* 8: 1169–1174.

Herencia F, Ferrandiz ML, Ubeda A *et al.* (1999). Novel anti-inflammatory chalcone derivatives inhibit the induction of nitric oxide synthase and cyclooxygenase-2 in mouse peritoneal macrophages. *FEBS Lett* 453: 129–134.

Hobbs A, Higgs A, Moncada S (1999). Inhibition of nitric oxide synthase as a potential therapeutic target. *Annu Rev Pharmacol Toxicol* 39: 191–220.

Hopkins SJ (2003). The pathophysiological role of cytokines. *Legal Med* 5: S45–S57.

Hougee S, Sanders A, Faber J *et al.* (2005). Decreased pro-inflammatory cytokine production by LPS-stimulated PBMC upon in vitro incubation with the flavonids apigenin, luteolin or chrysin, due to selective elimination of monocytes/macrophages. *Biochem Pharmacol* 69: 241–248.

Hsieh HK, Tsao LT, Wang JP *et al.* (2000). Synthesis and anti-inflammatory effect of chalcones. *J Pharm Pharmacol* 52: 163–171.

Huang TH-W, Tran VH, Duke RK *et al.* (2006). Harpagoside suppresses lipopolysaccharide-induced iNOS and COX-2 expression through inhibition of NF-κB activation. *J Ethnopharmacol* 104: 149–155.

Hwang D, Fischer NH, Jang B-C *et al.* (1996). Inhibition of the expression of inducible cyclooxygenase and proinflammatory cytokines by sesquiterpene lactones in macrophages correlates with the inhibition of MAP kinases. *Biochem Biophys Res Commun* 226: 810–818.

Ikeda Y, Murakami A, Ohigashi H (2005). Ursolic acid promotes the release of macrophage migration inhibitory factor via ERK2 activation in resting mouse macrophages. *Biochem Pharmacol* 70: 1497–1505.

Ivanovska N, Philipov S (1996). Study on the anti-inflammatory action of *Berberis vulgaris* root extract, alkaloid fractions and pure alkaloids. *Int J Immunopharmacol* 18: 553–561.

Jang M-H, Lim S, Han S-M *et al.* (2003) *Harpagophytum procumbens* suppresses lipopolysaccharide stimulated expressions of cyclooxygenase-2 and inducible nitric oxide synthase in fibroblast cell line L929. *J Pharmacol Sci* 93: 367–371.

Jang SI, Kim BH, Lee WY *et al.* (2004). Stylopine from *Chelidonium majus* inhibits LPS-induced inflammatory mediators in RAW 264.7 cells. *Arch Pharm Res* 27: 923–929.

Jantaratnotai N, Utaisincharoen P, Piyachaturawat P *et al.* (2006). Inhibitory effect of *Curcuma comosa* on NO production and cytokine expression in LPS-activated microglia. *Life Sci* 78: 571–577.

Joe B, Lokesh BR (1994). Role of capsaicin, curcumin and dietary n-3 fatty acids in lowering the generation of reactive oxygen species in rat peritoneal macrophages. *Biochim Biophys Acta* 1224: 255–263.

Joseph SB, Castrillo A, Laffitte BA *et al.* (2003). Reciprocal regulation of inflammation and lipid metabolism by liver receptors. *Nat Med* 9: 213–219.

Juergens UR, Stober M, Schmidt-Schilling L *et al.* (1998). Antiinflammatory effects of eucalyptol (1.8-cineole) in bronchial asthma: inhibition of arachidonic acid metabolism in human blood monocytes ex vivo. *Eur J Med Res* 3: 407–412.

Juergens UR, Stober M, Vetter H (1998). Inhibition of cytokine production and arachidonic acid metabolism by eucalyptol (1.8-cineole) in human blood monocytes in vitro. *Eur J Med Res* 3: 508–510.

Jung SH, Park SY, Kim-Pak Y *et al.* (2006). Synthesis and PPAR-γ ligand-binding activity of new series of 2′-hydroxychalcone and thiazolidinedione derivatives. *Chem Pharm Bull* 54: 368–371.

Kang B-Y, Chung S-W, Cho D *et al.* (2002). Involvement of p38 mitogen-activated protein kinase in the induction of interleukin-12 p40 production in mouse macrophages by berberine, a benzodioxoloquinolizine alkaloid. *Biochem Pharm* 63: 1901–1910.

Karin M (2005). Inflammation-activated protein kinases as targets for drug development. *Proc Am Thorac Soc* 2: 386–390.

Kelly D, Campbell JI, King TP *et al.* (2004). Commensal anaerobic gut bacteria attenuate inflammation by regulating nuclear cytoplasmic shuttling of PPARγ and RelA. *Nat Immunol* 5: 104–112.

Kharitonov S, Yates D, Robbins RA *et al.* (1994). Increased nitric oxide in exhaled air of asthmatic patients. *Lancet* 343: 133–135.

Kim HP, Son KH, Chang HW *et al.* (2004). Anti-inflammatory plant flavonoids and cellular action mechanisms. *J Pharmacol Sci* 96: 229–245.

Kim HW, Murakami K, Abe M *et al.* (2005). Suppressive effects of Mioga Ginger and Ginger constituents on reactive oxygen and nitrogen species generation, and the expression of inducible pro-inflammatory genes in macrophages. *Antioxid Redox Signal* 7: 1621–1629.

Kim J-Y, Jung K-S, Jeong H-G (2004a). Suppressive effects of the kahweol and cafestol on cyclooxygenase-2 expression in macrophages. *FEBS Lett* 569: 321–326.

Kim J-Y, Jung K-S, Lee K-J *et al.* (2004b). The coffee diterpene kahweol suppresses the inducible nitric oxide synthase expression in macrophages. *Cancer Lett* 213: 147–154.

Kim Y-H, Lee S-H, Lee J-Y *et al.* (2004c). Triptolide inhibits murine-inducible nitric oxide synthase expression by down-regulating lipopolysaccharide-induced activity of nuclear factor-kB and c-Jun NH2-terminal kinase. *Eur J Pharmacol* 494: 1–9.

Kim K-S, Lee S-D, Kim K-H *et al.* (2005). Suppressive effects of a water extract of *Ulmus davidiana* Planch (Ulmaceae) on collagen-induced arthritis in mice. *J Ethnopharmacol* 97: 65–71.

Kimura Y, Okuda H, Okuda T *et al.* (1987). Studies on the activities of tannins and related compounds, X. Effects of caffeetannins and related compounds on arachidonate metabolism in human polymorphonuclear leukocytes. *J Nat Prod* 50: 392–399.

Kirikae T, Ojima I, Kirikae F *et al.* (1996). Structural requirements of taxoids for nitric oxide and tumor necrosis factor production by murine macrophages. *Biochem Biophys Res Commun* 227: 227–235.

Klein TW (2005). Cannabinoid-based drugs as anti-inflammatory therapeutics. *Nat Rev Immunol* 5: 400–411.

Kracht M, Saklatvala J (2002). Transcriptional and post-transcriptional control of gene expression in inflammation. *Cytokine* 20: 91–106.

Kujubu DA, Fletcher BS, Varnum BC *et al.* (1991). TIS10, a phorbol ester tumor promoter-inducible mRNA from Swiss 3T3 cells, encodes a novel prostaglandin synthase/cyclooxygenase homologue. *J Biol Chem* 266: 12866–12872.

Kundu JK, Mossanda KS, Na HK, Surh YJ (2005). Inhibitory effects of the extracts of *Sutherlandia frutescens* (L.) R. Br. and *Harpagophytum procumbens* DC. on phorbol ester-induced COX-2 expression in mouse skin: AP-1 and CREB as potential upstream targets. *Cancer Lett* 218: 21–31.

Kuo C-L, Chi C-W, Liu T-Y (2004). The anti-inflammatory potential of berberine in vitro and in vivo. *Cancer Lett* 203: 127–137.

Kyriakis JM, Avruch J (2001). Mammalian mitogen-activated protein kinase signal transduction pathways activated by stress and inflammation. *Physiol Rev* 81: 807–869.

Lee CH, Chawla A, Urbiztondo N *et al.* (2003). Transcriptional repression of atherogenic inflammation: modulation by PPARδ. *Science* 302: 453–457.

Lee JC, Laydon JT, McDonnell PC *et al.* (1994). A protein kinase involved in the regulation of inflammatory cytokine biosynthesis. *Nature* 372: 739–746.

Lee JC, Young PR (1996). Role of CSB/p38/RK stress response kinase in LPS and cytokine signalling mechanisms. *J Leukoc Biol* 59: 152–157.

Lee D-U, Kang Y-J, Park M-K *et al.* (2003). Effects of 13-alkyl-substituted berberine alkaloids on the expression of COX-II, TNF-α, iNOS, and IL-12 production in LPS-stimulated macrophages. *Life Sci* 73: 1401–1412.

Li RW, David Lin G, Myers SP *et al.* (2003). Anti-inflammatory activity of Chinese medicinal vine plants. *J Ethnopharmacol* 85: 61–67.

Li W-G, Zhang X-Y, Wu Y-J *et al.* (2001). Anti-inflammatory effect and mechanism of proanthocyanidins from grape seeds. *Acta Pharmacol Sin* 22: 1117–1120.

Liang Y-C, Huang Y-T, Tsai S-H *et al.* (1999). Suppression of inducible cyclooxygenase and inducible nitric oxide synthase by apigenin and related favonoids in mouse macrophages. *Carcinogenesis* 20: 1945–1952.

Liang Y-C, Tsai S-H, Tsai D-C *et al.* (2001). Suppression of inducible cyclooxygenase and nitric oxide synthase through activation of peroxisome proliferator-activated receptor-γ by flavonoids in mouse macrophages. *FEBS Lett* 496: 12–18.

Lin CH, Chang CW, Wang CC *et al.* (2002). Byakangelicol, isolated from *Angelica dahurica*, inhibits both the activity and induction of cyclooxygenase-2 in human pulmonary epithelial cells. *J Pharm Pharmacol* 54: 1271–1278.

Lin C-C, Hsu Y-F, Lin T-C (2001). Antioxidant and free radical scavenging effects of the tannins of *Terminalia catappa* L. *Anticancer Res* 21: 237–243.

Lyss G, Knorre A, Schmidt TJ *et al.* (1998). The anti-inflammatory sesquiterpene lactone helenalin inhibits the transcription factor NF-kB by directly targeting p65. *J Biol Chem* 273: 33508–33516.

Magne N, Toillon R-A, Bottero V *et al.* (2006). NF-κB modulation and ionizing radiation: mechanisms and future directions for cancer treatment. *Cancer Lett* 231: 158–168.

Matsui S, Matsumoto H, Sonoda Y *et al.* (2004). Glycyrrhizin and related compounds down-regulate production of inflammatory chemokines IL-8 and eotaxin 1 in a human lung fibroblast cell line. *Int Immunopharmacol* 4: 1633–1644.

Mizushima Y, Tsukada M, Akimoto T (1972). A modification of rat adjuvant arthritis for testing antirrheumatic drugs. *J Pharm Pharmacol* 24: 781–785.

Moilanen E, Whittle B, Moncada S (1999). Nitric oxide as a factor in inflammation. In: *Inflammation: Basic Principles and Clinical Correlates,* Eds. JL Gallin and R. Snyderman. Lippincott, Williams & Wilkins, Philadelphia, pp. 787–800.

Monaco C, Andreakos E, Kiriakidis S *et al.* (2004). T cell-mediated signalling in immune, inflammatory and angiogenic processes: the cascade of events leading lo inflammatory diseases. *Curr Drug Targets Inflamm Allergy* 3: 35–42.

Moon TC, Murakami M, Kudo I *et al.* (1999). A new class of COX-2 inhibitor, rutaecarpine from *Evodia rutaecarpa. Inflamm Res* 48: 621–625.

Moos PJ, Fitzpatrick FA (1998). Taxane-mediated gene induction is independent of microtubule stabilization: induction of transcription regulators and enzymes that modulate inflammation and apoptosis. *Proc Nat Acad Sci USA* 95: 3896–3901.

Neto AG, Costa JM, Belati CC *et al.* (2005). Analgesic and anti-inflammatory activity of a crude root extract of *Pfaffia glomerata* (Spreng) Pedersen. *J Ethnopharmacol* 96: 87–91.

Osadebe PO, Okoye FB (2003). Anti-inflammatory effects

of crude methanolic extract and fractions of *Alchornea cordifolia* leaves. *J Ethnopharmacol* 89: 19–24.

Parente L, Perretti M (2003). Advances in the pathophysiology of constitutive and inducible cyclooxygenases: two enzymes in the spotlight. *Biochem Pharmacol* 65: 153–159.

Park K-Y, Lee S-H, Min B-K *et al.* (1999). Inhibitory effect of luteoline 4′-O-glucoside from *Kummerowia striata* and other flavonoids or interleukin-5 bioactivity. *Planta Med* 65: 457–459.

Park E-Y, Shin Y-W, Lee H-U *et al.* (2005). Inhibitory effect of ginsenoside Rb1 and compound K on NO and prostaglandin E2 biosynthesis of RAW264.7 cells induced by lipopolysaccharide. *Biol Pharm Bull* 28: 652–656.

Pascual G, Fong AL, Ogawa S *et al.* (2005). A SUMOylation-dependent pathway mediates transrepression of inflammatory response genes by PPAR-gamma. *Nature* 437: 759–763.

Pearson CM (1956). Development of arthritis, periarthritis and periostitis in rats given adjuvants. *Proc Soc Exp Biol Med* 91: 95–101.

Pearson G, Robinson F, Beers Gibson T *et al.* (2001). Mitogen-activated protein (MAP) kinase pathways: regulation and physiological functions. *Endocrinol Rev* 22: 153–183.

Pergola C, Rossi A, Dugo P *et al.* (2006). Inhibition of nitric oxide biosynthesis by anthocyanin fraction of blackberry extract. *Nitric oxide* 15: 30–39.

Pinna GF, Fiorucci M, Reimund JM *et al.* (2004). Celastrol inhibits pro-inflammatory cytokine secretion in Crohn's disease biopsies. *Biochem Biophys Res Commun* 322: 778–786.

Poli G, Leonarduzzi G, Biasi F *et al.* (2004). Oxidative stress and cell signalling. *Curr Med Chem* 11: 1163–1182.

Pop-Busui R, Sima A, Stevens M (2006). Diabetic neuropathy and oxidative stress. *Diabetes Metab Res Rev* 22: 257–273.

Porath D, Riegger C, Drewe J *et al.* (2005). Epigallocatechin-3-gallate impairs chemokine production in human colon epithelial cell lines. *J Pharmacol Exp Ther* 315: 1172–1180.

Rapizzi E, Fossati S, Moroni F *et al.* (2004). Inhibition of poly(ADP-ribose) glycohydrolase by gallotannin selectively up-regulates expression of proinflammatory genes. *Mol Pharmacol* 66: 890–898.

Rotelli AE, Guardia T, Juárez AO *et al.* (2003). Comparative study of flavonoids in experimental models of inflammation. *Pharmacol Res* 48: 601–606.

Sandoval-Chacon M, Thompson JH, Zhang X-J *et al.* (1998). Antiinflammatory actions of cat's claw: the role of NF-κB. *Aliment Pharmacol Ther* 12: 1279–1289.

Santos FA, Silva RM, Campos AR *et al.* (2004). 1,8-Cineole (eucalyptol), a monoterpene oxide attenuates the colonia damage in rats on acute TNBS-colitis. *Food Chem Toxicol* 42: 579–584.

Sautebin L (2000). Prostaglandins and nitric oxide as molecular targets for anti-inflammatory therapy. *Fitoterapia* 71: S48–S57.

Schneider I, Bucar F (2005). Lipoxygenase inhibitors from natural plant sources. Part 1: Medicinal plants with inhibitory activity on arachidonate 5-lipoxygenase and 5-lipoxygenase/cyclooxygenase. *Phytother Res* 19: 81–102.

Schwartsburd PM (2003). Chronic inflammation as inductor of procancer microenvironment: pathogenesis of dysregulated feedback control. *Cancer Metastasis Rev* 22: 95–102.

Shiratori K, Ohgami K, Ilieva I *et al.* (2005). Effects of fucoxanthin on lipopolysaccharide-induced inflammation in vitro and in vivo. *Exp Eye Res* 81: 422–428.

Siedle B, Garcia-Piñeres A, Murillo R *et al.* (2004). Quantitative structure-activity relationship of sesquiterpene lactones as inhibitors of the transcription factor NF-κB. *J Med Chem* 47: 6042–6054.

Silvan AM, Abad MJ, Bermejo P *et al.* (1996). Anti-inflammatory activity of coumarins from *Santolina oblongifolia*. *J Nat Prod* 59: 1183–1185.

Smith WL, Garavito RM, DeWitt DL (1996). Prostaglandin endoperoxide H synthases (cyclooxygenases)-1 and -2. *J Biol Chem* 271: 33157–33160.

Smith WL, Langenbach R (2002). Why there are two cyclooxygenase enzymes? *J Clin* Invest 107: 1491–1495.

Smolinski AT, Pestka JJ (2005). Comparative effects of the herbal constituent parthenolide (Feverfew) on lipopolysaccharide-induced inflammatory gene expression in murine spleen and liver. *J Inflamm* 29: 2–6.

Stewart KM, Cole D (2005). The commercial harvest of devil's claw (*Harpagophytum* spp.) in southern Africa: The devil's in the details. *J Ethnopharmacol* 100: 225–236.

Suh N, Honda T, Finlay H-J *et al.* (1998). Novel triterpenoids suppress inducible nitric oxide synthase (iNOS) and inducible cyclooxygenase (COX-2) in mouse macrophages. *Cancer Res* 58: 717–723.

Tak PP, Firestein GS (2001). NF-kB: a key role in inflammatory diseases. *J Clin Invest* 107: 7–11.

Takada Y, Kobayashi Y, Aggarwal BB (2005). Evodiamine abolishes constitutive and inducible NF-κB activation by inhibiting IκBalpha kinase activation, thereby suppressing NF-κB-regulated antiapoptotic and metastatic gene expression, up-regulating apoptosis, and inhibiting invasion. *J Biol Chem* 280: 17203–17212.

Tarrant TK, Patel DD (2006). Chemokines and leukocyte trafficking in rheumatoid arthritis. *Pathophysiology* 13: 1–14.

Tornhamre S, Schmidt TJ, Nasman-Glaser B *et al.* (2001). Inhibitory effects of helenalin and related compounds on 5-lipoxygenase and leukotriene C4 synthase in human blood cells. *Biochem Pharmacol* 62: 903–911.

Trentham DE, Townes AS, Kang AH (1977). Autoimmunity to type II collagen: an experimental model of arthritis. *J Exp Med* 146: 857–868.

Valko M, Rhodes CJ, Moncol J, Izakovic M, Mazur M

(2006). Free radicals, metals and antioxidants in oxidative stress-induced cancer. *Chem Biol Interact* 160: 1–40.

Vane JR, Bakhle YS, Botting RM (1998). Cyclooxygenases 1 and 2. *Annu Rev Pharmacol Toxicol* 38: 97–120.

Vigo E, Cepeda A, Gualillo O, Perez-Fernandez R (2004). In-vitro anti-inflammatory effect of *Eucalyptus globulus* and *Thymus vulgaris*: nitric oxide inhibition in J774A.1 murine macrophages. *J Pharm Pharmacol* 56: 257–263.

Vigo E, Cepeda A, Gualillo O *et al.* (2005). In-vitro anti-inflammatory activity of *Pinus sylvestris* and *Plantago lanceolata* extracts: effect on inducible NOS, COX-1, COX-2 and their products in J774A.1 murine macrophages. *J Pharm Pharmacol* 57: 383–391.

Walter L, Stella N (2004). Cannabinoids and neuro-inflammation. *B J Pharmacol* 41: 775–785.

Wang CC, Lai JE, Chen LG *et al.* (2000). Inducible nitric oxide synthase inhibitors of Chinese herbs. Part 2: naturally occurring furanocoumarins. *Bioorg Med Chem* 8: 2701–2707.

Warnock M, McBean D, Suter A *et al.* (2007). Effectiveness and safety of Devil's claw tablets in patients with general rheumatic disorders. *Phytother Res* 21: 1228–1233.

Whitehouse MW, Fairlie DP, Thong YH (1994). Anti-inflammatory activity of the isoquinoline alkaloid, tetrandrine, against established adjuvant arthritis in rats. *Agents Actions* 42: 123–127.

Williams RO (2004). Collagen-induced arthritis as a model for rheumatoid artritis. *Methods Mol Med* 98: 207–216.

Williamson EM, Okpako DT, Evans FJ (1996). Selection, preparation and pharmacological evaluation of plant material. In: *Pharmacological Methods in Phytotherapy Research*. Wiley, Chichester, UK, pp. 15–23.

Winter C, Risley E, Nuss G (1962). Carrageenan-induced edema in hind paw of rats as an assay for anti-inflammatory drug. *Proc Soc Exp Biol Med* 111: 207–210.

Wong CC, Seow WK, O'Callaghan JW *et al.* (1992). Comparative effects of tetrandrine and berbamine on subcutaneous air pouch inflammation induced by interleukin-1, tumour necrosis factor and platelet-activating factor. *Agents Actions* 36: 112–128.

Xie WL, Chipman JG, Robertson DL *et al.* (1991). Expression of a mitogen-responsive gene encoding prostaglandin synthase is regulated by mRNA splicing. *Proc Nat Acad Sci USA* 88: 2692–2696.

Xu GL, Yao L, Rao SY *et al.* (2005). Attenuation of acute lung injury in mice by oxymatrine is associated with inhibition of phosphorylated p38 mitogen-activated protein kinase. *J Ethnopharmacol* 98: 177–183.

Yang C-W, Chen W-L, Wu P-L *et al.* (2006). Anti-inflammatory mechanisms of phenanthroindolizidine alkaloids. *Mol Pharmacol* 69: 749–758.

Yang L-L, Liang Y-C, Chang C-W *et al.* (2002). Effects of sphondin, isolated from *Heracleum lacinatum,* on IL-1β-induced cyclooxygenase-2 expression in human pulmonary epithelial cells. *Life Sci* 72: 199–213.

Yin W, Wang T-S, Yin F-Z *et al.* (2003). Analgesic and anti-inflammatory properties of brucine and brucine N-oxide extracted from seeds of *Strychnos nux-vomica. J Ethnopharmacol* 88: 205–214.

Yoon J-H, Baek SJ (2005). Molecular targets of dietary polyphenols with anti-inflammatory properties. *Yonsei Med J* 46: 585–596.

You X, Pan M, Gao W *et al.* (2006). Effects of a novel tylophorine analog on collagen-induced arthritis through inhibition of the innate immune response. *Arthritis Rheum* 54: 877–886.

Zhou H-L, Deng Y-M, Xie Q-M (2006). The modulatory effects of the volatile oil of ginger on the cellular immune response in vitro and in vivo in mice. *J Ethnopharmacol* 105: 301–305.

19

Tests for antioxidant activity and their relevance to herbal medicinal products

Kakali Mukherjee, N Satheesh Kumar, Sujay Rai and Pulok K Mukherjee

Introduction

Free radicals are chemical species possessing one or more unpaired electrons and can be considered as a fragment of molecules that are extremely reactive and short lived. They are produced continuously in cells, either as accidental byproducts of metabolism or deliberately (for example, during phagocytosis). Unpaired electrons usually make a molecule more reactive than the corresponding non-radical. The molecule acts as an electron acceptor and essentially 'steals' electrons from other molecules. Free radicals are referred to as oxidising agents since they cause other molecules to donate their electrons (Halliwell, 1997). Free radicals can be formed by the homolytic cleavage of a covalent bond of a normal molecule, with each fragment retaining one unpaired electron; by the loss of a single electron from a normal molecule; or by the addition of a single electron to a normal molecule.

The most common cellular oxygen free radicals are superoxide radical (O_2^-), hydroxyl radical ($OH^{\cdot}$) and nitric oxide ($NO^{\cdot}$) (Simonian and Coyle, 1996). Other molecules, such as hydrogen peroxide (H_2O_2) and peroxynitrate ($ONOO^{\cdot}$) are not free radicals themselves but can lead to their generation through various chemical reactions.

Oxygen free radicals and related molecules are often classified together as reactive oxygen species (ROS), to signify their ability to promote oxidative changes within the cell.

All aerobic organisms produce free radicals, predominantly superoxide, formed as a side product during the reduction of molecular oxygen by mitochondria. An average cell utilises 10^{13} molecules of O_2 per day. It is estimated that 1% of respired molecular oxygen will form ROS, thus approximately 10^{11} ROS are produced by each cell in a day. Cells normally employ a number of defence mechanisms against damage induced by free radicals (Simonian and Coyle, 1996; Evans *et al.*, 2002). Oxidative stress is the term referring to the imbalance between generation of reactive oxygen species and the activity of the antioxidant defences.

There is increasing evidence to support the involvement of free-radical reactions in several human diseases since ROS play a role in a variety of normal regulatory systems, the de-regulation of which may play an important role in inflammation. ROS and other free radicals have long been known to be mutagenic and have more recently emerged as mediators of other phenotypic and genotypic changes causing mutations and neoplasia.

In the last decade, evidence has accumulated that the free-radical process known as lipid peroxidation plays a crucial and causative role in the pathogenesis of atherosclerosis, cancer, myocardial infarction and also in ageing (Harman, 1992). Participation of free-radical oxidative interactions in promoting tissue injury in conditions such as brain trauma, ischaemia, toxicity and also in neurodegenerative diseases such as Parkinson's disease, Alzheimer's dementia, multiple sclerosis and lipofuscinosis are now well documented (Cheeseman and Slater, 1993). The involvement of ROS in the pathogenesis of several lung diseases has also been suggested while the pioneering studies on the role of ROS reactions in the genesis and the expression of cellular and tissue damage has been carried out mainly in the liver, using acute rat poisoning with carbon tetrachloride (Cheeseman and Slater, 1993; Raja *et al.*, 2007).

Studies in experimental models have incriminated ROS as primary mediators in the pathogenesis of renal injury. Diabetes mellitus is also associated with oxidative reactions, particularly those that are catalysed by decompartmentalised transition metals, but their causative significance in diabetic tissue damage remains to be established (Cheeseman and Slater, 1993).

In 1956, Harman proposed the free-radical theory of ageing (Tripathi, 1995), the assumption that ageing results from random deleterious effects of tissue brought about by ROS and it is very likely that ROS contribute considerably to the development of stochastic disorders observed during the progress of ageing (Mukherjee *et al.*, 2007a).

In recent years, increasing experimental and clinical data have provided compelling evidence for the involvement of oxygen free radicals in the three main disorders of prematurity – chronic lung disease, retinopathy of prematurity and intraventicular haemorrhage, the hypothesis being that oxygen-centred radical and related reactive oxygen metabolites are formed too rapidly to be detoxified by antioxidant defence mechanisms (Rai *et al.*, 2006).

Defence against free radicals: antioxidants

Antioxidant defences fall in to two main categories, those whose role is to prevent the generation of free radicals and those that intercept any radicals that are generated. They exist in both the aqueous and membrane compartments of cells and can be enzymes or non-enzymes. Various animal studies have shown that antioxidants delay or protect against the oxidative damage produced by the free-radical reaction and a protective role against ailments mediated by free radicals is now well established (Cheeseman and Slater, 1993).

Antioxidants are exogenous (natural or synthetic) or endogenous compounds acting in several ways, including removal of O_2, scavenging reactive oxygen/nitrogen species or their precursors, inhibition of ROS formation and binding metal ions needed for catalysis of ROS generation and up-regulation of endogenous antioxidant defences. The protective efficacy of antioxidants depends on the type of ROS that is generated, the place of generation and the severity of the damage (Halliwell *et al.*, 1994; Halliwell, 1997). The natural antioxidant system can be classified into two major groups: endogenous enzymes and low-molecular-weight antioxidants.

Endogenous enzymes include extensively studied enzymes such as superoxide dismutase (SOD), catalase, glutathione peroxidases, DT diaphorase, and glutathione-regenerating enzyme systems (Sies, 1991). Some enzymatic systems such as SOD and catalase act specifically against ROS, while certain other enzyme systems reduce thiols. The low-molecular-weight antioxidants can be further classified into directly acting antioxidants (e.g. scavengers and chain-breaking antioxidants) and indirectly acting antioxidants (e.g. chelating agents). The directly acting antioxidants are extremely important for defence against oxidative stress. Direct scavenging of ROS is one of the many antioxidant actions required to restore oxidative equilibrium once it is lost in different pathologies. This subgroup of antioxidants currently contains several hundred compounds including ascorbic acid (vitamin C), retinoic acid (vitamin A), melatonin, lipoic acids, polyphenols, and carotenoids, being derived from dietary and herbal sources. The hypothesis that restoring redox equilibrium through activation of intracellular signals is also an important step of the antioxidation process is gaining increasing support (Shohami *et al.*, 1997). It is likely that the trapping of excess free radicals could restore redox equilibrium in the initial states of cellular oxidative stress.

Free radicals in various diseases

According to Halliwell and Gutteridge (1999), oxidative stress occurs in most human diseases, although this is not the same as saying that it is the cause of most diseases. The increase in free radicals may be secondary to the disease process. Free radicals are very short lived and difficult to study in vivo. Direct detection of free radicals is possible with electron spin resonance, but it is very expensive and complex (Clarkson and Thompson, 2000; Tarpey and Fridovich, 2001), so a variety of surrogate markers to ascertain free-radical activity must be used. Developing accurate methods to measure biomarkers for DNA damage and lipid peroxidation is challenging and methods in the current literature include urine levels of F2-isoprostanes as a biomarker for lipid peroxidation, measurement of oxidised low-density lipoprotein (LDL), use of a chemical mutagenic product of fat oxidation, and 8-oxo-deoxyguanosine, associated with a decline in mitochondrial function (Halliwell, 1999; Tarpey and Fridovich, 2001). There have also been efforts to detect changes in the levels of antioxidants such as SOD, glutathione or vitamin E in the body in response to oxidative stress, to identify many conditions associated with free-radical formation, but results have not been consistent. The implications of the presence of ROS in cardiovascular, pulmonary (Halliwell and Gutteridge, 1999), carcinogenesis (Kasai and Nishimura, 1984; Floyd, 1990) diabetes (Langenstroer and Pieper, 1992) and neurological diseases (Kontos, 2001) as well as inflammation (McCord, 2000) are currently under intense investigation.

It is easy to appreciate that the lungs are vulnerable to inhaled agents, e.g. ozone, nitrogen dioxide, sulphur dioxide and other toxins, that stimulate ROS production. ROS can stimulate lipid peroxidation and oxidation of DNA bases in the lungs. The irritant effect of smoke also activates lung macrophages and neutrophils with resultant production of additional ROS (Halliwell and Gutteridge, 1999). Chronic lung inflammation such as asbestosis, asthma and cystic fibrosis is also associated with elevated markers of oxidative stress so ROS may contribute to the ongoing pathology (Halliwell and Gutteridge, 1999).

The brain may be especially sensitive to oxidative damage. Oxidative stress can damage neurones and glial cells in a manner similar to other issues: via products of lipid peroxidation that are neurotoxic, DNA damage, etc. (Halliwell and Gutteridge, 1999). Reperfusion injury also occurs in the brain after a stroke and superoxide produced during reperfusion results in abnormalities of cerebral vascular responses and blood–brain barrier permeability. Extracellular glutamate levels in the brain increase rapidly during ischaemia, leading to increased production of $OH^{\cdot}$ radicals, calcium ion imbalance and increased neurotoxicity (Halliwell and Gutteridge, 1999). If bleeding occurs with the stroke, normally sequestered iron molecules are released and may initiate harmful free-radical chain reactions. Neurodegenerative diseases associated with ROS include Parkinson's, Alzheimer's, and many others (Halliwell and Gutteridge, 1999; Tarpey and Fridovich, 2001). It is possible that although the initiators of the disease state vary, free radicals are involved in a common pathway that leads to neural cell death.

The acute inflammatory response is typically beneficial to the organism, being a major defence against microorganisms and normally self-limited. However, the superoxide-producing neutrophil itself is destroyed in the process and healthy surrounding cells may also be damaged (McCord, 2000). With chronic inflammation, such as in rheumatoid arthritis, the overall impact of the continued generation of free radicals is deleterious. Degradation of hyaluronic acid (synovial fluid) is driven by the presence of OH. These radicals may be produced by phagocytic cells in the joint, by changes in tissue oxygenation caused by swelling, followed by reperfusion, or by some of the drugs used to treat RA. A role for ROS in the endothelial dysfunction associated with diabetes was proposed (Langenstroer and

Pieper, 1992) and levels of manganese superoxide dismutase have been reported to be decreased in streptozotocin-induced diabetes in rats. Normalising mitochondrial $O_2^{\cdot}$ has been shown to block pathways involved in hyperglycaemic damage. Consistent with these observations, SOD pretreatment improved vasodilation in isolated aortic rings from streptozotocin diabetic rats. Levels of $O_2^{\cdot}$ are also increased in hyperinsulinaemic rats, which is believed to be related to activation of NAD(P)H oxidase.

The progression of heart failure is associated with programmed cell death or apoptosis, which studies suggest occurs in response to ischaemia, reperfusion, pressure overload and in dilated cardiomyopathies (Chien, 1999). Oxidative stress may also be critical for the activation of apoptosis in dilated cardiomyopathies.

Free radicals in cardiovascular diseases

Cardiovascular disease is a heterogeneous group of disorders that affects the heart and blood vessels. The diseases are characterised by angina pectoris, hypertension, congestive heart failure, acute myocardial infarction (heart attacks), stroke and arrhythmia. There is now considerable biochemical, physiological and pharmacological data to support a connection between free-radical reactions and cardiovascular tissue injury. Evidence shows that these disease conditions are directly or indirectly related to oxidative damage and share common mechanisms of molecular and cellular damage. As these mechanisms are elucidated, it may be possible to improve the techniques for clinical and pharmacological intervention.

Ischaemia–reperfusion myocardial injury

Exposure of myocardial tissue to a brief, transient ischaemia, followed by reperfusion, has attracted much attention in recent years as an explanation for some cardiac diseases. Myocardial ischaemia occurs when myocardial oxygen demand exceeds oxygen supply. Unless reversed, this situation results in cell injury and, clinically, myocardial infarction. Logically, reperfusion of ischaemic myocardium is recognised as potentially beneficial, because mortality is directly proportional to infarct size, and this latter to the severity and duration of ischaemia. Reperfusion of the ischaemic myocardium can restore oxygen and substrates to the ischaemic myocardial cells, but this process may create another form of myocardial damage termed 'reperfusion injury' (Bolli, 1991, 1992; Ferrari *et al.*, 1993). Thus, restoration of a normal blood flow in the heart by methods such as angioplasty, thrombolytic agents or cardiopulmonary bypass can lead to specific lesions (arrhythmias, deficit in contractility, necrosis), the importance of which also depends on the duration of ischaemia.

Evidence suggests that this may be due, in part, to the generation of toxic ROS (Bolli, 1991; Fox, 1992 Starkopf *et al.*, 1995). The active involvement of ROS in the ischaemia–reperfusion damage is demonstrated by direct and indirect experimental evidences. Direct evidence arises from the possibility of measuring radicals in myocardial tissue by electron spin resonance (ESR) and spin trapping methodology (Garlick *et al.*, 1987; Pietri *et al.*, 1989); indirect evidence by the measurement of the products of free-radical attack on biological substrates (e.g. malondialdehyde as a measure of lipid peroxidation extent), and intracellular and extracellular antioxidant capacity (Dousset *et al.*, 1983; Ytrehus and Hegstad, 1991). Experimental findings suggest that in ischaemic tissue there is an impairment of antioxidant mechanisms (Starkopf *et al.*, 1997). Evidence to support this statement comes also from the cardioprotective effects of agents capable of inducing antioxidant enzymes in the heart and from the beneficial effects of several enzymatic free-radical scavengers, antioxidants and iron chelators in reperfused myocardium (Jeroudi *et al.*, 1994).

Free-radical hypothesis of atherosclerosis

Considerable in-vivo evidence, animal and human, supports the important role of ROS in atherosclerotic coronary heart disease (Parthasaratry and Rankin, 1992; White *et al.*, 1994). While the exact mechanisms for atherogenesis are not completely understood, recent studies suggest that oxidative modification of low-density lipoproteins (LDL) is a critical factor (Morel *et al.*, 1984). LDL may be oxidatively modified by all major cell types of the arterial wall via their extracellular release of reactive oxygen species (ROS) (Morel *et al.*, 1984). Hydroxyl radicals (thus formed) may initiate the peroxidation of long-chain polyunsaturated fatty acids within LDL, giving rise to conjugated dienes and lipid hydroperoxy radicals (LOO·) (Mukherjee, 2003). This process is self propagating, since LOO· can attack adjacent fatty acids until complete fatty acid chain fragmentation occurs. A number of highly reactive products then accumulate in the LDL particle, including malondialdehyde and lysophosphatides, which interact with the amino side chain of the apoprotein B 100 and modify it to form new epitopes that are not recognised by the LDL receptor.

Hypertension

Essential hypertension (EH) appears associated with increased superoxide anion and hydrogen peroxide production, as well as decreased antioxidant capacity (Kuman and Das, 1993; Jun *et al.*, 1996). The involvement of ROS in EH is also suggested by the observation of increased level of lipid peroxides and decreased concentrations of antioxidant vitamin E in plasma of EH patients. Recently, Simi *et al.* (1998) have shown that patients with EH have plasma concentrations of free-radical scavengers lower than healthy normotensive subjects. The elevated consumption of plasma antioxidants was accompanied by increased activity of extracellular antioxidant enzymes (glutathione peroxidase and SOD), suggesting that ROS production in EH overwhelms antioxidant defence capacity. Oxidative stress in patients with EH is accompanied with the decreased red blood cell counts (Simi *et al.*, 1998) and decreased (Tse *et al.*, 1994) SOD and glutathione peroxidase activity in neutrophils.

Chronic heart failure

Chronic heart failure is a state characterised by a number of processes that may promote ROS generation in vivo, including cytokine activation (Cross and Jones, 1991; Berry and Clark, 2000), recurrent hypoxia–reperfusion (Ferrari *et al.*, 1998), possibly genetic susceptibilities (Guzik *et al.*, 2000) and activation of the renin–angiotensin system (Berry and Clark, 2000). There are a number of potential cellular sources implicated in enhanced ROS generation in chronic heart failure. It has recently been demonstrated that patients with chronic heart failure may have increased leucocyte O_2^- production, which is, in turn, related to severity of disease (Ellis *et al.*, 2000). Other sources of enhanced ROS generation in human chronic heart failure are both the myocardium (Dieterich *et al.*, 2000) and peripheral blood vessels. Increased activity of myocardial NADPH oxidase has been reported in heart failure (Heymes *et al.*, 2003).

Myocardial damage

ROS have direct effects on cellular structure and function and may be integral signalling molecules in myocardial remodelling and failure. ROS result in a phenotype characterised by hypertrophy and apoptosis in isolated cardiac myocytes (Siwik *et al.*, 1999). ROS have also been shown to activate matrix metalloproteinase (MMP) in cardiac fibroblasts (Siwik *et al.*, 2001). Myocardial MMP activity is increased in the failing heart (Creemers *et al.*, 2001) and an MMP inhibitor has been shown to limit early left ventricular dilatation in a murine model of myocardial infarction (MI) (Rohde *et al.*, 1999). Hayashidani *et al.* (2003) showed significant improvement in the survival after MI in MMP-2 knockout mice, which was mainly attributable to the inhibition of early cardiac rupture and the development of subsequent LV dysfunction. Because MMP can be activated by ROS (Rajagopalan *et al.*, 1996), one proposed mechanism of ventricular remodelling is the activation of MMPs secondary to increased ROS production. Sustained MMP activation might influence the structural properties of the myocardium by providing an abnormal extracellular environment with which the myocytes interact. Kinugawa *et al.* (2000) demonstrated that the OH scavenger, dimethylthiourea, inhibits the activation of MMP-2 in association with the development of ventricular remodelling and failure. These data raise the interesting possibility that increased ROS after MI can be a stimulus for myocardial MMP activation, which might play an important role in the development of HF.

Left ventricular hypertrophy

In animal models of heart failure, levels of ROS are elevated and cardiac protection is observed with antioxidant treatment (Cargnoni *et al.*, 2000). The increase in ROS associated with left ventricular hypertrophy appears to be NAD(P)H oxidase-dependent. Myocardial NAD(P)H oxidase activity is elevated and expression of p22*phox*, gp91*phox*, p67*phox* and p47*phox* is increased in left ventricular tissue from guinea pigs after aortic banding (Li *et al.*,

2002). The gp91*phox* containing NAD(P)H oxidase has been shown to play an important role in the cardiac hypertrophic response to Ang II in mice (Bendall *et al.*, 2002). It has been suggested that the increase in ROS is responsible for impaired endothelial regulation of left ventricular relaxation observed in moderate pressure overload left ventricular hypertrophy (Maccarthy *et al.*, 2001).

Cardiac hypertrophy occurs in response to a sustained increase in cardiac work. The mechanisms underlying this progression from compensated hypertrophy to decompensated heart failure remain poorly understood and incompletely explored (Chien, 1999). There are data supporting at least a contributory role for alterations in ROS production in the pathophysiology of cardiac hypertrophy. There is substantial evidence from animal studies indicating that ROS, and particularly $O_2^{\cdot}$, production is increased in cardiac hypertrophy. Recently, Date *et al.* demonstrated attenuated cardiac hypertrophy in mice subjected to pressure overload following treatment with the free-radical scavenger, *N*-2-mercaptopropionyl glycine (Date *et al.*, 2002). This is the first evidence in an experimental model suggesting a causal role for ROS in the development of pressure overload hypertrophy. The precise source of ROS in this study was not apparent. In a similar study using a guinea pig model of pressure overload, an attenuation of LV hypertrophy was observed in animals treated with vitamin E. Taken together, these data support an important functional role for ROS, in particular NADPH oxidase derived ROS, in the development of pressure-overload hypertrophy.

Free radicals in hypercholesterolaemia

Increased levels of $O_2^{\cdot}$ generation and attenuated NO mediated responses have been demonstrated in aortic rings from cholesterol-fed rabbits (Mugge *et al.*, 1994). Treatment of the animals with polyethylene glycolated SODs improved endothelium-dependent vasodilation (White *et al.*, 1994). Supplementation with L-arginine has also been shown to reduce $O_2^{\cdot}$ levels and restore NO-mediated responses in cholesterol-fed animals (Boger *et al.*, 1995). $O_2^{\cdot}$ levels are also raised in WHHL (Watanabe heritable hyperlipidaemic) rabbits (Miller *et al.*, 1998). Multiple mechanisms appear to be involved in O_2^- production in association with hypercholesterolaemia. Stepp and colleagues (Stepp *et al.*, 2002) provided evidence that in canine carotid arteries eNOS, mechanisms dependent on xanthine oxidase and possibly NAD(P)H-oxidase were involved. Further evidence for the involvement of NAD(P)H oxidase was obtained in WHHL rabbits (Warnholtz *et al.*, 1999). In monkeys with atherosclerosis, disease severity is related to $O_2^{\cdot}$ levels, and regression of atherosclerosis is associated with decreases in $O_2^{\cdot}$ levels and NAD(P)H oxidase activity (Hathaway *et al.*, 2002).

Free radicals in skeletal muscle dysfunction

Oxidative stress could be the mechanistic basis also for muscle fatigue and reduced exercise tolerance in patients with heart failure (Wilson, 1995). This notion is supported by a positive correlation between ROS and exercise intolerance in these patients (Nishiyama *et al.*, 1998). Further, Tsutsui *et al.* (2001) demonstrated that the production of ROS was increased in the skeletal muscle homogenates obtained from a murine model of HF and increased ROS were identified as $OH^{\cdot}$ originating from $O_2^{\cdot}$, which was associated with a concomitant increase in the oxidation of lipids. These results are consistent with the previous studies that the oxidative capacity is reduced and O_2 utilisation is inadequate in skeletal muscle mitochondria from patients with heart failure (Mancini *et al.*, 1989). Skeletal muscle mitochondria from heart failure are associated with a decrease in the activities of complex I and complex III (Tsutsui *et al.*, 2001). As has been shown in the failing hearts (Ide *et al.*, 1999), the defects in electron transfer function may lead to ROS production. ROS may play an important role in the muscle atrophy commonly seen in patients with heart failure through the induction of apoptosis. In addition, ROS impair myoplasmic Ca^{2+} homeostasis and inhibit the oxidative energy production in the mitochondria, both of which may contribute to the muscle contractile dysfunction. An attempt to attenuate oxidative stress would improve, to some extent, the exercise capacity of patients with heart failure.

Tests for antioxidant activity

Antioxidant activity can be evaluated both in vitro and in vivo. There are potential models for evaluation of the antioxidant activity. Animals such as mice, rats, guinea pigs and rabbits can be used for in-vivo evaluation with the oxidative stress induced by some external chemical agent (e.g. carbon tetrachloride), physical, emotional, mental or environmental stress (e.g. torturing the animals, depriving animals from food, water and sexual activity, increasing noise or temperature of the animal housing). Even surgery can be performed for inducing oxidative stress in rats, e.g. cerebral ischaemia/reperfusion induced oxidative stress in which the induction of ischaemia in rats was performed by occluding bilateral common carotid arteries with clamps for 30 min followed by 24 h reperfusion (Jingtao *et al.*, 1999). Following any of the methods whereby the oxidative stress can be induced in the animals, they should be grouped as treated (at least two or more doses), control and normal animals. In the end of study the animals can be sacrificed to isolate the vital organs. Enzymes such as SOD, catalase and glutathione can be measured in these tissues, together with the extent of lipid peroxidation caused by the oxidative stress, using assays such as barbituric acid reactive substances (TBARS) (Mukherjee, 2002; Mukherjee and Mukherjee, 2005).

In-vitro methods consist of chemical methods in which free radicals can be generated using chemical reactions, e.g. nitric oxide method or chemicals which themselves act as the source of free radicals such as DPPH (2,2-diphenyl-1-picrylhydrazyl). In-vitro methods are also available in which generated free radicals can attack tissues isolated from the animal body leading to the oxidation of lipids present in the tissues, e.g. thiobarbituric acid-reactive substances (TBARS) assay. Details on some of the in-vitro methods used for the evaluation of antioxidant activity are given below.

DPPH radical scavenging assay

The antioxidant activity of the plant extract and pure compounds was assessed on the basis of radical scavenging effect of the stable DPPH free radical, which is purple. Antioxidants react with DPPH, and convert it to 1,1-diphenyl-2-(2,4,6-trinitrophenyl) hydrazine, which is colourless. Reaction mixtures containing test samples (dissolved in DMSO) and 300 μmol/L DPPH ethanolic solutions in 96-well microtitre plates are incubated at 37°C for 30 min, and absorbances measured at 515 nm. The degree of discolouration indicates the scavenging potentials of the antioxidant compounds and IC50 values can be calculated, i.e. the concentration of sample required to scavenge 50% DPPH free radicals (Gamez *et al.*, 1998). DPPH reagent (0.5% in methanol) can be sprayed on to preparative TLC plates to identify active antioxidant compounds in plant extracts. Active radical scavengers give yellow colour zones against a purple background (Mukherjee, 2006a).

Nitric oxide radical scavenging assay

Nitric oxide ($NO^{\cdot}$) is a free radical and scavengers of nitric oxide compete with oxygen, leading to reduced production of nitric oxide. NO is generated from sodium nitroprusside and measured by the Griess Illosvoy reagent (Garratt, 1964), which can be modified by using naphthylethylenediamine dihydrochloride (0.1% w/v) instead of 1-naphthylamine (5%). The extent of NO radical scavenging can be assessed by colorimetry whereby reaction mixtures containing 10 mmol/L sodium nitroprusside, phosphate buffer saline and extracts or standard solution are incubated at 25°C for 150 min. After incubation, 0.5 mL of the reaction mixture is mixed with 1 mL of sulphanilic acid reagent (0.33% in 20% glacial acetic acid) and allowed to stand for 5 min to complete diazotisation. Naphthyl ethylenediamine dihydrochloride is then added, mixed and allowed to stand for 30 min at 25°C and a pink coloured chromophore is formed in diffused light whose intensity is measured at 540 nm (Rai *et al.*, 2006a).

Scavenging of superoxide anion radicals assay

Various cellular enzymes can catalyse chemical reactions involving molecular oxygen, including admission formation of superoxide radicals, which can inactivate vital cell components. Superoxide can be generated by enzymatic oxidation of hypoxanthine with xanthine oxidase and can be detected colorimetrically by nitroblue tetrazolium (NBT) reduction. The reaction is started by adding 100 μL of phenazine methosulphate (PMS) solution (60 μmol/L PMS in 100 mmol/L phosphate buffer, pH 7.4) to the mixture, incubating at 25°C for 5 min, and measuring the absorbance at 560 nm. Decreased absorbance of the reaction mixture indicates increased superoxide anion scavenging activity (Liu and Ng, 2000).

Deoxyribose degradation assay

In this method hydroxyl radicals are generated by incubating a mixture containing KH_2PO_4-KOH, H_2O_2, $FeCl_2$-EDTA and deoxyribose (Paya *et al.*, 1992). The extent of deoxyribose degradation by the formed hydroxyl radical can be assessed by the thiobarbituric acid method. The typical reaction is started by adding Fe(II) at a final concentration of 6 μmol/L to a 0.5 mL final volume of 20 mmol/L phosphate buffer, 5 mmol/L of 2-deoxyribose, Cu(II) (5 μmol/L) (pH 7.2) and 100 μmol/L H_2O_2 with and without 10 μmol/L of ascorbate as an iron chelator. Reactions were carried out for 10 min at 25 °C ± 1°C and were stopped by adding of 0.5 mL of 50 mmol/L NaOH containing 4% (w/v) phosphoric acid. After boiling for 15 min, the absorbance of the solution containing the oxidation products is measured at 532 nm (Juliana Khouri *et al.*, 2007).

Thiobarbituric-acid-reactive substances assay

In this method the lipid peroxidation is measured in terms of malondialdehyde (MDA) content following the thiobarbituric acid method of Ohkawa *et al.* (1979). MDA is formed in vivo and in vitro through oxidation of unsaturated lipids by ROS, and other oxidative agents. Thiobarbituric acid reacts with MDA to form a pink chromogen, which can be detected spectrophotometrically at 532 nm (Halliwell and Gutteridge, 1989).

β-Carotene-linoleic acid (linoleate) assay

The antioxidant activity is measured by the ability of a compound to minimise the coupled oxidation of linoleic acid and β-carotene in an emulsified aqueous system. β-Carotene loses its orange colour when reacting with ROS (Al-Saikhan *et al.*, 1995), so colorimetery can be used to investigate the decline in colour caused by oxidative stress. In this method a stock solution of β-carotene and linoleic acid is prepared by dissolving 0.5 mg of β-carotene in 1 mL of chloroform and adding 25 μL of linoleic acid together with 200 mg of Tween 40, evaporating the chloroform and adding 100 mL of aerated water to the residue. To 2.5 mL of this mixture, 300 μL of extract is added and the mixture incubated in boiling water for 2 h together with two blanks, one containing the antioxidant BHT and the other without antioxidant, before measuring the absorbance at 470 nm.

DNA nicking assay

The ability of a test drug to prevent the DNA damage caused by agents such as 2,2′-azobis (2-methylpropionamide) dihydrochloride (APPH) is measured in this method. The test substance is mixed with DNA and APPH, dissolved in phosphate-buffered saline, is added to start the reaction. The resultant mix is developed on agarose gel, electrophoresis carried out and then staining with ethidium bromide. DNA bands are visualised under illuminated ultraviolet light and examined for DNA breakage (Wejewickreme and Kitts, 1997).

Herbal antioxidant products

The ethnomedical literature contains a large number of plants that can be used against diseases, in which ROS are thought to play a major role. A large number of plants and phytoconstituents possess antioxidant properties (Table 19.1) and many of them are now articles of commerce, claiming to prevent or reduce diseases associated with high levels of ROS. Antioxidants can also be used in the preservation of food products. An important source of antioxidants is the diet, which contains numerous plants with antioxidant activity, including the spices and condiments. The traditional medical literature describes the potential role of spices as a source of many vitamins and as domestic remedies for many human diseases (Mukherjee *et al.*, 2006b, 2006c) and the consumption of fruits and vegetables, olive oil, red wine and tea is inversely correlated with rates of incidence of many diseases.

Spices and herbs, particularly from the Lamiaceae family, demonstrate strong antioxidant properties

Table 19.1 Potent antioxidant plants and their phytoconstituents

Plants	Family	Part used	Phytoconstituents	Reference
Artemisia monata	Asteraceae	Aerial	Luteolin-7-O-rutinoside and Esculctin	Kim *et al.*, 2000
Andrographis paniculata	Acanthaceae	Arial parts	Andrographolide 14-deoxy-11-oxo-andrographolide, neo-andrographolide	Maiti *et al.*, 2006
Allium sativum	Liliaceace	Bulb	Garlicin, allicin, S-allylcysteine, S-allylmercaptocysteine, allin, allixin, N-acetyl-S-allylcysteine	Rekka and Kourounakis, 1994, Ide *et al.*, 1996; Imai *et al.*, 1994
Anoectochilus formosanus	Orchidaceae	Whole plant	Kinsenone (diarylpentanoid) and flavonoid glycosides	Wang *et al.*, 2002
Asparagus racemosus	Liliaceae	Rhizomes	Shatavarin, coniferin and undecanyl cetanoate	Mukherjee, 2002
Broussonetia papyrifera	Moraceae	Leaf	Broussoflavonols	Ko *et al.*, 1997
Bacopa monniera	Scrophulariaceae	Whole plant	BacosideA_3, bacosaponin C	Pawar *et al.*, 2001
Bulbine capitata	Asphodelaceae	Root	Isofuranonaphthoquinones	Bezabih *et al.*, 2001
Burkea africana	Leguminosae	Bark	Proanthocyanidins	Mathisen *et al.*, 2002
Cedrus decodara	*Pinaceae*	Heartwood	Matairesinol	Tiwari *et al.*, 2001
Crocus sativus	Iridaceae	Stigmas	Crocin	Pham *et al.*, 2000
Curcuma longa	Zingiberaceae	Rhizhomes	Curcumin, turmeric antioxidant protein	Sreejayam *et al.*, 1997; Selvam *et al.*, 1995
Chrysophyllum cainito	Sapotaceae	Seeds, fruits	Quercetin and other polyphenols	Luo *et al.*, 2002
Corylus colurna	Betulaceae	Leaves	Flavonoids	Benov and Georgiev, 1999
Crataegus monogyna	Rosaceae	Leaves, flowers and fruits	Flavonoids, proanthocyanidins, catechins	Bahorun *et al.*, 1994
Cyanchum wilfordii	Asclepiadaceae	Roots	Cynandione A and a biacetophenone	Lee *et al.*, 2000
Dalbergia odorifera	Fabaceae	Root	Benzophenone derivative and flavonoids	Wang *et al.*, 2000
Dirca palustris	Thymelaeaceae	Twigs	Five novel phenolic glycosides	Ramsewak *et al.*, 1999
Daphniphyllum calycinum	Daphniphyllaceae	Leaf	Flavonoid glycoside	Gamez *et al.*, 1998
Dracaena cinnabari	Ruscaceae (Dracaenaceae)	Whole plant	Homoisoflavonoids	Juranek *et al.*, 1993
Ephemerantha lonchophylla	Orchidaceae	Stem	Dihydrostilbene, phenantherene	Chen *et al.*, 1999b
Eucalyptus globulus	Myrtaceae	Leaves	Ellagic acid	Kim *et al.*, 2001
Eriobotrya japonica	Rosaceae	Leaves	Flavonoids; chlorogenic acid, quercetin-3-sambubioside, methyl chlorogenate kaempferol, quercetin-3-rhamnoside	Jung *et al.*, 1999b

(*continued overleaf*)

Table 19.1 (*continued*)

Plants	Family	Part used	Phytoconstituents	Reference
Emblica officinalis	Euphorbiaceae	Fruits	Emblicanin A and B, gallic acid, punigluconin and pedunculagin	Bhattacharaya *et al.*, 2000; Ghosal *et al.*, 1996; Bandyopadhyay *et al.*, 2000
Ficus bengalensis	Moraceae	Bark	Rhamnoside and cellobioside	Daniel *et al.*, 1998
Garcinia subelliptica	Clusiaceae	Wood	Three prenylated xanthones	Minami *et al.*, 1996
Garcinia kola	Clusiaceae	Seeds	Kolaviron (biflavones)	Farombi *et al.*, 2000
Camellia sinensis	Theaceae	Leaf	Epigallocatechin, gallocatechin and epigallocatechin gallate	Yokozawa *et al.*, 2000; Miura *et al.*, 1995
Hordeum vulgare	Poaceae	Leaves	Isovitexin derivatives	Arimoto *et al.*, 2000
Glycyrrhiza glabra	Leguminosae	Roots	Glabridin	Bellnky *et al.*, 1998; Vaya *et al* 1997
Ginkgo biloba	Ginkgoaceae	Leaf	Ginkgolides, bilobalide, sciadopitysin, ginkgetin, bilobetin	Joyeux *et al.*, 1995; Haramaki *et al.*, 1994
Helenium aromaticum	Compositae	Whole plant	Sesquiterpene lactones; helenalin, mexicanin-I, linifolin A, geigerinin	Jodynis-Liebert *et al.*, 2000
Hedyotis diffusa	Rubiaceae	Fresh aerial	New acylflavonol diglycoside; kaempferol and quercetin derivatives, flavonol and iridoid glycosides	Lu *et al.*, 2000
Hierochloe odorata	Poaceae	Aerial	Benzophenanthrone derivatives	Pukalskas *et al.*, 2002
Hibiscus syriacus	Malvaceae	Root bark	Lignans: hibiscuside, syringaresinol, E&Z feruloyltyramines and isoflavonoids	Lee *et al.*, 1999
Hypericum erectum	Hypericaceae	Aerial	Flavonoids-quercetrin, hyperoside, isoquercetrin, orientin	Jung *et al.*, 1999a
Helichrysum picardii	Asteraceae	Aerial	Gnaphalin	Puerta *et al.*, 1999
Iryanthera lancifolia	Poaceae	Pericarps	Two dihydrochalcones and two flavonolignans	Silva *et al.*, 1999
Iresine herbstii	Amaranthaceae	Aerial	Waxes, β-sitosterol, cam, pestrol and methoxy flavone	Kubinova *et al.*, 1998
Iberis amara	Brassicaceae	Seeds	6-O-sinapoyl sucrose	Fabre *et al.*, 2000
Lavandula angustifolia	Lamiaceae	Aerial	Phenolics-romarinic acid, caffeic acid, luteolin and methyl carnosoate	Hohmann *et al.*, 1999
Larix gmelini	Pinaceae	Wood	Dihydroquercetin	Kolhir *et al.*, 1996
Mahonia aquifolium	Berberidaceae	Root and leaf	Alkaloids	Misik *et al.*, 1995
Muscari racemosum	Liliaceae	Flower	homoisoflavonoids	Juranek *et al.*, 1993
Magnolia coco	Magnoliaceae	Stem	Lignans-sesamin, fargesin, syringaresinol	Chen *et al.*, 1999a

Table 19.1 *(continued)*

Plants	Family	Part used	Phytoconstituents	Reference
Myrica gale	Myricaceae	Fruit	Flavonoids- C-methylated dihydrochalcones, myrigalone A & B	Mathiesen *et al.*, 1995
Mangifera indica	Anacardiaceae	Leaves, bark, fruits	Mangiferin, myricetin, protocatechuic acid, quercetin, friedelin, gallic acid, homomangiferin, kaempferol and lupeol	Rai *et al.*, 2007
Nelumbo nucifera	Nymphaeaceae	Rhizomes, seed, leaves, flower	Gallic acid	Rai *et al.*, 2006a
Panax pseudoginseng	Araliaceae	Roots	Trilinolein	Chan and Tomlinson, 2000
Phyllostachys edulis	Poaceae	Leaves	Chlorogenic acid derivatives	Kweon *et al.*, 2001
Punica granatum	Punicaceae	Fruits	Flavonoids	Schubert *et al.*, 1999
Prunus cerasus	Rosaceae	Fruits	Cholorgenic acid methylester derivatives	Wang *et al.*, 1999
Prunus amygdalus	Rosaceae	Fruit skin	Catechin, protocatechinic acid and flavonoids	Sang *et al.*, 2002
Phaseolus aureus	Fabaceae	Seeds	Flavonoids	Kim *et al.*, 1998
Pteleopsis hylodendron	Combretaceae	Stem bark	Ellagic acid derivatives	Atta-Ur-Rahaman *et al.*, 2001
Psoralea corylifolia	Leguminosae	Seeds	Monoterpene phenol-bakuchiol	Haraguchi *et al.*, 2000
Pistacia weinmannifolia	Anacardiaceae	Leaves	Pistafolia A	Wei *et al.*, 2002
Picrorhiza kurroa	Scrophulariaceae	Roots and rhizomes	Picrovil	Rastogi *et al.*, 2000
Panax ginseng	Araliaceae	Roots	Ginsenosides	Facino *et al.*, 1999
Palm spp.	Arecaceae	Oil	Tocotrienols	Kamat *et al.*, 1997
Podocarpus nagi	Podocarpaceae	Root bark	Totarane diterpenoids	Haraguchi *et al.*, 1997
Rosmarinus officinalis	Lamiaceae	Leaves	Diterpenoids	Haraguchi *et al.*, 1995
Salvia officinalis	Lamiaceae	Leaves	Phenolics-abietane diterpenes, caffeoyl glycosides, rosmarinic acid	Zupko *et al.*, 2001
Saururus chinensis	Sauruaceae parts	Underground	Machilin-D	Abn *et al.*, 2001
Saururus cernuus	Saururaceae	Whole plant	Feruloylgeraniol derivative	Rajbhandari *et al.*, 2001
Silybum marianum	Asteraceae	Seeds	Silybin, silymarin	Borsari *et al.*, 2001; Psotova *et al.*, 2002; Farghali *et al.*, 2000; Pietrangelo *et al.*, 1995
Spinacia oleracea	Amaranthaceae	Leaves	p-Coumaric acid derivative and flavonoids	Bergman *et al*, 2001
Terminalia catappa	Euphorbiaceae	Leaves	Punicalagin and punicalin	Lin *et al.*, 2001

(*continued overleaf*)

Table 19.1 *(continued)*

Plants	Family	Part used	Phytoconstituents	Reference
Terminalia bellerica	Combetaceae	Fruits	Gallic acid, ellagic acid, ethyl gallate, galloyl glucose, chebulagic acid, bellericanin	Mukherjee *et al.*, 2007, Mukherjee *et al.*, 2006
Telekia speciosa	Asteraceae	Leaves and Roots	Sesquiterpene lactones	Jodynis-Liebert *et al.*, 2000
Vaccinium myrtillus	Ericaceae	Leaves	Anthocyanosides	Martin-Aragon *et al.*, 1999
Vitex rotundifolia	Verbenaceae	Fruits	Labdane and abietane-type diterpenoids	Ono *et al.*, 1999
Withania somnifera	Solanaceae	Root	Glycowithanolides	Bhattacharya *et al.*, 2001
Triticum aestivum	Poaceae	Leaves	Ferulic acid dehydrodimers	Garcta-Conesa *et al.*, 1997
Vitis vinifera	Vitaceae	Fruits and seeds	Proanthocyanidins and resveratrol	Pataki *et al.*, 2002; Martinez and Moreno, 2000
Zingiber cassumunar	Zingiberaceae	Rhizome	Cassumunin A & B (cucurminoids)	Nagano *et al.*, 1997
Zingiber officinalis	Zingiberaceae	Rhizome	6-gingerol	Rai *et al.*, 2006b

(Khan *et al.*, 1997) and a shortage of antioxidants in the diet might enable diseases caused by ROS to arise. Many vegetables and fruits used as foods are particularly rich in natural antioxidant nutrients, e.g. including vitamin C, the tocopherols and carotenoids. Phenolic antioxidants such as flavonoids, tannins, coumarins, xanthenes and more recently, procyanidins, have been shown to scavenge radicals in a dose-dependent manner and therefore are viewed as promising therapeutic potential for free-radical pathologies. A sufficient supply of antioxidants from the diet might help to prevent or delay the occurrence of pathological changes associated with oxidative stress. When diet fails to meet the antioxidant requirements, dietary supplement might be used to enhance health but more needs to be done to test this hypothesis by good clinical studies. Consumer demand for healthy food products provides an opportunity to develop food rich in antioxidants as new functional foods or nutraceuticals (Mukherjee *et al.*, 2007b).

Gingko biloba (ginkgo)

Gingko biloba extract is widely used in traditional medicine for a great number of therapeutical properties. A large number of studies confirm the antioxidant nature of the extract and its phytoconstituents. A study by Butnaru *et al.* (1997) in rats showed that the treatment with this extract before stress inhibited the post-stress growth MDA concentration and the process of stress ulcer formation. Gingko protects against cardiac ischaemia and reperfusion injury and these effects are shown to be dependent on its antioxidant properties (Haramaki *et al.*, 1994). Its in-vivo free-radical scavenging action and proof of its haematological properties in rats was confirmed (Louajri *et al.*, 2001). *G. biloba* extract and kaemferol isolated from it were demonstrated to be antioxidant in a lipid peroxidation assay. *G. biloba* extracts have properties indicative of potential neuroprotective ability (Sloley *et al.*, 2000). From the *n*-butanol extract of *G. biloba* leaves, flavonoids were isolated, which showed strong antioxidant activities in DPPH and cytochrome-c reduction assays using the HL-60 cell culture system (Tang *et al.*, 2001).

Bacopa monniera (brahmi)

B. monniera is a component of several popular drugs of the Ayurvedic system of medicine. Its ethanol extract showed strong protection against lipid peroxidation induced by ferrous sulphate and cumene hydroperoxide (Tripathi and Chaurasia, 1996). *B. monniera* alcohol extract exerted a hepatoprotective effect against morphine-induced liver toxicity, which was found to be related to its antioxidant nature (Sumathy *et al.*, 2001). The effect of a standardised extract of *B. monniera* was assessed on rat brain frontal cortical, striatial and hippocampal SOD, catalase and glutathione peroxidase activities and the results indicated a significant antioxidant effect.

Mangifera indica (mango)

The standardised aqueous extract of crude mango stem bark showed a powerful scavenger activity of hydroxyl radicals and hypochlorous acid and acted as an iron chelator. The extract also showed a significant inhibitory effect on the peroxidation of rat brain phospholipid and inhibited DNA damage by bleomycin or copper phenanthrolin system (Martiniz *et al.*, 2000). Oral administration of an *M. indica* extract (QF 808) was found to reduce ischaemia-induced neuronal loss and oxidative damage in gerbil brain (Martinez Sanchez *et al.*, 2001). QF 808 has the ability to scavenge free radicals involved in microsome peroxidation (Martiniz *et al.*, 2001). An aqueous decoction of mango bark has been developed in Cuba on an industrial scale to be used as a nutritional supplement, cosmetic and phytomedicine. It is useful in preventing the production of reactive oxygen species and oxidative tissue damage in vivo. Polyphenols including mangiferin were found to be the major constituents (Nunez Selles *et al.*, 2002). Mangiferin has shown to be able to maintain the cellular oxidant/antioxidant balance (Ghosal *et al.*, 1996; Rai *et al.*, 2007).

Curcuma longa (turmeric and curcumin)

Curcuma longa and a large number of its constituents exhibit potent antioxidant properties in several models. Curcumin and its sodium salt have been shown to have a strong antioxidant activity. Curcumin exhibited a significant time- and concentration-dependent effect on lipid peroxidation induced by radiation (Sreejayam *et al.*, 1997) and other curcumin analogues exhibited an antioxidant activity stronger than α-tocopherol (Sreejayam and Rao, 1994; Bonte *et al.*, 1997). Turmeric antioxidant proteins isolated from the aqueous extract of turmeric were found to prevent Ca^{2+}-stimulated ATPase from inactivation in the presence of promoters of lipid peroxidation, as well as the depletion of the thiol content during peroxidation (Selvam *et al.*, 1995).

Withania somnifera (ashwagandha)

Withania somnifera is used as an antistress adaptogen. Its glycowithanolides showed antioxidant effects in chronic footshock stress-induced perturbations of oxidative free-radical scavenging enzyme and lipid peroxidation in rats (Bhattacharya *et al.*, 2001). Administration of plant extract, along with equivalent doses of lead acetate for 20 days, significantly decreased lipid peroxidation and increased SOD and catalase, thus retaining normal peroxidative status of the tissues (Chaurasia *et al.*, 2000). The antioxidant effects depend on the presence of steroidal lactones, the withanolides (Dhuley, 1998).

Allium sativum (garlic)

The inhibitory property of garlic on ROS generation and lipid peroxidation has been reported in a number of in-vitro studies. Banerjee *et al.* (2002) showed that chronic garlic intake dependently augmented endogenous antioxidants, which might have important direct cytoprotective effects on the heart, especially in the event of oxidative stress-induced injury. Diallyl sulphide is a flavour component from garlic and is found to attenuate lipid peroxidation in mice infected with *Trichinella spiralis* (Grudzinski *et al.*, 2001). Antioxidant activity of the diallyl sulphide garlicin was due to its ability to scavenge peroxyl or alkoxyl radical intermediates of lipid peroxidation. Allicin, another component, may have multiple mechanisms of action, acting both as a stronger chain-breaking antioxidant and as an inhibitor of first chain reaction by scavenging an initiating radical species (Rekka *et al.*, 1994).

Punica granatum (pomegranate)

Punica granatum fermented juice and seed oil flavonoids exhibited antioxidant activities (Schubert *et al.*, 1999) and the methanol extract of pomegranate demonstrated potent antioxidant activity using various in-vitro models (Singh *et al.*, 2002). Three major anthocyanidins isolated from *Punica granatum* fruits showed free-radical scavenging activity and inhibitory effects on lipid peroxidation in rat brain homogenates (Noda *et al.*, 2002).

Ocimum sanctum (tulsi, holy basil)

An aqueous extract of the leaves of *Ocimum sanctum* has been found to protect mice against radiation lethality and bone marrow damage and had strong radical scavenging activity in vitro. The extract also protected against radiation-induced lipid peroxidation, where GSH and antioxidant enzymes play an important role in protection (Uma Devi and Ganasoundari, 1999). The hydroalcoholic extract, investigated against isoproterenol-induced myocardial infraction in rats, caused a significant reduction in GSH, SOD, LDH and TBARS levels, thus demonstrating antioxidant and cardioprotective effects (Sharma *et al.*, 2001).

Garcinia

G. kola, G. indica, G. subelliptica, G. atroviridis and several other *Garcinia* species were found to possess strong antioxidant activity and a large number of active constituents isolated from *G. kola* fruits possess inhibitory activity against lipid peroxidation (Adegoke *et al.*, 1998). Kola-viron, a mixture of Garcinia biflavonoids 1 and 2 and kolaflavonone isolated from *G. kola* seed extract, acts as an in-vivo natural antioxidant and effective hepatoprotective and is as effective as BHA in rats (Farombi *et al.*, 2000). Garcinol, a polyisoprenylated benzophenone derivative isolated from *G. indica* fruit rind, has shown potent free-radical scavenging activity and was able to scavenge both hydrophilic and hydrophobic ROS, the activity being stronger than that of DL-α-tocopherol. Oral administration prevented acute ulceration in rats induced by indometacin and water-immersion stress caused by radical formation (Mackeen *et al.*, 2000; Yamaguchi *et al.*, 2000).

Emblica officinalis

The fruits of *Emblica officinalis* contain polyphenolic compounds such as emblicanin A and B which have been reported to exhibit antioxidant activity in vitro and in vivo (Bhattacharya *et al.*, 2000). A study showed that emblicanin A and B preserve erthrocytes against oxidative stress induced by asbestos, a generator of superoxide radical (Scartezzini and Speroni, 2000). The active tannoids administered intraperitoneally for 7 days showed augmentation of brain SOD, catalase and reduction in lipid peroxidation. The results indicate that the antioxidant activity may reside in these tannoids rather than vitamin C itself (Ghosal *et al.*, 1996). Pretreatment with the butanol extract of the water fraction of *Emblica officinalis* fruits, orally administrated to rats for 10 consecutive days, was found to prevent indometacin-induced gastric ulcer; this activity was attributed to its antioxidant property (Bandyopadhyay *et al.*, 2000).

Salvia officinalis (sage)

Salvia is an important genus, widely cultivated and used in flavouring and folk medicine. It is a rich source of polyphenols, and a large number of these are apparently constructed from the caffeic acid building block (Lu and Foo, 2002). *S. officinalis* 50% methanol extract demonstrated considerable inhibition of lipid peroxidation in both enzyme-dependent and enzyme-independent systems (Hohmann *et al.*, 1999) and supercritical fluid extracts of *S. officinalis* also showed antioxidant activity (Dauksas *et al.*, 2001). *S. officinalis* leaves and terpenoids and flavonoids showed strong antioxidant properties using DPPH and by the oil stability index method (Miura *et al.*, 2002). Various constituents such as rosmarinic acid, abietene diterpenes and caffeoylglycosides have been identified as antioxidant principles (Zupko *et al.*, 2001). The extracts of other *Salvia* species also displayed considerable concentration-dependent antioxidative effects that were comparable with those of *S. officinalis* (Chen *et al.*, 2001; Choi *et al.*, 2001; Perry *et al.*, 2001; Zupko *et al.*, 2001).

Vitis vinifera (grapevine)

Resveratrol is a polyphenolic stilbene occurring in grapes and various other medicinal plants and has been the subject of a considerable amount of recent research. It has been identified as a potential cancer chemopreventive agent and its presence in red wine has been suggested to be linked to the low incidence of heart diseases in France (Burkitt and Duncan, 2000). It acts as a powerful antioxidant, both by classic hydroxyl radical scavenging and also via a novel glutathione-sparing mechanism. Various studies have demonstrated the effects of resveratrol on biological mechanisms involved in cardioprotection. These include modulation of lipid turnover, inhibition of eicosanoid production, prevention of low-density lipoprotein oxidation and inhibition of platelet aggregation.

Based on the quantity and diversity data available on the biological activity of resveratrol, it has to be considered to be a very promising chemoprotector and chemotherapeutic. Urgent investigation on its bioavailability and effects on in-vivo systems, especially in humans, are necessary (Olas *et al.*, 1999; Ignatowicz and Baer, 2001). Martinez and Moreno (2000) showed that resveratrol treatment caused a significant impairment of COX-2 induction, stimulated by lipopolysaccharides and phorbol esters or by O_2^- or H_2O_2 exposure. It also significantly decreased [^{3}H]arachidonic acid release induced by these agents. These results support the anti-inflammatory action of resveratrol.

Silybum marianum (milk thistle)

Silybum marianum fruits are reported to exert antioxidant and free-radical scavenging action. Silymarin and silybin, the flavonolignans present, were found to be the active constituents. Silymarin prevents doxorubicin-mediated damage to rat heart membrane primarily through free radical scavenging (Psotova *et al.*, 2002). Oral administration of silybin protected against iron-induced hepatotoxicity in vivo and can be used in chelation therapy of chronic iron overload (Pietrangelo *et al.*, 1995; Borsari *et al.*, 2001).

Conclusions

It is obvious that a large number of plants possess strong antioxidant potential and these include commonly used fruits, vegetables and spices. Concentration of total phenols in the plant show close correlation with the antioxidant activity, so it is useful to determine the total phenol content of the plants before antioxidant screening. A large number of plants have been tested, based on their uses in folklore and have been found to be active, and still there is scope for antioxidant screening of a large number of plants belonging to families rich in antioxidants. Fermented extracts have been found to be more potent and the production of low-molecular-weight compounds during fermentation is responsible for the action. There is scope for evaluation of antioxidant properties of fermented extracts of plants known to possess strong antioxidant properties.

Acknowledgements

The authors are thankful to the Department of Science & Technology, Government of India for financial support through WOS-A program to Dr. Kakali Mukherjee. Thanks are due to The All India Council for Technical Education, New Delhi, India for MODROB Project grant.

References

Abn BT, Lee SB, Lee RS *et al.* (2001). Low-density lipoprotein-antioxidant constituents of *Saururus chinensis*. *J Nat Prod* 64: 1562–1564.

Adegoke GO, Vijay Kumar M, Sanbaiab K (1998). Inhibitory effect of *Garcinia kola* on lipid peroxidation in rat liver homogenate. *Indian J Exp Biol* 36: 907–910.

Al-Saikhan MS, Howard LR, Miller JC, Jr. (1995). Antioxidant activity and total phenolics in different genotypes of potato (*Solanum tuberosum* L.). *J Food Sci* 60: 341–343, 347.

Arimoto T, Ichinose T, Yoshikawla T (2000). Effect of the natural antioxidant 2′-O-glycosylisovitexin on superoxide and hydroxyl radical generation. *Food Chem Toxicol* 38: 849–852.

Atta-Ur-Rahman A, Ngounou FN, Choudhary MI *et al.* (2001). New antioxidant and antimicrobial ellagic acid derivatives from *Pteleopsis hylodendron*. *Planta Med* 67: 335–339.

Bahorun T, Trotin F, Pommery J *et al.* (1994). Antioxidant activities of *Crataegus monogyna* extracts. *Planta Med* 60: 323–328.

Bandyopadhyay SK, Pakrashi SC, Pakrashi A (2000). The role of antioxidant activity of *Phyllanthus omblica* fruits on prevention from indomethacin induced gastric ulcer. *J Ethnopharmacol* 70: 171–176.

Banerjee SK, Maulik M, Mancahanda SC *et al.* (2002).

Dose-dependent induction of endogenous antioxidants in rat heart by chronic administration of garlic. *Life Sci* 70: 1509–1518.

Bellnky PA, Avtram M, Mahmood S *et al.* (1998). Structural aspects of the inhibitory effect of glabridin on LDL oxidation. *Free Radic Biol Med* 24: 1419–1429.

Benov L, Georgiev N (1999). The antioxidant activity of flavonoids isolated from *Corylus colurna*. *Phytother Res* 8: 92–94.

Bendall JK, Cave AC, Heymes C *et al.* (2002). Pivotal role of a gp91phox-containing NADPH oxidase in angiotensin II-induced cardiac hypertrophy in mice. *Circulation* 105: 293–296.

Bergman M, Varshavsky L, Gottlieb HE *et al.* (2001). The antioxidant activity of aqueous spinach extract: chemical identification of active fractions. *Phytochemistry* 58: 143–152.

Berry C, Clark AL (2000). Catabolism in chronic heart failure. *Eur Heart J* 21: 521–532.

Bezabih M, Abegaz BM, Dufall K *et al.* (2001). Antiplasmodial and antioxidant isofuranonaphthoquinones from the roots of *Bulbine capitata*. *Planta Med*, 67: 340–344.

Bhattacharya A, Ghosal S, Bhattacharya SK (2001). Antioxidant effect of *Withania somnifera* Glycowithanolides in chronic footshock stress induced perturbations of oxidative free radical scavenging enzymes and lipid peroxidation in rat frontal cortex and striatum. *J Ethnopharmacol* 74: 1–6.

Bhattacharya A, Kumar M, Ghosal S *et al.* (2000). Effect of bioactive tannoid priciples of *Emblica officinalis* on iron-induced hepatic toxicity in rats. *Phytomedicine* 7: 173–175.

Bolli R (1992). Postischemic myocardial injury. Pathogenesis, pathophysiology, and clinical relevance. In: Yellon DM, Jennings RB (eds). *Myocardial Protection: the pathophysiology of reperfusion and reperfusion injury*, Raven Press, New York: 105–149.

Bolli R (1991). Oxygen-derived free radicals and myocardial reperfusion injury: An overview. *Cardiovasc Drugs Ther* 5: 249–268.

Boger RH, Bode-Boger SM, Mugge A (1995). Supplementation of hypercholesterolaemic rabbits with l-arginine reduces the vascular release of superoxide anions and restores NO production. *Atherosclerosis* 117: 273–284.

Bonte F, Noel-Hudson MS, Wepiefre J (1997). Protective effect of curcuminoids on epidermal skin cells under free oxygen radical stress. *Planta Med* 63: 265–266.

Borsari M, Gabbi C, Ghelfi F *et al.* (2001). Silybin, a new iron-chelating agent. *J Inorg Biochem* 85: 123–129.

Burkitt MJ, Duncan J (2000). Effects of trans-reveratrol on copper-dependent hydroxyl-radical formation and DNA damage: evidence for hydroxyl-radical scavenging and a novel, glutathione-sparing mechanism of action. *Arch Biochem Biophys* 381: 253–263.

Butnaru M, Iacobovici A, Ilaulica I *et al.* (1997). [*Ginkgo biloba* extract (EGb 761) as a antioxidant factor of exogenous origin.] [in Romanian]. *Re Med Chir Soc Med Nat Iasi* 101: 192–196.

Cargnoni A, Ceconi C, Bernocchi P *et al.* (2000). Reduction of oxidative stress by carvedilol: role in maintenance of ischaemic myocardium viability. *Cardiovasc Res* 47: 556–566.

Chan P, Tomlinson B (2000). Antioxidant effects of Chinese traditional medicine: focus on trilinolein isolated from the Chinese herb Sandhi (*Panax pseudoginseng*). *J Clin Pharmacol* 40: 457–461.

Chaurasia SS, Panda S, Kar A (2000). *Withania somnifera* root extract in the regulation of load-induced oxidative damage in male mouse. *Pharmacol Res* 41: 663–666.

Chen CC, Chen HY, Shiao MS *et al.* (1999a). Inhibition of low density lipoprotein oxidation by tetralydrofurofuran lignans from Forsythia syspensa and magnolia coco. *Planta Med* 65: 709–711.

Chen HY, Shio MS, Huang YL *et al.* (1999b). Antioxidant principles from Ephemerantha lonchophylla. *J Nat Prod* 62: 1225–1227.

Chen YL, Yang SP, Shiao MS *et al.* (2001). Salvia miltiorrhiza inhibits intimal hyperplasia and monocyte chemotactic protein-1 expression after balloon injury in cholesterol-fed rabbits. *J Cell Biochem* 83: 484–493.

Cheeseman KH, Slater TF (1993). Free radical in medicine. *Br Med Bull* 49: 479–724.

Chien KR (1999). Stress pathways and heart failure. *Cell* 98: 555–558.

Choi JS, Kang HS, Jung HA *et al.* (2001). A new cyclic phenylactamide from Salvia miltiorrhiza. *Fitoterapia* 72: 30–34.

Clarkson P, Thompson HS (2000). Antioxidants: what role do they play in physical activity and health. *Am J Clin Nutr* 72: 637.

Creemers EE, Cleutjens JP, Smits JF *et al.* (2001). Matrix metalloproteinase inhibition after myocardial infarction: a new approach to prevent heart failure? *Circ Res* 89: 201–210.

Cross AR, Jones OTG (1991). Enzymatic mechanisms of superoxide production. *Biochim Biophys Acta* 1057: 281–298.

Daniel RS, Mathew BC, Devi KS (1998). Antioxidant effect of two flavonoids from the bark of *Ficus bengalensis* Linn in hyperlipidermic rats. *Indian J Exp Biol* 36: 902–906.

Date MO, Morita T, Yamashita N *et al.* (2002). The antioxidant N-2- mercaptopropionyl glycine attenuates left ventricular hypertrophy in in vivo murine pressure-overload model. *J Am Coll Cardiol* 39: 907–912.

Dauksas E, Venskutonis PR, Povilaityte V, Sivik B (2001). Rapid screening of antioxidant activity of sage (*Salvia officinalis* L.) extracts obtained by supercritical carbon dioxide at different extraction conditions. *Nahrung* 45: 338–341.

Dhuley JM (1998). Effect of *Ashwagandha* on lipid peroxidation in stress induced animals. *J Ethanopharmacol* 60: 173–178.

Dieterich S, Bieligk U, Beulich K *et al.* (2000). Gene expression of antioxidative enzymes in the human heart. Increased expressin of catalase in the end-stage failing heart. *Circulation* 101: 33–39.

Dousset JC, Trouilh M, Foglietti MJ (1983). Plasma malondialdehyde levels during myocardial infarction. *Clin Chim Acta* 129: 319–322.

Ellis GR, Anderson RA, Lang D *et al.* (2000). Neutrophil superoxide anion-generating capacity, endothelial function and oxidative stress in chronic heart failure: Effects of short- and long-term vitamin C therapy. *J Am Coll Cardiol* 36: 1474–1482.

Evans JL, Goldfine ID, Maddux BA, Grodsky GM (2002). Oxidative stress and stress-activated signaling pathways: a unifying hypothesis of type 2 diabetes. *Endocr Rev* 23: 599–622.

Fabre N, Urizzi P, Souchard JP *et al.* (2000). *Fitoterapia* 71: 425–428.

Facino RM, Carini M, Aldini G *et al.* (1999). Panax ginseng administration in the rat prevents myocardial ischemia-reperfusion damage induced by hyperbaric oxygen: Evidence for an antioxidant intervention. *Planta Med* 65: 614–619.

Farombi EO, Tahnteng JG, Agboola AO *et al.* (2000). Chemoprevention of 2-acetylaminofluorene-induced hepatotoxicity and lipid peroxidation in rats by kolaviron – a *Garcinia kola* seed extract. *Food Chem Toxicol* 38: 535–541.

Farghali H, Kamenikova L, Hynic S *et al.* (2000). Silymarin effects on intracellular calcium and cytotoxicity: a study in perfused rat hepatocytes after oxidative stress injury. *Pharmacol Res* 41: 231–237.

Floyd RA (1990). The role of 8-hydroxyguanine in carcinogenesis. *Carcinogenesis* 11(9): 1447–1450.

Ferrari R, Ceconi C, Curello S *et al.* (1993). Myocardial damage during ischemia and reperfusion. *Eur Heart J* 14: 25–30.

Ferrari R, Agnoletti L, Comini L *et al.* (1998). Oxidative stress during myocardial ischemia and heart failure. *Eur Heart J* 19: B2–B11.

Fox KAA (1992). Reperfusion injury: a clinical perspective. In: Yellon DM, Jennings RB (eds). *Myocardial Protection: the pathophysiology of reperfusion and reperfusion injury*. Raven Press, New York: 151–165.

Gamez EJ, Luyengi L, Lee SK *et al.* (1998). Antioxidant flavonoids glycosides from *Daphniphyllum calycinum*. *J Nat Prod* 61: 706–708.

Garcta-Conesa MT, Plumb GW, Waldron KW *et al.* (1997). Ferulic acid dehydrodimers from wheat bran: isolation, purification and antioxidant properties of 8-0-4-diferulic acid. *Redox Report* 3: 319–323.

Garlick PB, Davies MJ, Hearse DJ *et al.* (1987). Direct detection of free radicals in the reperfused rat heart using electron spin resonance spectroscopy. *Circ Res* 61: 757–760.

Garrat DC (1964). *The Quantitative Analysis of Drugs*, Vol. 3. Chapman & Hall Ltd, Japan, pp. 456–458.

Ghosal S, Tripathi VK, Chauhan S (1996). Active constituents of *Emblica officinalis*: Part I. The chemistry and antioxidative effects of two hydrolysable tannins, Emblicannin A and B. *Indian J Chem* 35B: 941–948.

Grudzinski IP, Frankiewicz-Jozko A, Bany J (2001). Diallyl sulfide – a flavour component from garlic (*Allium sativum*) attenuates lipid peroxidation in mice infected with *Trichinella spiralis*. *Phytomedicine* 8: 174–177.

Guzik TJ, West NEJ, Black E *et al.* (2000). Functional effect of the C242T polymorphism in the NAD(P)H oxidase p22phox gene on vascular superoxide production in atherosclerosis. *Circulation* 102: 1744–1747.

Halliwell B, Gutteridge JC (1999). *Free Radicals in Biology and Medicine*, 3rd edn. London: Oxford University Press.

Halliwell B (1997). Antioxidants: the basics – what they are and how to evaluate them. *Adv Pharmacol* 38: 3–20.

Halliwell B (1994). Free radicals, antioxidants, and human disease: curiosity, cause or consequence? *Lancet* 344: 721–724.

Halliwell B (1992). Reactive oxygen species and the central nervous system. *J Neurochem* 59: 1609–1623.

Halliwell B (1999). Establishing the significance and optimal intake of dietary antioxidants: The biomarker concept. *Nutr Rev* 57: 104–113.

Halliwell B, Gutteridge JMC (1989). *Free Radicals in Biology and Medicine*, 2nd edn. Clarendon Press, Oxford.

Haraguchi H, Inoue J, Tamura Y *et al.* (2000). Inhibition of mitochondrial lipid peroxidation by bakuchiol, a meroterpene from psoralea corylifolia. *Planta Med* 66: 569–571.

Haraguchi H, Ishikawa H, Kubo I (1997). Antioxidative action of diterpenoids from *Podocarpus nagi*. *Planta Med* 63: 213–215.

Haraguchi H, Satio T, Okamura N *et al.* (1995). Inhibition of lipid peroxidation and superoxide generation by diterpenoids from *Rosmarinus officinalis*. *Planta Med* 61: 333–336.

Haramaki N, Aggarwal S, Kawabata T *et al.* (1994). Effects of natural antioxidant *Ginkgo biloba* extract (EGB 761) on myocardial ischemia – reperfusion injury. *Free Rad Biol Med* 16: 789–794.

Harman D (1992). Role of free radicals in aging and disease. *Ann NY Acad Sci* 673: 126–134.

Hathaway CA, Heistad DD, Piegors DJ *et al.* (2002). Regression of atherosclerosis in monkeys reduces vascular superoxide levels. *Circ Res* 90: 277–283.

Hayashidani S, Tsutsui H, Ikeuchi M *et al.* (2003). Targeted deletion of MMP-2 attenuates early LV rupture and late remodeling after experimental myocardial infarction. *Am J Physiol Heart Circ Physiol* 285: H1229–1235.

Heymes C, Bendall JK, Ratajczak P *et al.* (2003). Increased myocardial NADPH oxidase activity in human heart failure. *J Am Coll Cardiol* 41: 2164–2171.

Hohmann J, Zupko I, Redei D *et al.* (1999). Protective effects of the aerial parts of *Salvia officinalis, Melissa officinalis* and *Lavandula angustigotia* and their constituents against enzyme-dependent and enzyme-independent lipid peroxiadation. *Planta Med* 65: 576–578.

Ide M, Matsuura H, Itakura Y (1996). Scavenging effect of aged garlic extract and its constituents on active oxygen species. *Phytother Res* 10: 340–341.

Ide T, Tsutsui H, Kinugawa S *et al.* (1999). Mitochondrial electron transport complex I is a potential source of oxygen free radicals in the failing myocardium. *Circ Res* 85: 357–363.

Ignatowicz E, Baer-Dubowska W (2001). Resveratrol, a natural chemopreventive agent against degenerative diseases. *Polish J Pharmacol* 53: 557–569.

Imai J, Idc N, Nagac S (1994). Antioxidant and radical scavenging effects of aged garlic extract and its constituents. *Planta Med* 60: 417–420.

Jeroudi MO, Hartley CJ, Bolli R (1994). Myocardial reperfusion injury: role of oxygen radicals and potential therapy with antioxidants. *Am J Cardiol* 73: 2B–7B.

Jingtao J, Sato S, Yamanaka N (1999). Changes in cerebral blood flow and blood brain barrier in the gerbil hippocampal CA1 region following repeated brief cerebral ischemia. *Med Electron Microsc* 32(3): 175–183.

Jodynis-Liebert J, Murias M, Blaoszyk E (2000). Effect of sesquiterpene lactones on antioxidant enzymes and some drug metabolizing enzymes in rat liver and kidney. *Planta Med* 66: 199–205.

Joyeux M, Lobstein A, Anton R *et al.* (1995). Comparative antilipoperoxidant, antinecrotic and scavenging properties of terpeues and biflavones from *Ginkgo* and some flavonoids. *Planta Med* 59: 126–129.

Jun T, Ke-Yan F, Catalano M (1996). Increased superoxide anion production in humans: a possible mechanism for the pathogenesis of hypertension. *J Hum Hypert* 10: 305–309.

Jung CM, Hwang BJ, Kwon HC (1999a). Antioxidative flavonoids from *Hypericum erectum. Korean J Pharmacogn* 30: 196–201.

Jung HA, Park JC, Chung HY *et al.* (1999b). Antioxidant flavonoids and chlorogenic acid from the leaves of *Eriobotrya japonica. Arch Pharm Res* 22: 213–218.

Juranek I, Suchy V, Stara D *et al.* (1993). Antioxidant activity of homoiso flavonoids from *Muscuri racemosum* and *Dracaena cinnabari. Pharmazie* 48(Apr): 310–311.

Kamat JP, Sarma HD, Devasagayam TP *et al.* (1997). Tocotrienols from palm oil as effective inhibitors of protein oxidation and lipid peroxidation in rat liver microsomes. *Mol Cell Biochem* 170: 131–137.

Kasai H, Nishimura S (1984). Hydroxylation of deoxyguanosine at the C-8 position by ascorbic acid and other reducing agents. *Nucl Acids Res* 12: 2137–2145.

Khan BA, Abraham A, Leelamma S (1997). Antioxidant effect of curry leaf, *Murraya koenigii* and mustard seeds *Brassica juncea* in rats fed with high fat diet. *Indian J Exp Biol* 35: 148–150.

Khouri J, Resck IS, Poças-Fonseca M *et al.* (2007). Grisolia anticlastogenic potential and antioxidant effects of an aqueous extract of pulp from the pequi tree (*Caryocar brasiliense* Camb). *Genet Mol Biol* 30: 442–448.

Kim BJ, Kim JH, Heo MY *et al.* (1998). Antioxidant and anti-inflammatory activities of Mung bean. *Cosmet Toiletr* 113: 71–74.

Kim JP, Lee TK, Yun RS *et al.* (2001). Ellagic acid rhamonsides from the stem bark of *Eucalyptus globulus. Phytochemistry* 57: 587–591.

Kim NM, Kim J, Chung HY *et al.* (2000). Isolation of lutcolin 7-0-rutinoside and cseulectin with potential antioxidant activity from the aerial parts of *Artemisia montana. Arch Pharm Res* 23: 237–239.

Kinugawa S, Tsutsui H, Hayashidani S *et al.* (2000). Treatment with dimethylthiourea prevents left ventricular remodeling and failure after experimental myocardial infarction in mice: role of oxidative stress. *Circ Res* 87: 392–398.

Ko HH, Yu SM, Ko FN *et al.* (1997). Bioactive constituents of *Morus australis* and *Broussonetia papyrifera. J Nat Prod* 60(Oct): 1008–1011.

Kolhir VK, ByKov VA, Baginskaja AI *et al.* (1996). Antioxidant activity of a dihydroquercetin isolated from *Larix gmelinii* (Rupr.) wood. *Phytother Res* 10: 478–482.

Kontos HA (2001). Oxygen radicals in cerebral ischemia. *Stroke* 32: 2712.

Kubinova R, Suchy V, Pizova M *et al.* (1998). Constituents of *Iresine herbstii. Ceska Slov Farm* 47: 268–270.

Kuman KV, Das UN (1993). Are free radicals involved in the pathobiology of human essential hypertension? *Free Radic Res Commun* 19: 59–66.

Kweon MH, Hwang HJ, Sung HC (2001). Identification and antioxidant activity of novel chlorogenic acid derivatives from bamboo (*Phyllostachys edulis*). *J Agric Food Chem* 49: 4646–4655.

Langenstroer P, Pieper GM (1992). Regulation of spontaneous EDRF release in diabetic rat aorta by oxygen free radicals. *Am J Physiol* 263: H257–H265.

Lee MK, Yeo H, Kim J *et al.* (2000). Cynandione A from *Cynanchum wilfordii* protects cultured cortical neurons from toxicity induced by H_2O_2, L-glutamate, and kainate. *J Neurosci Res* 59: 259–264.

Lee SJ, Yun YS, Lee IK *et al.* (1999). An antioxidant lignan and other constituents from the root bark of *Hibiscus Syriacus. Planta Med* 65: 658–660.

Li J, Gall NP, Grieve DJ *et al.* (2002). Activation of NADPH oxidase during progression of cardiac hypertrophy to failure. *Hypertension* 40: 477–484.

Lin CC, Hsu YF, Lin TC *et al.* (2001). Antioxidant and hepatoprotective effects of punicalegin and punicalin on acetaminophen-induced liver damage in rats. *Phytother Res* 15: 206–212.

Liu F, Ng TB (2000). Antioxidative and free radical scavenging activities of selected medicinal herbs. *Life Sci* 66: 725–735.

Louajri A, Harraga S, Godot V (2001). The effect of *Ginkgo biloba* extract on free radical production in hypoxic rats. *Biol Pharm Bull* 24: 710–712.

Lu CM, Yang JJ, Wang PY *et al.* (2000). A new acylated flavonol glycoside and antioxidant effects of *Hedyotis diffusa. Planta Med* 66: 374–377.

Lu Y, Foo LY (2002). Polyphenolics of saliva – a review. *Phytochemistry* 59: 117–140.

Luo XD, Basile MJ, Kennelly EJ (2002). Polyphenolic antioxidants from the fruits of *Chrysophyllum cainito* L. (Star Apple). *J Agric Food Chem* 50: 1379–1382.

Maccarthy PA, Grieve DJ, Li J *et al.* (2001). Impaired endothelial regulation of ventricular relaxation in cardiac hypertrophy. Role of reactive oxygen species and NADPH oxidase. *Circulation* 104: 2967–2974.

Mackeen MM, Khan MN, Samadi Z *et al.* (2000). Brine shrimp toxicity of fractionated extracts of Malaysian medicinal plants. *Nat Prod Sci* 6: 131–134.

Maiti K, Gantait A, Mukherjee K *et al.* (2006). Therapeutic potentials of andrographalide from *Andrographis paniculata*, a review. *J Nat Rem* 6: 1–13.

Mancini DM, Coyle E, Coggan A *et al.* (1989). Contribution of intrinsic skeletal muscle changes to 31P NMR skeletal muscle metabolic abnormalities in patients with chronic heart failure. *Circulation* 80: 1338–1346.

Martin-Aragon S, Basabe B, Benedi JM *et al.* (1999). In vitro and in vivo antioxidant properties of Vaccinium myrtillus. *Pharm Biol* 37: 109–113.

Mathisen E, Diallo D, Anderson OM *et al.* (2002). Antioxidants from the bark of Burkea africana, an African medicinal plant. *Phytother Res* 16: 148–153.

Mathiesen L, Malterud KE, Sund RB (1995). Antioxidant activity of fruit exudate and C-methylated dihydrochalcones from Myrica gale. *Planta Med* 59: 515–518.

Martinez Sanchez G, Chandelario-Jalil E, Giuliani A *et al.* (2001). *Mangifera indica* L. extract (QF808) reduces ischaemia-induced neuronal loss and oxidative damage in the gerbil brain. *Free Radic Res* 35: 465–473.

Martinez J, Moreno JJ (2000). Effect of resveratrol, a natural polyphenolic compound, on reactive oxygen species and prostaglandin production. *Biochem Pharmacol* 69: 865–870.

McCord JM (2000). The evolution of free radicals and oxidative stress. *Am J Med* 108: 652.

Miller Jr FJ, Gutterman DD, Rios CD *et al.* (1998). Superoxide production in vascular smooth muscle contributes to oxidative stress and impaired relaxation in atherosclerosis. *Circ Res* 82: 1298–1305.

Minami H, Kuwayama A, Yoshizawa T *et al.* (1996). Novel prenylated xanthones with antioxidant property from the wood of *Garcinia subelliptica*. *Chem Pharm Bull* 44: 2103–2106.

Misik V, Benzakova L, Malekova L *et al.* (1995). Lipoxygenase inhibition and antioxidant properties of protoberberine and aporphine alkaloids isolated from *Mahonia aquifolium*. *Planta Med* 61: 372–373.

Miura K, Kikuzaki H, Nakatani N (2002). Antioxidant activity of chemical components from sage (*Salvia officinalis* L.) and thyme (*Thymus vulfaris* L.) measured by the oil stability index method. *J Agric Food Chem* 50: 1845–1851.

Miura S, Watanabe J, Sano M *et al.* (1995). Effects of various natural antioxidant on the Cu(2)-mediated oxidative modification of low density lipoprotein. *Biol Pharm Bull* 18: 1–4.

Morel DW, DiCorleto PE, Chisolm GM (1984). Endothelial and smooth muscle cells alter low density lipoprotein by free radical oxidation. *Arteriosclerosis* 4: 357–364.

Mugge A, Brandes R, Boger RH *et al.* (1994). Vascular release of superoxide radicals is enhanced in hypercholesterolemic rabbits. *J Cardiovasc Pharmacol* 24: 994–998.

Mukherjee PK (2002). *Quality Control of Herbal Drugs: an approach to evaluation of botanicals*. Business Horizons: New Delhi, India, pp. 650–710.

Mukherjee PK (2003). Plant products with hypocholesterolemic potentials. *Adv Food Nutr Res* 47: 278–324.

Mukherjee PK, Mukherjee K (2005). Evaluation of botanicals – perspectives of quality safety and efficacy. In: *Advances in Medicinal Plants*, Vol 1, ND Prajapati, T Prajapati and S Jaypura (Eds). Asian Medicinal Plants, pp. 87–110.

Mukherjee PK, Wahile A (2006a). Perspectives of safety for natural health products. In: *Herbal Drugs – A Twenty First Century Perspective*. RK Sharma and R Arora (Eds) Jaypee Brothers Medicinal Publishers Ltd., New Delhi, pp. 50–59.

Mukherjee PK, Wahile A, Kumar V (2006b). Marker profiling for a few botanicals used for hepatoprotection in Indian systems of medicine. *Drug Inform J* 40: 131–139.

Mukherjee PK, Wahile A (2006c). Integrated approaches towards drug development from Ayurveda and other Indian systems of medicines. *J Ethanopharmacol* 103: 25–35.

Mukherjee PK, Kumar V, Mal M, Houghton PJ (2007a). Acetylcholinesterase inhibitors from plants. *Phytomedicine* 14: 289–300.

Mukherjee PK, Rai S, Kumar V *et al.* (2007b). Plants of Indian origin in drug discovery. *Expert Opin Drug Disc* 2(5): 633–657.

Nagano T, Oyama Y, Kajita N *et al.* (1997). New curcuminoids isolated from *Zingiber cassumunar* protect cells suffering from oxidative stress: a flow-cytometric study using rat thymocytes and H_2O_2. *Japan J Pharmacol* 75: 363–370.

Nishiyama Y, Ikeda H, Haramaki N *et al.* (1998). Oxidative stress is related to exercise intolerance in patients with heart failure. *Am Heart J* 135: 115–120.

Noda Y, Kaneyuki T, Mori A *et al.* (2002). Antioxidant activities of pomegranate fruit extract and its anthocyanidins: delphinidin, cyanidin, and pelargonidin. *J Agric Food Chem* 50: 166–171.

Nunez Selles AJ, Velez Castro HT, Aquero-Aquero J *et al.* (2002). Isolation and quantitative analysis of phenolic antioxidants, free sugars, and polyols from mango (*Mangifera indica* L.) stem bark aqueous decoction used in Cuba as a nutritional supplement. *J Agric Food Chem* 50: 762–766.

Ohkawa H, Ohishi N, Yagi K (1979). Assay for lipid peroxides in animal tissues by thiobarbituric acid reaction. *Ann Intern Med* 95: 351–358.

Olas R, Zhikowaka HM, Wachowicz R *et al.* (1999). Inhibitory effect of resveratrol on free radical generation in blood platelets. *Acta Biochim Polon* 46: 961–966.

Ono M, Yamamoto M, Masuoka C *et al.* (1999). Diterpenes from the fruits of *Vitex rotundifolia*. *J Nat Prod* 62: 1532–1537.

Parthasaratry S, Rankin SM (1992). Role of oxidized low density lipoproteins in atherogenesis. *Progr Lipid Res* 31: 127–143.

Pataki T, Bak I, Kovacs P *et al.* (2002). Grape seed proanthocyanidine improved cardiac recovery during reperfusion after ischemia in isolated rat hearts. *Am J Clin Nutr* 75: 894–899.

Pawar R, Gopalakrishnan C, Bhutani KK (2001). Dammarane triterpene saponin from Bacopa monniera as the superoxide inhibitor in polymorphonuclear cells. *Planta Med* 67: 752–754.

Paya M, Halliwell B, Hoult JR (1992). Interactions of a series of coumarins with reactive oxygen species. Scavenging of superoxide, hypochlorous acid and hydroxyl radicals. *Biochem Pharmacol* 44(2): 205–214.

Perry NS, Houghton PJ, Sampson J *et al.* (2001). In-vitro activity of *S. lavandulacfolia* (Spanish sage) relevant to treatment of Alzheimer's disease. *J Pharm Pharmacol* 53: 1347–1356.

Pham TQ, Cormier F, Farnworth E *et al.* (2000). Antioxidant properties of crocin from Gardenia jasminoides Ellis and study of the reactions of crocin with linoleic acid and crocin with oxygen. *J Agric Food Chem* 48: 1455–1461.

Pietrangelo A, Borella F, Casalgrandi G *et al.* (1995). Antioxidant activity of silybin in vivo during long-term iron overload in rats. *Gastroenterology* 109: 1941–1949.

Pietri S, Culcasi M, Cozzone PJ (1989). Real-time continuous-flow spin trapping of hydroxyl radical in the ischemic and post-ischemic myocardium. *Eur J Biochem* 186: 163–173.

Psotova J, Chlopcikova S, Grambal F *et al.* (2002). Influence of silymarin and its flavonolignans on doxorubicin-iron induced lipid peroxidation in rat heart microsomes and mitochondria in comparison with quenrcetin. *Phytother Res* 1: S63–S67.

Pukalskas A, Van Beek TA, Venskutonis BP *et al.* (2002). Identification of radical scavengers in sweet grass (*Hicrochloc odorata*). *J Agric Food Chem* 50: 2914–2919.

Rai S, Basak S, Mukherjee K *et al.* (2007). Oriental medicine *Mangifera indica* – a review. *Orient Pharm Exp Med* 7: 1–10.

Rai S, Wahile A, Mukherjee K *et al.* (2006a). Antioxidant activity of Nelumbo nucifera (Sacred Lotus) seeds. *J Ethanopharmacol* 104: 322–327.

Rai S, Mukherjee K, Mal M *et al.* (2006b). Determination of 6-gingerol in ginger (*Zingiber officinale*) using high-performance thin-layer chromatography. *J Separation Sci* 29: 2292–2295.

Raja S, Nazeer Ahamed KFH, Kumar V *et al.* (2007). Antioxidant effect of *Cytisus scoparius* against carbon tetrachloride treated liver injury in rats. *J Ethnopharmacol* 109: 41–47.

Rajagopalan S, Meng XP, Ramasamy S (1996). Reactive oxygen species produced by macrophage-derived foam cells regulate the activity of vascular matrix metalloproteinases invitro. Implications for atherosclerotic plaque stability. *J Clin Invest* 98: 2572–2579.

Rajbhandari I, Takamatsu S, Nagle DG (2001). A new dehydropteranylgeraniol antioxidant from *Saururus cernuus* that inhibits intracellular reactive oxygen species (ROS)-catalyzed oxidation within HL-60 cells. *J Nat Prod* 64: 693–695.

Ramsewak RS, Nair MG, Dewitt DC *et al.* (1999). Phenolic glycosides from *Dirca palustris*. *J Nat Prod* 62: 1558–1561.

Rastogi R, Srivastava AK, Srivastava M *et al.* (2000). Hepatocurative effect of picroliv and silymarin against aflatoxin B induced hepatotoxicity in rats. *Planta Med* 66: 709–713.

Rekka EA, Kourounakis PN (1994). Investigation of the molecular mechanism of the antioxidant activity of some *Allium sativum* ingredients. *Pharmazie* 49(Jul): 539–540.

Rohde LE, Ducharme A, Arroyo LH *et al.* (1999). Matrix metalloproteinase inhibition attenuates early left ventricular enlargement after experimental myocardial infarction in mice. *Circulation* 99: 3063–3070.

Sang S, Lapsley K, Jeong WS *et al.* (2002). Antioxidative phenolic compounds isolated from almond skins (*Prunus amygdalue* Batsch). *J Agric Food Chem* 50: 2459–2463.

Scartezzini P, Speroni E (2000). Review of some plants of Indian traditional medicine with antioxidant activity. *J Ethanopharmacol* 71: 23–43.

Schubert SY, Lanslay EP, Neeman I (1999). Antioxidant and eicosanoid enzyme inhibition properties of pomegranate seed oil and fermented juice flavonoids. *J Ethanopharmacol* 66: 11–17.

Selvam R, Subramanian L, Gayathri R *et al.* (1995). The antioxidant activity of turmeric. *J Ethanopharmacol* 47: 59–67.

Sharma M, Kishore K, Gupta SK *et al.* (2001). Cardioprotective potential of *Oimum sanctum* in isoproterenol induced myocardial infarction in rats. *Mol Cell Biochem* 225: 75–83.

Sies H (1991). Oxidative stress: from basic research to clinical application. *Am J Med* 91 (supp. 3C): 31–38.

Silva DH, Davino SC, Barros YM (1999). Dihydrochalcones and flavonolignans from *Iryanthera lanicifolia*. *J Nat Prod* 62: 1475–1478.

Simi D, Simi T, Mimi-Oka J *et al.* (1998). *Antioxidant status in patients with essential hypertension.* XIII World Congress of Cardiology, Monduzzi Editore Sp. A. Bologna, 421–425.

Simonian NA, Coyle JT (1996). Oxidative stress in neurodegenerative diseases. *Annu Rev Pharmacol Toxicol* 36: 83–106.

Singh RP, Chidambaramurthy KN, Jayaprakasha GK (2002). Studies on the antioxidant activity of pomegranate (*Punica granatum*) peel and seed extracts using in vitro models. *J Agric Food Chem* 50: 81–86.

Siwik DA, Tzortzis JD, Pimental DR *et al.* (1999). Inhibition of copperzinc superoxide dismutase induces cell growth, hypertrophic phenotype, and apoptosis in neonatal rat cardiac myocytes invitro. *Circ Res* 85: 147–153.

Siwik DA, Pagano PJ, Colucci WS (2001). Oxidative stress regulates collagen synthesis and matrix metalloproteinase activity in cardiac fibroblasts. *Am J Physiol* 280: C53–60.

Sloley BD, Urichuk LJ, Morley P *et al.* (2000). Identification of kaempferol as a monoamine oxidase inhibitor and potential neuroprotectant in extracts of *Ginkgo biloba* leaves. *J Pharm Pharmacol* 52: 451–459.

Sreejayam N, Rao MN, Priyadarsini KI *et al.* (1997). Inhibition of radiation induced lipid peroxidation by curcumin. *Int J Pharm* 151: 127–130.

Sreejayam Rao MMA (1994). Curcuminoids as potent inhibitor of lipid peroxidation. *J Pharm Pharmacol* 46: 1013–1016.

Starkopf J, Zilmer K, Vihalemm T *et al.* (1995). Time-course of oxidative stress during open-heart surgery. *Scand J Thorac Cardiovasc Surg* 29(4): 181–186.

Starkopf J, Tamme K, Zilmer M *et al.* (1997). The evidence of oxidative stress in cardiac and septic patients: a comparative study. *Clin Chim Acta* 262: 77–88.

Stepp DW, Ou J, Acherman AW *et al.* (2002). Native LDL and minimally oxidized LDL differentially regulate superoxide anion in vascular endothelium in situ. *Am J Physiol Heart Circ Physiol* 283: H750–H759.

Sumathy T, Subramanian S, Govidasamy S *et al.* (2001). Protective role of *Bacopa monnicra* on morphine induced hepatotoxicity in rats. *Phytother Res* 15: 643–645.

Tang Y, Lou F, Wang J, Li Y *et al.* (2001). Coumaroyl flavonol glycosides from the leaves of *Ginkgo biloba*. *Phytochemistry* 58: 1251–1256.

Tarpey MM, Fridovich I (2001). Methods of detection of vascular reactive species nitric oxide, superoxide, hydrogen peroxide and peroxynitrite. *Circ Res* 89: 224.

Tiwari AK, Srinivas PV, Kumar SP *et al.* (2001). Free radical scavenging active components from *Codrus decodara*. *J Agric Food Chem* 49: 4642–4645.

Tripathi YB, Chaurasia S, Tripathi E *et al.* (1995). *Bacopa monniera* Linn. as an antioxidant: mechanism of action. *Indian J Exp Biol* 34: 523–526.

Tripathi YB, Chaurasia S (1996). Effect of *Strychnos nux vomica* alcohol extract on lipid peroxidation in rat liver. *Int J Pharmacogn* 34: 295–299.

Tse WY, Maxwell SR, Thomason H *et al.* (1994). Antioxidant status in controlled and uncontrolled hypertension and its relationship to endothelial damage. *J Hum Hypertension* 8: 843–849.

Tsutsui H, Ide T, Hayashidani S *et al.* (2001). Enhanced generation of reactive oxygen species in the limb skeletal muscles from a murine infarct model of heart failure. *Circulation* 104(2): 134–136.

Uma Devi P, Ganasoundari A (1999). Modulation of glytathione and antioxidant enzymes by *Ocimum sanctum* and is role in protection against radiation injury. *Indian J Exp Biol* 37: 262–268.

Vaya J, Belinky PA, Avtram M (1997). Antioxidant consituents from licorice roots: isolation, structure elucidation and antioxidative capacity toward LDL oxidation. *Free Radic Biol Med* 23: 302–313.

Wang H, Nair MG, Strasburg GM *et al.* (1999). Novel antioxidant compounds from tart cherries (*Prunus cerasus*). *J Nat Prod* 62: 86–88.

Wang SY, Kuo YH, Chang HN *et al.* (2002). Profiling and characterization antioxidant activities in *Anocctochilus formosanus* hayata. *J Agric Food Chem* 50: 1859–1865.

Wang W, Weng X, Cheng D (2000). Antioxidant activities of natural phenolic components from *Dalbergia odorifera* T. Chen. *Food Chem* 71: 45–49.

Warnholtz A, Nickenig G, Schulz E *et al.* (1999). Increased NADH-oxidase-mediated superoxide production in the early stages of atherosclerosis. Evidence for involvement of the renin–angiotensin system. *Circulation* 99: 2027–2033.

Wei T, Sun H, Zhao X *et al.* (2002). Scavenging of reactive oxygen species and prevention of oxidative neuronal cell damage by a novel gallotannin, pistafolia A. *Life Sci* 70: 1889–1899.

White CR, Brock TA, Chang LY *et al.* (1994). Superoxide and peroxynitrite in atherosclerosis. *Proc Natl Acad Sci USA* 91(3): 1044–1048.

Wilson JR (1995). Exercise intolerance in heart failure. Importance of skeletal muscle. *Circulation* 91: 559–561.

Yamaguchi F, Saito M, Ariga T *et al.* (2000). Free radical scavenging activity and antiulcer activity of garcinol from *Garcinia india* fruit rind. *J Agric Food Chem* 48: 2320–2325.

Yokozawa T, Cho EJ, Hara Y (2000). Antioxidative activity of green tea treated with radical initiator z, 2′-azobis (2-amidinopropane) dihydrochloride. *J Agric Food Chem* 48: 5068–5073.

Ytrehus K, Hegstad AC (1991). Lipid peroxidation and membrane damage of heart. *Acta Physiol Scand* S599: 81–91.

Zupko I, Hohmann J, Redei D *et al.* (2001). Antioxidant activity of leaves of salvia species in enzyme-dependent and enzyme-independent systems of lipid peroxidation and their phenolic constituents. *Planta Med* 67: 366–368.

20

Herbal medicinal products affecting memory and cognitive disorders

Pulok K Mukherjee, KFH Nazeer Ahmed, V Kumar, N Satheesh Kumar and Peter J Houghton

Introduction

The human brain is very complex and is based on specialised cells designed to transmit information, called neurones. Neurones are an integral part and basic functional unit of the brain, which contains almost one billion of these cells. The neurones consists of a cell body containing a nucleus and an electricity-conducting fibre called an axon, which also gives rise to many branches before ending at nerve terminals. Neurones send signals by transmitting electrical impulses along their axons. When the signals reach the end of the axons, they trigger the release neurotransmitters, which then bind to receptors in adjacent neurones. This point of vital contact is called the synapse. The synaptic response involves the closing and opening of ion channels, which pass through the cell membranes and enable the ions to flow through them. This phenomenon creates an electrical current that provides tiny voltage changes across the membrane which leads to altered synaptic connectivity.

This network is capable of controlling a vast array of activities, including heart rate, body movement, perception, sexual function, emotions, learning and memory. The organisation and neurotransmitter content of intrinsic cerebral cortical and hippocampal neurones, and those of extrinsic inputs to these regions, are described below with respect to neuronal systems known to be affected in Alzheimer-type dementia. For the intrinsic neurones, particular attention is focused on the neuropeptides such as cholecystokinin, vasoactive intestinal polypeptide, somatostatin and neuropeptide Y, which are apparently stable post mortem and provide biochemical markers that can be used to judge the integrity of neuropeptide-containing cells in dementia (Emson and Lindvall, 1986).

Neurochemistry of cognition and cognitive dysfunction: cholinergic hypothesis

The first neurochemical was identified 70 years ago as acetylcholine. The neurones that release acetylcholine are called cholinergic neurones and control the heartbeat and voluntary muscles, causing them to contract. Acetylcholine also serves as a neurotransmitter in many regions of the brain and plays an important role in learning and memory function. Mammalian brain contains several groups of cholinergic projection neurones located within the basal forebrain and brainstem (Nagai *et al.*, 1983). Cholinergic axons exert their neurotransmitter effect through the mediation of nicotinic and muscarinic receptors. Cholinergic neurones and cholinergic neurotransmitter pathways are highly implicated in cognition and cognitive dysfunction (Scarpini *et al.*, 2003). The cholinergic neurones are centred on the medial septum, around the vertical limb of the diagonal band of Broca, around the horizontal limb of the diagonal band of Broca, and are also found around the nucleus basalis of Meynert (Parent *et al.*, 1989; Mesulam *et al.*, 1983).

All cholinergic neurones of the human basal forebrain and brain stem contain the cholinergic enzymes choline acetyltransferase and acetylcholinesterase (Hedreen *et al.*, 1984; Geula *et al.*, 1989). Much of the research on the participation of neurotransmitter systems in cognitive decline associated with ageing and Alzheimer's disease has concentrated on the role of acetylcholine, because of its correlation with the degree of cognitive dysfunction, and learning and memory deficits produced in humans, even though the role of interaction between acetylcholine and other neurotransmitters such as noradrenaline, dopamine, serotonin, γ-aminobutyric acid (GABA) and several neuropeptides affecting cognition are also important (Perry *et al.*, 1981; Coyle *et al.*, 1983). To improve cholinergic transmission, different strategies have been suggested including increased acetylcholine synthesis, the augmentation of presynaptic acetylcholine release, and stimulation of postsynaptic acetylcholine muscarinic and nicotinic receptors and reduction of acetylcholine synaptic degradation with cholinesterase inhibitors. Several aspects of the functional features of the cholinergic system are shown in Figure 20.1.

Assessment of neurodegeneration

Animal models used for the assessment

Drugs effective in neurodegenerative disease should have several aims: to improve the cognitive impairment, control the behavioural and neurological symptoms, delay the progression of the disease and to prevent the onset. To attain these targets, cell and animal models are needed in which pathogenetic hypothesis and potential effectiveness of new drugs are to be tested, exploiting links between the molecular and biochemical studies on the disease and the reality of human pathology. Animal models of Alzheimer's disease can provide insight into the neurological and pathological mechanisms of cognitive and behavioural changes in patients. Monitoring

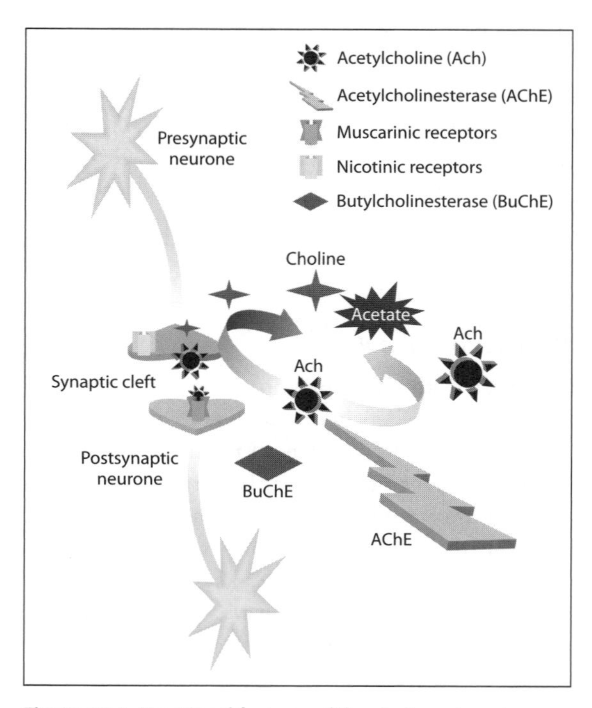

Figure 20.1 Functional features of the cholinergic system.

of behavioural changes in animal models could both provide insight into the neurobiology of these behavioural changes and help validate the felicity of the model to Alzheimer's disease. Animal models will play a critical role in further defining the events and processes underlying the final phenotypic expression.

Aged animals models

Aged animals (rats, mice and monkeys) have been investigated on a variety of learning and memory tasks. Aged rodents have been shown to have memory impairment on tasks such as the Morris water maze and passive avoidance tests. This behavioural impairment has provided a model that resembles the neuropsychiatric symptoms commonly observed in Alzheimer's disease. The senescence-accelerated mouse (SAM) exhibits age-related deficits in learning and memory in the Morris water maze and radial arm maze and decreased acetylcholine synthesis in hippocampus pyramidal neurones (Flicker *et al.*, 1983; Bartus *et al.*, 1985; Allain *et al.*, 1998). The effect of nerve growth factor (NGF) on cognition of aged rats has been assessed by intraventricular infusion of NGF, delayed alternation, Morris water maze, and sensory motor tasks. NGF has been most thoroughly assessed in this setting and has shown effects in rats (Koliatsos *et al.*, 1991; Tuszynski *et al.*, 1991; Frautschy *et al.*, 1996), which have provided a model for the assessment of cholinergic neurones and the cholinoprotective effects of compounds potentially useful in the treatment of Alzheimer's disease.

Brain lesion models

In concert with the recognition of the importance of the cholinergic deficit in Alzheimer's disease, early models of the disease concentrated on surgical or chemical lesions of the basal forebrain. Transection of the fornix results in degeneration of cholinergic cells in the basal forebrain. These experiments involved primarily rats, monkeys and baboons, which demonstrated deficits in attention and memory, tested in various maze paradigms such as passive active avoidance, Morris water maze and the eight-arm radial arm maze (Flicker *et al.*, 1983; Bartus *et al.*, 1985; Allain *et al.*, 1998). Lesion studies have focused primarily on the behavioural changes of the animals, with only limited attention to the pathological to the neuropsychiatric symptoms commonly observed in Alzheimer's disease. Ageing studies are all likely to contribute information important to our understanding of the disease, and none are likely to represent a completely isomorphic model that is fully predictive of the pathogenesis, course, and treatment of human Alzheimer's disease.

Amyloid beta protein infusion induced model of Alzheimer's disease

Artificially created amyloid (AS) deposits in normal rats, and transgenic mice overexpressing amyloid precursor protein (APP) are the models in which possible treatments are tested. They are aimed at preventing formation of AS deposits or its transformation in neuritic plaques. Synthetic amyloid beta protein ($A\beta_{1-42}$) application in vitro, using neuroglial and astrocytes, has also been used to screen various neuroprotective drugs. The injection of synthetic Aβ peptides β_{12-28}, β_{25-35} and β_{1-40} into the septum of adult rats induced a marked decrease in basal and potassium-evoked acetylcholine release in the hippocampus. These findings confirmed in vivo the neurotoxic effects of Aβ observed in primary neuronal cell cultures exposed to Aβ peptides (Koh *et al.*, 1990; Yankner *et al.*, 1990).

The multiple mechanisms through which Aβ peptides, involving oxidative stress, loss of cellular calcium homeostasis and mitochondrial dysfunction have been reviewed and, in both in-vitro and in-vivo experiments, it has been shown that Aβ neurotoxicity depends on its fibrillary aggregation forming a sheet (Giovannelli *et al.*, 1998). These preclinical experiments give support to the hypothesis of the pivotal pathogenetic role of AS deposit in Alzheimer's disease, throw some light on the molecular mechanisms of AS toxicity, and offer an experimental model for testing potentially useful drugs. Undoubtedly, there are limitations in the validity of intracerebral Aβ injections as a model of Alzheimer's disease.

Amyloid precursor protein transgenic mouse model

The development of transgenic mice, mimicking the genetic mutations occurring in familial Alzheimer's disease and showing some of the neurochemical and morphological alterations of the disease, is another example of the interactions between clinical and preclinical investigations into this disease. The clinical and genetic investigations have identified the early-onset, familial forms of the disease, and the genes in which autosomal dominant mutations take place. There is a clear recognition of autosomal dominant cases induced by mutations of *APP* (chromosome 21), *presenilin 1* (chromosome 14), or *presenilin 2* (chromosome 1), which allowed development of transgenic mouse models of Alzheimer's disease (Sarter *et al.*, 1992). These transgenic animals exhibit some of the pathological hallmarks of the disease, including neuritic plaques, although they have not evidenced neurofibrillary tangles and have limited cell death. These models facilitate investigation of the relationship of amyloid deposition to other aspects of the pathology of Alzheimer's disease, including inflammation, hormonal levels, trophic factor influences, calcium metabolism, amino acid toxicity and apoptosis. However, there has been limited behavioural testing of transgenic mice, but impairments of memory have been reported on the Morris water maze, spatial reference memory and Y-maze alternation tasks.

Apolipoprotein knockout models

Cognitive tasks analogous to the deficits observed in human Alzheimer's disease need to be developed for application to transgenic, knockout and other models currently used to investigate pathogenesis. Tests of language are obviously not applicable but assessment of attention, memory, spatial orientation and executive function are feasible (Hsiao *et al.*, 1996; Weiss and Kilts, 1998). A variety of transgenic and knockout apolipoprotein models are available to screen novel molecules for the treatment of the disease. The *E-4* allele of apolipoprotein (*ApoE-4*) confers an increased risk for Alzheimer's disease and a decreased age of onset. Review of the cognitive testing and behavioural measures of the various available animal models reveals the impoverished state of these assessments and the need to develop new evaluation technologies.

Brain inflammation models

Epidemiological and clinical studies (Mcgeer and Mcgeer, 1995), reporting the efficacy of non-steroidal anti-inflammatory drugs (NSAIDs) in reducing the incidence and progression of Alzheimer's disease, provided strong support for the critical involvement of inflammatory processes in the pathogenesis of the disease. Brain inflammation is considered to be a pathogenetic link in many neurodegenerative diseases, including Alzheimer's disease (Mcgeer and Mcgeer, 1998). The long-term lipopolysaccharide (LPS) infusion into the fourth ventricle was followed by astrocyte activation, an increase in microglia cells, an increase in the levels of interleukin (IL)-1β, tumour necrosis factor (TNF)-α, *APP* mRNA and the degeneration of hippocampal neurones.

In-vitro screening methods for acetylcholinesterase inhibition

Several methods have been reported for the screening of acetylcholinesterase inhibitory activity from herbal medicinal products (HMPs). Acetylcholinesterase inhibition was initially detected by the use of gut-bath pharmacological methods with isolated tissue preparations such as guinea pig ileum (Houghton *et al.*, 2006). These methods are costly in several respects, including time, animal tissue and amounts of compound needed, so they have been replaced by more sensitive chemical methods. Consideration of the relative merits of various methods that might be useful in studying the time course of acetylcholinesterase activity in very small tissue samples use a combined method reported by Koelle (1951) with a sulphydryl reagent studied by Ellman (1959). This Ellman method is extremely sensitive and is applicable to either small amounts of tissue or to low concentrations of enzyme.

The principle of this colorimetric method is the measurement of the rate of production of thiocholine, as acetylthiocholine is hydrolysed by the acetylcholinesterase enzyme. Thiocholine reacts with Ellman reagent [5,5′-dithiobis-(2-nitro-benzoic acid) (DTNB)] to produce 2-nitrobenzoate-5-mercaptothiocholine and 5-thio-2-nitrobenzoate (Figure 20.2). This product has a yellow chromophore that can be detected at 405 nm. The reaction with the thiol has been shown to be sufficiently rapid so as not to be rate limiting in the measurement of the enzyme, and in the concentrations used does not inhibit the enzymatic hydrolysis. The absorbance obtained using a standard volume of a known concentration of the substrate with a fixed dose of acetylcholinesterase is

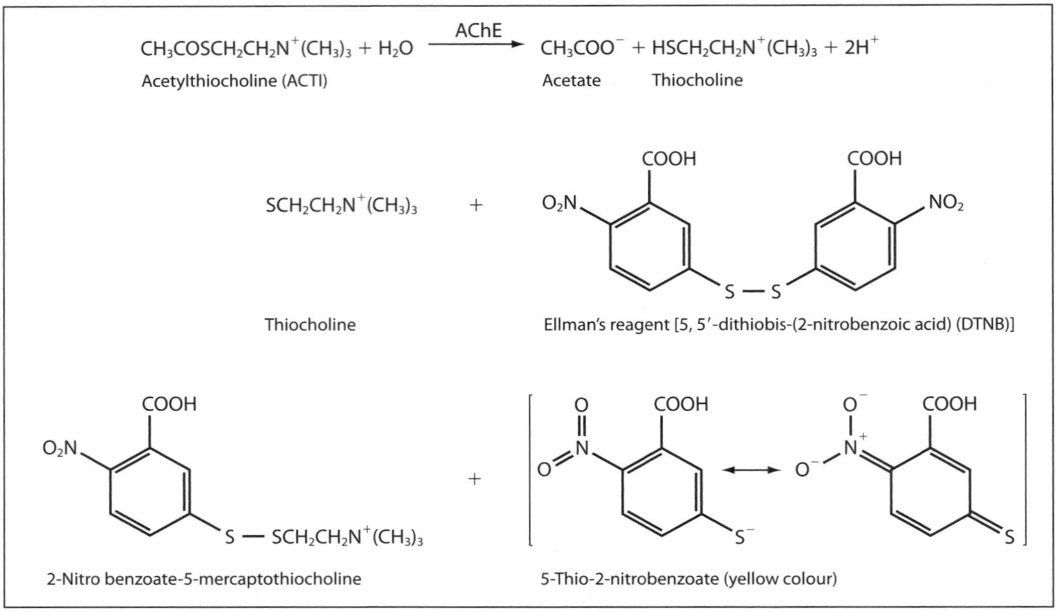

$$CH_3COSCH_2CH_2N^+(CH_3)_3 + H_2O \xrightarrow{AChE} CH_3COO^- + HSCH_2CH_2N^+(CH_3)_3 + 2H^+$$

Acetylthiocholine (ACTI) Acetate Thiocholine

$SCH_2CH_2N^+(CH_3)_3$ + Ellman's reagent

Thiocholine

Ellman's reagent [5, 5′-dithiobis-(2-nitrobenzoic acid) (DTNB)]

2-Nitro benzoate-5-mercaptothiocholine + 5-Thio-2-nitrobenzoate (yellow colour)

Figure 20.2 The detection of acetylcholinesterase activity by Ellman's method.

compared with that in the presence of an added compound or extract, a significant reduction indicating an inhibitory role for the substance added.

This visible spectroscopy procedure requires several millilitres of reaction mixture and it was sometimes difficult to obtain enough material to show an effect. The development of the method for use on a smaller scale, using microtitre well plates and a microplate reader, has been introduced and has enabled determinations to be performed with a much higher throughput. Microtitre plate assay method requires smaller amounts of reagents and test substances (Ingkaninan *et al.*, 2000; Brlihlmann *et al.*, 2004).

The Ellman reaction has also been adapted for thin-layer chromatography (TLC) bioautography assay for acetylcholinesterase inhibitory activity (Rhee *et al.*, 2001). The TLC plate is developed in the usual way. After development, enzyme-inhibitory activities of the developed spots were detected by spraying the substrate, dye and enzyme based on Ellman's method. After incubating the plates, white spots on a yellow background showed inhibition of acetylcholinesterase. A false-positive test is carried out, to confirm any acetylcholinesterase-inhibiting activity arising from inhibition of thiocholine hydrolysis caused by the enzyme. To detect false-positive reactions, the plate is sprayed with substrate, dye and enzyme without test compounds. After a few minutes incubation, a yellow background appeared, the occurrence of white spots indicating false-positive reactions.

A similar method for TLC detection has been introduced by Marston *et al.* (2002), which uses acetylnaphthol as the substrate and measures the amount of naphthol, the reaction product formed, by its chromogenic reaction with Fast Blue B salt (Mukherjee *et al.*, 2007a).

High-performance liquid chromatography (HPLC) with online coupled ultraviolet, mass spectrometric and biochemical detection methods for the identification of acetylcholinesterase inhibitors has also been developed (Ingkaninan *et al.*, 2000). This uses a reverse-phase column with the column eluate being split into two streams, one with an ultraviolet detector and the other connected to a biochemical detection system. This latter system consisted of the eluant being mixed with acetylcholinesterase and DTNB before the online introduction of acetylthiocholine. The intensity of the reaction product was measured at 405 nm by means of a spectrophotometer as an indication of the amount of thiocholine-DTNB product formed. A

HPLC method for the detection of acetylcholinesterase inhibition on immobilised acetylcholinesterase column and HPLC with online coupled ultraviolet, mass spectrometric and biochemical detection for acetylcholinesterase inhibitory activity has also been reported (Ingkaninan *et al.*, 2000).

Effect of HMPs on neurotransmission and enhancing cognition

HMPs have played a pivotal role in development of CNS-active drugs that affect neurotransmissions in the brain (Mukherjee *et al.*, 2002; Howes and Houghton, 2003; Howes *et al.*, 2003; Mukherjee, 2007e). The interest of CNS-active HMPs originated from opioid alkaloids, e.g. morphine from *Papaver somniferum* and the tropane alkaloid cocaine from *Erythroxylon coca*. Anticholinesterase agents such as physostigmine from *Physostigma venosum* have shown significant activity on the CNS (Mukherjee, 2002; Houghton *et al.*, 2006; Mukherjee *et al.*, 2007a; 2007b). This chapter deals with various medicinal plants, and compounds derived from them, which affect neurotransmission related to behaviour and memory dysfunction.

Acorus calamus L. (sweet flag, calamus)

Acorus calamus L. (Araceae) is a semi-aquatic, perennial, aromatic herb with creeping rhizomes. In Ayurveda, herbal medicines with rasayana effects (plants having adaptogen-like properties) are believed to be restorative, to attain longevity, intelligence and freedom from age-related disorders. *A. calamus* (AC) is regarded in Ayurvedic medicine as promoting rasayana effects and has been used to treat memory loss (Mukherjee and Wahile, 2006). *A. calamus* is used in Ayurvedic medicine on a regular basis for the treatment of loss of memory and other mental disorders (Howes and Houghton, 2003). AC extract has also been used as a traditional Chinese prescription and its beneficial effects on memory disorder, on learning performance, lipid peroxide content and anti-ageing effect in senescence have been reported (Mukherjee *et al.*, 2007c). The in-vitro acetylcholinesterase inhibitory effect of hydro-alcoholic extract and essential oil of AC rhizomes has been reported, based on Ellman's method. The essential oil showed stronger inhibition than the hydroalcoholic extract (Mukherjee *et al.*, 2007d). Methanol extracts of AC showed significant acetylcholinesterase enzyme inhibition at the concentration 200 μg/mL (Oh *et al.*, 2004). Mukherjee *et al.* (2007d) reported the in-vitro acetylcholinesterase inhibitory effect of β-asarone and α-asarone from the AC. β-Asarone is at least an order of magnitude more active than its *trans* isomer α-asarone, so the acetylcholinesterase-inhibitory activity of the oil can be ascribed to β-asarone. Since cognitive performance and memory are related to acetylcholine levels, the acetylcholinesterase-inhibitory effect of the plant may account for its traditional use.

Albizia lebbeck Benth. (lebbeck)

Albizia lebbeck Benth. (Mimosaceae), is a well-known Indian medicinal plant and it has been reported to possess nootropic activity. The saponin-rich *n*-butanol fraction separated from leaves of *A. lebbeck* has been shown to affect the normal and impaired memory function in rats (Pal *et al.*, 1995; Pratibha *et al.*, 2004). Semi-purified saponins at doses of 10, 25 and 50 mg/kg, when administered orally, enhanced the learning and memory of normal and amnesic rats induced by scopolamine. Administration of 10 and 25 mg/kg of the saponin-containing butanol fraction increased the step-down latencies in acquisition and retention period as measured by inflexion ratio on the second and ninth day at levels comparable with the standard nootropic agent piracetum (100 mg/kg) tested in both the passive avoidance 'step-through test' using a passive avoidance chamber and the elevated plus maze test.

The nootropic effect of the natural saponins was correlated with concentrations of various neurochemicals of the rat brain, since dopamine and GABA levels decreased, and serotonin and noradrenaline increased in the *A. lebbeck*-treated mice. The memory-enhancing property of the saponin fraction from *A. lebbeck* is considered to be due to inhibition of GABA and enhancement of noradrenaline in the brain (Chintawar *et al.*, 2002). Three active albizia saponins A, B, and C were isolated and identified (Pal *et al.*, 1995; Al-Showiman, 1998).

Amaranthus paniculatus L. (amaranth)

Amaranthus paniculatus L. (Amaranthaceae) is said to overcome the problems of psychological stress and affordability and its effects have been tested in stress-induced memory dysfunction. Stress was induced by gamma radiation in mice and methanolic extract of *A. paniculatus* at a dose of 600 mg/kg and 800 mg/kg was administered orally for 15 days. It was observed that mice supplemented with the extract, and trained in Hebb William's maze model D, took less time to reach the goal than those without any treatment. The mice treated with *A. paniculatus* were further exposed to gamma radiation by ^{60}Co-beam therapy; the surviving mice took less time to reach their goals than those without plant extract (Bhatia *et al.*, 2003). This finding is explained by presuming that mice supplemented with *A. paniculatus* have a lower concentration of free radicals formed by the radiation stress and so less damage occurs to the relevant parts of the brain, therefore leading to sustenance of the learning ability even after irradiation. The study has been correlated with the anti-oxidative property of nutrients and their effect on maintaining cholinergic neurone integrity, which is essential for maintaining the learning and memory process.

Azadirachta indica A. Juss. (neem)

A. indica (Meliaceae) is a well-known traditional herb in India and is reported to exert therapeutic effects relating to the CNS. Azardirachitin is a major constituents found in neem. The aqueous extract of leaves at the dose of 500 mg/kg for 7 days significantly improved the memory, which was impaired by cerebral hypoperfusion inducing ischaemic insult (Yanpallewar *et al.*, 2005). The memory task of the ischaemic rats was tested after 2 weeks of hypoperfusion period in the Morris water maze. The aqueous extract from *A. indica* significantly prevented the delay in escape latencies and increased the acquisition memory of rats.

Bacopa monniera L. (brahmi)

Bacopa monnieri L. (Scrophulariaceae) has a long history of use in India as an anti-ageing and memory-enhancing ethnobotanical therapy. It has been mentioned in religious, social and medical treatises of India since the time of Atharvan Ved (800 BC); the first clear reference to its CNS effect is to be found in *Charak Samhita*, written in the first century AD. It is mentioned in the authentic Ayurvedic treatise, *Susrutu Samhita*, which describes brahmi as efficacious in the loss of intellect and memory.

The alcoholic extract of brahmi showed a beneficial effect on the acquisition, consolidation and retention of three newly acquired behavioural responses in albino rats (Singh *et al.*, 1982). Alcoholic extract of brahmi (40 mg/kg) and its two important chemical constituents, bacosides A and B (10 mg/kg), were investigated for shock-motivated brightness discrimination reaction, active conditioned avoidance and conditioned taste aversion response. Preadministration for 3 days with bacosides A and B significantly improved the acquisition, consolidation and retention in all three behavioural paradigms. Beside this effect bacosides attenuated the retrograde amnesia produced by immobilisation-induced stress, and scopolamine (Singh and Dhawan, 1997).

In another experiment, standardised *B. monniera* extract was concluded to be beneficial in animal models of Alzheimer's disease and elevated levels of their central cholinergic markers such as choline acetyltransferase and acetylcholine (Bhattacharya *et al.*, 1999). Chronic administration of *B. monniera* given orally for 12 weeks improved the speed of early information processing, verbal learning rate and memory consolidation in humans (Stough *et al.*, 2001). This finding supported previous preclinical animal studies and clinical studies in children (Sharma *et al.*, 1987) and patients with anxiety neurosis. *B. monniera* interferes with cholinergic transmission and also has some serotonergic modulation (Singh and Singh, 1980).

Celastrus paniculatus Willd. (staff tree)

C. paniculatus (Celastraceae) seeds and seed oil have been used in Ayurvedic medicine for stimulating intellect and sharpening the memory. It has been reported to have beneficial effects in psychiatric patients (Warrier *et al.*, 1995; Nadkarni, 1996). Administration of the seed oil, rich in sesquiterpenes, to rats also reversed a scopolamine-induced memory deficit assessed in navigational memory performance, but this effect was not associated with acetylcholinesterase activity (Gattu *et al.*, 1997). The seed oil (3 g/kg) significantly improved the retention ability of the drug-treated rat passive avoidance paradigm and decreased levels of noradrenaline, dopamine, serotonin and their metabolites (Nalini *et al.*, 1995). Beside this, the memory-enhancing effect of *C. paniculatus* was correlated with the antioxidant-enhancing effect of the drug on brain tissue (Kumar *et al.*, 2002a; Godkar *et al.*, 2003). These data indicate that *C. paniculatus* oil causes an overall decrease in the turnover of the three central monoamines and implicates the involvement of these aminergic systems in the learning and memory process.

Centella asiatica L. (gota kola)

C. asiatica (Umbelliferae) is a reputed ancient Ayurvedic remedy to enhance memory and longevity (Kapoor, 1990). The pharmacological basis to explain the reputed anti-amnesic effects of *C. asiatica* has been explored experimentally. Studies have shown that the alcoholic extract has a tranquillising effect in rats, which was attributed to α-triterpene and brahmoside (Sakina and Dandiya, 1990). *Centella asiatica* ethanolic extract was also found to elicit a marked increase in neurite outgrowth in human SH-SY5Y cells in the presence of nerve growth factor. Asiatic acid in *Centella* ethanolic extract showed marked activity at 1 μg/mL. Neurite elongation by Asiatic acid was completely blocked by the extracellular-signal-regulated kinase (ERK) pathway inhibitor PD 098059 (10 μmol/L). Male Sprague–Dawley rats given *Centella* ethanolic extract in their drinking water (300–330 mg/kg daily) demonstrated more rapid functional recovery and increased axonal regeneration (larger-calibre axons and greater numbers of myelinated axons) compared with controls, indicating that the axons grew at a faster rate (Soumyanath *et al.*, 2005). Further studies showed that the extract of *C. asiatica* leaf possessed cholinomimetic action in vivo (Sakina and Dandiya, 1990) and that it may also influence cholinergic activity, and thus cognitive function.

Cognitive-enhancing effects have been observed in rats following oral administration of an aqueous extract of *C. asiatica,* this effect being associated with an antioxidant mechanism in the CNS (Kumar *et al.*, 2002b). The essential oil from *C. asiatica* leaf contains monoterpenes, e.g. α-pinene, β-pinene and γ-terpinene (Brinkhaus *et al.*, 2000), which are reported to inhibit acetylcholinesterase (Ryan and Byrne, 1988; Miyazawa *et al.*, 1997; Perry *et al.*, 2000). However, monoterpene acetylcholinesterase inhibitors are weak compared with the anticholinesterase alkaloid, physostigmine (Perry *et al.*, 2000). In view of the relatively weak anticholinesterase activity of monoterpenes reported to date, it is unlikely that they would be therapeutically effective in cognitive disorders. Asiatic acid, a triterpene from *C. asiatica* (L.) has been patented as a treatment for dementia and an enhancer of cognition by Hoechst (EP 0 383 171 A2).

Clitoria ternatea L.

The root of the Indian medicinal plant *C. ternatea* (Fabaceae) has a reputation for promoting intellectual behaviour (Misra, 1998). *C. ternatea* contains the triterpenes taraxerol and taraxerone as major phytoconstituents (Kumar *et al.*, 2007). Administration of *C. ternatea* root extract to rats showed an increase in acetylcholine and choline acetyltransferase in rat brain and they were shown to increase the acetylcholinesterase activity in cortical regions (Taranalli and Cheeramkuzhy, 2000). An aqueous extract of the root also increased acetylcholine levels in rat hippocampus, and it was hypothesised that this effect may be due to an increase in acetylcholine synthesis (Rai *et al.*, 2002).

Coptis chinensis Franch.

Coptis chinensis (Ranunculaceae) has been used in traditional Chinese medicine for several conditions. Studies have shown that methanol extract fraction of *C. chinensis* improved scopolamine-induced learning and memory deficit in rats (Hsieh *et al.*, 2000). The contained alkaloids berberine and palmatine have been shown to possess acetylcholinesterase inhibition in vitro (Park *et al.*, 1996).

Curcuma longa L. (turmeric)

Curcuma longa (Zingiberaceae) has also been used for culinary purposes. Turmeric has several components with immunomodulatory and antioxidant properties. Curcumin, an antioxidant present in turmeric, has been shown to protect the brain in vivo from ethanol-induced oxidative stress. It modulated glutathione-linked detoxification enzymes and reduced the lipid peroxidation in rat brain under oxidative stress (Rajakrishnan *et al.*, 1999). Some compounds from *C. longa*, including curcumin, demethoxycurcumin, bisdemethoxycurcumin and calebin-A (and some of its synthetic analogues), were shown to protect PC12 cells from β-amyloid insult in vitro, and this activity was suggested to be due to an antioxidant effect (Kim *et al.*, 2001).

In another study using a rat intraventricular Aβ infusion model, curcumin at a dose of 25 mg/kg reduced the isoprostane index of oxidative damage, amyloid plaque burden and Aβ-induced spatial memory deficits in the Morris water maze in rats. Curcumin has been shown to lower the oxidised proteins and interleukin-1β in the transgenic mouse model of Alzheimer's disease (Lim *et al.*, 2001).

Ocimum sanctum L. (tulsi)

In Ayurveda, *Ocimum sanctum* (Lamiaceae) is described as rasayana. These Ayurvedic rasayanas have been reported in literature to improve physical and mental health, increase non-specific resistance of body, promote physiological functions and augment cognition (Rege *et al.*, 1999). The aqueous extract of leaves of *Ocimum sanctum* at a dose of 500 mg/kg for 7 days significantly improved memory in rats, which was impaired by cerebral hypoperfusion-induced ischaemic insult. The memory task of the ischaemic rats was tested after 2 weeks of hypoperfusion period in the Morris water maze and those treated with *O. sanctum* extract had delayed escape latencies. This effect was correlated with their ability to reduce the lipid peroxidation, superoxide dismutase and increase in tissue sulphydryl groups and ascorbic acid contents of the hypoperfused brain tissue (Yanpallewar *et al.*, 2005).

Panax ginseng C.A. Mey. (ginseng)

Interest in the use of *Panax ginseng* (Araliaceae) comes from its purported 'adaptogen' or 'tonic' activity, which is thought to increase the body's capacity to tolerate external stresses, leading to increased physical or mental performance (Schulz *et al.*, 1998). *P. ginseng* alone was tested in young (3 months) and old (26 months) rats, on a battery of negatively reinforced learning tests (two-way active avoidance; passive avoidance/step-down; passive avoidance/step-through), and on the Morris water maze (Petkov *et al.*, 1993). Ginseng (17, 50, 150 mg/kg), administered orally to young rats, increased the number of avoidance responses in the two-way passive avoidance test at all doses tested.

Although an extensive literature documenting adaptogenic effects in laboratory animal systems exists, results from human clinical studies are conflicting and variable. However, there is evidence that extracts of ginseng can have an immunostimulatory effect in humans, and this may contribute to the adaptogen or tonic effects of these plants (Attele *et al.*, 1999). The major secondary products present in ginseng roots are an array of triterpene saponins, collectively called ginsenosides. The ginsenosides, of which there are at least 30, glycosylated derivatives of two major aglycones, panaxadiol and panaxatriol (Petkov *et al.*, 1993), are considered to be the most relevant for pharmacological activity. From laboratory studies, it has been suggested that the pharmacological target sites for these compounds involve the hypothalamus–pituitary–adrenal axis, owing to the observed effects on serum levels of adrenocorticotrophic hormone and corticosterone (Huang, 1999).

Salvia species (sage)

Several species of *Salvia* (Lamiaceae) have been reported to have potential activity in CNS.

Al-Yousuf *et al.* (2002) reported that *S. aegyptiaca* L. is used for treating various unrelated conditions that include nervous disorders, dizziness and trembling. This work examines some effects of the crude acetone and methanol extracts of the plant given at single oral doses of 0.25, 0.5, 1 or 2 g/kg, on the CNS in mice. It is concluded that the crude methanol and acetone extracts of *S. aegyptiaca* have CNS depressant properties, manifested as antinociception and sedation.

Perry *et al.* (2002) reported that *S. lavandulaefolia* Vahl. (Spanish sage) extracts and constituents have demonstrated anticholinesterase, antioxidant, anti-inflammatory, oestrogenic and CNS depressant (sedative) effects, all of which are currently relevant to the treatment of Alzheimer's disease. The essential oil inhibits the enzyme acetylcholinesterase from human brain tissue and bovine erythrocyte and individual monoterpenoid constituents inhibit acetylcholinesterase with varying degrees of potency.

In a study in healthy volunteers, essential oil administration produced significant effects on cognition. In a pilot open-label study involving oral administration of the essential oil to patients with Alzheimer's disease, a significant increase in diastolic and systolic blood pressure was observed in two patients; however, this may have been due primarily to pre-existing hypertension and there were no abnormalities in other vital signs or blood samples during the trial period (Perry *et al.*, 2003).

S. elegans Vahl, popularly known as *mirto*, is a shrub that has been widely used in Mexican traditional medicine for the treatment of different CNS diseases, principally anxiety.

The antidepressant and anxiolytic-like effects of hydroalcoholic (60%) extract of *S. elegans* (leaves and flowers) have been reported in mice. The extract, administered orally, was able to increase the percentage of time spent and the percentage of arm entries in the open arms of the elevated plus maze, as well as to increase the time spent by mice in the illuminated side of the light–dark test, and to decrease the immobility time of mice subjected to the forced swimming test. The same extract was not able to modify the spontaneous locomotor activity measured in the open-field test. These results provide support for the potential antidepressant and anxiolytic activity of *S. elegans* (Maribel *et al.*, 2006). Wake *et al.* (2000) also reported that *S. elegans* displayed differential displacement at nicotinic and muscarinic acetylcholine receptors, with the highest [3H](N)-scopolamine displacement.

In a double-blind, placebo-controlled, crossover study, 30 healthy participants received a different treatment in counterbalanced order on each occasion (placebo, 300, 600 mg dried sage leaf). On each day mood was assessed before the dose and at 1 h and 4 h afterwards. Both doses of sage led to improved ratings of mood in the absence of the stressor (that is, in pre-DISS mood scores) post-dose, with the lower dose reducing anxiety and the higher dose increasing 'alertness', 'calmness' and 'contentedness' on the Bond-Lader mood scales. Task performance was improved for the higher dose at both post-dose sessions, but reduced for the lower dose at the later testing session (Kennedy, 2006).

Withania somnifera L. (ashwagandha)

Withania somnifera (Solanaceae) root is one of the most highly regarded herbs in Ayurvedic medicine. *W. somnifera*, an Ayurvedic rasayana (memory-facilitating drug), was shown to attenuate amnesic effects in animal models of Alzheimer's disease by reversal of cholinergic dysfunction induced by ibotenic acid (Bhattacharya *et al.*, 1995; Mukherjee *et al.*, 2007e). Ayurvedic formulations based on *W. somnifera* induced a similar amnesia-reversal effect in rats (Bhattacharya *et al.*, 1998). The steroidal derivatives sitoindosides IX and from *W. somnifera*, augmented learning acquisition and memory in both young and old rats (Ghosal *et al.*, 1989). The root extract of *W. somnifera* reversed scopolamine-induced disruption of acquisition and attention and attenuated amnesia following electroconvulsive shock in mice. These effects are attributed to nootropic activity (Dhuley, 2001).

The mechanism of this memory-enhancing effect is attributed to enhanced acetylcholinesterase activity and reversed the ibotenic acid altered cholinergic marker such as acetylcholine and choline acetyl transferase. Therefore preferential action is on cholinergic neurotransmission in the cortical and basal forebrain areas involved in cognitive function. In another experiment *W. somnifera* (50 mg/kg) which contains sitoindosides VII–IX and withaferin A as the major bioactive entities, the relative abundance of these compounds in the extract being responsible for 28–30% significant enhancement of leaning as tested in passive avoidance test in chronically stressed rats (Bhattacharya *et al.*, 2003).

Acknowledgements

The authors wish to express their gratitude to the Department of Science & Technology (DST), Government of India, for providing financial assistance through the research project to the School of Natural Product Studies, Jadavpur University.

References

Allain H, Bentue-Ferrer D, Zekri O *et al.* (1998). Experimental and clinical methods in the development of anti-Alzheimer's drugs. *Fundam Clin Pharmacol* 12: 13–29.

Al-Showiman SS (1998). Furfural from some decorative plants grown in Saudi Arabia. *J Sci Indian Res* 57: 907–910.

Al-Yousuf MH, Bashir AK, Ali BH *et al.* (2002). Some effects of *Salvia aegyptiaca* L. on the central nervous system in mice. *J Ethnopharmacol* 81: 121–127.

Attele AS, Wu JA, Yuan CS (1999). Ginseng pharmacology: multiple constituents and multiple actions. *Biochem Pharmacol* 58: 1685–1693.

Bartus RT, Flicker C, Dean RL *et al.* (1985). Selective memory loss following nucleus basalis lesions: long term behavioral recovery despite persistent cholinergic deficiencies. *Pharmacol Biochem Behav* 23: 125–135.

Bhatia AL, Jain M (2003). *Amaranthus paniculatus* (Linn.) improves learning after radiation stress. *J Ethnopharmacol* 85: 73–79.

Bhattacharya SK, Kumar A, Ghosal S (1995). Effects of glycowithanolides from *Withania somnifera* on an animal model of Alzheimer's disease and perturbed cholinergic markers of cognition in rats. *Phytother Res* 9: 110–113.

Bhattacharya SK, Kumar A, Ghosal S (1999). Effect of *Bacopa monniera* on animal models of Alzhemier's disease and perturbed central cholinergic markers of cognition in rats. *Res Pharmacol Toxicol* 4: 1–12.

Bhattacharya SK, Muruganandam AV (2003). Adaptogenic activity of *Withania somnifera*: an experimental study using a rat model of chronic stress. *Pharmacol Biochem Behav* 75: 547–555.

Bhattacharya SK (1998). Effect of Trasina, an Ayurvedic herbal formulation, on experimental models of Alzheimer's disease and central cholinergic markers in rats. *J Altern Complement Med* 3: 327–367.

Brinkhaus B, Lindner M, Schuppan D (2000). Chemical, pharmacological and clinical profile of the East Asian medicinal plant *Centella asiatica*. *Phytomedicine* 7: 427–448.

Brlihlmann C, Marston A, Hostettmann K *et al.* (2004). Screening of non-alkaloidal natural compounds as acetylcholinesterase inhibitors. *Chem Biodiv* 1: 819–829.

Chintawar SD, Somani RS, Kasture VS *et al.* (2002). Nootropic activity of *Albizzia lebbeck* in mice. *J Ethnopharmacol* 81: 299–305.

Coyle JT, Price DL, DeLong MR (1983). Alzheimer's disease: A disorder of cortical cholinergic innervation. *Science* 219: 1184–1190.

Dhuley JN (2001). Nootropic-like effect of ashwagandha (*Withania somnifera* L.) in mice. *Phytother Res* 15: 524–528.

Ellman GL (1959). Tissue sulfhydryl groups. *Arch Biochem Biophy* 82: 70–77.

Emson PC, Lindvall O (1986). Neuroanatomical aspects of neurotransmitters affected in Alzheimer's disease. *Br Med Bull* 42: 57–62.

Flicker C, Dean RL, Watkins DL *et al.* (1983). Behavioral and neurochemical effects following neurotoxic lesions of a major cholinergic input to the cerebral cortex in the rat. *Pharmacol Biochem Behav* 18: 973–981.

Frautschy SA, Yang F, Calderon L *et al.* (1996). Rodent models of Alzheimer's disease: rat AB infusion approaches to amyloid deposits. *Neurobiol Aging* 17: 311–321.

Gattu M, Boss KL, Terry AV (1997). Reversal of scopolamine-induced deficits in navigational memory performance by the seed oil of *Celastrus paniculatus*. *Pharmacol Biochem Behav* 57: 793–799.

Geula C, Mesulam MM (1989). Cortical cholinergic fibers in aging and Alzheimer's diseases: a morphometric study. *Neuroscience* 33: 469–481.

Ghosal S, Srivastava RS, Bhattacharya SK *et al.* (1989). Immunomodulatory and CNS effects of sitoindosides IX and X, two new glycowithanolides from *Withania somnifera*. *Phytother Res* 2: 201–206.

Giovannelli L, Scali C, Faussone-Pellegrini MS, Pepeu G, Casamenti F (1998). Long-term changes in the aggregation state and toxic effects of γ-amyloid injected into the rat brain. *Neuroscience* 82: 349–357.

Godkar P, Gordon RK, Ravindran A *et al.* (2003). *Celastrus paniculatus* seed water soluble extracts protect cultured rat forebrain neuronal cells from hydrogen peroxide-induced oxidative injury. *Fitoterapia* 74: 658–669.

Hedreen JC, Struble RG, Whitehouse PJ *et al.* (1984). Topography of the magnocellular basal forebrain system in human brain. *J Neuropathol Exp Neurol* 43: 1–21.

Houghton PJ, Ren Y, Howes MR (2006). Acetylcholinesterase inhibitors from plants and fungi. *Nat Prod Rep* 23: 181–199.

Howes MJR, Perry NSL, Houghton PJ (2003). Plants with traditional uses and activities, relevant to the management of Alzheimer's disease and other cognitive disorders. *Phytother Res* 17: 1–8.

Howes MR, Houghton PJ (2003). Plants used in Chinese and Indian traditional medicine for improvement of memory and cognitive function. *Pharmacol Biochem Behav* 75: 513–527.

Hsiao K, Chapman P, Nilsen S *et al.* (1996). Correlative memory deficits, Abeta elevation, and amyloid plaques in transgenic mice. *Science* 274: 99–102.

Hsieh MT, Peng WH, Wu CR *et al.* (2000). The ameliorating effect of the cognitive enhancing Chinese herbs on scopolamine induced amnesia in rats. *Phytother Res* 14: 375–377.

Ingkaninan K, Best D, Heijden VD *et al.* (2000). High-performance liquid chromatography with on-line coupled UV, mass spectrometric and biochemical detection for identification of acetylcholinesterase inhibitors from natural products. *J Chromatography A* 872: 61–73.

Kapoor LD (1990). *Handbook of Ayurvedic Medicinal Plants.* Boca Raton (FL), CRC Press.

Kennedy DO, Pace S, Haskell C, Okello EJ, Milne A, Scholey AB (2006). Effects of cholinesterase inhibiting sage (*Salvia officinalis*) on mood, anxiety and performance on a psychological stressor battery. *Neuropsychopharmacology* 31: 845–852.

Kim HP, Pham HT, Ziboh VA (2001). Flavonoids differentially inhibit guinea pig epidermal cytosolic phospholipase A2. *Prostaglandins, Leukotrienes and Essential Fatty Acids* 65: 281–286.

Koelle GB (1951). The elimination of enzymatic diffusion artifacts in the histochemical localization of cholinesterases and a survey of their cellular distributions. *J Pharmacol Exp Therap* 103: 153–171.

Koh J, Yang LL, Cotman CW (1990). S-amyloid protein increases the vulnerability of cultured cortical neurons to excitotoxic damage. *Brain Res* 5: 315–320.

Koliatsos VE, Clatterbuck RE, Nauta HJW *et al.* (1991). Human nerve growth factor prevents degeneration of basal forebrain cholinergic neurons in primates. *Ann Neurol* 30: 831–840.

Kumar MHV, Gupta YK (2002a). Antioxidant property of *Celastrus paniculatus* Willd.: a possible mechanism in enhancing cognition. *Phytomedicine* 9: 302–311.

Kumar MHV, Gupta YK (2002b). Effect of different extracts of *Centella asiatica* on cognition and markers of oxidative stress in rats. *J Ethnopharmacol* 79: 253–260.

Kumar V, Mukherjee K, Kumar S *et al.* (2007). Validation of HPTLC method for the analysis of taraxerol in *Clitoria ternatea. Phytochem Anal* 9: 2.

Lim GP, Chu T, Yang F *et al.* (2001). The curry spice curcumin reduces oxidative damage and amyloid pathology in an Alzheimer transgenic mouse. *J Neurosci* 21: 8370–8377.

Maribel HR, Yolanda GB, Sergio M *et al.* (2006). Antidepressant and anxiolytic effects of hydroalcoholic extract from *Salvia elegans. J Ethnopharmacol* 107: 53–58.

Marston A, Kissling J, Hostettmann K (2002). A rapid TLC bioautographic method for the detection of acetylcholinesterase and butyrylcholinesterase inhibitors in plants. *Phytochem Anal* 13: 51–54.

McGeer EG, McGeer PL (1998). The importance of inflammatory mechanisms in Alzheimer's disease. *Exp Gerontol* 3: 371–378.

McGeer PL, McGeer EG (1995). The inflammatory response system of brain: implications for therapy of Alzheimer and other neurodegenerative diseases. *Brain Res Rev* 21: 195–218.

Mesulam MM, Mufson EJ, Levey AI *et al.* (1983). Cholinergic innervations of cortex by the basal forbrain: cytochemistry and cortical connections of the septal area, diagonal band nuclei nucleus basalis (substantia innominata) and hypothalamus in the rhesus monkey. *J Com Neurol* 214: 170–197.

Misra R (1998). Modern drug development from traditional medicinal plants using radioligand receptor-binding assays. *Med Res Rev* 18: 383–402.

Miyazawa M, Watanabe H, Kameoka H (1997). Inhibition of acetyl cholinesterase activity by monoterpenoids with a p-menthane skeleton. *J Agric Food Chem* 45: 677–679.

Mukherjee K, Saha BP, Mukherjee PK (2002). Psychopharmacological profiles of *Leucas Lavandulaefolia* Rees. *Phytother Res* 16: 696–699.

Mukherjee PK, Rai S, Kumar V *et al.* (2007e). Plants of Indian origin in drug discovery. *Expert Opin Drug Disc* 2: 633–657.

Mukherjee PK, (2002). *Quality Control of Herbal Drugs – an approach to evaluation of botanicals.* New Delhi, India, Business Horizons, pp. 692–694.

Mukherjee PK, Maiti K, Mukherjee K *et al.* (2006). Leads from Indian medicinal plants with hypoglycemic potentials. *J Ethnopharmacol* 106: 1–28.

Mukherjee PK, Wahile A, (2006). Integrated approaches towards drug development from Ayurveda and other Indian system of medicines. *J Ethnopharmacol* 103: 25–35.

Mukherjee PK, Kumar V, Mal M, Houghton PJ (2007a). Acetylcholinesterase inhibitors from plants. *Phytomedicine* 14: 289–300.

Mukherjee PK, Kumar V, Houghton PJ (2007b). Screening of Indian medicinal plants for acetylcholinesterase inhibitory activity. *Phytother Res* 21: 1142–1145.

Mukherjee PK, Kumar V, Mal M, Houghton PJ (2007c). *Acorus calamus*: scientific validation of Ayurvedic tradition from natural resources. *Pharm Biol* 45: 651–666.

Mukherjee PK, Kumar V, Mal M, Houghton PJ (2007d). *In vitro* acetylcholinesterase inhibitory activity of essential oil and its main constituents of *Acorus calamus. Planta Med* 73: 283–285.

Mukherjee PK, Ahamed KF, Kumar V *et al.* (2007e). Protective effect of biflavones from *Araucaria bidwillii* Hook in rat cerebral ischemia/reperfusion induced oxidative stress. *Behav Brain Res* 178: 221–228.

Nadkarni AK, (1996). *Indian Materia Medica.* Popular Prakashan Private Limited, Bombay, India, Vol. 1, pp. 296–666.

Nagai T, Mc Geer PL, Peng GH *et al.* (1983). Choline acetyltransferase immunohistochemistry in brains of Alzheimer's disease patients and controls. *Neuroscience Lett* 36: 195–199.

Nalini K, Karanth KS, Rao A *et al.* (1995). Effects of *Celastrus paniculatus* on passive avoidance performance and biogenic amine turnover in albino rats. *J Ethnopharmacol* 47: 101–108.

Oh MH, Houghton PJ, Whang WK, Cho JH (2004). Screening of Korean herbal medicines used to improve cognitive function for anti-cholinesterase activity. *Phytomedicine 11*: 544–548.

Pal BC, Achari B, Yoshikawa K, Arihara S (1995). Saponins from *Albizia lebbeck. Phytochemistry* 38: 1287–1291.

Parent A, Poirier LJ, Boucher R, *et al.* (1989). Morphological characteristics of acetylchoinesterase containing neurons in the CNS of DFP treated monkeys. *J Neurol Sci* 32: 9–28.

Park CH, Kim S, Choi W (1996). Novel anticholinesterase and antiamnesic activities of dihydroevodiamine, a constituent of *Evodia ruraecarpa*. *Planta Med* 62: 405–409.

Perry GW, Wilson DL (1981). Protein synthesis and axonal transport during nerve regeneration. *J Neurochem* 37: 1203–1217.

Perry NS, Houghton PJ, Jenner P, Keith A, Perry EK (2002). *Salvia lavandulaefolia* essential oil inhibits cholinesterase *in vivo*. *Phytomedicine* 9: 48–51.

Perry NSL, Houghton PJ, Theobald AE, *et al.* (2000). *In-vitro* inhibition of human erythrocyte acetylcholine esterase by *Salvia lavandulaefolia* essential oil and constituents terpenes. *J Pharm Pharmacol* 52: 895–902.

Perry NSL, Bollen CK, Perry EK, Ballard C (2003). Salvia for dementia therapy: review of pharmacological activity and pilot tolerability clinical trial. *Pharm Biochem Behavior* 75: 651–659.

Petkov VD, Kehayov R, Belcheva S, *et al.* (1993). Memory effects of standardized extracts of *Panax ginseng* (G115), *Ginkgo biloba* (GK 501) and their combination Gincosan1 (PHL-00701). *Planta Med* 59: 106–114.

Pratibha N, Saxena VS, Amit A *et al.* (2004). Anti-inflammatory activities of Aller-7, a novel polyherbal formulation for allergic rhinitis. *Int J Tissue React* 26: 43–51.

Rai KS, Murthy KD, Karanth KS, *et al.* (2002). *Clitoria ternatea* root extract enhances acetylcholine content in rat hippocampus. *Fitoterapia* 73: 685–689.

Rajakrishnan V, Viswanathan P, Rajasekharan KN *et al.* (1999). Neuroprotective role of curcumin from *Curcuma longa* on ethanol-induced brain damage. *Phytother Res* 13: 571–574.

Rege TN, Thatte UM, Dahanukar SA (1999). Adaptogenic properties of six rasayana herbs used in Ayurvedic medicine. *Phytother Res* 13: 275–291.

Rhee IK, Meent M, Ingkaninan K, Verpoorte R (2001). Screening for acetylcholinesterase inhibitors from Amaryllidaceae using gel thin layer chromatography in combination with bioactivity staining. *J Chromatography A* 915: 217–223.

Ryan MF, Byrne O (1988). Plant–insect co evolution and inhibition of acetylcholinesterase. *J Chem Ecol* 14: 1965–1975.

Sakina MR, Dandiya PC (1990). A psychoneuropharmacological profile of *Centella asiatica* extract. *Fitoterapia* 61: 291–296.

Sarter M, Hagan J, Dudchenko P (1992). Behavioral screening for cognition enhancers: from indiscriminate to valid testing: part I. *Psychopharmacology* 107: 144–159.

Scarpini E, Schelternsand P, Feldman H (2003). Treatment of Alzheimer's disease; current status and new perspectives. *Lancet Neurol* 29: 539–547.

Sharma R, Chaturvedi C, Tewari PV (1987). Efficacy of *Bacopa monniera* in revitalizing intellectual functions in children. *J Res Educ Indian Med* 1: 12.

Singh HK, Dhawan BN (1982). Effect of *Bacopa monnieri* Linn. (Brahmi) extract in avoidance responses in rats. *J Ethnopharmacol* 5: 205–214.

Singh HK, Dhawan BN (1997). Neuropsychopharmacological effects of the Ayurvedic nootropic *Bacopa monniera* Linn. (BRAHMI). *Int J Pharmacol* 29: S359–S365.

Singh RH, Singh L (1980). Studies on the anti-anxiety effect of themedyha rasayana drug Brahmi (*Bacopa monniera* Wettst.). *Res Ayur Siddha* 1: 133–148.

Soumyanath A, Zhong YP, Gold SA *et al.* (2005). *Centella asiatica* accelerates nerve regeneration upon oral administration and contains multiple active fractions increasing neurite elongation in-vitro. *J Pharm Pharmacol* 57: 1221–1229.

Stough C, Lloyd J, Clarke J *et al.* (2001). The chronic effects of extract of *Bacopa monniera* (brahmi) on cognitive function in healthy human subjects. *Psychopharmacology* 156: 481–484.

Taranalli AD, Cheeramkuzhy TC (2000). Influence of *Clitoria ternatea* extracts on memory and central cholinergic activity in rats. *Pharm Biol* 38(1): 51–56.

Tuszynski MH, Sang H, Yoshida K, Gage FH (1991). Recombinant human nerve growth factor infusions prevent cholinergic neuronal degeneration in the adult primate brain. *Ann Neurol* 30: 625–636.

Wake G, Court J, Pickering A, Lewis R, Wilkins R, Perry E (2000). CNS acetylcholine receptor activity in European medicinal plants traditionally used to improve failing memory. *J Ethnopharmacol* 69: 105–114.

Warrier PK, Nambiar VPK, Ramankutty C (1995). *Indian Medicinal Plants,* vol. 2. Orient Longman, India.

Weiss JM, Kilts CD (1998). Animal models of depression and schizohrenia. In: Schatzberg AF, Nemeroff CB, eds. *The American Psychiatric Press: textbook of psychopharmacology.* 2nd ed. Washington, D.C.: American Psychiatric Press, Inc. pp. 89–131.

Yankner B, Duffy LK, kirschner DA (1990). Neurotrophic and neurotoxic effects of amyloid-P-protein: reversal by tachykinin neuropeptides. *Science* 250: 279–282.

Yanpallewar S, Rai S, Kumar M *et al.* (2005). Neuroprotective effect of *Azadirachta indica* on cerebral post ischemic reperfusion and hypoperfusion in rats. *Life Sci* 76: 1325–1338.

Yanpallewar SU, Rai S, Kumar M (2004). Evaluation of antioxidant and neuroprotective effect of *Ocimum sanctum* on transient cerebral ischemia and long-term cerebral hypoperfusion. *Pharmacol Biochem Behav* 79: 155–164.

21

Evaluation of herbal medicinal products against herpes virus diseases

Debprasad Chattopadhyay, Sonali Das, Sekhar Chakraborty and Sujit K Bhattacharya

Introduction

Over the centuries herbal medicinal products formed the basis of medicaments in Africa, China, India and in many other civilisations (Chattopadhyay, 2006; Chattopadhyay and Bhattacharya, 2008). Traditional healers have long used herbal products to prevent or to cure infectious conditions but scientific interest in natural antivirals is more recent, spurred on by the rapid spread of emerging and re-emerging infectious diseases. Additionally the rapid rate of species extinction leads to irretrievable loss of structurally diverse and potentially useful phytochemicals, compounds which are often species/strain-specific with diverse structures and bioactivities, synthesised mainly for defence against predators (Chattopadhyay and Naik, 2007). This chapter will describe some promising extracts and compounds of herbal origin, having antiherpes virus activity, with in-vitro and some documented in-vivo activities, along with structure–activity relationship considerations.

The herpes virus

The herpes virus belongs to Herpesviridae, a family of DNA viruses that cause diseases in humans and animals. There are eight distinct viruses in this family, presented in Table 21.1, known to cause disease in humans. Viruses of the herpes group are morphologically indistinguishable, share many common features of intracellular development, but differ widely in biological properties. All human herpes viruses (HHV) contain a large double-stranded, linear DNA with 100–200 genes encased within an icosahedral protein capsid wrapped in a lipid bilayer envelope, called a virion. Following the binding of viral envelope glycoproteins to host cell-membrane receptors, the virion is internalised and dismantled, allowing viral DNA to migrate to the host cell nucleus, where viral DNA replication and transcription occurs.

One replication cycle of herpes virus depends upon a number of steps:

- virion entry
- expression of immediate-early (α) genes such as those for infected cell proteins (ICP) 0 and 4
- early (β_1, β_2) genes including DNA polymerase and thymidine kinase
- late genes (γ_1, γ_2) containing glycoprotein B (gB), C (gC) and ICP5
- unpaired DNA replication (Sandri-Goldin, 2006).

During symptomatic infection, infected cells transcribe *lytic* viral genes, but sometimes a small number of *latency associated transcript* (LAT) genes accumulate, which help the virus to persist in the host cell indefinitely. The primary infection is a self-limited period of illness, but long-term latency is symptom-free. Following reactivation, transcription of viral genes switches from LAT to multiple *lytic* genes that lead to enhanced replication and virion production.

Herpes viruses cause localised skin infections of the mucosal epithelia of the oral cavity, pharynx, oesophagus and the eye, or genitals, depending upon the type involved (Habif, 2004). Moreover, the herpes viruses establish latent infections that can be periodically reactivated, and sometimes produce serious infections of the CNS, such as acute encephalitis and meningitis, and can be fatal in immune-deficient patients (Sandri-Goldin, 2006). The immediate-early genes of herpes simplex virus (HSV) can also activate the genes of HIV (Ostrove *et al.*, 1987), varicella-zoster virus (Felser *et al.*, 1988) or human papillomavirus type 18 (Gius and Laimins, 1989), causing a significant risk factor for transmission of HIV/AIDS (Corey *et al.*, 2004). The herpes virus can also lead to scarification, a major cause of blindness in developing nations (Habif, 2004; Sandri-Goldin, 2006).

HSV-2 is also known as an oncogenic virus as it can convert infected cells into tumour cells (Habif, 2004). The search for selective antiherpes virus agents is an urgent need as the problems such as viral resistance, conflicting efficacy in recurrent infection and immunocompromised patients with available antiherpes drugs remain unresolved. Moreover, herpes viruses (HSV-1 and HSV-2) spread silently (asymptomatic), cause opportunistic infections in immunocompromised patients, and develop resistance to acyclovir.

Control of herpes virus infection

The herpes virus causes a lifelong infection with high morbidity, and is underdiagnosed because of its mild and asymptomatic nature. HSV alone affects more than one third of the world's population and is responsible for a wide array of human disease. Before the 1970s, when acyclovir was introduced as an antiviral drug, cutaneous HSV infection was managed with drying agents and other local care.

Table 21.1 Members of human herpesviridae

Type	Synonym	Subfamily	Pathophysiology
HHV-1	Herpes simplex virus-1 (HSV-1)	*Alphaherpesvirinae*	Oral and/or genital herpes (orofacial)
HHV-2	Herpes simplex virus-2 (HSV-2)	α (alpha)	Oral and/or genital herpes (genital)
HHV-3	Varicella zoster virus (VZV)	α (alpha)	Chickenpox and shingles
HHV-4	Epstein-Barr virus (EBV) Lymphocryptovirus	*Gammaherpesvirinae* γ (gamma)	Infectious mononucleosis, Burkitt's lymphoma, CNS lymphoma (in AIDS patients), post-transplant lymphoproliferative syndrome (PTLS), nasopharyngeal carcinoma
HHV-5	Cytomegalovirus (CMV)	*Betaherpesvirinae*	Infectious mononucleosis-like syndrome, retinitis, etc.
HHV-6, 7	Roseolovirus	α (beta)	Roseola infantum or exanthem subitum
HHV-8	Kaposi's sarcoma-associated herpes virus (KSHV), a rhadinovirus	γ (gamma)	Kaposi's sarcoma, primary effusion lymphoma, some multicentric Castleman's disease

Newer antiviral drugs such as famciclovir and valacyclovir with once-daily dosage benefits have emerged during the past several years but are more expensive. Although no cure is available to date, the nucleoside analogue acyclovir is widely used, as it is selectively phosphorylated by thymidine kinase enzyme in infected cells. However, acyclovir-resistant herpes virus has been isolated in immunocompromised patients and is not suitable in neonatal infections (Habif, 2004). Therefore, new antiherpes virus agents are highly desirable.

The development of antiherpetic agents from herbal sources is less explored probably because there are very few specific viral targets for small natural molecules. However, studies have shown that a variety of compounds inhibit the replication of herpes viruses, e.g. phloroglucinol (Arisawa *et al.*, 1990), anthraquinones (Sydiskis *et al.*, 1991), polysaccharides (Marchetti *et al.*, 1996), triterpenes and saponins (Simões *et al.*, 1999) and polyphenols (Kuo *et al.*, 2002; Chattopadhyay and Naik, 2007). A topical preparation from *Glycyrrhiza glabra* (liquorice root) containing triterpene glycyrrhetinic acid (Glycyrrhizin) used for the prevention and treatment of herpes outbreaks was found to inhibit acyclovir-resistant HSV-1, by induction of CD4+ T cells (Utsunomiya *et al.*, 1995).

Oryzacystatin from rice plant (*Oryzae sativa*) showed in-vitro and in-vivo anti-HSV-1 activity by inhibiting proteinase enzyme of herpes viruses (Aoki *et al.*, 1995). When 19 plant-derived compounds were tested by plaque reduction assay against HSV-2, it was found that eugenol, cineole, curcumin and carrageenan lambda type IV (ED_{50}=7.0 mg/mL), provided significant protection ($P<0.05$) in intravaginal HSV-2-mice infected and guinea pigs (Bourne *et al.*, 1999). All these findings indicated that the herbal products are still potential sources for new antiherpetic agents. Owing to their amazing structural diversity and broad range of bioactivities, herbal medicinal products can be explored as a source of complementary antiherpetic agents, as many of them inhibit several steps of replication cycle and certain cellular factors of herpes viruses (Chattopadhyay and Khan, 2008).

The objective of this chapter is to summarise the potential uses of natural products, especially derived from herbal sources, for the prevention and treatment of infections caused by herpes viruses, especially HSV-1 and HSV-2.

Screening models for herbal anti-HSV agents and their value in drug discovery

In-vitro primary screening assays

The most commonly used in-vitro method for preliminary screening of extracts or compounds is the study of cytopathic effect (CPE) by plaque reduction assay on HSV-infected cells. Here the Hep2 or Vero cells are grown in suitable cell culture media with incubation at 37°C for 24 h. Confluent cell monolayers are then infected with 100–200 plaque-forming units (PFU) of the virus. After 1 h incubation (to allow viral adsorption), the cells are washed with phosphate buffer saline and overlaid with agar in cell culture medium containing twofold dilutions of the extracts or test compounds, and recultured at 37°C, until plaques appeared. Finally the monolayer cells are fixed with formalin, stained, dried and the number of plaques are microscopically counted. The percentage inhibition of plaque formation [(mean number of plaques in control − mean number of plaques in test)/(mean number of plaques in control) × 100], or the effective concentration for 50% plaque reduction (EC_{50}; the lowest extract concentration that reduced plaque number by 50% in the treated cultures compared with untreated ones), or the 50% inhibitory concentration (IC_{50}; the extract concentration required to reduce the virus plaque number by 50%) is calculated. When different herbal preparations (cold aqueous, hot aqueous, ethanolic, acid ethanolic, and methanolic) were analysed by plaque reduction assay, it was observed that the ethanolic extract of *Rheum officinale* and methanol extract of *Paeonia suffruticosa* inhibited attachment and penetration of HSV-1; whereas the aqueous extract of *P. suffruticosa* and ethanolic extract of *Melia toosendan* inhibited attachment and replication of HSV-1 and HSV-2 (Hsiang *et al.*, 2001), indicating that these herbs have some potential for new anti-HSV leads.

The pioneering work of Vanden Berghe and his group showed that the inhibition of cytopathic effect on Vero cell monolayer infected with HSV can be measured by endpoint titration method (Vanden

Berghe *et al.*, 1993), which is also helpful to determine virucidal activity after preincubations of test compound and virus (Vlietinck *et al.*, 1997; Apers *et al.*, 2002). The 50% endpoint titration (Figure 21.1) was performed on confluent monolayers of Vero cells (10^4 cells per well) infected with serial tenfold dilutions (10^7 TCD_{50}/mL) of virus suspension and the first monolayer of cells was infected with multiplicity of infection of 10 to 10^{-4} by serial tenfold dilution. The virus was allowed to absorb for 1 h at 37°C, and then serial twofold dilutions of extract or test compound (in maintenance medium, supplemented with 2% fetal bovine serum and antibiotics) were added. The plates were incubated (37°C) and viral CPE was recorded by light microscopy for 7 days (Figure 21.1).

It is important to run cytotoxicity control (uninfected but treated cells), and cell control (uninfected untreated cell) at each treatment concentration, with the virus control (infected but untreated) at each viral dilution. Toxic doses (CT) of the test extract or compound are considered to be dilutions that cause destruction of monolayer of cells, so that no virus titre can be determined. The antiviral activity is expressed as the virus titre reduction at the maximum non-toxic dose of the test extract or substance, i.e. the highest concentration that does not affect the monolayers under test conditions. In this method virus titre reduction factors (RF, the ratio of the virus titre reduction in the absence and presence of the maximum non-toxic dose of the test sample) of 10^3 to 10^4 indicate a pronounced antiviral activity and are suitable as selection criteria for further investigation of the said extract or compound. It was observed that the antiviral activity should be present in at least two subsequent dilutions of the test substance, otherwise the activity is likely to be due to its toxicity, or the activity is only virucidal. The extracellular virucidal activity can also be determined by the titration method of the residual infectious virus at room temperature after incubation of the test compound with virus suspension (10^6 TCD_{50}/mL) during 1 h at 37°C (Vanden Berghe *et al.*, 1993; Apers *et al.*, 2001).

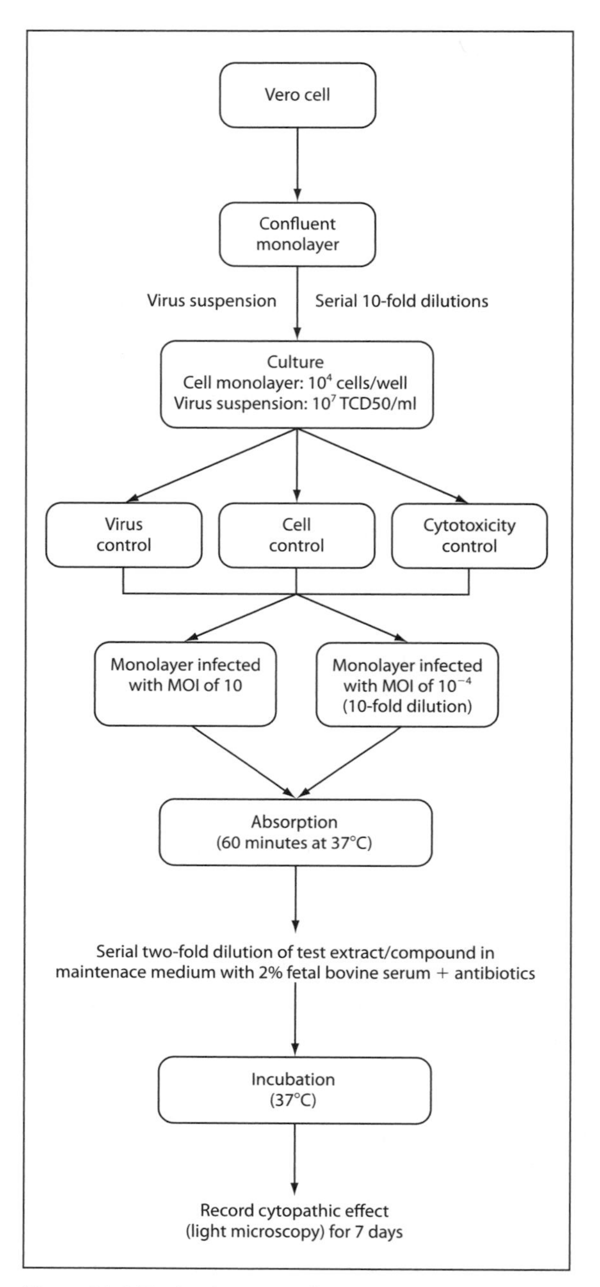

Figure 21.1 The in-vitro antiviral testing protocol.

Another rapid and sensitive in-vitro procedure of evaluating anti-HSV agents is based on spectrophotometrical assessment for viability of virus- and mock-infected cells via in situ reduction of a tetrazolium dye 3-(4,5-dimethylthiazol-2-yl)-2,5-diphenyltetrazolium bromide (MTT), and is proved to have similar sensitivity to the plaque reduction assay (Sudo *et al.*, 1994). The MTT test not only significantly simplifies the assay procedures, but also allows the evaluation of larger numbers of compounds at a time. Kira *et al.* (1995) reported the development of another highly sensitive assay system using a suspension cell line derived from human myeloma cells, that are sensitive to several HSV strains such as HSV-1: standard strain KOS, acyclovir-resistant A4D, clinical isolate Hangai and HSV-2 standard strain G; and many known antiherpes virus compounds (acyclovir, sorivudine, arabinoside, 9-(1,3-dihydroxy-2-propoxy)methyl guanine, phosphonoformate and dextran sulphate). This produced good results when tested against KOS and G strains of HSV. Kurokawa *et al.* (1999) reported the in-vitro anti-HSV activity of *Rhus javanica* extracts by plaque reduction assay against wild-type, acyclovir-phosphonoacetic acid-resistant, thymidine kinase-deficient HSV-1 and wild-type HSV-2 (EC_{50} 2.6–3.9μg/mL) and the in-vivo efficacy of the cutaneously infected mice with HSV-1.

High-throughput screening assays

High-capacity anti-HSV drug screening assay is available for the primary analysis of compounds in a 96-well microtitre assay. The basic assay methods involve infection of Vero cells with HSV-1 or HSV-2 in the presence of test compounds. The ability of the compounds to inhibit HSV-induced cell killing is measured 5 days post-infection using the tetrazolium dye MTS. Mitochondrial enzymes of viable cells convert MTS to a soluble, coloured formazan. The quantitation of the amount of the formazan product present in each well of the microtitre plate is then determined spectrophotometrically at 490/650 nm, while the toxicity of the test compounds to host cells is measured concurrently in the same microtitre plate. Data can be analysed by a statistical software program along with determinations of the efficacy (IC_{50}), toxicity (TC_{50}) and selectivity (therapeutic index, TI) of the compounds.

Several primary screens are also available for the evaluation of compounds against human cytomegalovirus (HCMV) using a method similar to the anti-HSV assay. The MRC-5 cells are infected with HCMV in the presence of drugs for a period of 7 days. Compound efficacy and toxicity are then measured using MTS. Standard plaque reduction assay as well as an ELISA is also available. For varicella zoster virus (VZV), the primary screen currently available is a standard plaque reduction assay, while for Epstein-Barr virus (EBV), a moderate-throughput polymerase chain reaction (PCR)-based assay is developed to identify inhibitors of EBV using P3HR1 cells, a cell line that is latently infected with EBV. Lytic virus replication spontaneously occurs in approximately 5% of the cell population resulting in the release of virus particles from the cells. The P3HR1 cells are incubated with compounds for a period of 6 days; supernatant virus is collected and quantitated using TaqMan PCR methodology. Compound toxicity is evaluated in parallel using MTS. A virus-induced CPE-inhibition assay is employed to evaluate compounds against HHV-6. Uninfected HSB-2 cells are co-cultured with HHV-6-infected HSB-2 cells in the presence of test compounds. After 6 days incubation, CPE inhibition is determined by microscopic inspection of the cultures.

Upon infection and replication of HHV-6 in HSB-2 cells, the cells increase in size and become light refractory. These changes are readily apparent by microscopic examination of the wells, which allows for the quantitation of the numbers of infected cells in each of the cultures. Compound toxicity is evaluated in parallel using MTS. An HHV-6 ELISA is also developed. A moderate-throughput PCR-based assay to identify inhibitors of HHV-8, using BCBL-1 cells, a cell line that is latently infected with HHV-8, is developed. Lytic virus replication is induced using the phorbol ester TPA, resulting in the release of virus particles from the cells. BCBL-1 cells are incubated with compounds for a period of 4 days. Supernatant virus is collected and quantitated using TaqMan PCR methodology. Compound toxicity is evaluated in parallel using MTS.

Secondary testing assays

Compounds or extracts that are evaluated for their ability to inhibit herpes virus infection need a variety of phenotypically distinct susceptible cell lines including Vero, MRC-5, HFF, BHK, HEp-2 as well as other human and mammalian cell lines. To evaluate compounds that inhibit replication of viruses a panel of virus isolates is needed, including clinical and/or drug-resistant herpes virus isolates. Currently there are ten HSV-1, five HSV-2, sixteen HCMV, five VZV, two EBV, two HHV-6 and two HHV-8 isolates used throughout the globe. To study the titre reduction of HSV-1, HSV-2, HCMV and VZV, supernatant virus from drug-treated cultures is collected and titrated to determine the level of reduction in virus produced as a result of drug treatment. This is an in-vitro model for estimating the log-fold reduction in virus that could be obtained by antiviral treatment in-vivo. The extracts or compounds can also be evaluated for their activity in combination with other drugs including other known herpes virus inhibitors, or HIV-1 inhibitors or any other compound of interest. Interactions (synergy, additivity, antagonism) of the compounds can be evaluated in terms of antiviral efficacy and toxicity.

Studies on the mechanism of action

Compounds can also be evaluated for activity when challenged with different amounts of virus such as HSV-1, HSV-2, HCMV and VZV ranging from very low to very high multiplicity of infection. Compounds are added or removed from cultures at various times pre- and post-infection. By comparison with other known herpes virus inhibitors, this allows the relative point in the virus life cycle that is being inhibited to be determined (immediate-early, early, late functions, DNA polymerisation, etc.). This standard technique is typically used early during the process of determining the mechanism of action, as it allows one to concentrate on a smaller target window of activity for further experimentation and gives an easy way to determine if a compound is acting by a unique or novel mechanism compared with other known inhibitors. Furthermore, time of removal studies allow one to determine the reversibility of activity. The effect of compounds on the production of viral DNA can be evaluated using various hybridisation techniques, PCR or TaqMan PCR. The effect of compounds on the production of immediate-early, early and late viral proteins can be evaluated using Western blots and/or flow cytometry. Resistant virus isolates are selected in tissue culture by serial passage of the virus in the presence of gradually increasing concentrations of the compound. Resistance selection can be evaluated using combinations of anti-HSV agents to judge the relative ability of the virus to become resistant to multiple agents.

In-vivo models

To test the in-vivo toxicity and efficacy of the herbal products in animals, several models have been developed. HSV infections of mice provide a good model for human disease, but other animals provide receptors for HSV entry and expression of viral glycoproteins that influence disease and pathogenicity in man, and these are discussed below. The most commonly used method of in-vivo toxicity determination is dermal toxicity testing of the extract or substance, usually done by the skin irritation test; while the efficacy of any extract or compound is measured by cutaneous lesion development in guinea pigs (Figure 21.2).

For dermal toxicity testing of any extract or formulations guinea pigs of either sex (200–250 g) are used. After removing body hair from the dorsal side of the animal, the naked skin (6 cm × 7 cm) is washed with warm water, dried and abraded with dermal (Seven-Star) needles. The extract or formulations of different potency are then applied to the abraded area of cohorts of animals (n = 5) usually at the rate of 2 g per animal. After 24 h, the extract is removed with warm water and the animals are examined for erythema and/or oedema 1 h later, up to the next 72 h.

To study the extract potency on HSV-1-induced cutaneous lesions, the abraded dorsal area of the animals is first divided into four quadrants and each of the quadrants is then infected with 30 μL of tenfold diluted HSV-1. The animals are observed for up to 10 days for typical herpes lesion development and, once the lesion develops, cohorts of fresh animals (n = 15) are infected as above and treated with the extract or formulations, control drug (acyclovir) or vehicle control to the infected area with sterile cotton swabs twice daily for 6 days (Figure 21.2). The extent of lesion should be scored daily as: 1.0–1.6 lesions on a quarter of the infected area; 1.7–2.4 lesions on a half of the infected area; 2.5–3.2 lesions on three-quarters of the infected area; and 3.3–4.0 lesions on the entire infected area (Zhang *et al.*, 2007).

A fast, simple reactivation model to study the ocular herpes virus infection and latency was successfully established by Gordon *et al.* (1990) in New Zealand female rabbits. Each unscarified rabbit eye was inoculated with a suspension of thymidine-kinase-positive HSV-1W strain (5×10^4 PFU/eye) into the lower fornix, following a topical anaesthesia with eye drops. The HSV-1W establishes latency and

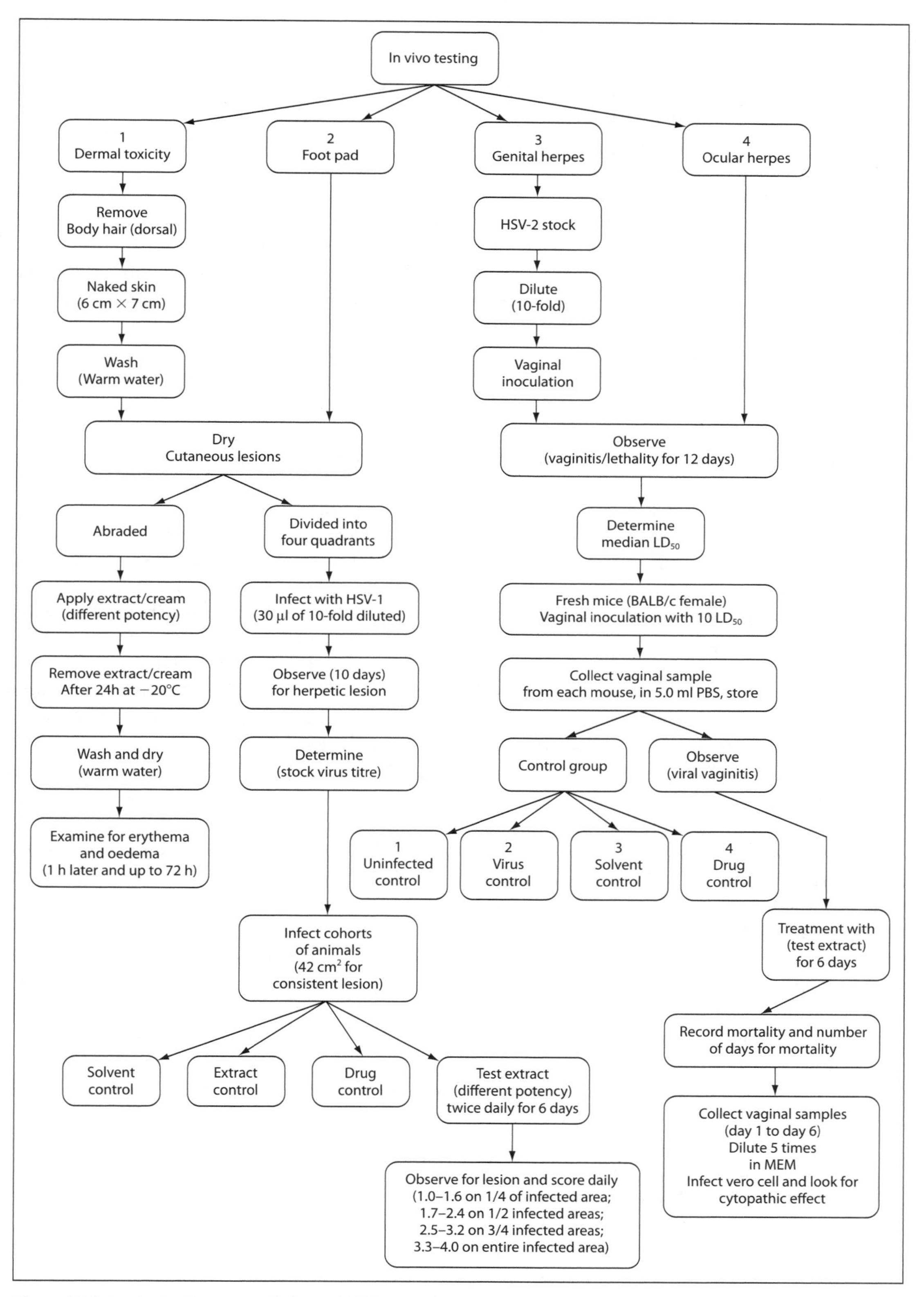

Figure 21.2 In-vivo testing protocols for anti-HSV extract/agents.

reactivates in a manner similar to mouse pathogenic strain HSV-1 McKrae (Gordon *et al.*, 1986). Successful inoculation (100%) of eyes was found on day 7 with typical herpetic dendritic ulcers and significant HSV-1 titre (10^4 PFU/mL) and viral shedding can be determined by neutralisation test. After satisfactory anaesthesia the globe was proptosed with a wooden cotton applicator and an operating microscope used to facilitate all surgical manipulations. Intrastromal injection by a no. 30 short bevel needle attached to a 0.25-mL tuberculin syringe is made into the central corneal stroma. One group receives deionised, sterile, endotoxin-free water, another group 100 μL air while the third group receives no injection, and for all three groups, the needle should be carefully withdrawn, and the proptosed globe gently returned to the orbit by gentle digital pressure. The anterior chamber injection with deionised sterile water is made at the limbus, inserted into the anterior chamber parallel to the iris plane. The needle is carefully withdrawn, and the insertion site pressed with a cotton swab for 30 s, to avoid aqueous loss. This pressure also returned the proptosed globe to its proper place in the orbit. For topical administration, 100 mL deionised, sterile water is washed on to the cornea of the proptosed globe by a pipette and the globe returned to the orbit by gentle digital pressure. Viral shedding (detection of latent HSV-1 after reactivation and induced shedding into the tear film) is determined by swabbing the eyes 2 days prior to treatment and for 7 consecutive days after treatment. Each eye swab is mixed with 0.3 mL MEM (modified Eagle's medium with Earle's salt, 10% newborn calf serum, 1% penicillin streptomycin, 1% Fungizone), vortexed, and the eluant is plated on to a Vero cell monolayer. After a 1-h adsorption period, an additional 1.5 mL media is added to the well, and the plate can be examined daily for 7 days for the progressive CPE characteristic of HSV-1. Random HSV-1 isolates can be confirmed by neutralisation (Gordon *et al.*, 1983, 1990).

To test the in-vivo efficacy of an extract or formulation against HSV-2, the genital-herpes model was developed in random-breed BALB/c female mice or in female *Sigmodon hispidus* (cotton) rats (Yim *et al.*, 2005) by intravaginal inoculation of HSV-2 in anaesthetised inbred 6-week-old mice or rats. After 1-week acclimatisation at room temperature (23 ± 3°C), the animals (10 animals for each dilution) are inoculated with HSV-2 (30 μL of 10^{-3} virus stock) to the vagina by a size 12 needle, and the animals observed for 12 days to see if they develop vaginitis or die, to determine the median lethal dose (LD_{50}).

To test the efficacy of the extract or formulation, fresh batches of animals are infected with 10 LD_{50} dose of the virus (10^5 PFU) as described above. Following inoculation, a vaginal cotton swab sample is collected from each animal, transferred to 0.5 mL of PBS and stored at −20°C. The animals are divided into test groups (different potency), positive control group (acyclovir), negative control group (solvent or base cream), and one no treatment (virus control) group as well as an additional group of uninfected control. Symptoms of viral vaginitis (topical oedema of the vaginal tract with turbid secretions) will be observed on the third day of infection.

Treatment began on day 3 post-infection, by applying the extract or formulations to the vaginal tract with cotton swabs, at a dose of 2 mg per mouse twice daily for a 6-day period (Zhang *et al.*, 2007). Mortality and the number of days for mortality to occur are recorded. From day 1 following the completion of the treatment, as well as from the animals immediately after death, vaginal swab samples should be collected (Figure 21.2). The vaginal samples are then diluted five times in MEM and used to infect Vero cells. Samples that gave positive CPE are considered positive for HSV-2 (Zhang *et al.*, 2007).

A polysaccharide lignin–carbohydrate complex from *Prunella vulgaris* (PPS-2b), when tested by the plaque reduction assay showed strong activities against HSV-1 and HSV-2, as the complex block HSV binding and penetration; while a cream with semi-purified fraction of *P. vulgaris* showed a significant reduction ($P < 0.01$) in skin lesions and animal ($P < 0.01$) mortality in a HSV-1 skin lesion guinea pigs model and HSV-2 genital infection model in BALB/c mice, indicating that this complex had potent anti-HSV activity (Zhang *et al.*, 2007).

In-vitro and in-vivo activity of crude herbal extracts

The search for natural antivirals was actually initiated by the Boots drug company (UK) in 1952. Since then many broad-based screening programmes have been undertaken throughout the world to evaluate the in-vitro and in-vivo antiviral activity of plant extracts and many of them revealed strong antiherpes virus activity, while some can be used as a lead for the development of antiherpes virus agents (Khan *et al.*, 2005; Yarnell and Abascal, 2005; Chattopadhyay *et al.*, 2006; Chattopadhyay and Khan, 2008). These reviews report the in-vitro and sometimes in-vivo antiherpes virus activities of many plant extracts, mainly against HSV-1 and HSV-2.

Garlic (*Allium sativum*) extracts showed strong inhibitory activity against HCMV (Khan *et al.*, 2005; Chattopadhyay and Bhattacharya, 2008; Chattopadhyay and Khan, 2008). Interestingly the intraperitoneal administration of black seed (*Nigella sativa*) oil to BALB/c mice strikingly inhibited HCMV in-vitro murine CMV titres in spleen and liver (Salem and Hossain, 2000) while the extract of *Terminalia chebula* not only significantly inhibited HSV in vivo, but also the replication of HCMV in vitro and murine CMV in immunosuppressed mice (Chattopadhyay and Khan, 2008).

Canadian researchers first reported the antiviral activities of grape, apple and strawberry juices against HSV and other viruses; while leaf extract of *Azadirachta indica* inhibited DNA viruses (Khan *et al.*, 2005). British Columbian ethnomedicines *Cardamine angulata*, *Conocephalum conicum*, *Polypodium glycyrrhiza* showed anti-HSV-1 activity (McCutcheon *et al.*, 1995); while strong anti-HSV activity was found with *Byrsonima verbascifolia* extract, a folk remedy for skin infections (Rao *et al.*, 1969). The aqueous extracts of *Nepeta nepetella*, *Dittrichia viscosa* and *Sanguisorba minor magnolii* of the Iberian peninsula inhibited vesicular stomatitis virus (VSV) and HSV-1 at 50–125 μg/mL (Glatthaar-Saalmuller *et al.*, 2001); while the Nepalese ethnomedicine *Nerium indicum* inhibited HSV and influenza A virus (Alche *et al.*, 2000). The Chinese antipyretic and anti-inflammatory folk medicine *Rheum officinale* and *Paeonia suffruticosa* prevented HSV attachment and penetration (Hsiang *et al.*, 2001). *Senecio ambavilla*, a folk remedy of La Reunion Island, had anti-HSV-1 and anti-poliovirus activities (Rajbhandari *et al.*, 2001). The extracts of *Aglaia odorata*, *Moringa oleifera* and *Ventilago denticulate*, folk medicines of Thailand, inhibited thymidine kinase-deficient and phosphonoacetate-resistant HSV-1 and delayed the development of skin lesions at 750 mg/kg per dose, increased the mean survival times and reduced the mortality of infected mice similar to acyclovir (Fortin *et al.*, 2002). The Taiwanese folk remedy *Boussingaultia gracilis* and *Serissa japonica* extract was shown to inhibit HSV and adenoviruses (ADV) 3, 8 and 11. (Chiang *et al.*, 2003). Interestingly the viral adsorption, replication and transcription of HSV-1 and HSV-2 were inhibited by *Ceratostigma willmattianum* extract, an ethnomedicine of China, with IC_{50} of 29.46 and 9.2 mg/L respectively (Chen *et al.*, 2004).

The extracts of *Senna petersiana*, a folk remedy for sexually transmitted diseases, have strong anti-HSV activity (Dong *et al.*, 2004). The aqueous extract of *Carissa edulis* (Forssk.) Vahl (Apocynaceae) root from Kenya, significantly (100%) inhibited plaque formation in Vero E6 cells infected with 100 PFU of wild-type HSV or resistant HSV strains at 50 μg/mL in vitro with minimal cell cytotoxicity (CC_{50} 480 μg/mL). The extract at an oral dose of 250 mg/kg significantly (50%) delayed the onset of HSV infections in a murine model using Balb/C mice, cutaneously infected with wild-type or resistant strains of HSV (Tshikalange *et al.*, 2005).

Methanol and hot-aqueous extracts of 25 different plant species, used in Yemeni traditional medicine when tested in two in-vitro viral systems using HSV-1 in Vero cells and influenza virus A in MDCK cells, showed greater activity against HSV-1 at non-cytotoxic concentrations.

In-vitro and in-vivo antiherpetic activity of compounds from herbal extracts

A list of some potential herbal extracts along with the isolated compounds having antiherpes virus activities with probable mode of action are presented in Table 21.2.

Phenolics and polyphenols

The simplest bioactive polyphenols are the phenylpropanoids, and in a high oxidation state these have a wide range of antiviral activities. The aqueous extract of *Geranium sanguineum* L. aerial roots containing polyphenolic complex catechins and condensed tannins was reported to inhibit both HSV-1 and

Table 21.2 Important antiherpetic extracts and compounds from diverse chemical groups

Natural product	Source	Antiviral activity (lg/mL)	Reference
Whole extract	*Aglaria odorata*	HSV-1	Fortin *et al.*, 2002
	Moringa oleifera		
	Ventilago denticulata		
	Boussingaultia gracilis	HSV-1, HSV-2	Chiang *et al.*, 2003
	Serissa japonica		
	Cretastigma willmaltianum	HSV-1(9.12[a],36.5)[d, f, m]	Chen *et al.*, 2004
	Senna petersiana	HSV-1	Dong *et al.*, 2004
	Triphasia trifolia	HSV-1, HSV-2	Likhitwitayawuid *et al.*, 2005
	Artocarpus lakoocha		
	Millettia erythrocalyx	HSV*	Likhitwitayawuid *et al.*, 2005
	Carissa edulis	HSV-1, HSV-2 (50)[a]	Tshikalange *et al.*, 2005
	Geranium sanguineum	HSV-1, HSV-2 (3.6–6)[b]	Serkedjieva and Ivancheva, 1999
Propolis		HSV-1, VZV, HSV-2	Huleihel and Isanu, 2002
Alkaloids			
Cepharanthine	*Stephania cepharantha*	HSV*	Nawawi *et al.*, 1999
FK-3000	*Stephania cepharantha*	HSV-1(7.8) [a, g]	Nawawi *et al.*, 1999
Harmine	*Ophiorrhiza nicobarica*	HSV-2 (300)[g, f]	Chattopadhyay *et al.*, 2006
Bis-benzylisoquinoline			
Protoberberine	*Stephania cepharantha* Hayata	HSV-1 (18) [a],	Nawawi *et al.*, 1999
N-methylcrotsparine		HSV-1, HSV-2 (7.8–9.9)[a] (90, 71, 81)[d]	Nawawi *et al.*, 1999
Phenolics			
Caffeic acid	*Plantago major*	HSV-1(15.3) [b], VZV*	Chiang *et al.*, 2002
	P. major	HSV-2 (87.3) [b, f]	Chiang *et al.*, 2002
Chlorogenic acid	*Aloe barbadensis*	HSV-1 (47.6) [a]	
		HSV-2 (86.5) [a,]	Sydiskis *et al.*, 1991
Procyanidin A1	*Vaccinium vitis-idaca*	HSV-2[*j]	Cheng and Lin-Chun, 2005
Procyanidin C1	*Crataegus sinaica*	HSV-1[*f]	Sahahat *et al.*, 2002
Prodelphinidine-o-gallate	*Myrica rubra*	HSV-2 (5.3) [a, f, j]	Cheng *et al.*, 2003
Rosmarinic acid	*Plantago major*	VZV*	Chiang *et al.*, 2002
Xanthohumol	*Humulus lupulus*	HSV*[g]	Buckwold *et al.*,2004
Polyphenols	*Geranium sanguineum L.*	HSV-1, HSV-2 (3.6–6.2)[b]	Serkedjieva and Ivancheva, 1999
Cochinolide B, tremulacin	*Homalium cochinchinensis*	HSV-1,HSV-2	Ishikawa *et al.*, 2004
Asiaticoside	*Centella asiatica*	HSV*	Yoosook *et al.*, 2000
Mangiferin	*Mangifera indica*	HSV-1*, HSV-2*	Yoosook *et al.*, 2000
Rutin, rutin sulphate	—	HSV-1 (3–8.8)[a,j]	Tao *et al.*, 2007
Phenolics	*Rheum officinale*	HSV-1[j]	Hsiang *et al.*, 2001
	Paeonia suffruticosa	HSV-1[f, j]	Hsiang *et al.*, 2001
	Melia toosendan	HSV-1[f, j]	Hsiang *et al.*, 2001
Flavonoids			
Catechin	*Citrus aurantium, Vitis vinifera*	HSV-1[m*]	Kaul *et al.*, 1985
Hesperidin	*Orange, grape*	HSV[m*]	Kaul *et al.*, 1985
Resveratrol	—	HSV[*, m]	Faith *et al.*, 2006
Oxyresveratrol	*Millettia erythrocalyx*	HSV*	Likhitwitayawuid *et al.*, 2005
Quercetin	*Caesalpinia pulcherrima*	HSV-1 (24.3)[b], (20)[e, f]	Chiang *et al.*, 2003a
Phloroglucinol methyl gallate	*Mallotus japonicus*	HSV*	Arisawa *et al.*, 1990
Apigenin	*Ocimum basillicum*	HSV-1*	Lyu *et al.*, 2005
Epiafzelechin	*Cassia javanica*	HSV-2*	Cheng *et al.*, 2006

Table 21.2 *(continued)*

Natural product	Source	Antiviral activity (lg/mL)	Reference
Terpenes/sterols			
Betulinic acid	*Ocimum basilicum, Rhus javanica*	HSV (2.6) [b]	Chiang *et al.*, 2005
Isoborneol	*Melaleuca alternifolia*	HSV-1, 2 (0.06)[a, f]	Farag *et al.*, 2004
Lupenone	*Euphorbia segetalis*	HSV-1, HSV-2*	Chattopadhyay, 2006
Moronic acid	*Myrceugenia euosma, R. javanica*	HSV (3.9)[b] HSV-2*	Kurokawa *et al.*, 1999
Glycyrrhetinic acid	*Glycyrrhizin glabra*	HSV-1	Utsunomiya *et al.*, 1995
Pulegone	*Minthostachys verticillata*	HSV-1(10)[c]	Primo *et al.*, 2001
Putranjivain A	*Euphorbia jolkini*	HSV-2, (6.3 μM) [a, f, j]	Cheng *et al.*, 2004
Ursolic acid	—	HSV-1[b,f]	Chiang *et al.*, 2005
Sclerocarpic acid (sesquiterpene)	*Glyptopetalum sclerocarpum*	HSV-1,HSV-2	Khan *et al.*, 2005
Scopadulcic acid B (diterpenoid)	*Scoparia dulcis* L.	HSV-1 (16.7) [d,f]	Chattopadhyay and Khan, 2008
Morin	*Maclura cochinchinensis*	HSV-2 (38.5–53)[b]	Bunyapraphatsara *et al.*, 2000
Quassinoids	—	EBV[*, f]	Chattopadhyay and Khan, 2008
28-deacetylsendanin (Limonoid)	*Melia azedarach*	HSV-1(1.46) [a, f, k]	Alche at al., 2000
Meliacine	*Melia azedarach*	HSV-1[*, f]	Alche *et al.*, 2000
Asiaticoside	*Centella asiatica* L.	HSV-1*, HSV-2*	Yoosook *et al.*, 2000
Mangiferin	*Mangifera indica* L.	HSV-1*, HSV-2*	Yoosook *et al.*, 2000
Cochinolide B, tremulacin	*Homalium cochinchinensis*	HSV-1*,HSV-2*	Ishikawa *et al.*, 2004
Essential oil	*Minthostachys verticillata*	HSV*	Primo *et al.*, 2001
	Artemisia arborescen	HSV-2 [a,f]	Saddi *et al.*, 2007
Black seed oil	*Nigella sativa*	MCMV*	Salem and Hossain, 2000
N-N-B5	*Nelumbo nucifera*	HSV-1, HSV-2 (50–62)[a, m]	Kuo *et al.*, 2005
Thiazolylsulphonamide	—	HSV[*, l]	Betz *et al.*, 2002
n-docosanol	—	HSV-1	Sacks *et al.*, 2001
Oryzacystatin	*Oryzae sativa*	HSV-1	Aoki *et al.*, 1995
Saponins			
8-Acetylharpagide, scorodioside	*Bupleurum nigidum*	HSV-1(500)[a]	
Saikosaponin	*Scrophularia scorodonia*	VSV*	Chattopadhyay, 2006
Saponin glycosides (spirostane, tomatidane)	*Solanum* spp.	HSV-1*	Ikeda *et al.*, 2000
Tannin			
Casuarinin	*Terminalia arjuna*	HSV-2 (1.5 μM)[a,j]	Cheng *et al.*, 2002
Eugeniin	*Geum japonicum*	HSV-1*, HSV-2*, EBV*	Chattopadhyay and Khan, 2008
	Syzygium aromaticum	HSV, VZV	Chattopadhyay and Khan, 2008
Samaragenin B	*Limonium sinensi*	HSV-1*	Kuo *et al.*, 2002
Ellagitannins	*Phyllanthus myrtifolius, P. urinaria*	EBV[*, m]	Ikeda *et al.*, 2000
Euglobal-G1,G2, G3	*Eucalyptus grandis*	EBV*	Chattopadhyay and Khan, 2008
n-docosanol	—	HSV-1*	Sacks *et al.*, 2001; Chattopadhyay and Khan, 2008
Lignans			
Lignan	*Rhus javanica*	HSV-2[m]	Sakagami *et al.*, 2005
Yatein	*Chamaecyparis obtusa*	HSV-1[*, f, m]	Kuo *et al.*, 2006

(*continued overleaf*)

Table 21.2 *(continued)*

Natural product	Source	Antiviral activity (lg/mL)	Reference
Carbohydrate			
Polysaccharide	*Selerotium glucanicum*	HSV-1*	Marchetti *et al.*, 1996
Anionic polysaccharide	*Prunella vulgaris*	HSV-1(100)[g], HSV-2(10)[g]	Xu *et al.*, 1999; Chiu *et al.*, 2004
Polysaccharide lignan complex	*Prunella vulgaris*	HSV-1, HSV-2 (20—100)[b,m]	Zhang *et al.*, 2007
Sulphated galactans	*Bostrychia montagnei*	HSV*,[f]	Duarte *et al.*, 2001
Galactofucan	*Undaria pinnatida*	HSV-1, HSV-2*	Thompson and Dagar, 2004
Proteins and peptides			
Mannose-specific lectins	*Listera ovata*	CMV (0.08)[b]	Balzarini *et al.*, 1992
GlcNAc) n-specific lectin	*Urtica dioica*	CMV (0.3—9)[b]	Balzarini *et al.*, 1992
Peptide	*Sorghum bicolor*	HSV-1[b,h]	Filho *et al.*, 2008

[a]IC_{50}, [b]EC_{50}, [c]ED_{50}, [d]TI, [e]SI, Inhibit: [f]virus replication/multiplication, [g]virus-induced cytopathic effects, [h]virus entry, [i]cellular fusion, [j]attachment and penetration, [k]thymidine kinase, [l]helicase-primase, [m]infected cell polypeptide/DNA polymerase/DNA replication/gene expression.
*IC_{50}/EC_{50}/ED_{50} not available.
HSV = herpes simplex virus; VZV = varicella zoster virus; CMV = cytomegalovirus; MCMV = murine cytomegalovirus; EBV = Epstein-Barr virus.

HSV-2 (EC_{50} 3.6–6.2 μg/mL) and at minimum inhibitory concentration (MIC)90 (120 μg/mL) it strongly inactivated HSV-1 Kupka strain in plaque reduction assay, and delayed the development of herpetic vesicles in guinea pigs (Serkedjieva and Ivancheva, 1999). Propolis, a crude extract of the balsam of various trees collected by bees, inhibits acyclovir-resistant HSV-1 and VZV because of the synergistic action of a mixture of terpenoids, flavonoids, benzoic acid esters and phenolic acid esters (Huleihel and Isanu, 2002). Interestingly the anticancer, anti-inflammatory and immunomodulatory agent caffeic acid phenethyl ester (CAPE), an active component of propolis from Brazilian honeybee hives, inhibited plaque formation in HSV at 10 mg/mL dose by 70%, while at higher concentrations it inhibited RNA, protein synthesis and proliferation of HSV (Huleihel and Isanu, 2002).

The aqueous extract of *Plantago major* L., a popular medicine of Ayurvedic, traditional Chinese medicine and *Chakma Talika Chikitsa* of Bangladesh showed anti-HSV activity. Caffeic acid, chlorogenic acid and rosmarinic acid from *P. major* exhibited strongest activity against both HSV-1 (EC_{50} 15.3 μg/mL) and HSV-2 (EC_{50} 87.3 μg/m) (Chiang *et al.*, 2002). Structure–activity relationship studies revealed that the site(s) and number of -OH groups on phenols are responsible for their antiviral activity. The *Myrica rubra* barks containing prodelphinidin-di-O-gallate inhibited HSV-2 attachment and penetration, and reduced viral infectivity by affecting the late stage of infection (Cheng *et al.*, 2003). Similarly *Homalium cochinchinensis* root bark containing cochinolide B, tremulacin and tremuloidin, inhibited HSV-1 and HSV-2 (Ishikawa *et al.*, 2004). The in-vitro anti-HSV activity of *Vaccinium vitis-idaea* Linn (Ericaceae) by XTT assay (IC_{50} 73.3 ± 14.5 μmol/L) and plaque reduction assay (IC_{50} 41.9 ± 2.0 μmol/L for HSV-1 and 62.8 ± 6.3 μmol/L for HSV-2) was found to be due to proanthocyanidin A-1. This compound blocks HSV-2 infection at a non-toxic dose (CC_{50} 282.1 ± 27.5 μmol/L) by inhibiting viral attachment and penetration and affects the late stage(s) of infection (Cheng and Lin-Chun, 2005). Similarly proanthocyanidins isolated from *Hamamelis virginiana* bark and oligomeric procyanidin C1 of *Crataegus sinaica* showed remarkable anti-HSV-1 activity in the plaque reduction assay (Shahat *et al.*, 2002).

It was observed that proanthocyanidin C1 non-specifically bound proteins, but selectively inhibited nuclear factor κB (NF-κB)-dependent gene expression, which modulates apoptosis (Cos *et al.*, 2004). A xanthohumol-enriched *Humulus lupulus* extract showed moderate antiviral activity against HSV-1, HSV-2 and CMV in the plaque reduction assay

(Buckwold *et al.*, 2004). An interesting structure–activity relationship study is noted with dimeric procyanidins and related polyphenols, where epicatechin-containing dimers show pronounced anti-HSV activities, and the ortho-trihydroxyl groups in the B-ring with the double interflavan linkages leads to a significant increase of anti-HSV activity.

The flavonoids and dimeric stilbenes from *Artocarpus gomezianus* Wall, phloroglucinols from *Mallotus pallidus* Airy Shaw, and coumarins from *Triphasia trifolia* (Burm.f.) inhibit both HSV-1 and HSV-2 owing to bis-hydroxyphenyl moiety (Likhitwitayawuid *et al.*, 2005), which can be the potential target for anti-HSV drug development. Sakagami *et al.* (2005) opine that the virucidal activity of polyphenols is due to their association with proteins and/or host cell surfaces, resulting in reduction or prevention of viral adsorption.

The health-promoting, disease-preventing dietary compounds called flavonoids are therapeutically useful or can be used as prototypes for drug development. Some recent reviews report that flavonoids can inhibit diverse viruses, including herpes viruses, both in vitro and in vivo by direct inactivation or blocking replication (Khan *et al.*, 2005; Chattopadhyay and Khan, 2008). Flavonoids such as quercetin, procyanidin, and pelargonidin are virucidal to HSV while catechin and hesperidins can inactivate HSV (Kaul *et al.*, 1985). Similarly quercetin, galangin, naringenin, kaempferol and 3-methyl kaempferol are potent antiherpetic compounds, as these agents inhibit viral attachment and penetration (Sarisky *et al.*, 2002). An extract of *Sapium sebiferum* containing methyl gallate and methyl-3,4,5-trihydroxybenzoate is a potent and specific inhibitor of herpes viruses; while phloroglucinol of *Mallotus japonicus* can only reduce HSV plaque formation (Arisawa *et al.*, 1990).

Hesperidin from orange (*Citrus aurantium* L.) and grape (*Vitis vinifera* L.) can inhibit HSV replication; catechin inhibits infectivity of HSV-1, but quercetin inhibits both, so the small structural differences of these compounds are critical to their activity. *Centella asiatica* L., *Maclura cochinchinensis* Cornor, and *Mangifera indica* L., used as herpes virus remedies in Thailand, can inhibit HSV-1 and HSV-2 virion production in plaque inhibition assay and combinations of these extracts with acyclovir resulted in synergistic or additive interaction in a dose-dependent manner, probably because of asiaticosidein in *C. asiatica* and mangiferin in *M. indica* (Yoosook *et al.*, 2000). Bunyapraphatsara *et al.* (2000) reported that the flavonoid morin, from *Maclura cochinchinensis*, had powerful anti-HSV-2 activity (EC_{50} 38.5–53.5 μg/mL), owing to its free hydroxyl groups.

Extracts of *Rhus succedanea* and *Garcinia multiflora* containing amentoflavone and robustaflavone, inhibited in-vitro growth of HSV, while VZV was inhibited by rhusflavanone and succedaneflavanone (Chattopadhyay, 2006). It was reported that the quercetin from *Caesalpinia pulcherrima* Swartz had a broad antiherpes virus activity (EC_{50} 24.3–50 mg/L), by inhibiting early stage of multiplication (Chiang *et al.*, 2003), suggesting its potential use for anti-HSV drug development. Similarly isoquercitrin of *Waldsteinia fragarioides* had significant anti-HSV activity (Khan *et al.*, 2005).

Eighteen flavonoids of five classes were tested against HSV-1 and HSV-2 and the result was that epicatechin (EC), epicatechin gallate (ECG) and quercetin (flavanols); genistein (isoflavone) and naringenin (flavanone) showed a high level of CPE inhibitory activity. EC, ECG, galangin and kaempferol showed strong anti-HSV activity, while catechin, epigallocatechin, epigallocatechin gallate, naringenin, apigenin, chrysin, baicalin, fisetin, myricetin, quercetin, and genistein had moderate effect on HSV-1 in plaque reduction assay. Hence, flavanols and flavonols appeared to be more active than flavones.

Vero cells treated with ECG and galangin before virus adsorption led to an enhancement of inhibition, indicating that an intracellular effect may also be involved (Lyu *et al.*, 2005). The potent antiviral flavonoids appear to block viral DNA/RNA polymerase, where the degree of inhibition depends on the structure and side chain. A recent study with *ent*-epiafzelechin-(4α-8)-epiafzelechin (EEE) from fresh leaves of *Cassia javanica* L. var. 'Agnes de Wit' revealed the inhibition of HSV-2 replication in a dose-dependent manner (IC_{50} 83.8 ± 10.9 μmol/L) by inhibiting penetration and replication at the late stage of its life cycle (Cheng *et al.*, 2006).

Tannins are polymeric phenolics (molecular weight 500–3000) and are grouped into hydrolysable and condensed tannins. It is believed that the consumption of tannin-containing beverages, such as green teas and red wines, can cure or prevent a variety of illnesses. Some recent reviews reported that tannins can stimulate phagocytic cells, inhibit tumours and a wide range of microbes by forming complexes with microbial proteins. They can inactivate virus adsorption, transport proteins, polysaccharides and viral enzymes (Chattopadhyay, 2006; Chattopadhyay and Naik, 2007). A detailed study on ellagitannins from *Phyllanthus myrtifolius* and *P. urinaria* (Euphorbiaceae) demonstrated the inhibition of Epstein-Barr virus DNA polymerase, probably because of the corilagin moiety of these tannins. *Terminalia arjuna* L. bark contains the virucidal hydrolysable tannin casuarinin which, at 25 μmol/L dose, reduced viral titres up to 10^5-fold (IC_{50} 3.6 ± 0.9 and 1.5 ± 0.2) in XTT and plaque reduction assay, and at C_{50} 89 ± 1.0 μmol/L it inhibited HSV-2 attachment and penetration (Cheng *et al.*, 2002).

Coumarins

Coumarins are reported to have antithrombotic, anti-inflammatory, antioxidant, anticarcinogenic, antiallergic, vasodilatory and hepatoprotective activities (Chattopadhyay and Bhattacharya, 2008); some being enzyme inhibitors or precursors of toxic substances, and are defences against infection. As coumarins can stimulate macrophages, they can exert an indirect effect on viral infections, e.g. recurrences of cold sores caused by HSV-1 (Khan *et al.*, 2005; Chattopadhyay, 2006). Hence, this plant can be a potential candidate as an anti-HSV agent. The coumarin derivatives 1,4-dihydropyridine-5-carboxylic acid and pyridine-5-carboxylic acid from some herbal products showed antiviral activities against CMV (AD-169 and Davis strain), HSV-1 (KOS, F, Mclntyre, TK-B2006, TK-VMW1837, TK-Cheng C158/77, TK-Field C137/101), HSV-2 (G, 196, Lyons), and VZV (TK OKA, TK YS, TK−07/1, TK−YS/R strains) (Patent WO 01/14370, Rephartox B.V.).

Hydroxylated coumarins are produced by many plants as defence in response to microbial infection, and so are a type of phytoalexin. A polyphenolic phytoalexin, resveratrol (3,5,4′-trihydroxystilbene) occurs in *cis*- (*Z*) and *trans*- (*E*) form. The *trans*-form can undergo isomerisation to the *cis*- form in presence of heat or ultraviolet irradiation in grapes, berries, plums, peanuts, *Vaccinium* species, pines and knotweed. Resveratrol is reported to inhibit HSV-1 and HSV-2 replication by suppressing NF-κB activation, an essential step of its lifecycle during infection (Gregory *et al.*, 2004). Further study by electromobility shift assays demonstrated that resveratrol suppressed NF-κB activation of both HSV types as well as acyclovir-resistant HSV-1 in a dose-dependent and reversible manner, impairing expression of essential immediate-early, early and late genes and synthesis of DNA (Faith *et al.*, 2006). Similarly oxyresveratrol of *Millettia erythrocalyx* and *Artocarpus lakoocha* inhibited herpes virus replication (Likhitwitayawuid *et al.*, 2005a).

Essential oils and terpenoids

Essential oils and terpenoids have antiviral activities against many viruses (Khan *et al.*, 2005). The monoterpene isoborneol can block HSV-1 replication within 30 min of exposure and can inhibit glycosylation of viral polypeptides and gB without affecting the glycosylation of host cell polypeptides; while pulegone inhibits HSV-1 replication (Primo *et al.*, 2001). On the other hand *Santalum album* oil had a dose-dependent anti-HSV-1 activity, but the essential oil of the Italian food plant *Santolina insularis* inhibited cell-to-cell transmission of herpes viruses (Khan *et al.*, 2005).

Terpinen-4-ol from *Mentha alternifolia* oil, used as an antimicrobial preservative in cosmetics, exhibited strong virucidal activity against HSV-1 and HSV-2 and, at a noncytotoxic dose, plaque formation was reduced by 98.2% (HSV-1) and 93.0% (HSV-2). The IC_{50} for plaque formation in RC 37 cell was 0.0008 (HSV-1) and 0.009% (HSV-2). Although the active antiherpes components of tree tea oil are not yet fully characterised, its application in recurrent herpes infection is promising.

The essential oils of *Artemisia douglasiana* and *Eupatorium patens* inhibit HSV-1 (65–125 ppm) while *Melissa officinalis* oil inhibits HSV-2 replication (Khan *et al.*, 2005; Chattopadhyay and Khan, 2008); while the volatile oil 1,8-cineole and terpinen-4-ol of *Melaleuca armillaris* are effective virucidal agents (Farag *et al.*, 2004). The essential oil obtained from *A. arborescens* is reported to inhibit HSV-1 (IC_{50} 24 μg/mL) and HSV-2 (4.1 μg/mL) at CC_{50}

132 μg/mL in MTT reduction assay and CC_{50}/IC_{50} ratio of 55 for HSV-1, and 32.2 for HSV-2 with a direct virucidal effect, inhibiting the virus and cell to cell virus diffusion (Saddi *et al.*, 2007).

The stem bark of *Glyptopetalum sclerocarpum*, containing a sesquiterpene sclerocarpic acid, showed antiviral activity against HSV-1 and HSV-2 (Chattopadhyay, 2006); while the quassinoids inhibit Epstein-Barr virus (Chattopadhyay and Khan, 2008). The diterpenoid scopadulcic acid B, isolated from *Scoparia dulcis* L., inhibits HSV-1 replication in vitro by interfering with early events of viral growth, while in hamsters it delayed the appearance of herpetic lesions and increased the survival time at 100–200 mg/kg/day dose (Chattopadhyay and Khan, 2008). Another diterpene putranjivain A of *Euphorbia jolkini* significantly reduced infectivity (IC_{50} 6.3 μmol/L), attachment and penetration and the late stage of HSV-2 replication (Cheng *et al.*, 2004).

It was observed that the triterpenes betulinic acid and moronic acid of *Rhus javanica* inhibited acyclovir-resistant, thymidine kinase-deficient and wild-type HSV-1 (EC_{50} of 2.6–3.9 μg/mL). Orally administered moronic acid fed to mice infected cutaneously with HSV-1 significantly retarded skin lesions and/or prolonged the mean survival times at non-cytotoxic dose by suppressing virus yields in the brain (Kurokawa *et al.*, 1999). Hence, moronic acid may be a good anti-HSV lead with a mechanism of action different from that of acyclovir.

Interestingly both aqueous and ethanolic extract of *Ocimum basilicum* along with purified apigenin, linalool and ursolic acid showed strong anti-HSV-1 activity. The ursolic acid showed the strongest activity against HSV-1 (EC_{50} 6.6 mg/L), while apigenin revealed the highest activity against HSV-2, by blocking the infection process and the replication phase (Chiang *et al.*, 2005), indicating its potential candidature as an antiherpes agent. Again the tetracyclic triterpenes lupenone of *Euphorbia segetalis* strongly inhibited plaque formation of HSV-1 and HSV-2 (Chattopadhyay, 2006).

It was found that a tetranortriterpenoid (limonoid) meliacine, isolated from *Melia azedarach* L. leaves, inhibited HSV-1 replication in vitro. Meliacine exerts potent anti-HSV-1 activity by inhibiting ICPs, DNA synthesis, nucleocapsids assembly and late stages of HSV life cycle. Ultrastructural analysis of infected cells showed that meliacine treatment results in accumulation of unenveloped nucleocapsids in the cytoplasmic vesicles of infected cells, suggesting that it also blocks the syntheses of viral DNA and its maturation (Alche *et al.*, 2000). Corneal herpetic stromal keratitis, a leading cause of human blindness, when developed in Balb/c mice by HSV-1 (KOS strain) and treated with meliacine topically, significantly reduced the development of keratitis and the histological damage in corneas. The results revealed that the viral titres in eyes of infected and treated mice were twofold lower than the corresponding controls (Alche *et al.*, 2000). Another limonoid terpene, 28-deacetylsendanin, of *Melia azedarach* fruit, showed anti-HSV-1 activity (IC_{50} 1.46 μg/mL) at 400 μg/mL.

Triterpenoid saponins of the oleanane group inhibit DNA synthesis, while the ursane group inhibits capsid protein synthesis of HSV-1. Apers *et al.* (2001) observed that alcoholic extract of *Maesa lanceolata* leaves contains a maesasaponin VI2 which showed virucidal effect against HSV (reduction factor 10^3 at 50 μg/mL), owing to diacylation of replicating enzymes. On the other hand, the saponin glycosides (spirostane, tomatidane, solasodane, nuatigenin, ergostane and furostane dimers) of some *Solanum* species inhibit HSV-1, probably because of their oligosaccharide moiety (Khan *et al.*, 2005).

Lignans

Larrea tridentates, *Rhinacanthus nasutus* and *Kadsura matsudai* extracts showed antiherpes activities owing to the lignan nordehydroguanoferate; while *Rhus javanica* lignans exhibited anti-HSV-2 activity similar to acyclovir. The cones of various pine trees (*Pinus* spp.) inhibited the proliferation of HSV, owing to lignin–carbohydrate complexes. It was observed that the anti-HSV activity was maximal when lignin was added at the time of virus adsorption (Sakagami *et al.*, 2005). A bioassay-guided study with the Chinese herb *Chamaecyparis obtusa*, yielded yatein, a lignan that significantly inhibited HSV-1 multiplication in HeLa cells. It was found that yatein can impede the levels of gB and gC mRNA expression in HeLa cells, can arrest DNA replication, inhibit the expression of α gene, *ICP0* and *ICP4* genes, arresting DNA synthesis and expression of structural protein of HSV-1(Kuo *et al.*, 2006).

Alkaloids

Many alkaloids have antiviral activities. The methanol extract of *Stephania cepharantha* root tubers, used in Chinese and Mongolian traditional medicine, contains isoquinoline alkaloids with in-vivo antitumour, anti-inflammatory, antiallergic and immunomodulatory activity and with potent anti-HSV-1 activity (IC_{50} 18 μg/mL). Further study revealed that cepharanthine from *S. cepharantha* inhibited HSV-1 (Nawawi *et al.*, 1999; Chattopadhyay, 2006). *N*-methylcrotsparine showed antiviral activity against HSV-1, thymidine kinase-deficient (acyclovir-resistant) HSV-1, and HSV-2 by plaque reduction assay; while the alkaloid FK-3000 was a more promising anti-HSV candidate (Nawawi *et al.*, 1999). Cepharanthine has strong antiviral activity against both RNA and DNA viruses. The ethanol extracts of lotus (*Nelumbo nucifera* Gaertn.) seed, used throughout south Asia for over a thousand years for gastrointestinal and bleeding disorders, significantly inhibits HSV-1 and HSV-2 replication at 100 μg/mL, with IC_{50} 50 μg/mL and IC_{50} 62.0 ± 8.9 μg/mL respectively; while its subfraction NN-B-5 from the bioactive butanol part showed the highest activity at 50 μg/mL by inhibiting thymidine kinase-deficient HSV-1 replication in HeLa cells (Kuo *et al.*, 2005).

Ophiorrhiza nicobarica, part of the folklore of Shompen and Nicobarese tribes of the Nicobar Islands, contains a β-carboline alkoloid harmine, which was found to inhibit plaque formation of HSV-1 and HSV-2, and delayed the eclipse phase of HSV replication at 300 μg/mL (Chattopadhyay *et al.*, 2006).

Lectins, polypeptides and polysaccharides

Lectins are natural proteins that target the sugar moieties of various glycoproteins and are widespread in higher plants. Mannose-specific lectins of *Cymbidium hybrid*, *Epipactis helleborine* and *Listera ovata* showed a marked anti-HCMV activity, while the (GlcNAc) n-specific lectin from *Urtica dioica* was inhibitory to CMV-induced cytopathicity at an EC_{50} of 0.3–9 μg/mL (Balzarini *et al.*, 1992). The antimicrobial peptides are often positively charged and contain disulphide bonds. Recently a 2-kDa peptide from seeds of *Sorghum bicolor* L. was shown to dose-dependently inhibit the replication of HSV-1, with EC_{50} and EC_{90} values of 6.25 and 15.25 μmol/L, respectively. The IC_{50} value of the 2-kDa peptide against Vero cells was 250 μmol/L. Preincubation of HSV-1 with various concentrations of the 2-kDa peptide showed dose-dependent CPE reduction at 6.25-50 μmol/L. Similar results were observed when the 2-kDa peptide was assayed against bovine herpes virus, an enveloped virus such as HSV-1, but there was only weak activity against non-enveloped poliovirus type 1 (Filho *et al.*, 2008).

The sulphated galactans from a marine alga *Bostrychia montagnei* were found to inhibit herpes virus multiplication in cell culture and replication in vitro (Duarte *et al.*, 2001), while the polysaccharide of *Cedrela tubiflora* leaves inhibited HSV-2 replication at non-cytotoxic doses, indicating that the anti-HSV activity of polysaccharides correlates with molecular weight and sulphate content.

Recently Thompson and Dragar (2004) reported that a seaweed *Undaria pinnatida,* containing a sulphated polysaccharide galactofucan, had anti-HSV-1 activity, inhibiting viral binding and entry into the host cell (IC_{50} 32 μg/mL), and was highly active against HSV-2 (IC_{50} 0.5 μg/mL; $P < 0.001$). A water-soluble anionic polysaccharide from *Prunella vulgaris* L. (Labiatae) inhibited HSV-1 at 100 μg/mL and HSV-2 at 10 μg/mL by plaque inhibition assay (Xu *et al.*, 1999) while the anionic polysaccharide of the same herb collected from Japan showed specific anti-HSV activity (IC_{50} 10 μg/mL) by competing for cell surface receptor (Chiu *et al.*, 2004).

Conclusions

The diseases caused by human herpes viruses (HSV, VZV, CMV, EBV and Kaposi's sarcoma-associated herpes virus) are of global concern. A 'cure' or development of effective vaccines are not yet possible; hence, cost-effective natural or complementary antivirals to prevent resistance development with reduced toxicity is of immediate need, especially since current antiherpes virus drugs are expensive, with high toxicity.

Compounds have been discovered with specific in-vitro and in-vivo activity and low toxicity. Some interfere with particular herpes virus enzymes, e.g. DNA polymerase inhibition by eugenol, eugeniin and ellagitannins, RNA and protein synthesis (CAPE, procyanidin C1), and DNA replication, e.g. prodelphinidine-di-O-gallate, ursolic acid, cellular fusion (essential oils, epicatechin gallate, galangin), attachment and penetration, e.g. casuarinin, putranjivain A, virus entry and target-cell binding, e.g. flavones. Although no plant-derived drug is currently in clinical use to treat herpes virus diseases, there are some promising herbal product/natural product-derived candidates in preclinical and clinical trials. Interestingly most of these compounds can block virus entry into host cells and/or specific cellular enzymes, alone or sometimes in combination with acyclovir, which is a very important aspect in the context of viral drug resistance and limited lifespan of antiviral drugs. The compounds having an alternative mechanism of action, unlike synthetic antivirals, are potential candidates to tackle the threats posed by drug-resistant herpes viruses, as it is quite difficult to eliminate herpes virus diseases by the available antivirals.

Acknowledgement

The authors wish to acknowledge Dr Sujit K Bhattacharya, the Additional Director General, Indian Council of Medical Research, New Delhi and the Officer-in Charge, ICMR Virus Unit, Kolkata, for their kind help and encouragement during the preparation of this manuscript.

References

Alche LE, Berra A, Veloso MJ, Coto CE (2000). Treatment with meliacine, a plant derived antiviral, prevents the development of herpetic stromal keratitis in mice. *J Med Virol* 61: 474–480.

Apers S, Baronikova S, Sindambiwe JB *et al.* (2001). Antiviral, haemolytic and molluscicidal activities of triterpenoid saponins from *Maesa lanceolata*: establishment of structure-activity relationship. *Planta Med* 67: 528–532.

Apers S, Cimanga K, Vanden Berghe D *et al.* (2002). Antiviral activity of Simalikalactone D, a quassinoid from *Quassia africana*. *Planta Med* 68: 20–24.

Aoki H, Akaike T, Abe K *et al.* (1995). Antiviral effect of oryzacystatin, a proteinase inhibitor in rice, against herpes simplex virus type 1 *in vitro* and *in vivo*. *Antimicrob Agents Chemother* 39: 846–849.

Arisawa M, Fujita A, Hayashi T, Hayashi K, Ochiai H, Morita N (1990). Cytotoxic and antiherpetic activity of phloroglucinol derivatives from *Mallotus japonicus* (Euphorbiaceae). *Chem Pharm Bull* 38: 1624–1626.

Balzarini J, Neyts J, Schols D *et al.* (1992). The mannose specific plant lectins from *Cymbidium hybrid* and *Epipactis helleborine* and the (N-acetylglucosamine) n-specific plant lectins from *Urtica dioca* are potent and selective inhibitors of HIV and cytomegalovirus replication *in vitro*. *Antiviral Res* 18: 191–207.

Bourne KZ, Bourne N, Reising SF, Stanberry LR (1999). Plant products as topical microbicide candidates: assessment of in vitro and in vivo activity against herpes simplex virus type 2. *Antiviral Res* 42: 219–226.

Buckwold VE, Wilson RJ, Nalca A *et al.* (2004). Antiviral activity of Hop constituents against a series of DNA and RNA viruses. *Antiviral Res* 61: 57–62.

Bunyapraphatsara N, Dechsree S, Yoosook C, Herunsalee A¸ Panpisutchai Y (2000). Anti-herpes simplex virus activity of *Maclura cochinchinensis*. *Phytomedicine* 6: 421–424.

Chattopadhyay D (2006). Ethnomedicinal antivirals: Scope and opportunity. Chapter 15. In: *Modern Phytomedicine: turning medicinal plants into drugs*, pp. 313–338. Ahmad I, Aquil F, Owais M (Eds.). Wiley-VCH Verlag GmbH & Co. Weinheim, Germany.

Chattopadhyay D, Arunachalam G, Mandal AB, Bhattacharya SK (2006). Dose dependent therapeutic antiinfectives from ethnomedicines of Bay Islands. *Chemotherapy* 52: 151–157.

Chattopadhyay D, Naik TN (2007). Antivirals of ethnomedicinal origin: structure-activity relationship and scope. *Mini Rev Med Chem* 7: 275–301 (Review).

Chattopadhyay D, Bhattacharya SK (2008). Ethnopharmacology: A new engine for the development of antivirals from naturaceuticals. In: *Handbook of Ethnopharmacology*, Eddouks M Ed. Research Signpost, Trivandrum, India, pp. 129–197.

Chattopadhyay D, Khan MTH (2008). Ethnomedicines and ethnomedicinal phytophores against herpes viruses. *Biotechnology Annual Review*, 14 (Chapter 12): 297–349.

Chen T, Jia W, Yang F *et al.* (2004). Experimental study on the antiviral mechanism of *Ceratostigma willmattianum* against herpes simplex virus type 1 *in vitro*. *Zhongguo Zhong Yao Za Zhi [China J Chinese Materia Medica]* 29: 882–886.

Cheng HY, Lin CC, Lin TC (2002). Antiherpes simplex virus type 2 activity of Casuarinin from the bark of *Terminalia arjuna* Linn. *Antiviral Res* 55: 447–455.

Cheng HY, Lin TC, Ishimaru K, Yang CM, Wang KC, Lin CC (2003). In vitro antiviral activity of prodelphinidin B-2 3, 3′-di-O-gallate from *Myrica rubra*. *Planta Med* 69: 953–956.

Cheng HY, Lin TC, Yang CM, Wang KC, Lin LT, Lin CC (2004). Putranjivain A from *Euphorbia jolkini* inhibits both virus entry and late stage replication of herpes simplex virus type 2 *in vitro*. *J Antimicrob Chemother* 53: 577–583.

Cheng HY, LinChun C (2005). The antiherpes simplex viruses activity of extracts and compounds of natural products. *J Trad Med* 22 (supp.1): 129–132.

Cheng HY, Yang CM, Lin TC, Shieh DE, Lin CC (2006). ent-Epiafzelechin-(4α-8)-epiafzelechin extracted from *Cassia javanica* inhibits HSV-2 replication. *J Med Microbiol* 55: 201–206.

Chiang LC, Cheng HY, Liu MC *et al.* (2003). In vitro anti-herpes simplex viruses and anti-adenoviruses activity of twelve traditionally used medicinal plants in Taiwan. *Biol Pharm Bull* 26: 1600–1604.

Chiang LC, Ng LT, Cheng PW *et al.* (2005). Antiviral activities of extracts and selected pure constituents of *Ocimum basilicum. Clin Exp Pharmacol Physiol* 32: 811–816.

Chiu LC-M, Zhu W, Ooi VE-C (2004). A polysaccharide fraction from medicinal herb *Prunella vulgaris* down-regulates the expression of herpes simplex virus antigen in Vero cells. *J Ethnopharmaco*l 93: 63–68.

Corey L, Wald A, Celum CL, Quinn TC (2004). The effects of herpes simplex virus-2 on HIV-1 acquisition and transmission: a review of two overlapping epidemics. *J Acquir Immune Defic Syndr* 35: 435–445.

Cos P, de Bruyne T, Hermans N *et al.* (2004). Proanthocyanidins in health care: current and new trends. *Curr Med Chem* 11: 1345–1359.

Dong Y, Li H, Yao Z *et al.* (2004). The respiratory syncytial virus (RSV) effect of Radix Glycyrrhizae *in vitro. Zhong Yao Cai* 27: 425–417.

Duarte ME, Noseda DG, Noseda M *et al.* (2001). Inhibitory effect of sulfated galactans from the marine alga *Bostrychia montagnei* on herpes simplex virus replication *in vitro. Phytomedicine* 8: 53–58.

Faith SA, Sweet TJ, Bailey E *et al.* (2006). Resveratrol suppresses nuclear factor-kappaB in herpes simplex virus infected cells. *Antiviral Res* 72: 242–251.

Farag RS, Shalaby AS, El-Baroty GA *et al.* (2004). Chemical and biological evaluation of the essential oils of different *Melaleuca* species. *Phytother Res* 18: 30–35.

Felser J, Kichington PR, Inchauspe G *et al.* (1988). Cell line containing varicella-zoster virus open reading frame 62 and expressing the 'IE' 175 protein complement ICP4 mutants of herpes simplex virus type 1. *J Virol* 62: 2076–2082.

Fortin H, Vigor C, Lohezic LDF *et al.* (2002). In vitro antiviral activity of thirty-six plants from La Reunion Island. *Fitoterapia* 73: 346–350.

Filho IC, Cortez DAG, Ueda-Nakamura T *et al.* (2008). Antiviral activity and mode of action of a peptide isolated from *Sorghum bicolor. Phytomedicine* 15: 202–208.

Glatthaar-Saalmuller B, Sacher F Esperester A *et al.* (2001). Antiviral activity of an extract derived from roots of *Eleutherococcus* senticosus. *Antivir Res* 50: 223–228.

Gius D, Laimins LA (1989). Activation of human papillomavirus type 18 gene expression by herpes simplex virus type 1 viral transactivators and phorbol ester. *J Virol* 63: 555–563.

Gordon YJ, Armstrong JA, Brown SI, Becker Y (1983). The role of herpes virus type 1 thymidine kinase in experimental ocular infections. *Am J Ophthalmol* 95: 175–181.

Gordon YJ, Araullo-Cruz TP, Romanowski E *et al.* (1986). The development of an improved reactivation model for the study of HSV-1 latency. *Invest Ophthalmol Vis Sci* 27: 1230–1234.

Gordon YJ, Romanowski E, Araullo-Cruz T (1990). A fast, simple reactivation method for the study of HSV-1 latency in the rabbit ocular model. *Invest Ophthalmol Vis Sci* 31: 921–924.

Gregory D, Hargett D, Holmes D, Money E, Bachenheimer SL (2004). Efficient replication by HSV-1 involves activation of the IκB kinase-IkappaB-RelA/p65 pathway. *J Virol* 78: 13582–13590.

Habif T (2004). Warts, herpes simplex, and other viral infections. In: *Clinical Dermatology*, 4th edn. Ed. Thomas Habif. New York, Mosby, pp. 381–388.

Hsiang CY, Hsieh CL, Wu SL, Lai IL, Ho TY (2001). Inhibitory effect of anti-pyretic and anti-inflammatory herbs on herpes simplex virus replication. *Am J Chin Med*. 29: 459–467.

Huleihel M, Isanu V. (2002). Anti-herpes simplex virus effect of an aqueous extract of Propolis. *Isr Med Assoc J* 4: 923–927.

Ikeda T, Ando J, Miyazono A *et al.* (2000). Anti-herpes virus activity of *Solanum* steroidal glycosides. *Biol Pharm Bull* 23: 363–364.

Ishikawa T, Nishigaya K, Takami K *et al.* (2004). Isolation of Salicin derivatives from *Homalium cochinchinensis* and their antiviral activities. *J Nat Prod* 67: 659–663.

Kaul TN Jr Middletown E, Ogra PL (1985). Antiviral effect of flavonoids on human viruses. *J Med Virol* 15: 71–79.

Khan MT, Ather A, Thompson KD, Gambari R (2005). Extracts and molecules from medicinal plants against herpes simplex viruses. *Antivir Res* 67: 107–119.

Kira T, Kakefuda A, Awano H, *et al.* (1995). Development of anti-HSV screening system using suspension cell line and screening several nucleoside analogues in this method. *Antiviral Res* 26: 309.

Kuo YC, Lin LC, Tsai WJ *et al.* (2002). Samaragenin B identified from *Limonium sinensis* suppressed herpes simplex virus type 1 replication in Vero cells by regulation of viral macromolecular synthesis. *Antimicrob Agents Chemother* 46: 2854–2864.

Kuo YC, Lin YL, Liu CP, Tsai WJ (2005). Herpes simplex virus type 1 propagation in HeLa cells interrupted by *Nelumbo nucifera. J Biomed Sci* 12: 1021–1034.

Kuo YC, Kuo YH, Lin YL, Tsai WJ (2006). Yatein from *Chamaecyparis obtusa* suppresses herpes simplex virus type 1 replication in HeLa cells by interruption the immediate-early gene expression. *Antiviral Res* 70: 112–120.

Kurokawa M, Basnet P, Ohsugi M, *et al.* (1999). Anti-herpes simplex virus activity of moronic acid purified from *Rhus javanica* in vitro and in vivo. *J Pharmacol Exp Ther* 289: 72–78.

Likhitwitayawuid K, Supudompol B, Sritularak B, *et al.* (2005). Phenolics with anti-HSV and anti-HIV activities from *Artocarpus gomezianus*, *Mallotus pallidus*, and *Triphasia trifolia. Pharm Biol* 43: 651–657.

Likhitwitayawuid K, Sritularak B, Benchanak K *et al.*

(2005a). Phenolics with antiviral activity of *Millettia erythrocalyx* and *Artocarpus lakoocha*. *Nat Prod Res* 19: 177–182.

Lyu S-Y, Rhim J-Y, Park W-B (2005). Antiherpetic activities of flavonoids against herpes simplex virus type 1 (HSV-1) and type 2 (HSV-2) *in vitro*. *Arch Pharm Res* 28: 1293–1301.

Marchetti M, Pisani S, Pietropaola V *et al.* (1996). Antiviral effect of a polysaccharide from *Sclerotium glucanicum* towards herpes simplex virus type 1 infection. *Planta Med* 62: 303–307.

McCutcheon AR, Roberts TE, Gibbons E *et al.* (1995). Antiviral screening of British Columbian medicinal plants. *J Ethnopharmacol* 49: 101–110.

Nawawi A, Ma C, Nakamura N, Hattori M *et al.* (1999). Anti-herpes simplex virus activity of alkaloids isolated from *Stephania cepharantha*. *Biol Phar Bull* 22: 268–274.

Ostrove JM, Leonard J, Weck KE *et al.* (1987). Activation of the human immunodeficiency virus by herpes simplex virus type 1. *J Virol* 61: 3726–3732.

Primo V, Rovera M, Zanon S *et al.* (2001). Determination of the antibacterial and antiviral activity of the essential oil from *Minthostachys verticillata* (Griseb.) Epling. *Rev Arg Microbiol* 33: 113–117.

Rajbhandari M, Wegner U, Julich M *et al.* (2001). Screening of Nepalese medicinal plants for antiviral activity. *J Ethnopharmacol* 74(3): 251–255.

Rao AR, Kumar SSV, Paramasivam TB *et al.* (1969). Study of antiviral activity of tender leaves of margosa tree (*Melia azadirachta*) on vaccinia and variola virus – a preliminary report. *Indian J Med Res* 57: 495–502.

Saddi M, Sanna A, Cottiglia F *et al.* (2007). Antiherpes activity of *Artemisia arborescence* essential oil and inhibition of lateral diffusion in Vero cells. *Ann Clin Microbiol Antimicrob* 6: 10.

Shahat AA, Cos P, De Bruyne T *et al.* (2002). Antiviral and antioxidant activity of flavonoids and proanthocyanidins from *Crataegus sinaica*. *Planta Med* 68: 539–541.

Sakagami H, Hashimoto K, Suzuki F *et al.* (2005). Molecular requirements of lignin–carbohydrate complexes for expression of unique biological activities. *Phytochemistry* 66: 2108–2120.

Salem ML, Hossain MS (2000). Protective effect of black seed oil from *Nigella sativa* against murine cytomegalovirus infection. *Int J Immunopharmacol* 22: 729–740.

Sandri-Goldin RM, ed. (2006). *Alpha Herpes Viruses: Molecular and Cellular Biology.* Caister Academic Press.

Sarisky RT, Crosson P, Cano R *et al.* (2002). Comparison of methods for identifying resistant herpes simplex virus and measuring antiviral susceptibility. *J Clin Virol* 23: 191–200.

Serkedjieva J, Ivancheva S (1999). Antiherpes virus activity of extracts from the medicinal plant *Geranium sanguineum* L. *J Ethnopharmacol* 64: 59–68.

Simões CMO, Amoros M, Girre L (1999). Mechanism of antiviral activity of triterpenoid saponins. *Phytother Res* 21: 317–325.

Sudo K, Konno K, Yokota T, Shigeta S (1994). A sensitive assay system screening antiviral compounds against herpes simplex virus type 1 and type 2. *J Virol Methods* 49: 169–178.

Sydiskis RJ, Owen DG, Lohr JL *et al.* (1991). Inactivation of enveloped viruses by anthraquinones extracted from plants. *Antimicrob Agents Chemother* 35: 2463–2466.

Thompson KD, Dragar C (2004). Antiviral activity of *Undaria pinnatifida* against herpes simplex virus. *Phytother Res* 18: 551–555.

Tshikalange TE, Meyer JJ, Hussein AA (2005). Antimicrobial activity, toxicity and the isolation of a bioactive compound from plants used to treat sexually transmitted diseases. *J Ethnopharmacol* 96: 515–519.

Utsunomiya T, Kobayashi M, Herndon DN *et al.* (1995). Glycyrrhizin (20 beta-carboxy-11-oxo-30-norolean-12-en-3 beta-yl-2-O-β-d-glucopyranuronosyl-alpha-d-glucopyranosiduronic acid) improves the resistance of thermally injured mice to opportunistic infection of HSV-1. *Immunol Lett* 44 (1): 59–66.

Vanden Berghe DAR, Haemers A, Vlietinck AJ (1993). Antiviral agents from higher plants and an example of structure-activity relationship of 3-methoxyflavones. In: Colegate S M, Milyneux R J., eds. *Bioactive Natural Products: Detection, Isolation, and Structural Determination*. Boca Raton: CRC Press, pp. 405–440.

Vlietinck A J, de Bruyne T, vanden Berghe DA (1997). Plant substances as antiviral agents. *Curr Org Chem* 1: 307–344.

Yarnell E, Abascal K (2005). Herbs for treating herpes zoster infections. *Altern Complement Ther* 11: 131–134.

Yim KC, Carroll CJ, Tuyama A *et al.* (2005). The cotton rat provides a novel model to study genital herpes infection and to evaluate preventive strategies. *J Virol* 79: 14632–14639.

Yoosook C, Bunyapraphatsara N, Boonyakiat Y, Kantasuk C (2000). Anti-herpes simplex virus activities of crude water extracts of Thai medicinal plants. *Phytomedicine* 6: 411–419.

Xu HX, Lee SH, Lee SF, White RL, Blay J (1999). Isolation and characterization of an anti HSV polysaccharide from *Prunella vulgaris*. *Antiviral Res* 44: 43–54.

Zhang Y, But P-H, Ooi E-CV *et al.* (2007). Chemical properties, mode of action, and *in vivo* anti-herpes activities of a lignin–carbohydrate complex from *Prunella vulgaris*. *Antiviral Res* 75: 242–249.

22

Herbal medicinal products for tinnitus: perspectives and evaluation

Cynthia L Darlington, Yiwen Zheng and Paul F Smith

The nature of tinnitus

Tinnitus is a chronic, auditory disorder characterised by a 'ringing' or 'buzzing' in the ears. The two main subtypes of tinnitus are 'objective' and 'subjective' tinnitus: whereas 'objective' tinnitus can be heard by someone else and is usually associated with a vascular problem in the ear, 'subjective' tinnitus is an auditory illusion. While objective tinnitus can be treated by surgery, there is no known cure for subjective tinnitus. Subjective tinnitus can be caused by damage to the inner ear as a result of physical trauma, excessive noise, vascular insufficiency, a viral or bacterial infection, Ménière's disease or exposure to ototoxic chemicals (e.g. aspirin or cancer chemotherapeutic agents such as cisplatin) (Eggermont and Roberts, 2004). Tinnitus can occur on its own or in combination with vestibular symptoms (e.g. as in Ménière's disease). Either way, it is a debilitating condition that can affect all aspects of life and sometimes even leads to suicide. Parnes (1997) estimated that approximately 1% of the population has chronic tinnitus that causes distress and that 90% of patients with hearing loss experience some tinnitus (Parnes, 1997). Almost 40% of people aged 60 or over have tinnitus (Abutan *et al.*, 1993) and as many as 50% of all tinnitus sufferers also have depression (George and Kemp, 1991).

The mechanisms that underlie the development of subjective tinnitus are unclear. However, animal studies suggest that exposure to intense sound, resulting in cochlear hair cell damage, causes hyperactivity in the brainstem cochlear nucleus, which receives auditory information directly from the inner ear (Kaltenbach *et al.*, 2000a, 2000b). Similar changes in cochlear nucleus neurones have been reported following outer hair cell loss as a result of treatment with cisplatin (Medlamed *et al.*, 2000). Other studies have confirmed that this type of hyperactivity can be found in higher auditory centres in the brain, including the superior olive, the inferior colliculus and even the auditory cortex, following noise- or chemically induced trauma to the cochlea (Eggermont and Kenmochi, 1998; Rauschecker *et al.*, 1999; Bauer *et al.*, 2000; Komiya and Eggermont, 2000).

Such neuronal hyperactivity is similar to the epileptiform discharge that occurs in the trigeminal nucleus during trigeminal neuralgia and in the dorsal horn of the spinal cord during phantom limb pain, and it has therefore been suggested that subjective tinnitus is a form of sensory epilepsy (Moller, 2000). Consistent with this hypothesis, antiepileptic drugs are sometimes used to treat tinnitus (Simpson and Davies, 1999). However, they are not always effective and can have serious adverse side-effects (Smith and Darlington, 2005). For this reason, many other drugs have been tested and the search for more effective treatments continues. Because of the shortcomings of the conventional medications used to treat tinnitus, herbal remedies have been investigated, particularly *Ginkgo biloba* extracts. This chapter evaluates their efficacy and safety in comparison with other drug treatments.

Conventional medications for tinnitus

A diverse range of drugs has been used to treat tinnitus, but no single therapy is accepted by all clinicians. Only some of these drug treatment options are based on an understanding of the mechanisms of tinnitus; many others have been discovered serendipitously (Smith and Darlington, 2005). Unfortunately, there are many spurious claims for clinical effects.

Intratympanic gentamicin therapy has been used to treat tinnitus associated with Ménière's disease. Diamond *et al.* (2003) concluded that a subjective improvement in tinnitus occurred in approximately 57% of patients. Similarly, Lange *et al.* (2004) reported a significant reduction in tinnitus in 50% of patients treated with intratympanic gentamicin 2–4 years earlier. By contrast, a 5-year follow-up study of patients who had received intratympanic gentamicin therapy showed no significant effect on any hearing measure, even though 74% still reported complete relief from vertigo (Atlas and Parnes, 2003).

Other kinds of intratympanic drug therapy have been investigated. Sakata *et al.* (2001) used intratympanic injection of 4% lidocaine in an attempt to depress cochlear hair cell function and relieve tinnitus. Lidocaine relieved tinnitus in 81% of patients; however, vertigo developed as a result of the infusion. Intratympanic administration of steroids has also been used. Cesarani *et al.* (2002) studied 50 patients who received transtympanic infusion of dexamethasone, 3 times per day for 3 months. Two weeks after the last administration, tinnitus had disappeared in 34% of patients, 40% experienced a significant decrease in its intensity, and 26% reported no effect. Shulman and Goldstein (2000) also reported relief from tinnitus in 7 of 10 patients after intratympanic steroid therapy. Intratympanic administration of acetylcholinesterase inhibitors and acetylcholine receptor agonists has also been investigated, with varying success (DeLucchi, 2000).

Because benzodiazepines activate the benzodiazepine-binding site on the $GABA_A$ receptor, increasing hyperpolarisation, benzodiazepine treatment is an obvious strategy to reduce neuronal hyperactivity associated with tinnitus. Benzodiazepines such as alprazolam have proven useful, but it is often difficult to determine how much of the therapeutic effect is attributable specifically to the relief of tinnitus and how much is due to a general anxiolytic effect (Simpson and Davies, 1999).

The benzodiazepine antiepileptic drug, clonazepam, as well as the antiepileptic drugs gabapentin and phenytoin, have also been used to treat tinnitus (Gananca *et al.*, 2002; Goldstein and Shulman, 2003). A retrospective survey of 25 years of clinical use suggested that tinnitus was improved in approximately 32% of patients treated with clonazepam. However, adverse side-effects, such as drowsiness, depression, nightmares and reduced libido, were reported in 16.9% of patients although they decreased with continued therapy (Gananca *et al.*, 2002).

Shulman *et al.* (2002) have argued that for patients with tinnitus of central origin, benzodiazepines can provide long-term relief in 90% of cases. In an imaging study using single photon emission computed tomography, Shulman *et al.* (2000) found that patients with severe tinnitus exhibited a reduction in benzodiazepine-binding sites in the medial temporal cortex, suggesting a possible neural basis for the therapeutic effects of benzodiazepines. By contrast, drugs that act as agonists at the $GABA_B$ receptor, such as baclofen, have not proven effective and have been associated with severe adverse side-effects (Simpson and Davies, 1999).

Antidepressants have also been used to treat tinnitus. If tinnitus causes depression in a particular patient, then the relief of the depression will usually result in some relief from the tinnitus as well (Simpson and Davies, 1999). This finding demonstrates that tinnitus is not just a sensory problem but a phenomenon that involves the entire CNS, including emotional areas of the brain such as the limbic system. Folmer and Shi (2004) studied 30 patients who developed depression after the onset of their tinnitus and received selective serotonin reuptake inhibitor therapy as treatment. At 20.6 months, the patients showed a statistically significant reduction in their tinnitus severity scores, which correlated with a decrease in their depressive symptoms.

One of the more unusual treatments for tinnitus is the intravenous administration of local anaesthetics, which was discovered in 1937 (Simpson and Davies, 1999). Although lidocaine was shown to reduce tinnitus, its in-vivo instability and adverse side-effects (e.g. nausea, dizziness, potentially fatal cardiovascular effects) have limited its use. There has been some controversy about whether lidocaine actually achieved its effects as a result of blocking sodium channels or as a result of some other non-specific effect of the drug, since other agents with similar actions have not produced the same effect.

Recently, there have been a number of reports of the use of systemically administered lidocaine for the treatment of tinnitus. Marzo *et al.* (2004) reported that intravenous lidocaine successfully treated incapacitating tinnitus caused by inner-ear tertiary syphillis. Savastano (2004) reported that intradermal injection of lidocaine relieved tinnitus with no adverse side-effects. Otsuka *et al.* (2003) reported that intravenous lidocaine relieved tinnitus either partially or completely in 70.9% of cases studied over a 24-year period. However, it is not clear how or where lidocaine is acting to achieve these effects, although recent studies using intratympanic injection suggest that it may be working either as a vasodilator or sodium-channel blocker in the inner ear (Simpson and Davies, 1999).

Various other vasodilators have been investigated for the treatment of tinnitus but recent studies have failed to confirm their efficacy (Simpson and Davies, 1999). Because prostaglandins stimulate vasodilation, the synthetic prostaglandin E1 (PGE1) analogue, misoprostol, has been investigated and found to be effective in relieving tinnitus in about 33% of patients (Simpson and Davies, 1999). Yilmaz *et al.* (2004) studied 28 patients receiving misoprostol and 12 patients receiving placebo: 64% of the patients receiving misoprostol reported a reduction in tinnitus loudness (33% for placebo), with 33% showing an improvement according to their subjective tinnitus score (17% for placebo).

Finally, diuretics have been used to treat tinnitus associated with Ménière's disease, which is believed to be caused by hypertension of the endolymphatic fluid. The loop diuretic, frusemide, has been effective in treating Ménière's-associated tinnitus (Simpson and Davies, 1999). However, other attempts to regulate osmotic pressure, using mannitol and glycerol, have had little success (Simpson and Davies, 1999).

Herbal remedies

The published peer-reviewed literature on herbal medicines to treat tinnitus is dominated by the use of *Ginkgo biloba* extracts. From extensive PubMed and other database searches, we could find virtually no other published papers in peer-reviewed journals on the effects of herbal medicines in tinnitus.

Ginkgo biloba extracts

Ginkgo biloba (Ginkgoaceae) is an ancient Chinese tree that has been cultivated for thousands of years. Purified extracts, marketed under the trade names Rokan, Tanakan, Tebonin and Ginkgold, are used throughout the world, although they are especially popular in Europe and in the USA (Drew and Davies, 2001). *G. biloba* extracts have been licensed in Germany for the treatment of cerebral vascular insufficiency. They are available as over-the-counter medications in western Europe and as herbal preparations in the USA, Australia and New Zealand (see Maclennan *et al.*, 2002 for a review).

EGb-761 is a standardised extract containing 24% flavonoids, 7% proanthocyanidins and 6% terpenoids. The flavonoids are mainly flavonol-glycosides with antioxidant properties, while the terpenoid fraction contains ginkgolides, sesquiterpene and bilobalide. Ginkgolide B in particular has potent platelet-activating factor receptor antagonist properties. Many of the CNS effects of EGb-761 have been attributed to the combination of its antioxidant and platelet-activating factor receptor antagonist actions. However, it is also a vasodilator, which might be the only rationale for speculating that it would be useful in the management of tinnitus (Maclennan *et al.*, 2002).

Hilton and Stuart (2004) critically evaluated the clinical evidence for the efficacy of *G. biloba* in treating tinnitus and concluded that there were insufficient reliable data on which to base a conclusion, as a result of the methodological flaws of the available studies. Very few studies have used double-blind, placebo-controlled designs. Interestingly, when these sorts of controls have been employed, the results have usually been negative (Meehan *et al.*, 2004). In an effort to focus on the best-designed clinical trials, Ernst and Stevinson (1999) performed a meta-analysis of only those clinical trials that employed standardised *Ginkgo* extracts that were compared with either placebo or another active medication, and where the primary complaint was tinnitus. Only five trials fulfilled these criteria.

Meyer (1986a) studied 103 patients with tinnitus using a randomised, double-blind, placebo-controlled design. Patients received EGb 761 (Tanakan) daily for 1–3 months and their tinnitus severity was assessed using a three-point scale. The EGb 761 group experienced a decrease in tinnitus severity but Ernst and Stevinson (1999) point out that the paper, available in French only, lacked a clear description of the methods used.

In another study, Meyer (1986b) studied 259 patients with tinnitus over 1 year. Patients receiving EGb 761 (Tanakan) daily for at least 1 month were compared with those receiving nicergoline or almitrine-raubasine. According to a specialist analysis, tinnitus appeared to show greater improvement in the EGb 761 group compared with the other two treatments. However, Ernst and Stevinson (1999) criticised this study for lack of random allocation of patients to the different treatment groups and lack of methodological detail in the published report; for example, it was not clear whether the patients and experimenters were blind to the treatment groups.

Holgers *et al.* (1994) recruited 80 patients into an open trial in which all of them received a *G. biloba* extract daily (Seredrin). This was followed by a double-blind, placebo-controlled phase of the trial using only the 20 patients who appeared to respond to the extract. However, according to patients' subjective reports, there were no significant effects of the *G. biloba* extract at the end of the trial.

Morgenstern and Bierman (1997) performed a randomised, double-blind study of 99 patients with chronic tinnitus, who received a *G. biloba* extract (Tebonin) or placebo daily for 12 weeks. The loudness of the tinnitus was evaluated using audiometry. They reported a significant reduction in loudness (from 42 to 39 dB) in the ginkgo-treated group. Juretzek (1998) treated 60 patients with chronic tinnitus with daily injections of EGb 761 for 10 days, and then randomly allocated them to oral EGb 761 or placebo for 3 months. The second phase of the design was double blind and tinnitus was assessed using audiometry. Juretzek also reported a significant reduction in tinnitus in the EGb 761 group compared with placebo.

The first large, double-blind, placebo-controlled study of the effect of *G. biloba* extracts on tinnitus was reported by Drew and Davies (2001). They recruited 1121 people between 18 and 70 years and matched 978 according to sex, age and the duration of their tinnitus. For 12 weeks, participants received either the ginkgo extract LI 1370 (Lichtwer Pharma, Berlin, Germany) or placebo. Subjects assessed their tinnitus in terms of loudness and how much it disrupted their daily life, using rating scales. However, there was no significant difference in either measure compared with placebo. In the most recent randomised, placebo-controlled, double-blind clinical trial, Rejai *et al.* (2004) also found no therapeutic effect of *G. biloba* compared with placebo in 66 patients with tinnitus. The primary outcome measures were the tinnitus handicap inventory, the Glasgow health status inventory and the average hearing threshold at 0.5, 1, 2 and 4 kHz. In a meta-analysis of clinical trials by the same authors, they found that only 21.6% of patients with tinnitus reported benefit from *G. biloba* versus 18.4% of patients who reported benefit from a placebo (Rejai *et al.*, 2004).

Because *G. biloba* extracts have vasodilatory effects, when they are combined with drugs such as aspirin, they can increase bleeding. Nonetheless, most of the evidence for haemorrhagic responses following the use of *G. biloba* extracts is based on anecdotal and case reports. Kohler *et al.* (2004) compared bleeding time, coagulation parameters and platelet activity in response to 2 × 120 mg/day EGb 761, or placebo, for 7 days and found no significant difference in any of these measures.

To date, only one study has investigated the effects of EGb 761 on salicylate-induced tinnitus using a conditioned-behaviour paradigm in rats (Jastreboff *et al.*, 1997). Daily oral administration of 25, 50 and 100 mg/kg EGb 761 was found to reduce tinnitus behaviour compared with vehicle. It should be noted, however, that these are very high doses and it is unlikely that they could be used in humans without adverse side-effects (even 25 mg/kg/day for a 70 kg adult corresponds to 1750 mg/day, which is more than five times the average daily dose used in humans).

Clearly, the investigation of the effects of *G. biloba* extracts on tinnitus has suffered from a lack of systematic clinical trials employing double-blind and placebo-controlled designs. While some clinical trials have yielded positive results (e.g. Meyer, 1986a, 1986b; Morgenstern and Biermann, 1997; Juretzek, 1998), these studies are few and have been limited either by design flaws (e.g. Meyer, 1986a, 1986b), the small size of the significant effects (e.g. Morgenstern and Biermann, 1997), or else the results have not been published in peer-reviewed journals (Juretzek, 1998). By contrast, the two most systematic clinical trials, which are double-blind and placebo-controlled, and are published in peer-reviewed journals, have yielded negative results.

Other herbal medicines

Very little has been published on the use of other herbal medicines to treat tinnitus. Yang (1989) has reported a blind trial in which patients with tinnitus were given either 'Western medicines' (i.e. diazepam, nicotinic acid, bromides, vitamin B, ATP, carbamazepine or lidocaine) and traditional Chinese medicine (TCM) or the Western medicines alone. TCM consisted of Rhizoma Gastrodiae, Ramulus Uncariae cum Uncis, Poria cocos, Flos Chrysanthemi, Akebia Quinata, Radix Polygoni Multflori, Fructus Liquidambris, Radix Rehmanniae, Rhizoma Alismatis, Radix Scrophulariae, Fructus Lycii, Radix Glycyrrhizae, Semen Plantaginis and Semen Vaccariae. Relief from tinnitus was observed in 84.4% of those receiving Western medicine and TCM and 55% of those receiving Western medicine only. Unfortunately, given the mixture of drug and herbal remedies the patients received, it is difficult to attribute an improvement in tinnitus to any particular agent, and in any case, there was no placebo control group.

It is important to recognise that in TCM, tinnitus is believed to be caused by changes in the relationship between the ear and the internal organs, such as the kidney, the liver, the gall bladder, the spleen and the stomach. TCM aims to treat tinnitus by achieving a balance of the yin and yang, external and internal, hot and cold, weak and strong. From the viewpoint of TCM, tinnitus is only one of the symptoms the patient presents with and the doctor needs to observe a series of symptoms using inspection, by listening and smelling, inquiring and palpation, to make the right diagnosis. For example, it is believed that normal kidney function will be reflected by normal hearing and a kidney dysfunction (*Shen kui*) will result in hearing loss or tinnitus. If the tinnitus is caused by kidney dysfunction, the patient tends also to experience vertigo and dizziness, a sore back, the tongue has a red look with no 'fur' or little fur and there is a weak pulse. There are many different types of tinnitus in TCM and most recently, tinnitus has been divided into five types at the Third Chinese Zhong Xi Yi Je He Otolaryngology Society Annual Meeting in 2002: *Wai Gan Fen Re Xing* (related to respiratory infection), *Gan Hou Shang Rao Xing* (related to abnormal liver function), *Tan Re Yu Jie Xing* (related to the 'hot' state in TCM), *Shen Jing Kui Xu Xing* (related to kidney dysfunction) and *Pi Qi Xu Ruo Xing* (related to abnormal spleen function).

Japanese herbal medicines have also been used to treat tinnitus. Okamoto *et al.* (2005) used *Yoku-kan-san* (TJ-54) to successfully treat tinnitus associated with undifferentiated somatoform disorder, presenting with headache and insomnia. Unfortunately, this was only a case report and therefore no controls were employed.

Importance of animal models for testing herbal remedies

A major problem for the development of new drug treatments for tinnitus is the paucity of animal models of the disorder. It is difficult to determine whether an animal such as a rat or a mouse is actually experiencing tinnitus, and many studies of the neurophysiological and neurochemical mechanisms of tinnitus simply assume that an animal has tinnitus following cochlear lesions produced by intense sound, surgery or chemical toxicity. This is not a valid assumption given that similar conditions in humans do not necessarily produce tinnitus.

To overcome this problem, a number of researchers have developed animal models of tinnitus in which rats are trained to respond differentially in a conditioned avoidance task depending upon whether they hear certain frequencies of background noise (Simpson and Davies, 1999; Bauer, 2003; Ruttiger *et al.*, 2003). For example, rats trained to make a particular response in the presence of a 10-kHz background noise, will continue to make the trained response, in the absence of the background noise, if tinnitus has been induced by the administration of a drug such as salicylate. In humans, salicylates produce tinnitus of approximately 10 kHz (Eggermont and Roberts, 2004), and rats treated with salicylates respond in behavioural tasks as if they hear a continuous background noise at around 10 kHz (Bauer, 2003; Ruttiger *et al.*, 2003). Using this type of conditioned-behavioural model, it is possible to screen new drugs for their potential application to the treatment of tinnitus.

Unfortunately, at present, such animal models have not been used extensively for the investigation of the neural mechanisms of tinnitus or for potential drug treatments. In addition to more well-controlled clinical trials, it is vital that herbal medicines be tested in realistic animal models of tinnitus.

Conclusions

It is clear from the studies reviewed here that the published literature on herbal medicines and tinnitus is small and in most cases focused on *G. biloba* extracts, where some evidence for efficacy has been found. Nevertheless, even the research on *G. biloba* and tinnitus lacks a substantial number of systematic, well-controlled clinical trials, in which double-blind protocols have been used. Unfortunately, most of the trials that have been well designed have failed to demonstrate efficacy for *G. biloba* in the treatment of tinnitus.

The only reasonable conclusion that can be reached at present is that the available data indicate that conventional medications offer more therapeutic benefit for patients with tinnitus than herbal alternatives. Given that clinical trials are expensive to run and are usually not undertaken unless there is substantial preclinical evidence to suggest that they may establish the efficacy of a new drug, it is probably very important that researchers and clinicians, who are interested in potential herbal treatments for tinnitus, use conditioned-behavioural models of tinnitus in animals to screen herbal agents. This would provide a clear path for the development of herbal remedies to treat tinnitus before initiating clinical trials.

References

Abutan BB, Hoes AW, Vandalsen CL, *et al.* (1993). Prevalence of hearing impairment and hearing complaints in older adults: A study in general practice. *Fam Pract* 10: 391–395.

Atlas J, Parnes LS (2003). Intratympanic gentamicin for intractable Meniere's disease: 5 year follow-up. *J Otolaryngol* 32: 288–293.

Bauer CA, Brozoski, TJ, Holder, TM, Casparg, DM *et al.* (2000). Effects of chronic salicylate on GABAergic activity in rat inferior colliculus. *Hearing Res* 147: 175–182.

Bauer CA (2003). Animal models of tinnitus. *Otolaryngol Clin N Am* 36: 267–285.

Cesarani A, Capobianco S, Soi D, Giuliano DA, Alpini D (2002). Intratympanic dexamethasone treatment for control of subjective idiopathic tinnitus: our clinical experience. *Int Tinnitus J* 8: 111–114.

DeLucchi E (2000). Transtympanic pilocarpine in tinnitus. *Int Tinnitus J* 6: 37–40.

Diamond C, O'Connell DA, Hornig JD, Liu R (2003). Systematic review of intratympanic gentamicin in Meniere's disease. *J Otolaryngol* 32: 351–361.

Drew S, Davies E (2001). Effectiveness of *Ginko biloba* in

treating tinnitus: double-blind, placebo controlled trial. *BMJ* 322: 1–6.

Eggermont JJ, Kenmochi M (1998). Salicylate and quinine selectively increase spontaneous firing rates in secondary auditory cortex. *Hearing Res* 117: 149–160.

Eggermont JJ, Roberts LE (2004). The neuroscience of tinnitus. *Trends Neurosci* 27: 676–682.

Ernst E, Stevinson C (1999). *Ginkgo biloba* for tinnitus: A review. *Clin Otolaryngol* 24: 164–167.

Folmer RL, Shi YB (2004). SSRI use by tinnitus patients: interactions between depression and tinnitus severity. *Ear Nose Throat J* 83: 107–108.

Gananca MM, Caovilla HH, Gananca FF *et al.* (2002). Clonazepam in the pharmacological treatment of vertigo and tinnitus. *Int Tinnitus J* 8: 50–53.

George RN, Kemp S (1991). A survey of New Zealanders with tinnitus. British *J Audiol* 25: 331–336.

Goldstein BA, Shulman A (2003). Tinnitus outcome profile and tinnitus control. *Int Tinnitus J* 9: 26–31.

Hilton M, Stuart E (2004). *Ginkgo biloba* for tinnitus. *Cochrane Database Syst Rev* 2: CD003852.

Holgers K-M, Axelsson A, Pringle I (1994). *Ginkgo biloba* extract for the treatment of tinnitus. *Audiology* 33: 85–92.

Jastreboff PJ, Zhou S, Jastreboff MM *et al.* (1997). Attenuation of salicylate-induced tinnitus by *Ginkgo biloba* extract in rats. *Audiol Neurootol* 2: 197–212.

Juretzck W (1998). Zusmmenfass und der Ergebnisse einder plazebokontrollierten Doppelblindstudie zur Therapie des Tinnitus mit dem Ginkgo-Extrakt Egb 761. *Schwabe Arneimittel* Internal Report 21.7.

Kaltenbach JA, Zhang J, Afman CE (2000a). Plasticity of spontaneous neural activity in the dorsal cochlear nucleus after intense sound exposure. *Hearing Res* 147: 282–292.

Kaltenbach JA, Zhang J, Finlayson P (2000b). Tinnitus as a plastic phenomenon and its possible neural underpinnings in the dorsal cochlear nucleus. *Hearing Res* 206: 200–226.

Kohler S, Funk P, Kieser M (2004). Influence of a 7 day treatment with *Ginkgo biloba* special extract EGb 761 on bleeding time and coagulation: a randomised, placebo-controlled, double-blind study in healthy volunteers. *Blood Coagul Fibrinolysis* 15: 303–309.

Komiya H, Eggermont JJ (2000). Spontaneous firing activity of cortical neurons in adult cats with reorganised tonotopic maps following pure-tone trauma. *Acta Otolaryngol* 120: 750–756.

Lange G, Maurer J, Mann W (2004). Long-term results after interval therapy with intratympanic gentamicin for Meniere's disease. *Laryngoscope* 114: 102–105.

Maclennan K, Darlington CL, Smith PF (2002). The CNS effects of *Ginkgo biloba* extracts and ginkgolide B. *Prog Neurobiol* 67: 236–258.

Marzo S, Stankiewicz JA, Consiglio AP (2004). Lidocaine for the relief of incapacitating tinnitus. *Ear Nose Throat J* 83: 236–238.

Medlamed SB *et al.* (2000). Cisplatin-induced increases in spontaneous neural activity in the dorsal cochlear nucleus and associated outer hair cell loss. *Audiology* 39: 24–29.

Meehan T, Eisenhut M, Stephens D (2004). A review of alternative treatments for tinnitus. *Audiol Med* 2: 74–82.

Meyer B (1986a). Etude multicentrique randomisee a double insuface au placebo du traitement des acouphenes par l'extrait de *Ginkgo biloba. Presse Med* 15: 1562–1564.

Meyer B (1986b). Etude multicentrique des acouphenes. *Ann Oto-Laryngol* 103: 185–188.

Moller AR (2000). Similarities between severe tinnitus and chronic pain. *J Am Acad Audiol* 11: 115–124.

Morgenstern C, Biermann E (1997). Ginkgo-Spezialextrakt Egb 761 in der Behandlung des Tinnitus aurium. *Fortschr Med* 115: 7–11.

Okamoto H, Okami T, Ikeda M, Takeuchi T (2005). Effects of Yoku-kan-san on undifferentiated somatoform disorder with tinnitus. *Eur Psychiatr* 20: 74–75.

Otsuka K, Pulec JL, Suzuki M (2003). Assessment of intravenous lidocaine for the treatment of subjective tinnitus. *Ear Nose Throat J* 82: 781–784.

Parnes SM (1997). Current concepts in the clinical management of patients with tinnitus. *Eur Arch Oto-Rhino-Laryngol* 254: 406–409.

Rauschecker JP (1999). Auditory cortical plasticity: A comparison with other sensory systems. *Trends Neurosci* 22: 74–80.

Rejai D, Sivakumar A, Balaji N (2004). *Ginkgo biloba* does not benefit patients with tinnitus: a randomized placebo-controlled double-blind trial and meta-analysis of randomized trials. *Clin Otolaryngol Allied Sci* 29: 226–231.

Rüttiger L, Ciuffani, J, Zenner, H-P, Knipper, M (2003). A behavioral paradigm to judge acute sodium salicylate-induced sound experience in rats: a new approach for an animal model on tinnitus. *Hearing Res* 180: 39–50.

Sakata H, Kojima Y, Koyama S, Furuya N, Sakata E (2001). Treatment of cochlear tinnitus with intratympanic infusion of 4% lidocaine into the tympanic cavity. *Int Tinnitus J* 7: 46–50.

Savastano M (2004). Lidocaine intradermal injection – a new approach in tinnitus therapy: a preliminary report. *Adv Ther* 21: 13–20.

Shulman A, Goldstein BA (2000). Intratympanic drug therapy with steroids for tinnitus control: a preliminary report. *Int Tinnitus J* 6: 10–20.

Shulman A, Strashun AM, Goldstein BA (2002). GABA(A)-benzodiazepine-chloride receptor-targeted therapy for tinnitus control: preliminary report. *Int Tinnitus J* 8: 30–36.

Shulman A, Strashun AM, Seibyl JP *et al.* (2000). Benzodiazepine receptor deficiency and tinnitus. *Int Tinnitus J* 6: 98–111.

Simpson J, Davies WE (1999). Recent advances in the

pharmacological treatment of tinnitus. *Trends Pharmacol Sci* 20: 12–18.

Smith PF, Darlington CL (2005). Drug treatments for tinnitus: Serendipitous discovery versus rational design. *Curr Opin Invest Drugs* 6: 712–716.

Yang DJ (1989). Tinnitus treated with combined traditional Chinese medicine and Western medicine. *Zhong Xi Yi Jie He Za Zhi* 9: 270–271.

Yilmaz I, Akkuzu B, Cakmak O, Ozuoglu LN (2004). Misoprostol in the treatment of tinnitus: a double-blind study. *Otolaryngol Head Neck Surg* 130: 604–610.

23

Traditional herbs for healthcare – turmeric: a case history

Wandee Gritsanapan and Werayut Pothitirat

Introduction

Turmeric is the rhizome of *Curcuma longa* L. which has been widely used for centuries in traditional medicines for treatment of several diseases. It is also popular as a yellow colouring agent, spice and food preservative in India, China and South East Asia, especially Thailand. Its medicinal properties have been attributed mainly to the volatile oil and yellow pigment curcuminoids, including curcumin, demethoxycurcumin and bisdemethoxycurcumin.

Curcumin, the main bioactive component of turmeric, has a wide spectrum of biological actions including antioxidant, anticarcinogenic, anti-inflammatory, antimutagenic, antimicrobial and hypocholesteraemic activities. In cosmetics, turmeric powder and its extract are popularly used in anti-ageing products. Turmeric is being used in primary healthcare in many countries because of its several medicinal uses, ease of cultivation, cheapness and lack of toxicity. Turmeric varies in quality and quantity of active components, so it is important to establish standardisations of turmeric and its extract. Ethnomedical uses, bioactivities, active components, analytical methods and standards for the active components in the standardised ethanolic turmeric extracts are discussed in this chapter.

Turmeric is an example of a traditional herb that is now popularly used as a dietary supplement, and also for more direct medical effects such as antioxidant, anti-inflammatory, anticarcinogenic, hypotensive and hypocholesteraemic.

In Thailand, the government has set up a national plan for development of medicinal plants to build up self-reliance on drug supplies. This chapter reviews chemical constituents and biological activities of turmeric, as an example of traditional herbs for healthcare.

Botanical origin and production of turmeric

Botanical origin and distribution

Turmeric *Curcuma longa* L. belongs to the Zingiberaceae (synonyms are *Curcuma domestica* Val., *C. rotunda* L., *C. xanthorrhiza* Naves and *Amomum curcuma* Jacq). Its common vernacular names are curcuma, common tumeric, yellow root, Indian saffron and Khamin chan. Turmeric is native to southern Asia and is widespread as a domestic spice plant throughout the tropics, including Africa (World Health Organization, 1999). In Thailand, turmeric is cultivated throughout the country, mostly in the south (ASEAN Countries, 1993) although India dominates the international trade producing 400 000 tonnes annually from 130 000 hectares (De Padua *et al.*, 1994). The part of this plant used is the dried, bright orange to yellow rhizome, containing volatile oil and yellow pigments, the curcuminoids.

Ethnomedical uses

Turmeric has long been used as a yellow food colouring, spice and is one of the principal ingredients in curry powder (Tyler, 1994). It is extensively used in Ayurveda, Unani and Siddha medicines as a home remedy for various diseases (Ammon and Wahl, 1991; Eigner and Scholz, 1999) and, in north India, in the mountains, is used to protect the skin against sunburn (Scartezzini and Speroni, 2000).

In India, turmeric is taken orally for poor digestion, for fevers, skin conditions, vomiting in pregnancy and liver disorders (Chopra *et al.*, 1982). Externally, it is used for conjunctivitis, skin infection, cancer, sprains, arthritis, haemorroids and eczema (Nadkarni and Nadkarni, 1976; Chopra *et al.*, 1982). Indian women apply turmeric to the skin to reduce hair growth (Goh and Ng, 1987).

In China, different uses are attributed to the rhizome and tuber. It is normally used for diseases associated with abdominal pains (Araujo and Leon, 2001). Turmeric rhizome is said to be a blood and *Qi* (vital energy) stimulant with analgesic properties. It is used to treat chest and abdominal pain and distension, jaundice, frozen shoulder and amenorrhoea caused by blood stasis, and postpartum abdominal pain owing to stasis. It is also used for wounds and injuries. The tuber has similar properties but is used in hot conditions as it is more cooling and has been used to treat viral hepatitis (Chang and But, 1987).

In Thailand, turmeric has been used in traditional recipes for a long time as follows (Farnsworth and Bunyapraphatsara, 1992).

- *Treatment of ringworm and mosquito bite:* for ringworm, mix powdered turmeric with rainwater and apply on the infected area two times daily. For treatment of mosquito bite, scrape the turmeric rhizome and rub on the affected area, it will relieve itching and inflammation; or mix powdered turmeric with water and apply frequently on the area.
- *Carminative and for treatment of peptic ulcers:* pills are made by mixing powdered turmeric with honey and administered orally three times a day.
- *Antidiarrhoea and antidysentery:* bruise the rhizomes into small pieces and then add warm water in a ratio of 1:1. Take two teaspoonfuls of this mixture three to four times a day. Salt may be added to improve the taste. Alternatively, roast the rhizome, then bruise into small pieces, add lime water, then squeeze the mixture and take one to two cups of the liquid.
- *Treatment of wounds:* boil powdered turmeric with coconut oil or lard until yellow oil is obtained. Apply the oil on the wounds, or bruise turmeric rhizome and squeeze the juice out for treatment of wounds, or mix turmeric with a few millilitres of lime water and alum or potassium nitrate, and then apply on the wounds. This recipe may also be used for inflammations.
- *Use as cosmetic:* for use as a cosmetic, Thai women in rural areas apply turmeric powder to their faces and body skin to make them a beautiful gold colour. Turmeric powder mixed with honey and ripe tamarind pulp is used for

scrubbing face and body skin for whitening and anti-ageing effects.

Active constituents and nutritative composition

The rhizome usually contains 4–6% of a pale yellow to orange-yellow volatile oil, composed mainly of turmerone (58%), ar-turmerone, zingiberene (25%), cineole, borneol (Kelkar and Sanjiva, 1933; Institute of Materia Medica, 1982), and yellow colouring matter including curcumin (1.8–5.4%), demethoxycurcumin and bisdemethoxycurcumin (Figure 23.1) (Institute of Materia Medica, 1982). Curcumin has a melting point of 176–177°C, forms a reddish-brown salt with alkali and is soluble in ethanol, alkali, ketone, acetic acid and chloroform.

Medicinal properties of turmeric are due to the volatile oil as a carminative and antifungal agent, while the yellow curcuminoids have potent antioxidative and anti-inflammatory properties. In Thailand, turmeric is mainly used in forms of capsule/tablet of turmeric powder for carminative and antiflatulent medicines. The crude ethanolic extract containing curcuminoids and volatile oil is used in drug and cosmetic preparations. Chemical components isolated from turmeric are summarised in Table 23.1.

Variation of active constituents

Turmeric derived from different sources shows variation in the major constituents. The geographical, climate, aged and harvesting conditions all have an effect on curcuminoid and volatile oil content.

Our study on the variation of bioactive components in the powder of *C. longa* rhizomes from 13 locations in Thailand showed that turmeric rhizomes from the south, where the humidity is high, with year-round rain and no extremes of temperature, contained the highest content of curcuminoids (8.99% dry weight). The lowest content of curcuminoids (5.60% dry weight) is found in the samples from the central part of Thailand where the climate is warm and dry. In contrast, the southern samples display a low content of volatile oil (7% v/w of dried powder), while northern and northeastern samples contain a high content of volatile oil (8.20% and 8.00% v/w of dried powder, respectively) (Pothitirat and Gritsanapan, 2006).

Extraction and isolation of curcuminoids from turmeric

Several methods of extraction and isolation of curcuminoids from *C. longa* rhizome have been developed. Usually, separation of curcuminoids has

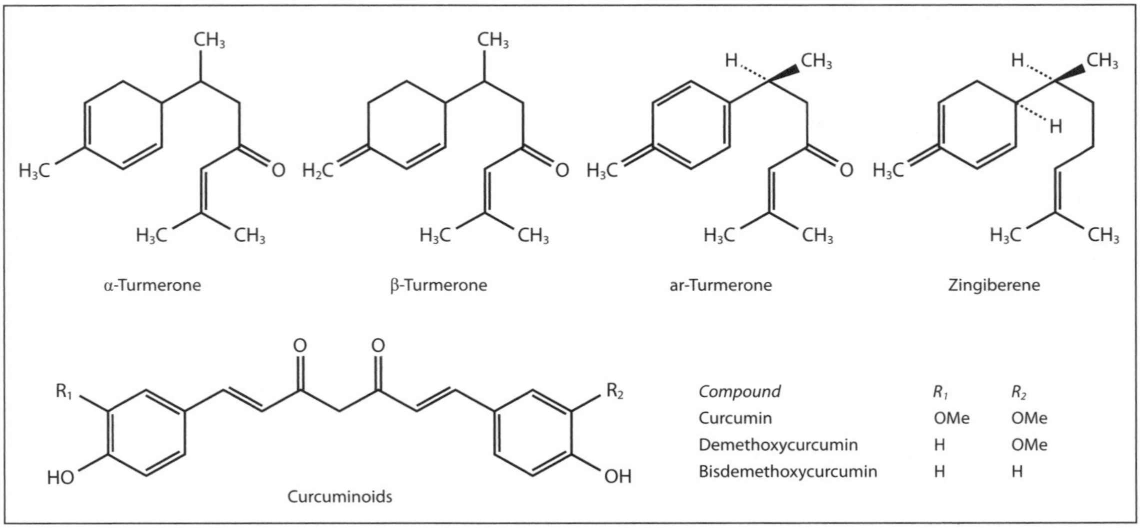

α-Turmerone

β-Turmerone

ar-Turmerone

Zingiberene

Curcuminoids

Compound	R_1	R_2
Curcumin	OMe	OMe
Demethoxycurcumin	H	OMe
Bisdemethoxycurcumin	H	H

Figure 23.1 Some constituents in turmeric rhizome.

Table 23.1 Chemical constituents in turmeric rhizome

Chemical	Reference
Curcuminoids	
Curcumin	Su *et al.*, 1982; Uehara *et al.*, 1992
5′-Methoxycurcumin	Masuda *et al.*, 1993
Bisdemethoxycurcumin	Jentzsch *et al.*, 1970; Toda *et al.*, 1985
Demethoxycurcumin	Jentzsch *et al.*, 1970; Toda *et al.*, 1985
Mono-demethoxycurcumin	Sanagi *et al.*, 1993
Cyclocurcumin	Kiuchi *et al.*, 1993
4-Hydroxy-cinnamoyl-methane	Park and Boo, 1991
4-Hydroxy-feruloxyl-methane	Park and Boo, 1991
Bis-(4-Hydroxy-cinnamoyl)-methane	Park and Boo, 1991
Bis-(*p*-Hydroxy-cinnamoyl)-methane	Toda *et al.*, 1985; Rao *et al.*, 1982
Di-feruloyl methane	Matthes *et al.*, 1980
Di-*p*-coumaroyl methane	Matthes *et al.*, 1980
Feruloyl-p-coumaroyl methane	Matthes *et al.*, 1980
p-Hydroxy-cinnamoyl-methane	Punyarajun *et al.*, 1981
p-Coumaroylmethane	Kiso *et al.*, 1983
Essential oil	
α- and β-atlantone	Su *et al.*, 1982
Bisabolene, β-bisabolene	Su *et al.*, 1982
Bisacumol	Ohshiro *et al.*, 1990
Bisacurone	Ohshiro *et al.*, 1990
Borneol, iso-borneol	Su *et al.*, 1982
Campesterol	Moon *et al.*, 1976
Camphene	Chen *et al.*, 1983
Camphor	Chen *et al.*, 1983; Fang *et al.*, 1982
Caryophyllene	Chen *et al.*, 1983; Fang *et al.*, 1982
1,8-Cineol, cineol	Chen *et al.*, 1983; Fang *et al.*, 1982
Curcumene, α-curcumene	Chen *et al.*, 1983; Fang *et al.*, 1982
Curcumenol	Ohshiro *et al.*, 1990
Curcumenone	Ohshiro *et al.*, 1990
Curdione, dehydro-curdione	Chen *et al.*, 1983; Fang *et al.*, 1982
Curlone	Golding *et al.*, 1982; Golding *et al.*, 1992
Curzerenone	Chen *et al.*, 1983; Fang *et al.*, 1982
p-Cymene	Malingre, 1975
Eugenol	Chen *et al.*, 1983; Fang *et al.*, 1982
Germacron-13-al	Ohshiro *et al.*, 1990
Procurcumadiol	Ohshiro *et al.*, 1990
Sabinene	Su *et al*, 1982
β-Sesquiphellandrene	Ahn and Lee, 1989
Terpinene	Chen *et al.*, 1983; Fang *et al.*, 1982
Terpineol	Fang *et al.*, 1982
Turmerin	Uehara *et al.*, 1992; Mitra, 1975
α-Turmerin	Ohshiro *et al.*, 1990
β-Turmerone	Uehara *et al.*, 1992
α-Turmerone	Golding *et al.*, 1982; Golding *et al.*, 1992
ar-Turmerone	Chen *et al.*, 1983; Fang *et al.*, 1982
Turmerone	Chen *et al.*, 1983; Fang *et al.*, 1982
ar-(+)-s-turmerone	John and Krishna, 1985
Turmeronal A	Imai *et al.*, 1990
Turmeronal B	Imai *et al.*, 1990
Zedoarondiol	Ohshiro *et al.*, 1990
Zingiberene	Uehara *et al.*, 1992; Mitra, 1975

(*continued overleaf*)

Table 23.1 *(continued)*

Chemical	Reference
Polysaccharide	
Ukonan A	Tomoda *et al.*, 1990
Ukonan B	Tomoda *et al.*, 1990
Ukonan C	Tomoda *et al.*, 1990
Ukonan D	Tomoda *et al.*, 1990
Peptide	
Turmerin	Srinivas *et al.*, 1992
α-Turmerin	Ohshiro *et al.*, 1990
Fatty acid and sterol	
Syringic acid	Merh *et al.*, 1986
Cholesterol	Fang *et al.*, 1982
β-Sitosterol	Fang *et al.*, 1982
Stigmasterol	Fang *et al.*, 1982
Others	
Protocatechuic acid	Merh *et al.*, 1986
o-Coumaric acid	Merh *et al.*, 1986
p-Coumaric acid	Schultz and Herrmann, 1980
2-Hydroxy-methyl anthraquinone	Ogbeide *et al.*, 1985

been achieved by thin-layer chromatography (TLC) and column chromatography (CC). The stationary phase most used is silica gel. The different solvent systems are shown in Table 23.2.

Ramussen *et al.* (2000) reported the simple and efficient separation of curcuminoids using dihydrogen phosphate impregnated silica gel TLC plates. Janaki and Bose (1967) reported the isolation of curcuminoids involving prior extraction of rhizomes with hexane to remove much of the volatile and fatty components and then extract with benzene. The concentrate extract readily crystallised on cooling and was further purified by crystallisation from ethanol to yield orange-yellow needles, but the yield of curcuminoids was poor (1.1%). Peter-Almeida *et al.* (2005) reported the first crystallisation of the curcuminoid pigment crystals containing 56.9% of curcumin and other curcuminoid pigments. Successive crystallisations improved the purity of curcumin but there was a loss in yield. In the third successive crystallisation, 92% pure curcumin was obtained with no bisdemethoxycurcumin detected. Krishnamurthy *et al.* (1976) reported the hot and cold percolation extraction methods with good yields with a high recovery of curcumin.

The best processing conditions to maximise the yield of essential oil and curcuminoids have been reported (Manzan *et al.*, 2003). Autoclave pressure and distillation time were the variables studied for the steam distillation process. The highest yields of essential oil (0.46%) and curcuminoids (0.16%) are obtained at a pressure of 1.0×10^5 Pa and a time of 2 h. On the other hand, with extraction by volatile solvents, the best yield of essential oil (5.49%) is obtained when using 0.175, 0.124, 0.088 mm turmeric powder particles at 40°C, for 6 h of extraction.

In recent years, supercritical fluid extraction has gained commercial importance as an efficient method of extraction for natural products. It has been also investigated for the extraction of essential oils and curcuminoids from *C. longa* (Marsin *et al.*, 1993; Hisashige *et al.*, 1994). Baumann *et al.* (2000) claimed efficient extraction of curcuminoids using supercritical CO_2 modified by 10% ethanol. Although supercritical fluid extraction is known to be a clean technology giving acceptable yields and purity, its major disadvantage lies in its high operating pressures. The scale-up problems could also be severe when the extraction is to be done at large scales.

Table 23.2 Different solvent systems for thin-layer and column chromatography for separation of curcuminoids from *C. longa*

Solvent system	Proportion	Reference
1. chloroform : acetic acid	90 : 10	Janben and Gole, 1984
2. chloroform : acetic acid	80 : 20	Janben and Gole, 1984
3. chloroform : ethanol	90 : 10	Janben and Gole, 1984
4. ethyl acetate : n-hexane	3 : 17	Punyarajun, 1981
5. hexane : methanol	90 : 10	Punyarajun, 1981
6. benzene : methanol	95 : 5	Punyarajun, 1981
7. benzene : methanol	90 : 10	Punyarajun, 1981
8. benzene : ethanol	95 : 5	Punyarajun, 1981
9. chloroform : benzene : methanol	80 : 15 : 5	Tewtrakul *et al.*, 1992
10. chloroform : methanol : formic acid	96 : 4 : 0.6	Chavalittumrong and Dechatiwongse, 1988
11. benzene : methanol	80 : 6	Guenther, 1952
12. toluene : ethyl acetate	93 : 7	Wagner *et al.*, 1983
13. chloroform : ethanol : glacial acetic acid	94 : 5 : 1	Wagner *et al.*, 1983
14. toluene : ethyl acetate	97 : 3	Peter-Almeida *et al.*, 2005
15. toluene : ethyl acetate	90 : 10	Peter-Almeida *et al.*, 2005
16. chloroform : methanol	95 : 5	Peter-Almeida *et al.*, 2005
17. dichloromethane : methanol	99 : 1	Peter-Almeida *et al.*, 2005
18. dichloromethane : methanol	95 : 5	Peter-Almeida *et al.*, 2005

Dandekar and Gaikar (2002) reported a microwave-assisted extraction (MAE) technique for selective and rapid extraction of curcuminoids. Turmeric powder irradiated for 2 and 4 min with microwaves showed marginally higher extraction of curcuminoids in 60 min by acetone.

High-speed countercurrent chromatography preparation with or without pH-zoning was used to separate multigram quantities of curcumin and other curcuminoids from turmeric powder (Patel *et al.*, 2000).

Braga *et al.* (2003) compared yield, composition, and antioxidant activity of turmeric extracts obtained using various techniques such as hydrodistillation, low-pressure solvent extraction, Soxhlet extraction, and supercritical extraction using carbon dioxide and co-solvents. The result showed that the largest yield (27%) was obtained from the Soxhlet extraction using ethanol while the lowest yield was found in the hydrodistillation process (2.1%). For the supercritical extraction, the best co-solvent was a mixture of ethanol and isopropyl alcohol. The maximum amount of curcuminoids (8.43%) was obtained using Soxhlet extraction (ethanol/isopropyl alcohol). The extracts obtained by Soxhlet extraction and low-pressure extraction exhibited the strongest antioxidant activities.

From our studies (Pothitirat and Gritsanapan, 2004), we compared three extraction methods; maceration, percolation and Soxhlet extraction, using 95% ethanol as a solvent for extraction of the ethanolic extract. It was shown that percolation is the recommended method for the highest content of total curcuminoids (59.09 ± 11.73% of the crude extract), a moderate time consumption, and low cost.

Quantitative analysis of curcuminoids in turmeric

A variety of methods for quantification of curcuminoids have been reported. Most of them are spectrophotometric methods (The Medicine Commission, 1973; ASTA Method, 1985). Although ultraviolet (UV) spectrophotometry is a rapid and economical method, it is not possible to quantify the individual curcuminoids and it lacks precision because of interference by other pigments present in the plant.

Recently, there have been many methods to determine the content of individual curcuminoids. Karasz *et al.* (1973), Tonnesen and Karlsen (1986) and Navas and Ramos (1992) reported a direct fluorometric method for analysis of curcumin in food products. Hiserodt *et al.* (1996) reported LC-MS and GC-MS methods for the separation of curcuminoids. These involve an octadecyl stationary phase using a mobile phase consisting of ammonium acetate with 5% acetic acid and acetonitrile. The presence of inorganic salts may contaminate the mass spectrometer ion source. Sun *et al.* (2002) reported the capillary electrophoresis with amperometric determination of curcumin using a running buffer composed of 15 mmol/L phosphate buffer (pH 9.7), separation voltage at 16 kV and detection at 1.2 V. However, this method does not describe the separation and identification of demethoxycurcumin and bisdemethoxycurcumin.

Many HPLC methods have been reported for quantification (Tonnesen and Karlsen, 1983; Smith and Witowska, 1984; Russell, 1988). Guddadarangavanahally *et al.* (2002) reported a HPLC method for separation and quantification of curcumin, demethoxycurcumin and bisdemethoxycurcumin using a tertiary mobile phase comprising methanol; 2% acetic acid and acetonitrile. The advantage of HPLC is that individual curcuminoids could be estimated from the varieties of turmeric rhizomes. HPTLC and TLC-densitometric methods have been developed for the simultaneous quantitation of three curcuminoid components in turmeric. The results indicated that the accuracy and precision of these methods are reliable. The methods were found to be suitable for rapid analysis and can be performed without any special sample pretreatment (Tewtrakul *et al.*, 1992; Gupta *et al.*, 1999; Pothitirat and Gritsanapan, 2005).

Pothitirat (2006) compared the analysis methods for total curcuminoids in 95% ethanolic extracts of *C. longa* collected from ten locations in Thailand using a UV spectrophotometer, TLC-densitometer, and HPLC. The results are shown in Table 23.3.

UV spectrophotometry is simple, fast and convenient, but it cannot determine individual curcuminoid content, but is used for analysis of total curcuminoid content in the *Thai Herbal Pharmacopoeia* (THP, 1995) and *The Standard of ASEAN Herbal Medicine* (ASEAN countries, 1993). TLC-densitometric method is also suitable for screening of the contents of each curcuminoid and total curcuminoids in *C. longa*. This method is fast and economical because one TLC plate (20 × 10 cm) can determine 15–18 samples in the same period. However, accuracy of this method is less than HPLC. HPLC gives the maximum accuracy although it consumes more time and solvents and the content of each curcuminoid and of total curcuminoids can be determined.

Standardisation of *C. longa* raw material and its ethanolic extract

Standardisation of dried rhizomes of *C. longa* has been recommended in WHO monograph, *The Thai Herbal Pharmacopoeia* and *The Standard of ASEAN Herbal Medicine* as summarised in Table 23.4. Chemical identification test of turmeric can be done by extracting 10 mg of powdered drug by shaking with 2 mL of acetic anhydride and a few drops of sulphuric acid, the solution giving a blood-red colour under UV 366 nm (ASEAN countries, 1993).

Standardisation of the ethanolic turmeric extract was reported by Pothitirat (2006) as shown in Table 23.5.

Table 23.3 Total curcuminoid contents in ethanolic turmeric extract of *C. longa* rhizomes collected from different locations in Thailand determined by UV-spectophotometry, TLC-densitometry and HPLC (Pothitirat, 2006)

		Total curcuminoid content (%w/w of extract)					
		UV		TLC		HPLC	
Location	Sample	Content	Average	Content	Average	Content	Average
North	1	22.78±0.09	22.88±0.16	37.75±1.11	37.81±1.60	21.76±0.48	21.89±0.37
	2	22.98±0.16		37.86±1.34		22.02±0.35	
Northeast	3	24.15±0.09	22.34 ±1.99	39.45±2.02	35.33±4.70	24.49±0.79	20.84±4.06
	4	20.53±0.12		31.22±0.60		17.19±0.80	
Central	5	14.14±0.87	20.30±0.27	32.61±2.06	33.71±2.28	16.93±0.63	18.82±1.96
	6	21.67±0.15		36.60±2.30		20.99±2.15	
	7	20.11±0.26		32.81±1.38		17.97±0.88	
	8	20.49±0.11		32.80±0.49		19.37±1.20	
South	9	23.62±0.22	25.19±1.73	36.31±1.11	40.20±4.32	20.38±1.82	24.87±5.09
	10	26.76±0.17		44.08±0.40		29.37±0.90	
Average		21.72±3.24		35.95±3.93		20.90±3.83	

Table 23.4 Specification of dried rhizome of *C. longa* recommended by WHO, Standard of ASEAN Herbal Medicine and Thai Herbal Pharmacopoeia (THP)

	WHO	ASEAN Herbal Medicine	THP
Volatile oil	> 4 %v/w	> 6 %v/w	> 6 %v/w
Total curcuminoids	> 3 %w/w	> 5 %w/w	> 5 %w/w
Foreign organic matter	< 3 %w/w	< 5 %w/w	< 5 %w/w
Ash content			
Total ash	< 8 %w/w	same as WHO	same as WHO
Acid-insoluble ash	< 1 %w/w	same as WHO	same as WHO
Extractives			
Water-soluble extractives	> 9 %w/w	same as WHO	same as WHO
Alcohol-soluble extractives	> 10 %w/w	same as WHO	same as WHO
Moisture content	< 10 %v/w	same as WHO	same as WHO
Pesticide residues	< 0.05 mg/kg	—	—
Heavy metals			
Lead	< 10 mg/kg	—	—
Cadmiun	< 0.3 mg/kg	—	—
Microbial contamination			
Preparation of decoction			
Salmonella spp.	negative	—	—
Aerobic bacteria	< 10^7/g	—	—
Fungi	< 10^5/g	—	—
E. coli	< 10^2/g	—	—
Preparation for internal use			
Aerobic bacteria	< 10^5/g or mL	—	—
Fungi	< 10^4/g or mL	—	—
Enterobacteria and certain Gram-negative bacteria	< 10^3/g or mL	—	—
E. coli	0/g or mL	—	—

Table 23.5 Specifications of ethanolic turmeric extract of C. longa rhizome (Pothitirat, 2006)

Description Colour/odour/characteristic	Orange-brown/characteristic/semi solid
Extract ratio	Crude drug: 95 % ethanol extract 3–5:1
Identification By colour test By TLC	 Blood-red colour, of the solution of the extract in acetic anhydride, treated with concentrated sulphuric acid, detected under UV366 Stationary phase: Silica gel 60 F_{254} Mobile phase: chloroform:benzene:methanol (80:15:5) Detector: UV366 (hRf: Curcumin = 69; Demethoxycurcumin = 51; Bisdemethoxycurcumin = 39)
Standardisation	Assay method: UV-vis spectrophotometer (λmax= 420 nm) Total curcuminoids >13 %w/w Assay method: HPLC (λmax = 425 nm) Curcumin > 8 % w/w; total curcuminoids >16 % w/w Assay method: TLC densitometer (λmax = 420 nm) Curcumin >11 % w/w; total curcuminoids >30 % w/w
Loss on drying	Not more than 10% w/w
Solubility	Insoluble in water, soluble in 95% ethanol
Heavy metals	Cd <3.00 ppm; Pb <0.50 ppm; As <0.05 ppm
Pesticides Organochlorine Organophosphorus	 Not detected Not detected
Microbial limits Total aerobic count Total fungi count *Escherichia coli* *Pseudomonas aeruginosa* *Staphylococcus aureus* *Salmonella* spp. *Clostridium* spp.	 $<5 \times 10^5$ cfu/g $<5 \times 10^3$ cfu/g None None None None None

Biological activities and pharmacological actions

For the last few decades, extensive work has been done to establish the biological activities and pharmacological actions of turmeric and its extracts. Biological activities of curcuminoids and volatile oil from turmeric have been studied both in vitro and in vivo. Curcumin has been shown to have a wide spectrum of biological actions including anti-inflammatory, antioxidant, anticarcinogenic, antimutagenic, anticoagulant, antifertility, antidiabetic, antifungal, antiprotozoal, antiviral, antifibrotic, antivenom, antiulcer, hypotensive and hypocholesteraemic activities (Chattopadhyay *et al.*, 2004).

Anti-inflammatory activity

Curcumin is effective against carrageenin-induced oedema in rats (Ghatak and Basu, 1972; Srihari *et al.*, 1982; Srivastava and Srimal, 1985; Brouet and Ohshima, 1995) and mice (Srimal and Dhawan, 1985) and was reported to be an anti-inflammatory agent with ED_{50} 2.10 μg/kg in rat (Ghatak and Busa, 1972), and LD_{50} 2 g/kg in mice (Srimal and Dhawan, 1973). It can inhibit 12-lipoxygenase and phospholipase D (Satoskar *et al.*, 1986; Yamamuta *et al.*, 1997). Demethoxycurcumin and bisdemethoxycurcumin can inhibit oedema induced by TPA on mouse ears (Masuda *et al.*, 1993). From our study (Pitakwongsaporn, 2000), we found that curcuminoids 0.026% w/w in creams containing 6% and 20% w/w of turmeric volatile oil can protect skin irritation because of anti-inflammatory activity of curcuminoids. The volatile oil (Chandra and Gupta, 1972) and the petroleum ether, alcohol and water extracts of *C. longa* showed anti-inflammatory effects (Yegnanarayan *et al.*, 1976). The anti-inflammatory action of curcumin is mediated through down-regulation of cyclo-oxygenase-2 and inducible nitric oxide synthetase (Surh *et al.*, 2001). Curcumin also enhances wound healing in diabetic rats and mice (Sidhu *et al.*, 1999) and in H_2O_2-induced damage in human keratinocytes and fibroblasts (Phan *et al.*, 2001).

Antibacterial and antifungal activities

Volatile oil from *C. longa* rhizome inhibits bacteria such as *Escherichia coli, Staphylococcus aureus* and *Pseudomonas aeruginosa* (Lyengar *et al.*, 1994.) and fungi such as *Trichoderma viride, Aspergillus flavus, Microsporum gypseum* and *Trichophyton mentagophytes* (Banerjee and Nigam, 1978). The ethanolic extract of *C. longa* inhibits *Clostridium botulinum* (minimum inhibitory concentration (MIC) 500 μg/mL), *Bacillus subtilis, Staph. aureus, Salmonella typhi, E. coli, Agrobacterium tumefaciens*, and *Mycobacterium tuberculosis* at LD_{50} 500 μg/mL. Curcumin was reported to inhibit growth of *Staph. aureus* (Todd *et al.*, 1949) and *Helicobacter pylori* in vitro at MIC 6.25–50 μg/mL (Mahady *et al.*, 2002). Turmeric oil (1 : 5000) can inhibit *Staph. albus* and *Staph. aureus* (Chopra *et al.*, 1941). Caichompoo *et al.* (2001) reported that turmeric oil exhibits a good inhibiting activity against dermatophytes and shows significantly better inhibition against *Cryptococcus* than *Candida,* but for bacteria, the oil shows unsatisfactory activity except against *Streptococcus pyogenes*. MICs of freshly distilled and 18 months-aged oils were nearly the same at 7.8 and 7.2 μg/mL respectively.

Crude ethanol extract can inhibit fungi, yeasts and bacteria but the activity is less than turmeric oil. Curcumin, demethoxycurcumin and bisdemethoxycurcumin show low activities against all organisms (Caichompoo, 1999). Furthermore, our studies demonstrate antidermatophytic effects for various concentrations, i.e. 3–15% w/w of turmeric oil, in cream preparations. These results reveal that turmeric oil and the crude ethanolic turmeric extract could be developed as medicinal and cosmetic products for skin diseases (Pitakwongsaporn, 2000).

Antipeptic ulcer

Turmeric powder was reported to decrease gastric juice in rabbits (Muderji *et al.*, 1981). Turmeric powder in capsule dosage form (250 mg/capsule), hexane extract and ar-turmerone show activity against HCl-induced peptic ulcer (Nutakul, 1994; Permpipat *et al.*, 1996). It has also been studied for antiulcer activity of curcumin in an acute ulcer model in rats by preventing glutathione depletion, lipid peroxidation and protein oxidation. Both oral and intraperitoneal administrations of curcumin blocked gastric ulceration in a dose-dependent manner. It accelerated the healing process and protected gastric ulcer through attenuation of MMP-9 activity and amelioration of MMP-2 activity (Swarnakar *et al.*, 2005). It is suggested that curcumin treatment results in a faster closure of wounds, better regulation of granulation tissue formation and induction of growth factors and acts at different levels to enhance wound repair (Maheshwari *et al.*, 2006).

Another experiment reported that healing rates were increased by 23.3% and 24.2% in rabbits and rats, respectively (Gujral *et al.*, 1953). It was found that turmeric increases the mucin content of the gastric juice, suggesting that the therapeutic effect of turmeric for gastric disorders may possibly be due to its mucous stimulatory effect (Muderji *et al.*, 1981). Curcumin was reported to be effective in preventing and ameliorating gastric lesions experimentally induced by aspirin and phenylbutazone. Curcumin increases gastric mucin, therefore its activity on gastric ulcers is likely to come from the stimulation of mucin production (Sinha *et al.*, 1975).

Anticancer activity

Recent studies have shown that curcumin acts as a potent anticarcinogenic compound and has a dose-dependent chemopreventive effect in several animal tumour bioassay systems, including colon, duodenal, stomach, oesophageal and oral carcinogenesis. It has been shown to reduce tumour promotion induced by phorbol ester (Huang *et al.*, 1988) on mouse skin, on carcinogen-induced tumorigenesis in the forestomach (Huang *et al.*, 1994). The molecular basis of anticarcinogenic and chemopreventive effects of curcumin is attributed to its effect on several targets including transcription factors, growth regulators, adhesion molecules, apoptotic genes, angiogenesis regulators and cellular signalling molecules (Aggarwal *et al.*, 2003). Among various mechanisms, induction of apoptosis plays an important role in its anticarcinogenic effect (Chen and Huang, 1998). Curcumin, demethoxycurcumin and bis-demethoxycurcumin were compared for their cytotoxic, tumour-reducing and antioxidant activities. It was found that bis-demethoxycurcumin is a more effective cytotoxic agent and was able to significantly inhibit Ehrlich ascites tumour in mice (Ruby *et al.*, 1995). Curcumin administration during both the initiation and post-initiation periods significantly inhibits colon tumorigenesis (Kawamori *et al.*, 1999).

Antioxidant activity

Curcumin exhibits strong antioxidant activity, comparable with vitamins C and E (Toda *et al.*, 1985). It was shown to be a potent scavenger of a variety of reactive oxygen species including superoxide anion radicals, hydroxyl radicals (Reddy and Aggarwal, 1994) and nitrogen dioxide radicals (Unnikrishnan and Rao, 1995; Sreejayan and Rao, 1997). Curcumin was also shown to inhibit lipid peroxidation in different animal models (Reddy and Lokesh, 1992; Sreejayan and Rao, 1994). Studies in our laboratory have shown that the ethanolic extract, crude curcuminoids, curcumin and demethoxycurcumin show high free-radical scavenging activity when tested by the DPPH scavenging assay. Curcumin, which is a major component in the extract, plays an important role as a free-radical scavenger of *C. longa* with EC_{50} of 6.38 ± 0.18 µg/mL, while demethoxycurcumin and bisdemethoxycurcumin promote the activity with EC_{50} of 10.50 ± 0.42 and 149.43 ± 0.03 µg/mL, respectively (Pothitirat, 2006).

It is suggested that dietary supplementation with curcumin may be beneficial in neurodegenerative diseases such as Alzheimer's disease (Calabrese *et al.*, 2003; Yang *et al.*, 2005). In a focal cerebral ischaemia model of rats, curcumin showed significant neuroprotective effect through inhibition of lipid peroxidation, increase in endogenous antioxidant defence enzymes and reduction in peroxynitrite formation (Thiyagarajan and Sharma, 2004). Curcumin promotes beneficial effects and appears to have a significant potential for treatment of various diseases which are a result of oxidative stress. These protective effects of curcumin are attributed mainly to its antioxidant properties and it could be further developed as a pharmaceutical (Maheshwari *et al.*, 2006).

Antimutagenic activity

Curcumin promotes antimutagenic effect. At 100 and 200 mg/kg body weight doses, curcumin has been shown to reduce the number of aberrant cells in cyclophosphamide-induced chromosomal aberration in Wistar rats (Shukla *et al.*, 2002). Turmeric also prevents mutation in urethane models (el Hamss *et al.*, 1999).

Antifertility activity

Aqueous and petroleum ether extracts of turmeric show antifertility effect in rats when fed orally (Garg, 1974). Curcumin inhibits 5α-reductase, which converts testosterone to 5α-dihydrotestosterone, thereby inhibiting the growth of flank organs in hamster (Liao *et al.*, 2001). Also, curcumin can inhibit human sperm motility and has the potential to develop as a novel intravaginal contraceptive (Rithaporn *et al.*, 2003).

Antidiabetic activity

Curcumin was reported to prevent galactose-induced cataract formation at very low dose (Suryanarayana *et al.*, 2003). Curcumin and turmeric decrease blood sugar level in alloxan-induced diabetes in rat (Arun and Nalini, 2002). Also, it decreases advanced glycation and product-induced complications in diabetes mellitus (Sajithlal *et al.*, 1998).

Toxicity

From our study on acute toxicity in mice, the ethanolic extract and crude curcuminoid extract from *C. longa* rhizomes showed no sign of toxicity (LD_{50} 5 g/kg body weight) and no abnormal sign was observed upon gross examination of visceral organs. There was also no difference in average body weight of treated and controlled animals (Pothitirat, 2006). In Wistar rats, guinea pigs and monkeys, fed with turmeric at much higher doses (2.5 g/kg body weight) than normally consumed by human, no changes were observed in the appearance, kidney, liver and heart weights (Holder *et al.*, 1978). For safety evaluation, the average intake of turmeric by Asians (0.5–1.5 g/person/day) produces no toxic symptoms (Eigner and Scholz, 1999). Human clinical trials also indicate that curcumin has no toxicity when administered at doses of 1–10 g/day (Aggarwal *et al.*, 2003; Chainani-Wu, 2003).

Pharmacokinetic studies on curcumin

Curcumin is poorly absorbed from the intestine after oral administration (Ravindranath and Chandrasekhara, 1980, 1981, 1982). In rats, it was shown that oral consumption of curcumin resulted in approximately 75% being excreted in the faeces and only traces appeared in the urine (Wahlstrom and Blennow, 1978). Curcumin, after being metabolised in the liver, is mainly excreted through bile (Chattopadhyay *et al.*, 2004). Intraperitoneal administration of curcumin showed a similar result for the level of faecal excretion of curcumin (Holder *et al.*, 1978). The results suggest poor absorption of curcumin from the intestine. Curcumin has been shown to be biotransformed to dihydrocurcumin and tetrahydrocurcumin, then these products are converted to monoglucuronide conjugates (Pan *et al.*, 1999).

Clinical studies and medicinal applications of turmeric and curcumin

In Nepal, powdered turmeric is used to treat wounds, bruises, inflamed joints and sprains (Surh, 2002). In India, current traditional medicines apply turmeric powder for treatment of biliary disorders, anorexia, cough, diabetic wounds, hepatic disorders, rheumatism and sinusitis (Jain and DeFillips, 1991). In 18 patients with rheumatoid arthritis, turmeric powder showed significant improvement in morning stiffness and joint swelling after 2 weeks with oral doses of 120 mg/day (Sinha *et al.*, 1974). The powder used in combination with other plants was reported for purification of blood and for menstrual and abdominal problems (Eigner and Scholz, 1990).

In Thailand, a clinical trial on the effect of turmeric on peptic ulcer was carried out in 12 patients. Two turmeric capsules (250 mg each) were given orally, 4 times a day, 1 h before meals and at bedtime. The ulcers were completely healed in 5 patients within 4 weeks, and the other 7 patients within 4–12 weeks (Prucksunand *et al.*, 1986). For treatment of gastritis in 25 patients, 2 capsules of turmeric powder (300 mg/capsule) were given orally 5 times/day for 4 weeks, 48%, 72% and 76% of patients recovered in 4, 8 and 12 weeks, respectively after the beginning of treatment (Prucksunand *et al.*, 2001). A randomised double-blind study of turmeric powder for dyspepsia was carried out in hospitals in Thailand. One hundred and six adult patients who had acid dyspepsia or flatulent dyspepsia were included in the study. Each patient received 2 capsules of placebo or flatulence drug or turmeric

(250 mg/capsule) 4 times/day for 7 days. Fifty-three per cent of the patients receiving placebo, 83% of patients receiving flatulence drug and 87% of patients receiving turmeric responded to the treatment. The differences in efficacy between placebo and turmeric were statistically significant (Thamlikitkul *et al.*, 1989).

Turmeric products on the Thai market

In Thailand, turmeric is available in forms of dried powder for raw material and spice; curcuminoids extract for raw material; capsules/tablets of powdered turmeric or curcuminoids as dietary supplement and herbal drugs for carminative and anti-flatulence; cream preparations for antifungal, anti-acne and mosquito repellant; anti-ageing cosmetic products in forms of night cream, facial and body scrub, lotion and soap.

Future prospects of turmeric

Turmeric has long been traditionally used as a food, medicine and as a cosmetic. Much research has been done on various biological activities which indicate its possible medicinal applications. Toxicity studies also show that turmeric is safe and produces no serious toxic symptom (Aggarwal *et al.*, 2003; Chainani-Wu, 2003). Moreover, curcuminoids and curcumin show a wide spectrum of biological actions. Therefore, turmeric and curcuminoids should be further developed in the form of modern medicines, especially curcumin, which might be developed as a novel anti-inflammatory, antioxidant and anticarcinogenesis drug.

Conclusions

Turmeric is a popular medicinal herb as yellow colouring agent, food flavour spice, and household medicine for various diseases. Biological activities of turmeric have been reported both in vitro and in vivo. Pharmacological actions of turmeric and curcumin, the main component, have been established. These include anti-inflammatory, antioxidant, anticarcinogenic, antimutagenic, antibacterial, antifungal, hypotensive, and hypocholesteraemic activities. Turmeric has been used to reduce post-operative inflammation. Medicinal uses of turmeric arise from volatile oil and yellow curcuminoids which comprise mainly curcumin, demethoxycurcumin and bisdemethoxycurcumin.

Turmeric is one of the most valuable plants used in primary healthcare in Thailand and other countries because of its low cost, it is easily grown and has no side-effects. It is one of the medicinal plants listed in the Thai Herbal Essential Drug List and has been selected as one of the 12 plant species to be developed as product champions of Thailand. However, the quality of turmeric products depends on the quality of the raw materials so standardisation of turmeric rhizome and its extract needs to be introduced and applied commercially. According to *The Standard of ASEAN Herbal Medicine* and *The Thai Herbal Pharmacopoeia*, dried turmeric should contain not less than 6% v/w of volatile oil and not less than 5% w/w of total curcuminoids, while WHO recommends not less than 4% and 3% of volatile oil and total curcuminoids, respectively. For the ethanolic extract of the rhizomes of *C. longa* cultivated in Thailand, an extract ratio (crude drug: 95% ethanolic extract) of 3–5 : 1, should contain total curcuminoids not less than 13% w/w when analysed by the UV-visible spectrophotometer; or not less than 8 and 16% w/w of curcumin and total curcuminoids, respectively when analysed by HPLC; or not less than 11% and 30% w/w of curcumin and total curcuminoids, respectively, when analysed by a TLC-densitometer.

Recently, turmeric has been valued worldwide as a functional food because of its health promotion properties. Safety evaluation studies indicate that turmeric and curcumin are well tolerated at very high doses without any toxic effects. Standardisations of turmeric and its extract, crude curcuminoids, and turmeric oil have been investigated.

References

Aggarwal BB, Kumar A, Bharti AC (2003). Anticancer potential of curcumin: preclinical and clinical studies. *Anticancer Res* 23: 363–398.

Ahn BZ, Lee JH (1989). Cytotoxic and cytotoxicity-potentiating effects of the *Curcuma* root on L 1210 cell. *Korean J Pharmacog* 20: 223–226.

Ammon HPT, Wahl MA (1991). Pharmacology of *Curcuma longa*. *Planta Med* 57: 1–7.

Araujo CAC, Leon LL (2001). Biological activities of *Curcuma longa* L. *Mem Inst Oswaldo Cruz* 96: 723–728.

Arun N, Nalini N (2002). Efficacy of turmeric on blood sugar and polyol pathway in diabetic albino rats. *Plant Foods Hum Nutr* 57: 41–52.

ASEAN Countries (1993). *Standard of ASEAN Herbal Medicine*, Vol. I. Jakarta: Aksara Buana Printing.

ASTA Method (1985). *Official Analytical Methods of the American Spice Trade Association*, 3rd edn. NJ: American Spice Trade Association.

Banerjee A, Nigam SS (1978). Antifungal efficacy of the essential oils derived from the various species of the genus *Curcuma* Linn. *J Res Indian Med Yoga Homeopath* 13: 63–70.

Baumann W, Rodrigues SV, Viana LM (2000). Pigment and their solubility in and extractability by supercritical CO_2. Part 1 The case of curcumin. *Braz J Chem Eng* 17: 323–328.

Braga MEM, Leal PF, Carvalho JOE, Meireles MAA (2003). Comparison of yield, composition, and antioxidant activity of turmeric (*Curcuma longa* L.) extracts obtained using various techniques. *J Agric Food Chem* 51: 6604–6611.

Brouet I, Ohshima H (1995). Curcumin, an antitumor promoter and anti-inflammatory agent, inhibits induction of nitric oxide synthase in activated macrophages. *Biochem Biophys Res Commun* 206: 533–540.

Caichompoo W (1999). *Antimicrobial Activities of Volatile Oil and Curcuminoids from Curcuma Longa*. Thesis of Master of Science (Pharmaceutical Chemistry and Phytochemistry), Faculty of Graduate Studies, Mahidol University, Bangkok.

Caichompoo W, Gritsanapan W, Wuthi-udomlert M, Luauratana O (2001). Antimicrobial activities of turmeric oil from *Curcuma longa* Linn. rhizome. *J Mahasarakram Univ* 19: 11–19.

Calabrese V, Butterfield DA, Stella AM (2003). Nutritional antioxidants and the heme oxygenase pathway of stress tolerance: novel targets for neuroprotection in Alzheimer's disease. *Ital J Biochem* 52: 177–181.

Chainani-Wu N (2003). Safety and antiinflammatory activity of curcumin: a component of turmeric (*Curcuma longa*). *J Altern Complement Med* 9: 161–168.

Chandra D, Gupta SS (1972). Antiinflammatory and antiarthritic activity of volatile oil of *Curcuma longa* (Haldi). *Indian J Med Res* 60: 138–142.

Chang HM, But PP (1987). *Pharmacology and Applications of Chinese Material Medica* vol. 2. Singapore: World Scientific.

Chattopadhyay I, Biswas K, Bandyopadhyay U, Banerjee RK (2004). Turmeric and curcumin: Biological actions and medicinal applications. *Curr Sci* 87: 44–53.

Chavalittumrong P, Dechatiwongse T (1988). Quality evaluation of turmeric. *Thai J Pharm Sci* 13: 317–325.

Chen YH, Yu JG, Fang HJ (1983). Studies on Chinese *curcuma* III: Comparison of the volatile oil and phenolic constituents from the rhizome and the tuber of *Curcuma longa*. *Chung Yao T'ung Pao* 8: 27–29.

Chen HW, Huang HC (1998). Effect of curcumin on cell cycle progression and apoptosis in vascular smooth cells. *Br J Pharmacol* 124: 1029–1040.

Chopra RN, Chopra IC, Hemda KL, *et al.* (1982). *Chopra's Indigenous Drugs of India*, 2nd edn. Calcutta: Academic.

Chopra RN, Gupta JC, Chopra GS (1941). Pharmacological action of the essential oil of *Curcuma longa*. *Indian J Med Res* 29: 769–772.

Dandekar DV, Gaikar VG (2002). Microwave assisted extraction of curcuminoids from *Curcuma longa*. *Sep Sci Technol* 37: 2669–2690.

De Padua LS, Bunyapraphatsara N, Lemmens RH, eds (1994). *PROSEA: Plant Resources of South-East Asia No. 12(1) Medicinal and poisonous plant 1*. Leiden: Backhuys Publishers.

Department of Medical Science Ministry of Public Health (1993). *Manual for Cultivation Production and Utilization of Herbal Medicines in Primary Health Care*, 2nd edn. Nonthaburi.

Eigner D, Scholz D (1990). Das Zauberbuchlein der Gyani Dolma. *Pharm Unserer Zeit* 19: 141–152.

Eigner D, Scholz D (1999). *Ferula asa-foetida* and *Curcuma longa* in traditional medicinal treatment and diet in Nepal. *J Ethnopharmacol* 67: 1–6.

el Hamss R, Analla M, Campos-Sanchez J *et al.* (1999). A dose dependent anti-genotoxic effect of turmeric. *Mutat Res* 446: 135–139.

Faculty of Pharmacy Mahidol University (1996). *Specification of Thai Medicinal Plants Volume 1*. Bangkok: Aksornsampan Press.

Fang HJ, Yu JG, Chen YH, Hu Q (1982). Studies on Chinese curcuma. II. Comparison of the chemical components of essential oils from rhizome of five species of medicinal *Curcuma* plants. *Yao Hsueh Hsueh Pao* 17: 441–447.

Garg SK (1974). Effect of *Curcuma longa* (rhizomes) on fertility in experimental animals. *Planta Med* 26: 225–227.

Ghatak N, Busa N (1972). Sodium curcuminate as an effective anti-inflammatory agent. *Indian J Exp Biol* 10: 235–236.

Goh CL, Ng SK (1987). Allergic contact dermatitis to *Curcuma longa* (turmeric). *Contact Derm* 17: 186.

Golding BY, Pombo E, Samuel CJ (1982). Turmerones: isolations from turmeric and their structure determination. *Chem Commun* 6: 363–364.

Golding BY, Pombo E (1992). Structure of alpha- and beta-turmerone. *J Chem Soc Perkin Trans I* 12: 1519–1524.

Guenther E (1952). *The Essential Oils,* Vol. 5. New York: Van Nostrand Reinhold.

Gujral ML, Chowdhury NK, Saxena PN (1953). Effect of indigenous remedies on the healing of wounds and ulcers. *J Indian Med Assoc* 22: 273–276.

Gupta AP, Gupta MM, Kumar S (1999). Simultaneous determination of curcuminoids in *Curcuma* samples using high performance thin layer chromatography. *J Liq Chromatogr Rel Technol* 22: 1561–1569.

Hisashige M, Shiroma T, Giho H, Hashimoto K (1994). Method for the extraction of curcumin, a known food additive, from *Curcuma longa*, Japan. *Kokai Tokyo Koho*: TP 06, 09479 [9409, 479] (Cl. C07c49/255).

Hiserodt R, Hartman TG, Ho CT, Rosen RT (1996). Characterization of powdered turmeric by liquid chromatography-mass spectrometry and gas chromatography-mass spectrometry. *J Chromatogr* 740: 51–63.

Holder GM, Plummer JL, Ryan AJ (1978). The metabolism and excretion of curcumin (1,7-bis-(4-hydroxy-3-methoxyphenyl)-1,6-heptadiene-3,5-dione) in the rat. *Xenobiotica* 8: 761–768.

Huang MT, Lou YR, Ma W *et al.* (1994). Inhibitory effects of dietary curcumin on forestomach, duodenal, and colon carcinogenesis in mice. *Cancer Res* 54: 5841–5847.

Huang MT, Smart RC, Wong CQ, Conney AH (1988). Inhibitory effect of curcumin, chlorogenic acid, caffeic acid, and ferulic acid on tumor promotion in mouse skin by 12-O-tetradecanoylphorbol-13-acetate. *Cancer Res* 48: 5941–5946.

Imai S, Morikiyo M, Furihata K (1990). Turmeronol A and Turmeronol B, new inhibitors of soybean lipoxygenase. *Agric Biol Chem* 54: 2367–2371.

Institute of Materia Medica (1982). *Chinese Materia Medica,* Vol. 2. Beijing: Ren-Min-Wei Sheng.

Jain SK, DeFillips RA (1991). *Medicinal Plants of India.* Michigan, Ann Arbor.

Janaki N, Bose JL (1967). An improved method for the isolation of curcumin from turmeric, *Curcuma longa* L. *J Indian Chem Soc* 44: 985–989.

Janben A, Gole TH (1984). Thin-layer chromatographic determination of curcumine (Turmeric) in spices. *Chromatographia* 18: 546–549.

Jentzsch K, Spiegl P, Kamitz R (1970). Qualitative and quantitative studies of curcuma dyes in different Zingiberaceae drugs 2: Quantitative studies. *Sci Pharm* 38: 50–58.

John TK, Krishna RGS (1985). Absolute configuration of naturally occurring −-xanthorrhizol. *Indian J Chem Ser B* 24: 35–37.

Karasz AB, DeCocca F, Bokus L (1973). Detection of turmeric in foods by rapid fluorimetric method and by improved spot test. *J Assoc Off Anal Chem* 56: 626–628.

Kawamori T, Lubet R, Steele VE *et al.* (1999). Chemopreventive effect of curcumin, a naturally occurring anti-inflammatory agent, during the promotion/progression stages of colon cancer. *Cancer Res* 59: 597–601.

Kelkar NC, Sanjiva B (1933). Essential oil from the rhizomes of *Curcuma longa* L. *J Indian Inst Sci* 17A: 7–24.

Kiso Y, Suzuki Y, Watanabe N *et al.* (1983). Antihepatotoxic principles of *Curcuma longa* rhizomes. *J Med Plant Res* 49: 185–187.

Kiuchi F, Goto Y, Sugimoto N, *et al.* (1993). Nematocidal activity of turmeric: synergistic action of curcuminoids. *Chem Pharm Bull (Tokyo)* 41: 1640–1643.

Krishnamurthy N, Mathew AG, Nambudiri ES *et al.* (1976). Oil and oleoresins of turmeric. *Trop Sci* 18: 37–39.

Liao S, Lin J, Dang MT *et al.* (2001). Growth suppression of hamster flank organs by topical application of catechins, alizarin, curcumin, and myristoleic acid. *Arch Dermatol Res* 293: 200–205.

Lyengar MA, Rao MPR, Bairy I (1994). Antimicrobial activity of the essential oil of *Curcuma longa* leaves. *Indian Drugs* 32: 249–250.

Mahady GB, Pendland SL, Yun G, Lu ZZ (2002). Turmeric (*Curcuma longa*) and curcumin inhibit the growth of *Helicobacter pylori*, a group 1 carcinogen. *Anticancer Res* 22: 4179–4181.

Maheshwari RK, Singh AK, Gaddipati J, Srimal RC (2006). Multiple biological activities of curcumin: A short review. *Life Sci* 78: 2081–2087.

Malingre TM (1975). *Curcuma xanthorrhiza*, Temoe lawak, a plant with cholagog activity. *Pharm Weekbl* 10: 601.

Manzan ACCM, Toniolo FS, Bredow E, Povh NP (2003). Extraction of essential oil and pigments from *Curcuma longa* (L.) by steam distillation and extraction with volatile solvents. *J Agric Food Chem* 51: 6802–6807.

Marsin SM, Ahmad UK, Smith RM (1993). Application of supercritical fluid extraction and chromatography to the analysis of turmeric. *J Chromatogr Sci* 31: 20–25.

Masuda T, Jitoe A, Isobe J *et al.* (1993). Anti-oxidative and anti-inflammatory curcumin-related phenolics from rhizomes of *Curcuma domestica*. *Phytochemistry* 32: 1557–1560.

Matthes HWD, Luu B, Ourisson G (1980). Cytotoxic components of *Zingiber zerumbet*, *Curcuma zedoaria* and *C. domestica*. *Phytochemistry* 19: 2643–2650.

Merh PS, Daniel M, Sabnis SD (1986). Chemistry and taxonomy of some members of the Zingiberales. *Curr Sci* 55: 835–839.

Mitra CR (1975). Important Indian spices I *Curcuma longa* (Zingiberaceae). *Riechst Aromen Koerperpflegem* 25: 15.

Moon CK, Park NS, Koh SK (1976). Studies on the lipid

components of *Curcuma longa*. I. The composition of fatty acids and sterols. *Soul Taehakkyo Yakhak Nonmumjip* 1: 132.

Muderji B, Zaidi SH, Singh GB (1981). Spices and gastric function: Part I – Effect of *Curcuma longa* on the gastric secretion in rabbits. *J Sci Indian Res* 20: 25–28.

Nadkarni KM, Nadkarni AK (1976). *Indian Material Medica*, Vol 1. Bombay: Popular Prakashan Private.

Navas DA, Ramos PMC (1992). Fluorometric determination of curcumin in yogurt and mustard. *J Agric Food Chem* 40: 56–59.

Nutakul W (1994). NMR analysis of antipeptic ulcer principle from *Curcuma longa* L. *Bull Dept Med Sci* 36: 211–218.

Ogbeide ON, Eduaveguavoen OI, Parvez M (1985). Identification of 2-(hydroxymethyl) anthraquinone in *Curcuma domestica*. *Pak J Sci* 37: 15–17.

Ohshiro M, Kuroyanagi M, Ueno A (1990). Structures of sesquiterpenes from *Curcuma longa*. *Phytochemistry* 29: 2201–2205.

Pan MH, Huang TM, Lin JK (1999). Biotransformation of curcumin through reduction and glucoronidation in mice. *Drug Metabol Dispos* 27: 486–494.

Park SN, Boo YC (1991). Cell protection from damage by active oxygen with curcuminoids. *Patent: Fr Demande Patent* 2, 655, 054.

Patel K, Krishna G, Sokoloski E, Ito V (2000). Preparative separation of curcuminoids from crude curcumin and turmeric powder by pH-zone refining countercurrent chromatography. *J Liq Chromatogr Rel Technol* 23: 2209–2218.

Permpipat U, Chuthaputti A, Kiatying-Angsulee N (1996). Antipeptic ulcer activity of turmeric (*Curcuma longa* L.). *Thai J Pharm Sci* 20: 27–38.

Peter-Almeida L, Cherubino APF, Alves RJ *et al.* (2005). Separation and determination of the physico-chemical characteristics of curcumin, demethoxycurcumin and bisdemethoxycurcumin. *Food Res Int* 38: 1039–1044.

Phan TT, See P, Lee ST, Chan SY (2001). Protective effects of curcumin against oxidative damage on skin cell *in vitro*: its implication for wound healing. *J Trauma* 51: 927–931.

Pitakwongsaporn P (2000). *The Study of Antifungal Activity, Stability and Skin Irritation of Turmeric Cream.* Thesis of Master of Science (Pharmaceutical Chemistry and Phytochemistry), Faculty of Graduate Studies, Mahidol University, Bangkok.

Pothitirat W, Gritsanapan W (2004). Extraction method for high curcuminoid content from *Curcuma longa*. *Mahidol Univ J Pharm Sci* 31: 44–47.

Pothitirat W, Gritsanapan W (2005). Quantitative analysis of curcumin, demethoxycurcumin and bisdemethoxycurcumin in the crude curcuminoid extract from *Curcuma longa* in Thailand by TLC-densitometry. *Mahidol Univ J Pharm Sci* 32: 23–30.

Pothitirat W (2006). *Standardization and Antioxidant Activity of Curcuma longa Rhizome Extracts*. Thesis of Master of Science (Pharmaceutical Chemistry and Phytochemistry), Faculty of Graduate Studies, Mahidol University, Bangkok.

Pothitirat W, Gritsanapan W (2006). Variation of bioactive components in *Curcuma longa* in Thailand. *Curr Sci* 91: 1397–1400.

Prucksunand C, Indrasukhsri B, Leethochawalit M *et al.* (2001). Phase II clinical trial on effect of the long turmeric (*Curcuma longa* Linn) on healing of peptic ulcer. *Southeast Asian J Trop Med Public Health* 32: 208–215.

Prucksunand C, Indrasukhsri B, Leethochawalit M *et al.* (1986). Effect of the long turmeric (*Curcuma longa* Linn.) on healing of peptic ulcer: A preliminary report of 10 cases study. *Thai J Pharmacol* 8: 139–151.

Punyarajun S (1981). Determination of the curcuminoid content in *Curcuma*. *Warasarn Phesatchasat* 8: 29–31.

Ramussen HB, Christensen SB, Kvist LP, Karazmi A (2000). A simple and efficient separation of the curcumins, the antiprotozoal constituents of *Curcuma longa*. *Planta Med* 66: 396–397.

Rao TS, Basu N, Siddiqui HH (1982). Anti-inflammatory activity of curcumin analogues. *Indian J Med Res* 75: 574–578.

Ravindranath V, Chandrasekhara N (1980). Absorption and tissue distribution of curcumin in rats. *Toxicology* 16: 259–265.

Ravindranath V, Chandrasekhara N (1981). In vitro studies on the intestinal absorption of curcumin in rats. *Toxicology* 20: 251–257.

Ravindranath V, Chandrasekhara N (1982). Metabolism of curcumin-studies with [3H] curcumin. *Toxicology* 22: 337–344.

Reddy AC, Lokesh BR (1992). Studies on spice principles as antioxidants in the inhibition of lipid peroxidation of rat liver microsomes. *Mol Cell Biochem* 111: 117–124.

Reddy S, Aggarwal BB (1994). Curcumin is a non-competitive and selective inhibitor of phosphorylase kinase. *FEBS Letters* 341: 19–22.

Rithaporn T, Monga M, Rajasekharan M (2003). Curcumin: a potential vaginal contraceptive. *Contraception* 68: 219–223.

Ruby AJ, Kuttan G, Babu KD *et al.* (1995). Antitumour and antioxidant activity of natural curcuminoids. *Cancer Lett* 94: 79–83.

Russell RL (1988). High performance liquid chromatographic separation and spectral characterization of the pigments in turmeric and Anatto. *J Food Sci* 53: 1823–1826.

Sajithlal GB, Chittra P, Chandrakasan G (1998). Effect of curcumin on the advanced glycation and cross-linking of collagen in diabetic rats. *Biochem Pharmacol* 56: 1607–1614.

Sanagi MM, Ahmad UK, Smith RM (1993). Application of supercritical fluid extraction and chromatography to the analysis of turmeric. *J Chromatogr Sci* 31: 20–25.

Satoskar RR, Shan SJ, Shenoy SG (1986). Evaluation of anti-inflammatory property of curcumin (diferuloyl methane) in patients with postoperative inflammation. *Int J Clin Pharmacol Ther Toxicol* 24: 651–654.

Scartezzini P, Speroni E (2000). Review on some plants of Indian traditional medicine with antioxidant activity. *J Ethnopharmacol* 71: 23–43.

Schultz JM, Herrmann K (1980). Occurrence of hydroxybenzoic acids and hydroxycinnamic acid in spices. IV. Phenolics of spices. *Z Lebensm-Unters Forsch* 171: 193–199.

Shukla Y, Arora A, Taneja P (2002). Antimutagenic potential of curcumin on chromosomal aberrations in Wistar rats. *Mutat Res* 515: 197–202.

Sidhu GS, Mani H, Gaddipati JP *et al.* (1999). Curcumin enhances wound healing in streptozotocin induced diabetic rats and genetically diabetic mice. *Wound Repair Regen* 7: 362–374.

Sinha M, Mukherjee BP, Mukherjee B *et al.* (1975). Study of the mechanism of action of curcumin: an antiulcer agent. *Indian J Pharm* 7: 98–99.

Sinha M, Mukherjee BP, Mukherjee B, Dasgupta SR (1974). Study on the 5-hydroxytryptamine contents in guinea pig stomach with relation to phenylbutazone induced gastric ulcers and the effects of curcumin thereon. *Indian J Pharmacol* 6: 87–96.

Smith RM, Witowska BA (1984). Comparison of detectors for the determination of curcumin in turmeric by high-performance liquid chromatography. *Analyst* 109: 259–261.

Sreejayan N, Rao MNA (1994). Curcuminoids as potent inhibitors of lipid peroxidation. *J Pharm Pharmaco* 46: 1013–1016.

Sreejayan N, Rao MNA (1997). Nitric oxide scavenging by curcuminoids. *J Pharm Pharmaco* 49: 105–107.

Srihari RT, Basu N, Siddqui HH (1982). Anti inflammatory activity of curcumin analogues. *Indian J Med Res* 75: 574–578.

Srimal RC, Dhawan BN (1973). Pharmacology of diferuloyl methane (curcumin), a non-steroidal anti-inflammatory agent. *J Pharm Pharmacol* 25: 447–452.

Srimal RC, Dhawan BN (1985). *Development of Unani Drugs from Herbal Sources and the Role of Elements in their Mechanism of Action*. New Delhi: Hamdard National Foundation Monograph.

Srinivas L, Shalini VK, Shylaja M (1992). Turmerin: a water soluble antioxidant peptide from turmeric (*Curcuma longa*). *Arch Biochem Biophys* 292: 617–623.

Srivastava R, Srimal RC (1985). Modification of certain inflammation-induced biochemical changes by curcumin. *Indian J Med Res* 81: 215–223.

Su HCF, Horvat R, Jilani G (1982). Isolation, purification and characterization of insect repellents from *Curcuma longa* L. *J Agric Food Chem* 30: 290–292.

Sun X, Gao C, Cao W *et al.* (2002). Capillary electrophoresis with amperometric detection of curcumin in Chinese herbal medicine pretreated by solid-phase extraction. *J Chromatogr A* 962: 117–125.

Surh YJ (2002). Anti-tumor promoting potential of selected spice ingredients with antioxidative and anti-inflammatory activities: a short review. *Food Chem Toxicol* 40: 1091–1097.

Surh YJ, Chun KS, Cha HH *et al.* (2001). Molecular mechanism underlying chemopreventive activities of anti-inflammatory phytochemicals: down regulation of COX-2 and iNOS through suppression of NF-kB activation. *Mutat Res* 480–481: 243–268.

Suryanarayana P, Krishnaswamy K, Reddy GB (2003). Effect of curcumin on galactose-induced cataractogenesis in rats. *Mol Vis* 9: 223–230.

Swarnakar S, Ganguly K, Kundu P *et al.* (2005). Curcumin regulates expression and activity of matrix metalloproteinases-9 and -2 during prevention and healing of indomethacin-induced gastric ulcer. *J Biol Chem* 280: 9409–9415.

Tewtrakul S, De-Eknamkul W, Ruangrungsi N (1992). Simultaneous determination of individual curcuminoids in turmeric by TLC-densitometric method. *Thai J Pharm Sci* 16: 251–259.

THP (1995). *Thai Herbal Pharmacopoeia,* Vol. 1. Bangkok: Prachachon.

Thamlikitkul V, Dechatiwongse T, Chantrakul C *et al.* (1989). Randomized double blind study of *Curcuma domestica* Val. for dyspepsia. *J Med Assoc Thailand* 72: 613–620.

The Medicine Commission (1973). *British Pharmacopoeia. A19*. London: HMSO.

Thiyagarajan M, Sharma SS (2004). Neuroprotective effect of curcumin in middle cerebral artery occlusion induced focal cerebral ischemia in rats. *Life Sci* 74: 969–985.

Toda S, Miyase T, Arichi H (1985). Natural antioxidants III. Antioxidative components isolated from rhizome of *Curcuma longa* L. *Chem Pharm Bull* 33: 1725–1728.

Todd AR, Rinderknecht H, Geiger WB *et al.* (1949). Antibacterial action of curcumin and related compounds. *Nature* 164: 456–457.

Tomoda M, Shimizu N, Gonda R, Kanari M (1990). Studies on the polysaccharides having activity on the reticuloendothelial system from several oriental crude drugs. *J Pharmacobio Dyn* 13: S-47.

Tonnesen HH, Karlsen J (1983). High-performance liquid chromatography of curcumin and related compounds. *J Chromatogr* 259: 367–371.

Tonnesen HH, Karlsen J (1986). Studies on curcumin and curcuminoids. VII: Chromatographic separation and quantitative analysis of curcumin and related compounds. *Z Lebensm Unters Forsch* 182: 215–218.

Tyler VE (1994). *Herbs of Choice*. New York: Pharmaceutical Products Press.

Uehara SI, Yasuda I, Takeya K, Itokawa H (1992). Comparison on the commercial turmeric and its cultivated plant by their constituents. *Shoyakugaku Zasshi* 46: 55–61.

Unnikrishnan MK, Rao MN (1995). Curcumin inhibits nitrogen dioxide induced oxidation of hemoglobin. *Mol Cell Biochem* 146(1): 35–37.

Wagner H, Bladt S, Zgainski EM (1983). *Plant drug analysis. A thin layer chromatography atlas.* New York, Springer.

Wahlstrom BO, Blennow G (1978). A study on the fate of curcumin in the rat. *Acta Pharmacol Toxicol* 43: 86–92.

World Health Organization (1999). *WHO Monographs on Selected Medicinal Plants* Vol. I. Malta.

Yamamuta H, Hanada K, Kawasaki K, Nishijima M (1997). Inhibitory effect of curcumin on mammalian phospholipase D activity. *FEBS Letters* 417: 196–198.

Yang F, Lim GP, Begum AN, *et al.* (2005). Curcumin inhibits formation of amyloid beta oligomers and fibrils, binds plaques, and reduces amyloid *in vivo*. *J Biol Chem* 280(7): 5892–5901.

Yegnanarayan R, Saraf AP, Balwani JH (1976). Comparison of anti-inflammatory activity of various extracts of *Curcuma longa* (Linn). *Indian J Med Res* 64: 601–608.

24

Safety and efficacy of Hachimi-jio-gan: a Chinese preparation to counteract oxidative damage

Takako Yokozawa, Noriko Yamabe and Ki Sung Kang

Introduction

Oxidative stress induced by free radicals has been considered as an important factor in many common and life-threatening human diseases over the last few decades, including diabetes. Hence, a therapeutic strategy to increase the antioxidant capacity would fortify long-term effective treatment with herbal medicines.

Oxidative stress and disease

Reactive oxygen species (ROS) are produced externally and endogenously (Nishikawa *et al.*, 2000; Fialkow *et al.*, 2007). In the latter instance they are essential for cell signalling, and thus ROS-mediated tissue injury is regarded as a final common pathway for a number of diseases including atherosclerosis, diabetes, and cancer, and also ageing. Many studies have been made on the connections between diabetes and ROS, being closely related to increased oxidative stress regarding the pathogenesis and development of its complications (Rahbar and Figarola, 2003). Diabetes affects approximately 170 million individuals worldwide, and is expected to alter the lives of at least 366 million individuals over the next 25 years. Moreover, diabetes is known as the single most common cause of end-stage renal disease, leading to serious mental, physical, and financial issues.

Intensive hyperglycaemic control in patients with type 1 diabetes has been promoted to delay the onset and slow the progression of diabetic complications (The Diabetes Control and Complication Trial Research Group, 1993). Hyperglycaemia itself leads to the overproduction of free radicals by the non-enzymatic glycation of proteins through the Maillard reaction, and these free radicals exert deleterious effects on the function of β-cells, making them vulnerable to oxidative stress (Brownlee *et al.*, 1984; Njoroge and Monnier, 1989). Nishikawa *et al.* (2000), showed that the TCA cycle was the source of increased ROS-generating substrates induced by hyperglycaemia, and that the normalisation of mitochondrial ROS could prevent diabetic, pathological changes. Hence, a therapeutic strategy for diabetes incorporating an increase in the antioxidant capacity seems reasonable.

Herbal medicines

General

Up to now, we have performed in-vitro and in-vivo studies using 12 Chinese prescriptions in expectation of the possibility of curing diabetic nephropathy (Yokozawa *et al.*, 2001a), and demonstrated the effects of a 5-week administration of four prescriptions: *Wen-Pi-Tang*, *Keishi-bukuryo-gan*, *Sairei-to*, and *Hachimi-jio-gan*, in an animal model of diabetic nephropathy by measuring biochemical parameters that are affected by persistent hyperglycaemia (Nakagawa *et al.*, 2001). In these prescriptions, Hachimi-jio-gan (HJG) is used clinically to improve several disorders associated with diabetes (Goto *et al.*, 1989; Furuya *et al.*, 1999), and it has been used widely for the treatment of renal dysfunction in human subjects (Yamada, 1992), although scientific evidence supporting a pharmacological basis for its therapeutic effects has not been fully elucidated. Therefore, this chapter discusses the novel therapeutic potential of HJG, one of the constituent crude drugs Corni Fructus, and the effects of its fractions against oxidative stress in animal models.

Hachimi-jio-gan extract

The composition of HJG is shown in Table 24.1. The eight plants in the proportions stated were boiled gently in 10 times their volume of water for 60 min, filtered, and the filtrate was spray-dried to obtain the extract. The composition of the extract obtained was measured by HPLC fitted with a diode array detector. Morroniside, loganin, and paeoniflorin were seen to be the major components with penta-O-galloylglucose, benzoylmesaconine, cinnamic acid, benzoylpaeoniflorin, cinnamaldehyde, and 16-ketoalisol A as minor constituents.

Corni Fructus, a constituent of HJG

Corni Fructus (CF), the extract from the fruit of *Cornus officinalis*, has been used as a traditional medicine in Japan and China (Fan and Xiang, 2001) and contains iridoids and polyphenols (Hatano *et al.*, 1989). It has a plasma glucose-lowering action in normal rats (Liou *et al.*, 2004) and Vareed *et al.* (2006) reported that CF has been used for improving liver and kidney functions. The total iridoid glycosides had the effect of preventing the overexpression of transforming growth factor (TGF)-β_1 and matrixes in glomeruli with a diabetic model (Xu and Hao, 2004) but the mechanisms of Corni Fructus against

Table 24.1 Composition of Hachimi-jio-gan

Botanical name	Common name	Family name	Part used	Content (%)
Rehmannia glutinosa Libosch. var. *purpurea* Makino	Rehmanniae Radix	Scrophulariaceae	Root	27.27
Cornus officinalis Sieb. et Zucc.	Corni Fructus	Cornaceae	Fruit	13.64
Dioscorea japonica Thunb.	Dioscoreae Rhizoma	Dioscoreaceae	Rhizome	13.64
Alisma orientale Juzep.	Alismatis Rhizoma	Alismataceae	Rhizome	13.64
Poria cocos Wolf	Hoelen	Polyporaceae	Sclerotium	13.64
Paeonia suffruticosa Andrews	Moutan Cortex	Paeoniaceae	Bark	11.36
Cinnamomum cassia Blume	Cinnamomi Cortex	Lauraceae	Bark	4.54
Aconitum carmichaeli Debx	Aconiti Tuber	Ranunculaceae	Tuber	2.27

glucose- and oxidative stress-associated metabolic disorders in diabetes have not been fully investigated.

CF extract was fractionated on Sephadex LH-20 column chromatography with water containing increasing proportions of methanol and finally 60% acetone to give four fractions: S1 (94.52 g), S2 (1.20 g), S3 (2.15 g), and S4 (1.55 g). The fractions were further separated to give 7-*O*-galloyl-D-sedoheptulose (Zhang *et al.*, 1999), mevaloside (Tschesche *et al.*, 1971), loganic acid (El-Naggar and Beal, 1980), and 5-hydroxymethyl-2-furfural (5-HMF) (Liu *et al.*, 2004), morroniside (Inouye *et al.*, 1973; Otsuka *et al.*, 2001) and loganin (Garcia and Chulia, 1986).

Evaluation of efficacy

Effect on diabetic oxidative stress

Efficacy of HJG

A rat model with diabetes induced by streptozotocin, which destroys pancreatic β-cells as a result of damage caused by radicals and a deficit in antioxidative defences, was used. HJG was dissolved in distilled water and orally administered at doses of 50, 100, and 200 mg/kg body weight/day via gavage (Yokozawa *et al.*, 1997). Rats with diabetes induced by streptozotocin and treated with HJG did not show body weight changes during the 10-day experimental period, whereas a duplicate untreated group showed loss of weight, thus showing that HJG successfully ameliorated diabetic oxidative stress (Table 24.2) and also significantly reduced the serum levels of glucose and glycosylated protein which were markedly elevated in rats with streptozotocin-induced diabetes (Figures 24.1a, b), while the serum creatinine level of groups given HJG were slightly lower than the control value. The elevated thiobarbituric acid (TBA)-reactive substance levels in serum and renal mitochondria of diabetic rats were markedly reduced by the administration of HJG, and a notable reduction was observed in the serum level from the lowest dose. From these results, it was supposed that HJG played a role in ameliorating glucose metabolism and attenuating oxidative stress under diabetes through scavenging free radicals and inhibiting lipid peroxidation, so it may be a beneficial therapy for pathological conditions associated with diabetic oxidative stress.

Which is the major contributor among the eight crude drugs comprising HJG?

It was previously discovered that HJG had effects on metabolic disorders, especially on advanced glycation end-product (AGE) formation and elevated oxidative stress in diabetic nephropathy (Nakagawa *et al.*, 2001) and that one of its constituent plants, Rehmanniae Radix extract, attenuated renal dysfunction in diabetic nephropathy, mainly because of its suppression of oxidative stress (Yokozawa *et al.*, 2004). However, further chemical characterisation of the other components is needed and morroniside, loganin and paeoniflorin were detected by HPLC as the major compounds in HJG, morroniside and loganin being found in Corni Fructus (CF)

Table 24.2 Effect of Hachimi-jio-gan on body weight changes in diabetes

Groups	Dose (mg/kg body weight/day)	Body weight Initial (g)	Final (g)	Gain (g/10 days)
Normal	—	220.8 ± 3.8*	284.4 ± 8.9*	63.6 ± 5.6*
Diabetes control	—	177.0 ± 3.1	205.4 ± 8.3	28.4 ± 6.1
Hachimi-jio-gan	50	172.7 ± 4.3	205.0 ± 8.3	28.8 ± 5.1
Hachimi-jio-gan	100	188.0 ± 2.4	213.8 ± 5.5	25.8 ± 4.8
Hachimi-jio-gan	200	178.3 ± 2.6	209.6 ± 6.1	31.3 ± 3.8

*$P<0.05$ compared with diabetic control rats.

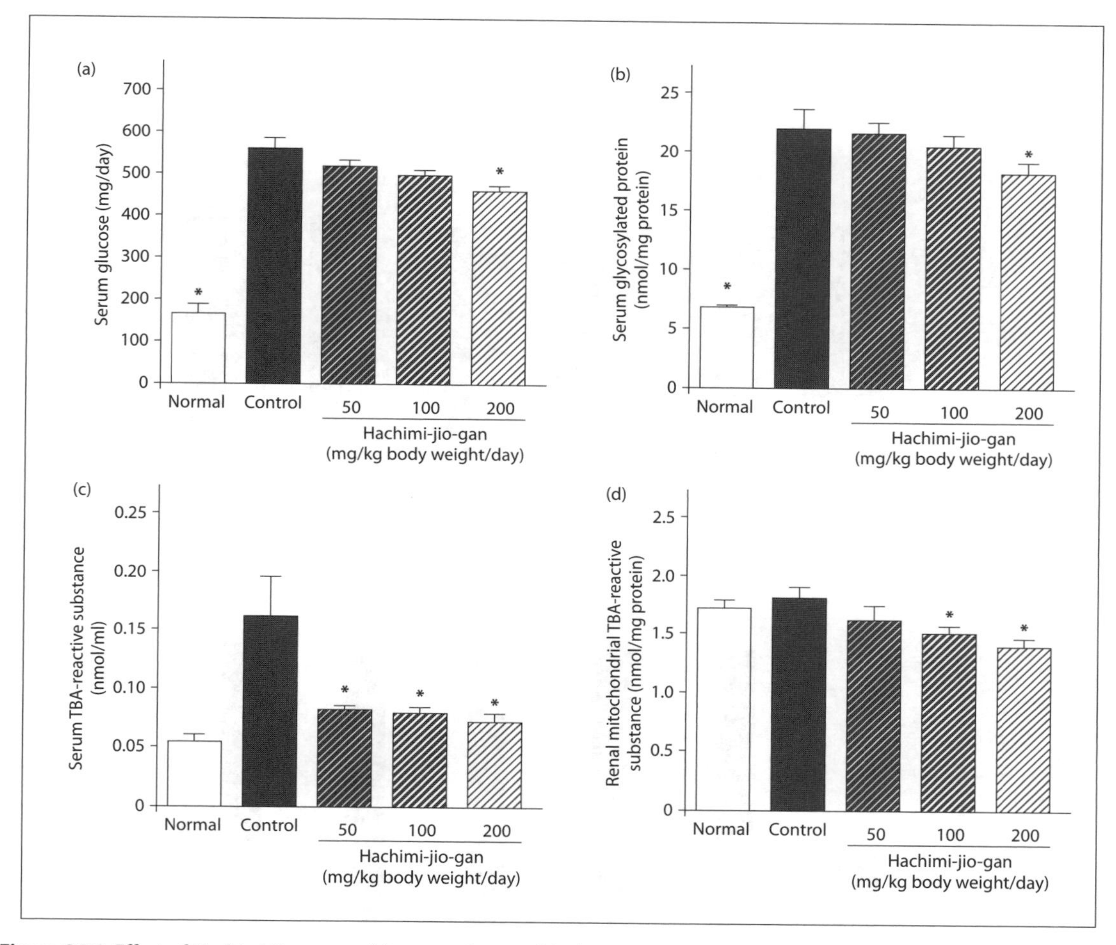

Figure 24.1 Effect of Hachimi-jio-gan on (a) serum glucose; (b) glycosylated protein; (c) TBA-reactive substance; and (d) renal mitochondrial TBA-reactive substance levels at 10 days. *$P < 0.05$ compared with diabetic control rats.

Table 24.3 Effect of Corni Fructus fractions on body weight changes, kidney weight, and food and water intake in diabetes

Groups	Body weight Initial (g)	Final (g)	Gain (g/10 days)	Kidney weight (mg/100 g BW)	Food intake (g/day)	Water intake (ml/day)
Normal	246.6 ± 4.3*	297.8 ± 7.1*	51.2 ± 4.4*	0.70 ± 0.02*	21.5 ± 1.3*	42.7 ± 3.8*
Diabetes control	199.0 ± 4.7	206.5 ± 6.0	11.4 ± 2.2	1.13 ± 0.02	30.0 ± 1.4	137.6 ± 3.1
S1D2 (20 mg/kg body weight/day)	199.3 ± 5.7	224.5 ± 7.3	17.5 ± 3.8	1.02 ± 0.03*	27.0 ± 0.9	120.9 ± 3.8*
S2 (20 mg/kg body weight/day)	197.9 ± 6.0	211.1 ± 10.3	14.3 ± 3.9	1.03 ± 0.03*	28.3 ± 1.5	125.7 ± 3.4*
S3 (20 mg/kg body weight/day)	197.6 ± 6.3	202.6 ± 9.3	5.0 ± 5.2	1.06 ± 0.02	28.5 ± 0.6	134.8 ± 6.7
S4 (20 mg/kg body weight/day)	197.5 ± 3.6	201.1 ± 6.8	3.6 ± 5.1	1.05 ± 0.03	29.6 ± 0.6	128.9 ± 6.3

*$P<0.05$ compared with diabetic control rats.

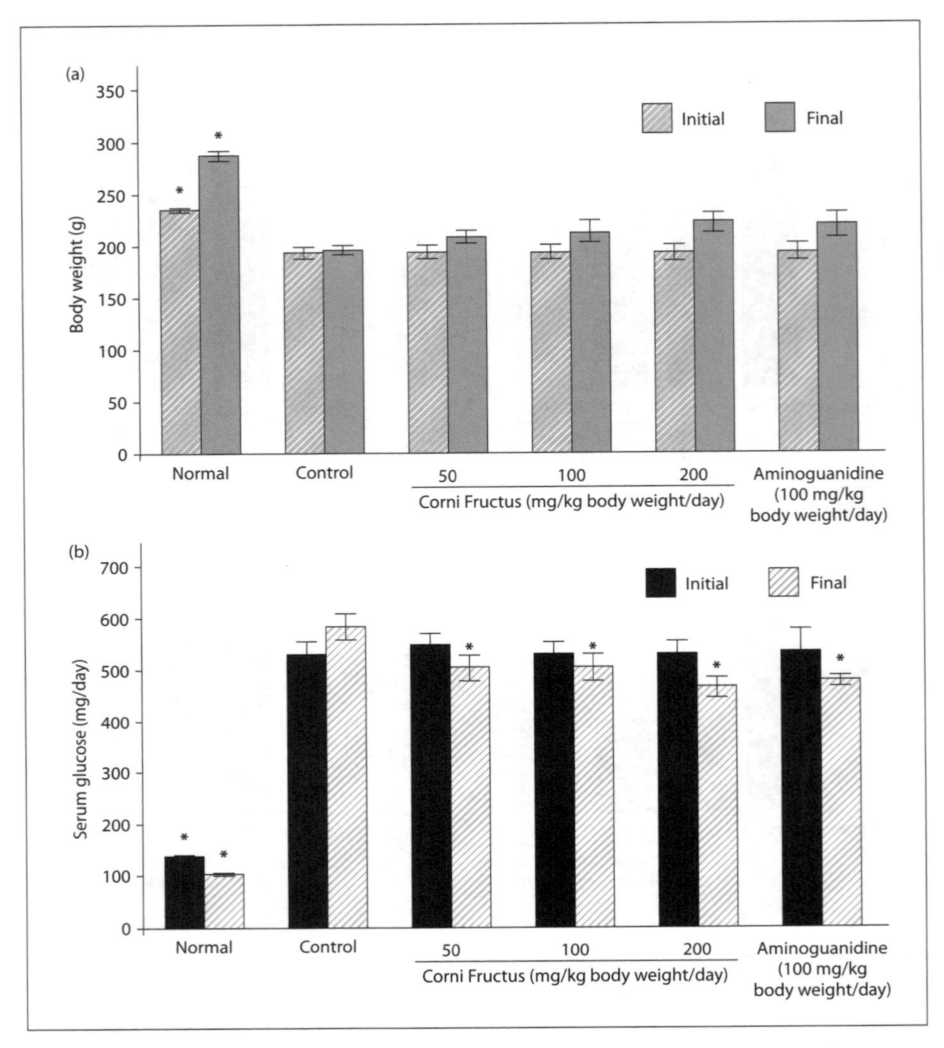

Figure 24.2 Effect of Corni Fructus and aminoguanidine on (a) body weight changes and (b) serum glucose levels in STZ-induced diabetic rats during the 10-day experimental period. *$P < 0.05$ compared with each value of diabetic control rats.

(Nakagawa *et al.*, 2001). Therefore, on the assumption that CF is a major contributor to the effects of HJG, the present study was carried out.

Efficacy of Corni Fructus and its fractions

A similar study to that performed for HJG in streptozotocin-induced diabetic rats was carried out for CF using doses of 50, 100, and 200 mg/kg body weight/day and comparing effects with those given by the inhibitor of AGE formation, aminoguanidine (100 mg/kg body weight/day) over 10 days. In addition, an iridoid and three polyphenol fractions, all shown to possess high ROS scavenging activity of CF were also tested.

The extract of CF dose-dependently increased the body weight and ameliorated hyperglycaemia (Figures 24.2a,b) as well as glucose-associated metabolic disorders in the serum and kidney, e.g. AGE levels (Figures 24.3a,c). The effects seen were similar to those of HJG. Some of the polyphenol fractions had greater hydroxyl radical scavenging activity than the iridoid (Figures 24.4a–c) and led to a decrease in body weight gain compared with the diabetic control value (Table 24.3), although these fractions significantly

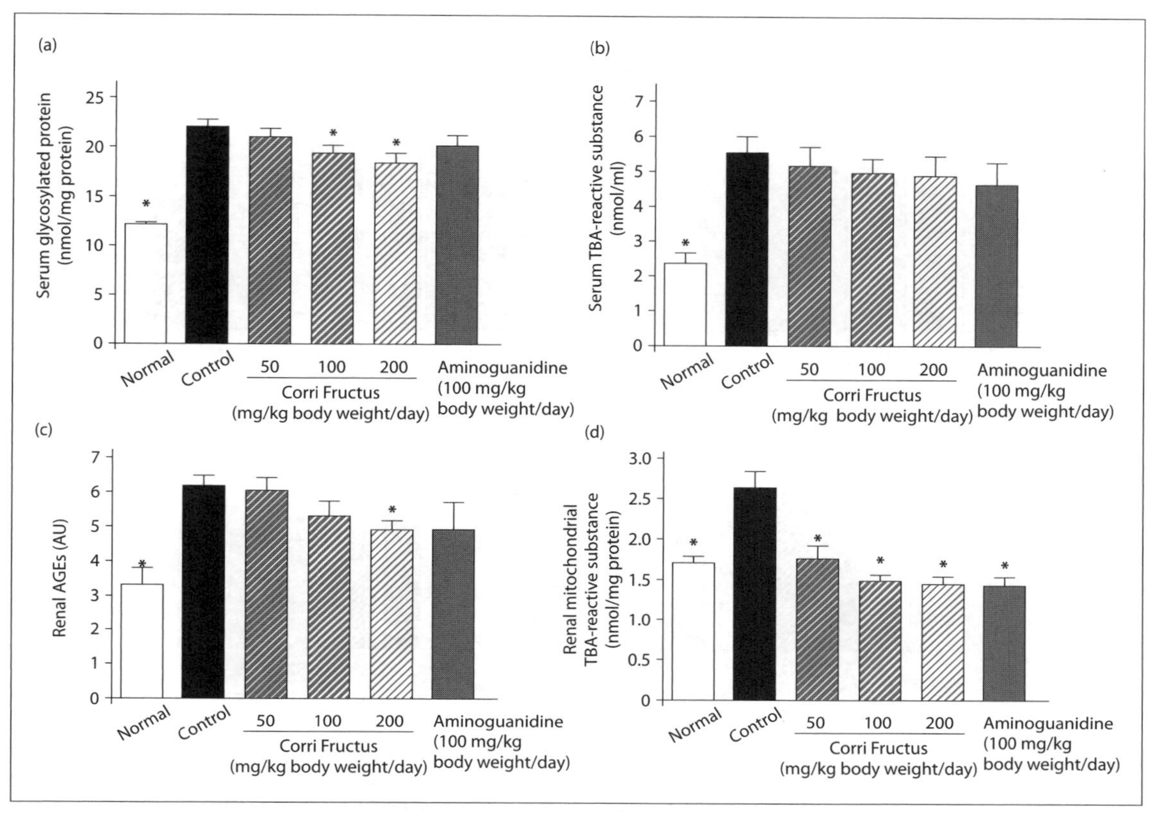

Figure 24.3 Effect of Corni Fructus and aminoguanidine on (a) serum glycosylated protein; (b) TBA-reactive substance; (c) renal AGE; and (d) mitochondrial TBA-reactive substance levels in STZ-induced diabetic rats at 10 days. *$P < 0.05$ compared with diabetic control rats.

inhibited the increase of serum and renal TBA-reactive substance levels (Figures 24.4c,e), suggesting that these two fractions may have radical scavenging activities but may include some toxic ingredients.

Increased oxidative stress also participates in renal structural changes, i.e. oxidative substances affect glomerular endothelial cells directly, infiltrating into the various parts of renal tissue, because of the abundant blood flow in the diabetic kidney. There is no doubt that microalbuminuria is an important indicator of the early stage of diabetic nephropathy because glomerular damage increases the albumin filtration rate, but proximal tubular reabsorption of this increased albumin is decreased via a decline in its endocytosis caused by a loss of megalin expression (Cui *et al.*, 1996). In the study on CF, diabetic rats also showed renal dysfunction, i.e. increased serum creatinine, urea nitrogen, and proteinuria and decreased creatinine levels, reflecting a decline in glomerular filtration rate. However, the rats given CF showed an up-regulated renal function and decreased uraemic toxin levels (Table 24.4), with certain antioxidative activities such as nitric oxide scavenging (Table 24.5). Aminoguanidine, the positive control, had almost the same effects as those of CF except concerning renal function, shown by the serum creatinine levels, and these differences might reflect AGE clearance. Aminoguanidine is reported to inhibit nitric oxide production and to trap reactive di-carbonyls, impeding conversion to AGEs, prevent cross-linking, and inhibit free-radical formation.

Therefore, it may be hypothesised that differences between CF and aminoguanidine are that CF can improve AGE clearance with an activated renal function, while aminoguanidine mainly inhibits AGE formation via its antioxidant properties. In addition,

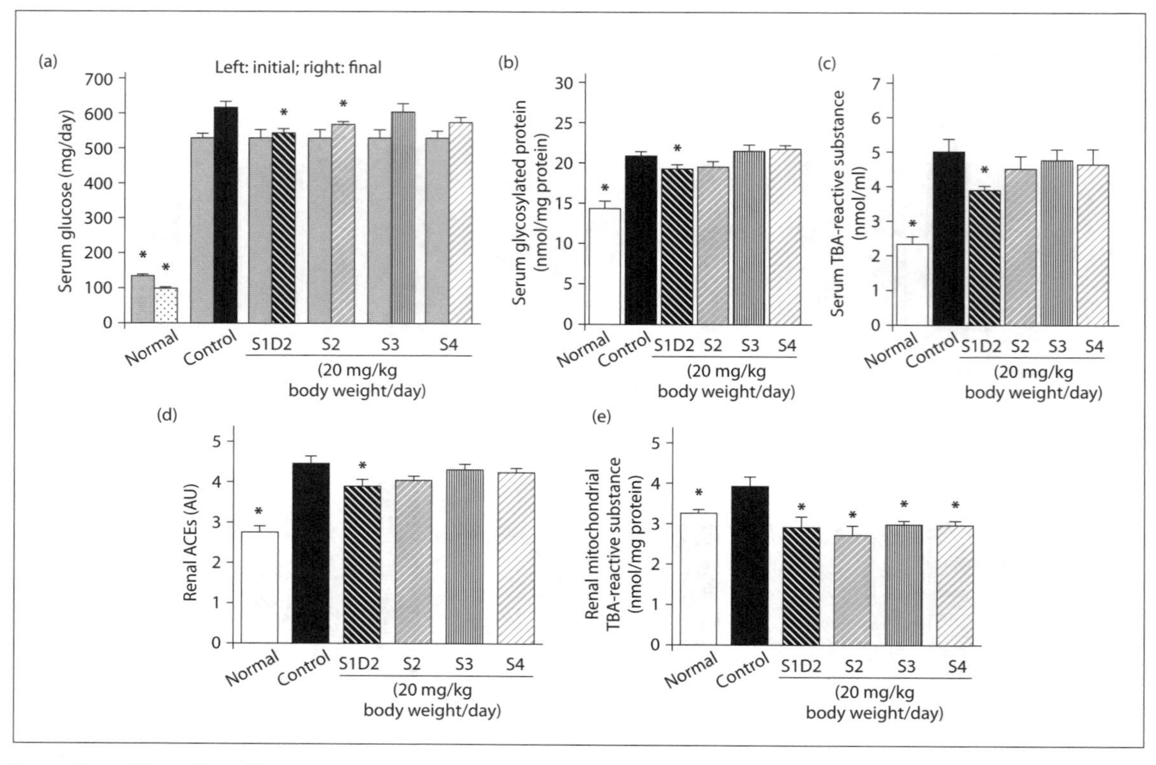

Figure 24.4 Effect of Corni Fructus fractions on (a) serum glucose; (b) glycosylated protein; (c) TBA-reactive substance; (d) renal AGE; and (e) mitochondrial TBA-reactive substance levels in STZ-induced diabetic rats at 10 days. *P < 0.05 compared with diabetic control rats.

similar results were observed with the treatment of two fractions of CF, S1D2 and S2, in terms of renal function parameters (Table 24.6).

These two fractions were identified as the compounds morroniside and 7-*O*-galloyl-D-sedoheptulose. The biological activities of morroniside have recently been studied (Xu and Hao, 2004; Xu *et al.*, 2004, 2006), which might be positively correlated with the activities of HJG. However, the biological activity 7-*O*-galloyl-D-sedoheptulose is as yet only poorly understood detected as a compound from Corni Fructus (Zhang *et al.*, 1999).

Table 24.4 Effect of Corni Fructus on renal function parameters in diabetes

Items	Normal	Diabetes control	Corni Fructus (50 kg/kg body weight/ day)	Corni Fructus (100 kg/kg body weight/ day)	Corni Fructus (200 kg/kg body weight/ day)	Aminoguanidine (100 kg/kg body weight/ day)
s-Urea nitrogen (mg/dl)	18.5±0.7*	33.6±2.1	27.8±1.5*	23.1±1.6*	20.9±1.1*	24.7±3.1*
s-Cr (mg/dl)	0.341±0.010*	0.404±0.021	0.348±0.012*	0.351±0.015*	0.338±0.017*	0.364±0.007
Ccr (ml/kg body weight/min)	7.68±0.14*	5.27±0.59	6.82±0.63*	7.47±0.48*	8.92±0.22*	5.73±1.28
Urine protein (mg/day)	13.3±0.9	16.8±2.2	12.5±3.1	12.1±2.7	10.3±0.9	9.7±1.1*

*P<0.05 compared with diabetic control rats.

Table 24.5 Antioxidative effects of Corni Fructus in diabetic serum

Groups	Nitrite/nitrate (μmol/L)	Inhibition of NBT reduction (% diabetic control)
Normal	15.7±1.9*	84.7±2.1
Diabetes control	32.6±5.7	100.0±5.7
Corni Fructus (50 mg/kg body weight/day)	26.4±7.4	97.5±2.1
Corni Fructus (100 mg/kg body weight/day)	19.0±3.4	93.7±1.0
Corni Fructus (200 mg/kg body weight/day)	10.5±0.5*	91.5±3.0
Aminoguanidine (100 mg/kg body weight/day)	8.3±0.3*	91.1±5.5

*$P<0.05$ compared with diabetic control rats.

Table 24.6 Effect of Corni Fructus fractions on renal function parameters in diabetes

Groups	s-Urea nitrogen (mg/dl)	s-Cr (mg/dl)	Ccr (ml/kg body weight/min)	Urinary protein (mg/day)
Normal	22.4±1.0*	0.369±0.004	7.75±0.07*	9.9±1.3
Diabetes				
Control	38.5±2.4	0.370±0.007	6.62±0.20	11.2±0.3
S1D2 (20 mg/kg body weight/day)	33.1±1.7	0.368±0.012	6.78±0.45	9.1±0.9
S2 (20 mg/kg body weight/day)	33.9±1.2	0.368±0.008	7.25±0.10*	9.3±0.6
S3 (20 mg/kg body weight/day)	36.8±2.1	0.369±0.009	6.68±0.25	11.8±0.9
S4 (20 mg/kg body weight/day)	34.9±3.8	0.371±0.018	6.68±0.35	9.8±0.5

*$P<0.05$ compared with diabetic control rats.

Table 24.7 Effect of Hachimi-jio-gan on body weight changes in diabetic nephropathy

Groups	Dose (mg/kg body weight/day)	Body weight Initial (g)	Final (g)	Gain (g/15 weeks)
Normal	—	292.0±6.6*	449.3±9.9*	157.3±4.4*
Diabetic nephropathy				
Control	—	263.8±6.4	303.5±9.8	39.9±7.4
Hachimi-jio-gan	50	259.2±6.4	301.4±11.9	42.9±6.3
Hachimi-jio-gan	100	260.4±8.4	305.1±14.2	44.3±10.6
Hachimi-jio-gan	200	259.3±6.0	305.9±10.0	46.1±8.5

*$P<0.05$ compared with diabetic nephropathy control rats.

Table 24.8 Effect of Hachimi-jio-gan on serum biochemical features in diabetic nephropathy

Items	Normal	Diabetic nephropathy control	Hachimi-jio-gan (50 mg/ kg body weight/ day)	Hachimi-jio-gan (100 mg/ kg body weight/ day)	Hachimi-jio-gan (200 mg/ kg body weight/ day)
Glycosylated protein (nmol/mg protein)	13.2±0.7*	25.8±1.4	24.1±0.8	20.6±1.3*	20.3±0.7*
Urea nitrogen (mg/dL)	20.7±0.5*	68.0±6.9	56.2±3.1	57.0±2.5	47.0±5.0*
Albumin (g/dL)	3.43±0.33*	2.31±0.08	2.45±0.10	2.45±0.09	2.63±0.04
TBA-reactive substance (nmol/mL)	2.44±0.47*	5.49±0.29	5.82±0.28	5.42±0.31	4.33±0.14*

*$P<0.05$ compared with diabetic nephropathy control rats.

Effect of HJG on type 1 diabetic nephropathy

Typical characteristics

Diabetic nephropathy is characterised as advanced kidney disease caused by longitudinal hyperglycaemia and its metabolic abnormalities. The study carried out involved long-term administration for 15 weeks, to show the effect of HJG on advanced kidney disease in diabetic nephropathy. Rats underwent subtotal nephrectomy and streptozotocin injection and showed metabolic abnormalities and renal lesions resembling diabetic nephropathy in humans (Yokozawa *et al.*, 2001b). The control rats, i.e. nephrectomised and treated with streptozotocin but not with extract, showed a decrease in body weight gain compared with normal rats, but the 15-week administration of HJG led to a slight increase in body weight gain, suggesting that there might be no or exceedingly little toxicity derived from long-term treatment with HJG (Table 24.7).

Over the experimental period, the serum glucose and urinary protein excretion levels were markedly higher in the rat model employed in this study than in normal rats (Figures 24.5a,b), indicating that disorders of glucose metabolism and changes in the capillary filtration barrier result in the increased permeability of the glomerular basement membrane (GBM). In addition, this rat model showed a significant decrease in creatinine clearance (Figure 24.5c), an effective index for expressing the glomerular filtration rate, which decreases exponentially until patients eventually develop nephritic syndrome (Bell, 1991). However, the present investigation demonstrated that the administration of HJG for 15 weeks reduced the serum glucose and urinary protein excretion levels, but increased creatinine clearance (Figure 24.6), suggesting that the good control of glucose metabolism has an important role in the prevention of diabetic complications, including diabetic nephropathy. In addition, the decreased serum albumin level in this animal model was reversed by the administration of HJG (Table 24.8). On the basis of these results, it was found that streptozotocin injection into subtotally nephrectomised rats resulted in progressive diabetic nephropathy but HJG prevented or delayed this.

Protein glycation reaction

Chronic hyperglycaemia results in irreversible tissue damage caused by the protein glycation reaction which leads to the formation of glycosylated proteins and AGEs, and stimulation of the polyol pathway (Cooper *et al.*, 1998; Yabe-Nishimura, 1998). The glycosylated serum protein level increased in the animal model used, implying that the oxidation of sugars was stimulated (see Table 24.8), enhancing

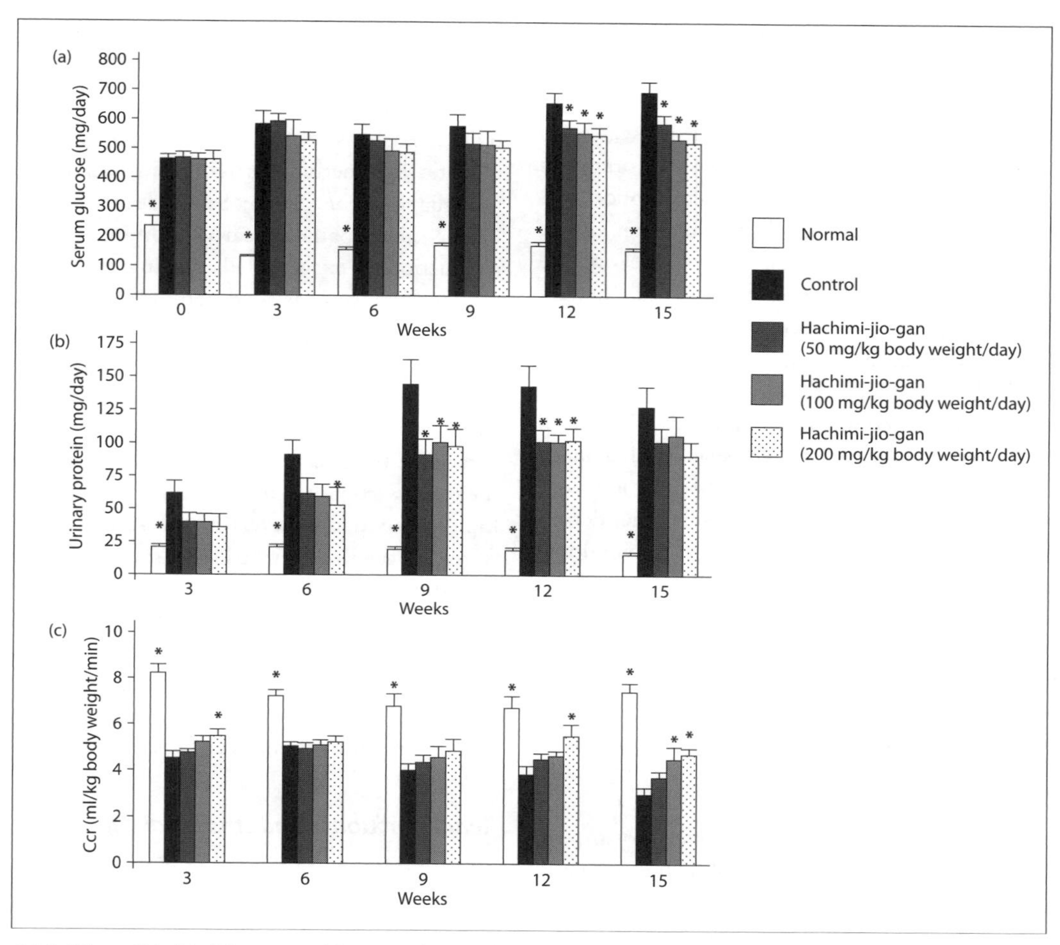

Figure 24.5 Effect of Hachimi-jio-gan on (a) serum glucose; (b) urinary protein; and (c) Ccr levels in experimental rats for 15 weeks. *$P < 0.05$ compared with each value of diabetic nephropathy control rats.

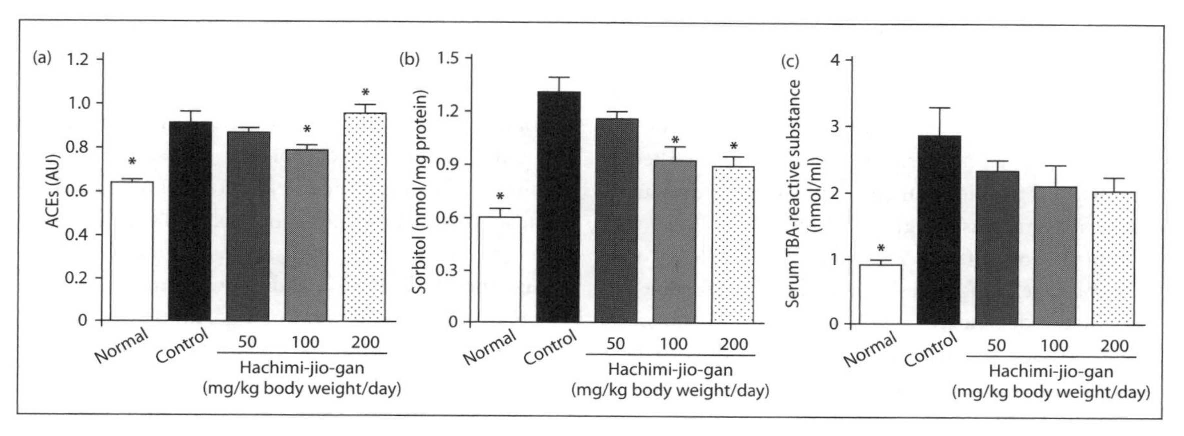

Figure 24.6 Effect of Hachimi-jio-gan on (a) renal AGE; (b) sorbitol; and (c) TBA-reactive substance levels at 15 weeks of the experimental period. *$P < 0.05$ compared with diabetic nephropathy control rats.

damage to both sugars and proteins in the circulation and vascular walls, continuing and reinforcing the cycle of oxidative stress and damage. In addition, accumulation of AGEs in the kidney was also observed (Figure 24.6a), and this excessive formation and accumulation can alter the structure and function of tissue proteins. In people with diabetes and/or chronic renal failure, AGEs accumulate in the kidney and are responsible for pathological changes (Vlassara *et al.*, 1994). AGEs also stimulate free-radical mechanisms and induce membrane peroxidation, which in turn increases membrane permeability. Therefore, AGE accumulation in the kidney has been regarded as an index of progressive renal damage associated with diabetic nephropathy and is recognised as playing a central role in various other degenerative processes, e.g. dialysis-related amyloidosis, and Alzheimer's disease (Niwa, 1997; Raj *et al.*, 2000). HJG reduced the levels of glycosylated serum proteins and AGEs significantly and dose-dependently (see Table 24.8 and Figure 24.6a), suggesting that it can inhibit oxidative damage and irreversible renal damage caused by protein glycation reactions.

Polyol pathway

In the polyol pathway, glucose is reduced to sorbitol by aldose reductase and sorbitol dehydrogenase. Increased polyol pathway activity results in the depletion of myoinositol and changes in the cellular redox potential, which has been proposed as a causative factor in the development of diabetic nephropathy. Moreover, it has been hypothesised that the glycation reaction leads to the production of AGEs by increasing the supply of fructose, which is a reactive glycation agent with stronger reducing activity than glucose (Goldfarb *et al.*, 1991; Hamada *et al.*, 1996; Cooper *et al.*, 1998). Our results showed that renal sorbitol levels were markedly elevated in rats with diabetic nephropathy compared with normal rats (Figure 24.6b). However, the administration of HJG significantly reduced the sorbitol level, suggesting that the disturbance of the glucose-dependent metabolic pathway, and irreversible tissue damage caused by such disturbance under conditions of diabetic nephropathy, would be ameliorated by decreasing the activity of the polyol pathway and inhibiting the protein glycation reaction.

Oxidative stress

The metabolic disorders associated with diabetic nephropathy induced lipid peroxidation caused by oxidative stress, which plays a potential role in diabetic glomerulosclerosis and renal fibrosis (Giugliano *et al.*, 1996; Salahudeen *et al.*, 1997). Under this pathological condition, free-radical production is exacerbated, leading to severe cytotoxic effects, such as lipid peroxidation and protein denaturation in cell membranes, followed by alterations in membrane receptors, fluidity, and properties. In the present study, the serum and renal TBA-reactive substance levels were measured to determine the effects of HJG on oxidative stress and the results are shown in Table 24.8 and Figure 24.6c. Lipid peroxidation levels in the serum and kidney were markedly elevated in rats with diabetic nephropathy compared with normal rats, while a 15-week course of HJG reduced these levels, suggesting that the administration of HJG would ameliorate the oxidative stress associated with diabetic nephropathy, and, thus improve the renal lesions caused by oxidative stress.

Renal functional and structural changes

The clinical manifestations of diabetic nephropathy, notably proteinuria, hypertension and renal insufficiency, are related to the severity of renal lesions (Winetz *et al.*, 1982; Adler, 1997). In the animal model used, the histopathological characteristics of diabetic nephropathy, glomerular sclerosis, and tubulointerstitial lesions were observed, especially the diffuse expansion of mesangial regions and basement membrane thickening of renal tubules. Recently, it has been suggested that diffuse mesangial expansion in the glomerulus plays a critical role in the obliteration of the capillary lumen, ultimately leading to the cessation of glomerular function. The greatly expanded mesangial matrix results in a reduction of the surface area available for filtration (Giugliano *et al.*, 1996), leading to the accumulation of urea nitrogen and creatinine in the serum, and a subsequent decrease in the creatinine clearance rate. The elevated serum urea nitrogen level was considered to be related to the renal lesions of glomerulosclerosis, while its reduction by HJG indicated amelioration of the renal lesions (Table 24.9 and

Figure 24.7). A substantial body of evidence suggests that progressive renal insufficiency is the ultimate expression of the pathological consequences of accumulating abnormalities of the glomerulus and tubulointerstitium (Winetz *et al.*, 1982; Yaqoob *et al.*, 1994; Adler, 1997). HJG had a significant protective effect against renal lesions (Table 24.9), suggesting that it would improve associated renal dysfunction. The results of the present study confirm that HJG has a protective effect in diabetic nephropathic rats through the amelioration of metabolic disorders, oxidative stress, and renal dysfunction associated with renal lesions.

Effect of HJG on type 2 diabetic pancreas

Glycaemic control

Otsuka Long-Evans Tokushima fatty (OLETF) rats were used as a model of human type 2 diabetes. HJG-treated groups did not show any differences in weight from untreated rats, but the serum glucose level in diabetic rats was reduced from the latter half of the administration period (Table 24.10). Oral administration of HJG could ameliorate these changes dose-dependently in insulin content and wet weight of the pancreas. Liou *et al.* (2002, 2004) reported that CF plays an important role in the

Table 24.9 Histopathological evaluation of the kidney

Items	Normal	Diabetic nephropathy control	Hachimi-jio-gan (50 mg/kg body weight/day)	Hachimi-jio-gan (100 mg/kg body weight/day)	Hachimi-jio-gan (200 mg/kg body weight/day)
Glomerular sclerosis	0*	2.88±0.87	1.38±0.18*	0.79±0.17*	0.43±0.24*
Tubulointerstitial changes	0*	2.88±0.13	2.25±0.25	2.33±0.21	2.29±0.18
Mesangial matrix expansion	0*	2.38±0.18	2.00±0.01	1.83±0.17*	1.43±0.20*
Arteriolar sclerosis	0*	2.13±0.23	2.00±0.27	1.50±0.22	1.43±0.20
Total	0*	11.82±2.66	7.38±0.69*	6.45±0.80*	5.58±1.04*

*$P<0.05$ compared with diabetic nephropathy control rats.

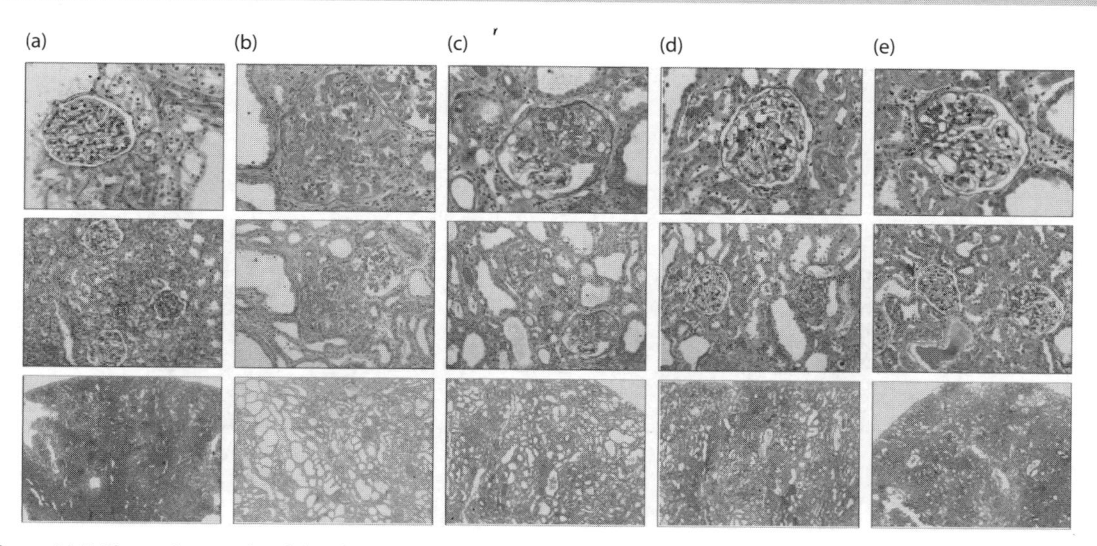

Figure 24.7 Photomicrographs of the glomeruli (upper panel, ×200), tubulus (middle panel, ×100), and interstitium (lower panel, ×20) obtained from (a) normal rats; (b) diabetic nephropathy rats in the control; and (c) Hachimi-jio-gan-treated (50 mg/kg body weight per day; (d) 100 mg/kg body weight per day; and (e) 200 mg/kg body weight per day) groups.

plasma glucose-lowering action associated with an increase in insulin secretion, via the release of acetylcholine from nerve terminals, which stimulates muscarinic cholinoceptors in the pancreatic islets. Taken together, HJG led to an increase in the pancreatic insulin level and might also stimulate insulin secretion, but the detailed mechanism requires further investigation.

Pancreatic fibrosis

An experiment was designed to elucidate the effect of HJG on the development of pancreatic fibrosis in relation with the effect on diabetic nephropathy. HJG was administered to rats from 32 weeks old to the age of 54 weeks old, HJG reduced the levels of TGF-β1 and fibronectin protein in the pancreas (Figure 24.8), and led to a reduction in pancreatic fibrosis via histological evaluation (Figure 24.9). Thus, these findings suggest that the hyperglycaemic control induced by HJG may, at least in part, be derived from the amelioration of pancreatic disorders such as pancreatic fibrosis.

Pancreatic oxidative stress

When they are exposed to oxidative stress, β-cells may be sensitive to ROS attack because they have a

Table 24.10 Effect of Hachimi-jio-gan on serum glucose levels during 32 weeks of administration

Groups	Serum glucose levels (mg/dL) Before	8 weeks	16 weeks	24 weeks	32 weeks
LETO					
Control	147.6±4.3*	142.3±4.4*	143.0±3.4*	143.3±4.7*	170.6±4.9*
OLETF					
Control	189.1±6.2	196.9±8.7	181.8±7.2	185.1±4.9	236.0±7.1
Hachimi-jio-gan (50 mg/kg)	188.6±8.6	187.8±7.5	178.9±10.9	174.6±3.1	229.0±9.7
Hachimi-jio-gan (100 mg/kg)	190.2±6.4	188.2±6.6	171.4±8.1	170.2±3.6*	227.5±6.8
Hachimi-jio-gan (200 mg/kg)	189.5±6.3	191.8±6.0	165.8±4.2	164.2±3.0*	216.6±5.2

*$P<0.05$ compared with each value of OLETF control rats.
LETO = Long-Evans Tokushima Otsuka rats; OLETF = Otsuka Long-Evans Tokushima Fatty rats.

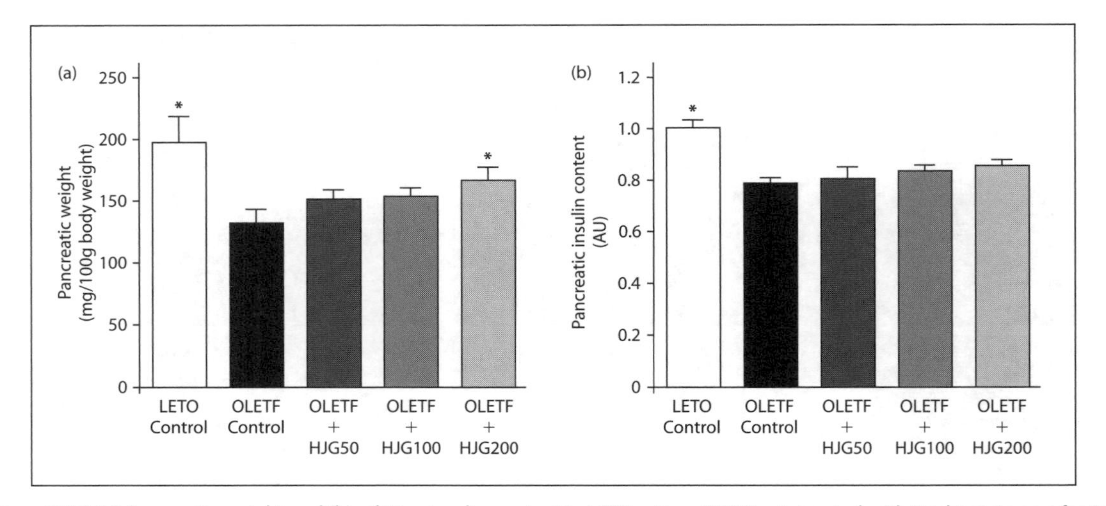

Figure 24.8 (a) Pancreatic weight and (b) relative insulin content in LETO rats or OLETF rats treated with Hachimi-jio-gan for 32 weeks. *$P < 0.05$ compared with the value of OLETF control rats. LETO = Long-Evans Tokushima Otsuka; OLETF = Otsuka Long-Evans Tokushima Fatty; HJG = Hachimi-jio-gan.

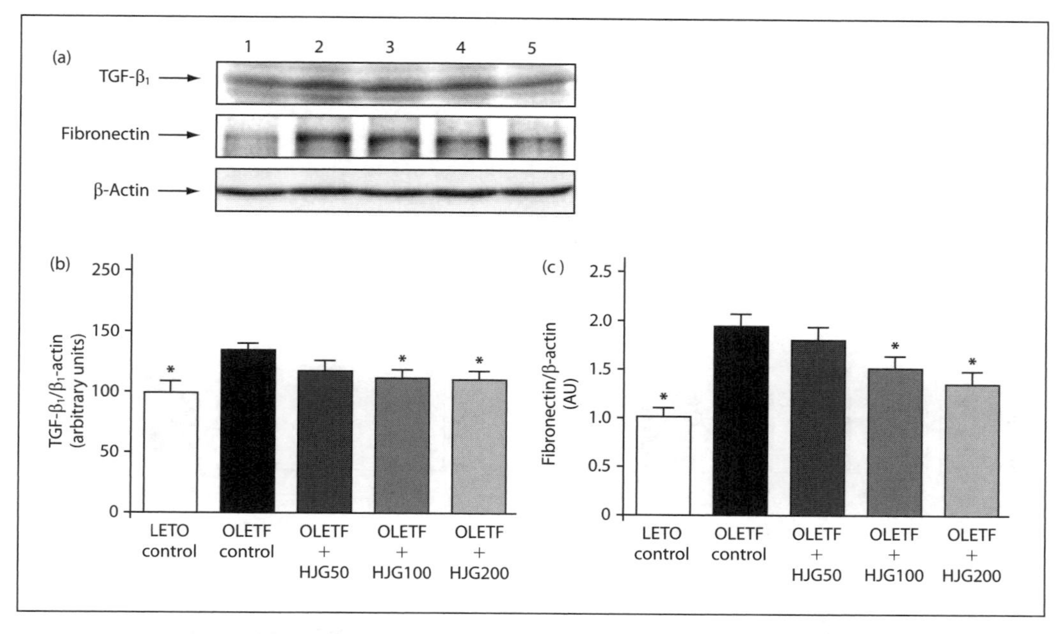

Figure 24.9 Effect of Hachimi-jio-gan on pancreatic protein expression-associated fibrosis. (a) Representative response of protein expression for TGF-β1, fibronectin, or β-actin in the pancreas isolated from LETO rats or OLETF rats treated with Hachimi-jio-gan for 32 weeks. Lane 1 = LETO control rats; lane 2 = untreated OLETF control rats; lanes 3, 4, and 5 Hachimi-jio-gan (50, 100, and 200 mg/kg, respectively)-treated OLETF rats. (b,c) Quantification of TGF-β1 and fibronectin protein levels by the ratio to β-actin; each column with a bar represents the mean plus SEM. *$P < 0.05$ compared with the values of OLETF control rats. LETO = Long-Evans Tokushima Otsuka; OLETF = Otsuka Long-Evans Tokushima Fatty; HJG = Hachimi-jio-gan.

poor antioxidative defence status compared with the liver and other tissues (Tiedge *et al.*, 1997). Eldor *et al.* (2006) reported that β-cell-specific activation of nuclear factor-kappa beta (NF-κB) is a key event in the progressive loss of β-cells in diabetes, and inhibition of the NF-κB pathway could be a potentially effective strategy for β-cell protection because it protects pancreatic β-cells from cytokine-induced apoptosis, while there are increased numbers of cytokine-sensitive genes including inducible nitric oxide synthase (iNOS) and cyclo-oxygenase-2 (COX-2), which possess binding sites for members of the NF-κB family of transcription factors; thus, it is likely that oxidative stress plays a major role in β-cell deterioration in type 2 diabetes.

Pancreatic NF-κB, inhibitor binding protein κB-α (IκB-α), iNOS, and COX-2 levels by western blot analyses were measured as indicators of oxidative stress. Total levels of pancreatic NF-κB and COX-2, except for iNOS, proteins in OLETF diabetic rats showed increases (Figure 24.10). However, oral administration of HJG reduced pancreatic NF-κB, iNOS, and COX-2 protein levels dose-dependently; and, in particular, HJG-treated rats showed a greater reduction in iNOS protein than LETO rats (Figure 24.10). It had been noted that islet-constitutive NOS activity, which is stimulated by the entry of extracellular Ca^{2+} into β-cells as well as the production of NADPH generated from glucose metabolism, appeared to be more rapidly adjusted to the glucose concentration than iNOS activity, which suggested the independence of cytokine action (Zawalich and Rasmussen, 1990; Henningsson *et al.*, 2002). However, iNOS is known to produce nitric oxide which inhibits glucose-stimulated insulin release from the pancreas. Although the intimate mechanisms behind glucose-stimulated iNOS activity and expression are presently unclear, the present data showed no increase in iNOS in OLETF control rats compared with LETO control rats, and so

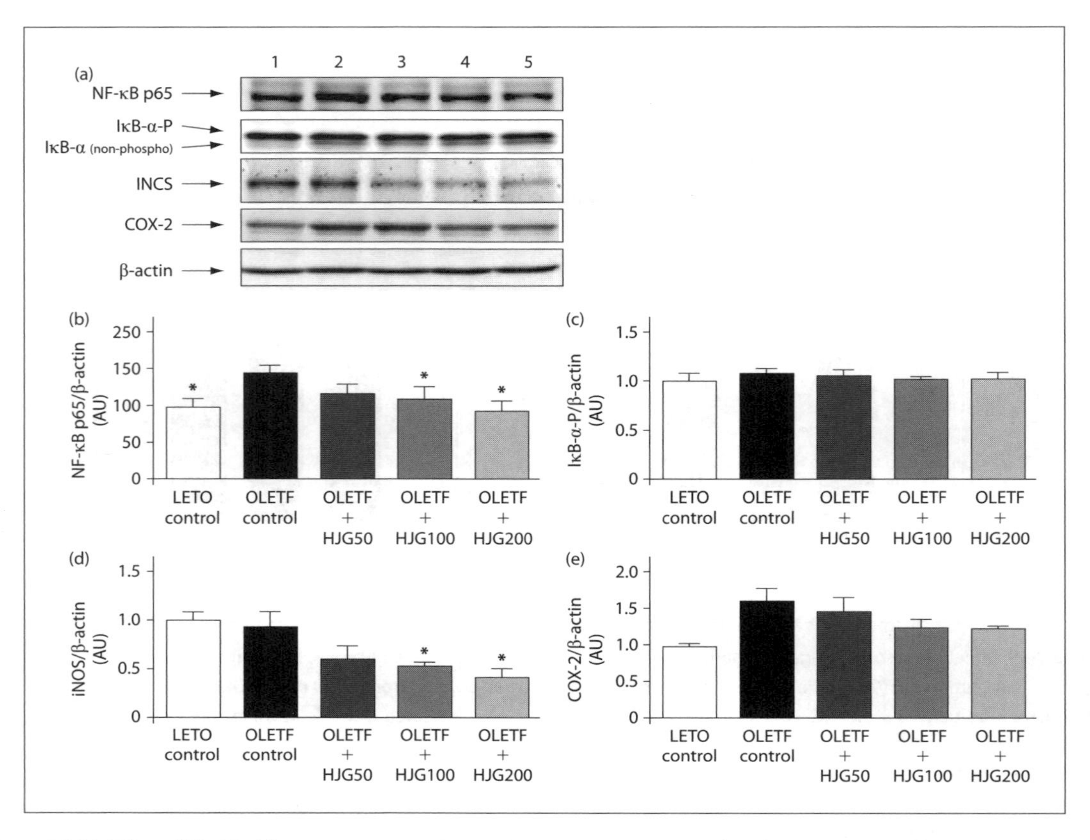

Figure 24.10 Effect of Hachimi-jio-gan on pancreatic protein expression-associated oxidative stress. (a) The representative response of protein expression for NF-κB p65, phosphorylated and non-phosphorylated IκB-α, iNOS, COX-2, or β-actin in the pancreas isolated from LETO rats or OLETF rats treated with Hachimi-jio-gan for 32 weeks. Lane 1 = LETO control rats; lane 2 = untreated OLETF control rats; lanes 3, 4, and 5 = Hachimi-jio-gan (50, 100, and 200 mg/kg, respectively)-treated OLETF rats. (b–e) Quantification of NF-κB p65, phosphorylated IκB-α, iNOS, and COX-2 protein levels by the ratio to β-actin; each column with a bar represents the mean plus SEM. *$P < 0.05$ compared with the value of OLETF control rats. LETO = Long-Evans Tokushima Otsuka; OLETF = Otsuka Long-Evans Tokushima Fatty; HJG = Hachimi-jio-gan.

we hypothesised that HJG would stimulate pancreatic insulin secretion via the inhibition of iNOS expression.

Conclusions

Oxidative stress is an important factor in many common and life-threatening human diseases because ROS-mediated tissue injury is regarded as a common pathway for a number of diseases. We investigated whether HJG could ameliorate advanced kidney disease in type 1 diabetic nephropathy and pancreatic fibrosis, and oxidative damage in type 2 diabetes. The results indicated that Hachimi-jio-gan could have a protective role in diabetic renal and pancreatic damage caused by oxidative stress. Morroniside and 7-O-galloyl-D-sedoheptulose in Corni Fructus were suggested to be important contributors to the effect of HJG against diabetic oxidative damage. However, it was discovered that some of the powerful antioxidant fractions might participate in the toxicity. Needless to say, herbal medicine would make full use of the efficacy of each crude drug synergistically to cure diseases and, this study on HJG provides novel information on bioactive ingredients of this herbal product.

References

Adler S (1997). Structure-function relationships in diabetic nephropathy: Lessons and limitations. *Kidney Int* 60: S42–S45.

Bell DS (1991). Diabetic nephropathy: Changing concepts of pathogenesis and treatment. *Am J Med Sci* 301: 195–200.

Brownlee M, Vlassara H, Cerami A (1984). Non-enzymatic glycosylation and the pathogenesis of diabetic complications. *Ann Intern Med* 101: 527–537.

Cooper ME, Gilbert RE, Epstein M (1998). Pathophysiology of diabetic nephropathy. *Metabolism* 47 (supp. 1): 3–6.

Cui S, Verroust PJ, Moestrup SK, Christensen EI (1996). Megalin/gp330 mediates uptake of albumin renal proximal tubule. *Am J Physiol* 271: F900–F907.

El-Naggar LJ, Beal JL (1980). Iridoids, a review. *J Nat Prod* 43: 649–707.

Eldor R, Yeffet A, Baum K *et al.* (2006). Conditional and specific NF-κB blockade protects pancreatic beta cells from diabetogenic agents. *Proc Natl Acad Sci USA* 103: 5072–5077.

Fan C, Xiang QY (2001). Phylogenetic relationships within Cornus (Cornaceae) based on 26S rDNA sequences. *Am J Bot* 88: 1131–1138.

Fialkow L, Wang Y, Downey GP (2007). Reactive oxygen and nitrogen species as signaling molecules regulating neutrophil function. *Free Rad Biol Med* 42: 153–164.

Furuya Y, Kawakita T, Tajima S (1999). Effect of Hachimi-jio-gan (Ba-Wei-Di-Huang-Wan) on insulin resistance in non-insulin dependent diabetes mellitus model mice. *J Trad Med* 16: 123–128.

Garcia J, Chulia AJ (1986). Loganin and new iridoid glucosides in *Gentiana pedicellata*. *Planta Med* 4: 327–329.

Giugliano D, Ceriello A, Paolisso G (1996). Oxidative stress and diabetic vascular complications. *Diabetes Care* 19: 257–267.

Goldfarb S, Ziyadeh FN, Kern EF, Simmons DA (1991). Effects of polyol-pathway inhibition and dietary myo-inositol on glomerular hemodynamic function in experimental diabetes mellitus in rats. *Diabetes* 40: 465–471.

Goto M, Inoue H, Seyama Y *et al.* (1989). Comparative effects of traditional Chinese medicines (dai-saiko-to, hatimi-zio-gan and byakko-ka-ninzin-to) on experimental diabetes and hyperlipidemia. *Nippon Yakugaku Zasshi* 93: 179–186.

Hamada Y, Araki N, Koh N *et al.* (1996). Rapid formation of advanced glycation end products by intermediate metabolites of glycolytic pathway and polyol pathway. *Biochem Biophys Res Commun* 228: 539–543.

Hatano T, Ogawa N, Kira R *et al.* (1989). Tannins of cornaceous plants. I. Cornusiins A, B and C, dimeric monomeric and trimeric hydrolyzable tannins from *Cornus officinalis*, and orientation of valoneoyl group in related tannins. *Chem Pharm Bull* 37: 2083–2090.

Henningsson R, Salehi A, Lundquist I (2002). Role of nitric oxide synthase isoforms in glucose-stimulated insulin release. *Am J Physiol* 283: C296–C304.

Inouye H, Tobita S, Akiyama Y *et al.* (1973). The monoterpene glucosides and related natural substances. XXI: The stereochemistry of morroniside and its derivatives. *Chem Pharm Bull* 21: 846–854.

Kaneto H, Xu G, Song KH *et al.* (2001). Activation of the hexosamine pathway leads to deterioration of pancreatic β-cell function through the induction of oxidative stress. *J Biol Chem* 276: 31099–31104.

LeRoith D (2002). β-Cell dysfunction and insulin resistance in type 2 diabetes: role of metabolic and genetic abnormalities. *Am J Med* 113: 3S–11S.

Liou SS, Liu IM, Hsu SF *et al.* (2004). Corni Fructus as the major herb of Die-Huang-Wan for lowering plasma glucose in Wistar rats. *J Pharm Pharmacol* 56: 1443–1447.

Liou SS, Liu IM, Hsu JH *et al.* (2002). Release of acetylcholine by Die-Huang-Wan to enhance insulin secretion for lowering plasma glucose in Wistar rats. *Auton Neurosci* 100: 21–26.

Liu ZL, Slininger PJ, Dien BS *et al.* (2004). Adaptive response of yeasts to furfural and 5-hydromethylfurfural and new chemical evidence for HMF conversion to 2,5-bis-hydromethylfuran. *J Indian Microbiol Biotechnol* 31: 345–352.

Moran A, Zhang HJ, Olson LK *et al.* (1997). Differentiation of glucose toxicity from beta cell exhaustion during the evolution of defective insulin gene expression in the pancreatic islet cell line, HIT-T15. *J Clin Invest* 99: 534–539.

Nakagawa T, Yokozawa T, Terasawa K (2001). A study of Kampo medicines in a diabetic nephropathy model. *J Trad Med* 18: 161–168.

Nishikawa T, Edelstein D, Du DL *et al.* (2000). Normalizing mitochondrial superoxide production blocks three pathways of hyperglycemic damage. *Nature* 404: 787–790.

Niwa T (1997). β2-Microglobulin dialysis amyloid and its formation: Role of 3-deoxyglucosone and advanced glycation end products. *Nephron* 76: 373–391.

Njoroge FG, Monnier VM (1989). The chemistry of the Maillard reaction under physiological conditions: a review. *Prog Clin Biol Res* 304: 85–107.

Otsuka H, Kijima K (2001). An iridoid gentiobioside, a benzophenone glucoside and acylated flavone C-glycosides from *Triterospermum japonicum* (Sieb. et Zucc.) Maxim. *Chem Pharm Bull* 49: 699–702.

Rahbar S, Figarola JL (2003). Novel inhibitors of advanced glycation endproducts. *Arch Biochem Biophys* 419: 63–79.

Raj DSC, Choudhury D, Welbourne TC, Levi M (2000). Advanced glycation end products: A neurologist's perspective. *Am J Kidney Dis* 35: 365–380.

Salahudeen AK, Kanji V, Reckelhoff JF, Schmidt AM (1997). Pathogenesis of diabetic nephropathy: A radical approach. *Nephrol Dial Transplant* 12: 664–668.

The Diabetes Control Complications Trial Research Group (1993). The effect of intensive treatment of diabetes on the development and progression of long-term complications in insulin-dependent diabetes mellitus. *N Engl J Med* 329: 977–986.

Tiedge M, Lortz S, Drinkgern J, Lenzen S (1997). Relation between antioxidant enzyme gene expression and antioxidative defense status of insulin-producing cells. *Diabetes* 46: 1733–1742.

Tikellis C, Cooper ME, Thomas MC (2006). Role of rennin-angiotensin system in the endocrine pancreas: Implications for the development of diabetes. *Int J Biochem Cell Biol* 38: 737–751.

Tschesche R, Struckmeyer K, Wulff G (1971). Glycoside with lactone forming aglycones. IV. Mevaloside, the glucoside of (-) (R) mevalonic acid lactone from the leaves of the medlar and a simple preparation of (-) (R)-mevalonic acid lactone. *Chem Ber* 104: 3567–3572.

Vareed SK, Reddy MK, Schutzki RE, Nair MG (2006). Anthocyanins in *Cornus alternifolia*, *Cornus controversa*, *Cornus kousa* and *Cornus florida* fruits with health benefits. *Life Sci* 78: 777–784.

Vlassara H, Striker LJ, Teichberg S, Fuh H, Li YM, Steffes M (1994). Advanced glycation end products induce glomerular sclerosis and albuminuria in normal rats. *Proc Natl Acad Sci USA* 91: 11704–11708.

Winetz JA, Golbetz HV, Spencer RJ, Lee JA, Myers BD (1982). Glomerular function in advanced human diabetic nephropathy. *Kidney Int* 21: 750–756.

Xu HQ, Hao HP (2004). Effects of iridoid total glycoside from *Cornus officinalis* on prevention of glomerular overexpression of transforming growth factor beta 1 and matrixes in an experimental diabetes model. *Biol Pharm Bill* 27: 1014–1018.

Xu HQ, Hao HP, Zhang X, Pan Y (2004). Morroniside protects cultured human umbilical vein endothelial cells from damage by high ambient glucose. *Acta Pharmacol Sci* 25: 412–415.

Xu HQ, Shen J, Liu H, Shi Y, Li L, Wei M (2006). Morroniside and liganin extracted from *Cornus officinalis* have protective effects on rat mesangial cell proliferation exposed to advanced glycation end products by preventing oxidative stress. *Can J Physiol Pharmacol* 84: 1267–1273.

Yabe-Nishimura C (1998). Aldose reductase in glucose toxicity: A potential target for the prevention of diabetic complications. *Pharmacol Rev* 50: 21–33.

Yamada T (1992). *Kinki Yoryaku*. Kyouwa-Kikaku, Tokyo, pp. 1–7.

Yaqoob M, McClelland P, Patrick AW *et al.* (1994). Evidence of oxidative injury and tubular damage in early diabetic nephropathy. *Q J Med* 87: 601–607.

Yokozawa T, Dong E, Oura H, Kashiwagi H, Nonaka G, Nishioka I (1997). Magnesium lithospermate B suppresses the increase of active oxygen in rats after subtotal nephrectomy. *Nephron* 75: 88–93.

Yokozawa T, Kim HY, Yamabe N (2004). Amelioration of diabetic nephropathy by dried Rehmanniae Radix (Di Huang) extract. *Am J Chin Med* 32: 829–839.

Yokozawa T, Nakagawa T, Terasawa K (2001a). Effects of Oriental medicines on the production of advanced glycation end products. *J Trad Med* 18: 107–112.

Yokozawa T, Nakagawa T, Wakaki K, Koizumi F (2001b). Animal model of diabetic nephropathy. *Exp Toxic Pathol* 53: 359–363.

Zawalich WS, Rasmussen H (1990). Control of insulin secretion: a model involving Ca^2, cAMP and diacylglycerol. *Mol Cell Endocrinol* 70: 119–137.

Zhang Y, Chen Y, Zhao S (1999). A sedoheptulose gallate from the fruits of *Cornus officinalis*. *Acta Pharm Sin* 34: 153–155.

Part 3

Product development

25

Essential oils in the treatment of skin diseases: aspects of efficacy and toxicology

Lara O Orafidiya

Introduction

Essential oils, also referred to as volatile or ethereal oils, are highly volatile substances secreted in oil cells, glandular hairs or in secretion ducts or cavities of odoriferous plants. They have been in use since antiquity, having been employed as food and drink flavours, perfumes, deodorants, disinfectants, embalming antiseptics and medicines. Scientifically obtained evidence on the important biological activities of many essential oils has lent credence to their traditional and folkloric application in therapeutics. Intense scientific research efforts have also led to a tremendous increase in the number and types of essential oils as well as their potential uses and applications. In addition, modern distillation technology has resulted in the establishment of international markets and industries. As such, essential oils can now be regarded as industrial raw materials. However, only few products containing essential oils as active therapeutic agents are available in the market. This is because most current research efforts are focused on assaying the biological activity of both old and newly discovered essential oils and only a few attempts have been made at determining the effective concentration/dose of essential oils with proven activity as well as carrying out clinical trials to determine their efficacy and safety for human use.

The formulation of essential oils into dosage forms demands additional considerations compared with conventional orthodox medicinal agents. Essential oils are multi-chemical in their composition with only a few of the constituents being responsible for the desired biological effects, although the presence of other constituents may enhance activity. Hence, factors that affect the efficacy of the active compounds are critical in the choice of dosage forms and excipients employed in formulation. For some essential oils, the active constituents are highly volatile compounds, requiring controlled procedures for incorporation of the oils into preparations so as to ensure efficacy of the products. While the unoxidised constituents are the active compounds in some essential oils, products of oxidation reaction of some constituents are toxic. Hence, the inclusion of antioxidants in essential oil-containing products is inevitable.

Essential oils were earlier used without much consideration for possible toxic or untoward effects on the users. However, recent research efforts into some of the commonly used essential oils, including perfumes, have revealed toxic potentials that have resulted in the control of their use by appropriate regulatory bodies. While the concentrations of essential oils permissible in certain preparations have been pegged, the inclusion of some essential oils, such as peppermint oil, in oral preparations is being discouraged. The toxicity of some of these essential oils has been traced to one or two of their constituents, the permissible concentrations of which are specified for the oils to be included in products. Essential oils have also been shown to cause sensitisation as well as phototoxicity which, hitherto, could not have been traced to them. Some observed reactions are due to indirect contact with the offending oils through inhalation or even skin contact with the oil vapour dispersed in the environment. The toxicity of some essential oils has been traced to poor storage by consumers leading to oxidation of some of the constituents; the reaction products of which elicit toxic or allergenic effects. Extensive toxicity studies are, therefore, still desirable for essential oils with potential therapeutic and other applications to be fully utilised as medicinal or chemical agents.

Essential oils as remedies for skin diseases

The earliest applications of essential oils in home remedies as well as in alternative and complementary medicines have been for the treatment of skin disorders. Many essential oils have demonstrated antibacterial, antifungal, wound-healing, antiparasitic, antiprotozoal antiviral, anti-inflammatory, hair-growth stimulating and insect-repellent properties (Hammer *et al.*, 1999; Oyedele *et al.*, 2000; Oladimeji *et al.*, 2000; Orafidiya *et al.*, 2003, 2004a). However, their efficacies at concentrations at which they can be used on humans without eliciting side-effects are mostly still being studied.

Many essential oils have demonstrated considerable broad-spectrum, antimicrobial activity comparable with existing antimicrobial agents. The essential oil obtained from the leaves and terminal branches of *Melaleuca alternifolia* (Maiden and Betche) Cheel (tea tree oil) was about the first to be subjected to antimicrobial screening. Penfold and Grant (1925) had rated the oil and some of its components such as cineole, cymene, linalool and terpinen-4-ol up to 16 times more active than phenol. Tea tree oil has remarkable activity against skin-infecting bacteria such as commensal skin staphylococci and micrococci as well as *Pseudomonas aeruginosa*. Tea tree oil also reduces skin carriage of meticillin-resistant *Staph. aureus* (MRSA). Clinical trial studies on the efficacy of tea tree oil in handwashes for hospital and healthcare settings have confirmed the antiseptic properties of the oil, with its aroma enhancing users' compliance (Messager *et al.*, 2005).

Baiju and Modax (2007) recently studied the antimicrobial activity of combinations of low concentrations of nine essential oils with fruit acids (citric and lactic acids). Although the test oils showed synergistic effects with citric acid, cinnamon leaf (*Cinnamomum zeylanicum* Blume) and citronella leaf (*Cymbopogon nardus* L.) essential oils exhibited superior activity against *Escherichia coli*, MRSA and *Pseudomonas aeruginosa* but only cinnamon oil exhibited high activity against *Candida albicans*. A hand soap containing a synergistic combination of cinnamon oil and citric acid was formulated and found to be significantly more effective than triclosan (a standard disinfectant) soap. The authors concluded that skin and surface cleansers containing cinnamon oil and citric acid in combination might provide rapid and broad-spectrum activity.

Acne vulgaris (acne) is caused by blockage, inflammation and subsequent bacterial colonisation of the pilosebaceous follicles of the face and upper trunk. In-vitro susceptibility studies on the essential oils of citronella grass (*Cymbopogon nardus* L.), lemongrass (*Cymbopogon citratus* [DC. ex Nees] Otto Stapf), kaffir lime (*Citrus hystrix* DC), holy basil (*Ocimum sanctum* L.), sweet basil (*Ocimum basilicum* L.), plai (*Zingiber cassumunar* Roxb.) and ginger (*Zingiber officinale* Roscoe) against *Propionibacterium acnes* (*P. acnes*) showed citronella grass oil as the most effective in inhibiting the growth of the microorganism. In addition, holy basil, plai and citronella oils demonstrated appreciable anti-inflammatory activity that could help to relieve acne blemishes (Lertsatitthanakorn *et al.*, 2006). Ocimum oil (from the leaves of *Ocimum gratissimum* L.), at 2%, reduced acne lesions faster in subjects than 10% benzoyl peroxide and 1% clindamycin standard products, while the activity of the oil lotion was greatly enhanced in combination with aloe vera gel (Orafidiya *et al.*, 2002, 2004b). On the other hand, 5% tea tree oil was less effective in reducing lesions than 5% benzoyl peroxide, although like the ocimum oil preparations, it was better tolerated than the benzoyl peroxide product (Bassett *et al.*, 1990). However, Biju *et al.* (2005) have observed the effect of pH on the anti-bacterial activity of tea tree oil against *P. acne, Staph. aureus* and *Staph. epidermidis.* Formulations containing 5% tea tree oil exhibited maximum effect at pH 5.5.

Microbial colonisation of wounds retards healing. Ocimum oil at 2% v/v has demonstrated marked antimicrobial activity against *Staph. aureus, P. aeruginosa* and *Proteus* spp. isolated from wounds and boils on human subjects, and *Trichophyton mentagrophytes* isolated from wounds on rabbits. Studies in rabbits showed that wounds colonised by *S. aureus* and *T. mentagrophytes,* previously treated with 0.5% cetrimide cream, did not heal until the 2% ocimum oil preparation, to which the microbes were susceptible, was applied (Orafidiya *et al.*, 2003). Apart from antimicrobial effects, the wound-healing property of ocimum oil has been attributed to accelerated scab formation, wound contraction and granulation, and early onset of epithelialisation in rabbits (Orafidiya *et al.*, 2003). However, in pigs, whose skin physiology is similar to that of humans, ocimum oil reduced wound contraction, but remarkably accentuated re-epithelialisation with the formation of epithelial pegs, conditions that may result in less scarification and may be useful in the management of keloids (Adesina, 2005). Another factor that may contribute to the wound-healing property of ocimum oil is its ability to increase cutaneous capillary permeability (Orafidiya *et al.*, 2005). Anecdotally, some essential oils are used to reduce malodour from infected cancerous wounds in palliative care (Warnke *et al.*, 2005).

Essential oils that have demonstrated considerable fungitoxicity against dermatophyte strains that cause *Tinea pedis* include those of *Melaleuca alternifolia* (Maiden and Betche) Cheel, *Thymus pulegioides* L., *Eucalyptus pauciflora* Sieber ex Spreng, *Cymbopogon citratus* (DC ex Nees) Otto Stapf, *Chenopodium ambrosioides* L., *Artemisia nilagirica* (Clarke) Pamp., *Mentha arvensis* L., *Ocimum gratissimum* L. *and Caesulia axillaries* Roxb. (Kishore *et al.*, 1993). These essential oils, along with others such as that of *Santolina chamaecyparissus* L., are equally effective against *Candida* species that cause cutaneous mycoses; while tea tree oil may also be effective in the treatment of mild-to-moderate dandruff, a condition attributed to the yeast *Pityrosporium ovale*. The fungicidal activity of essential oils against *Trichophyton mentagrophytes* and *T. rubrum* has been shown to be enhanced by heat and sodium chloride. The effect was attributed to increase in mycelial adsorption of antifungal constituents of the essential oils in the presence of sodium chloride while hyphal damage by the oils occurred at 27°C (Inouye *et al.*, 2007). The authors concluded that thermotherapy in combination with essential oils and sodium chloride might be effective in the treatment of *Tinea pedis* in a foot bath.

Shahi *et al.* (2000) observed that the essential oil of *Eucalyptus pauciflora* Sieber ex Spreng showed strong activity against *Epidermophyton floccosum, Microsporum audouinii, M. canis, M. gypseum, M. nanum, Trichophyton mentagrophytes, T. rubrum, T. tonsurans and T. violacea*, all of which are human pathogenic fungi. A 1% ointment formulation of the oil was tested on patients presenting with either *Tinea pedis, T. corporis* or *T. cruris*. At the end of the treatment period, 60% of the patients recovered fully with no relapse 2 months after, while 40% showed significant improvement from the disease. The authors proposed to carry out multicentre clinical trials of the ointment to exploit its commercialisation. Inouye *et al.* (2006) studied the vapour activity of 72 essential oils against *T. mentagrophytes*. The oils exhibited potent vapour activity depending on their major components of phenols > aldehydes > alcohols > ketones > esters > ethers/oxides. Hydrocarbon-rich oils had the weakest activity. A similar pattern of activity was observed when the constituents were tested separately. In general, the antimicrobial activity of most essential oils has been attributed to a variety of monoterpene or phenolic constituents, e.g. linalool, thymol, carvacrol, terpinen-4-ol, terpineol, eugenol, α-pinene, Δ-3-carene and nerolidol (Tyler *et al.*, 1981).

Studies, including clinical trials, have proved the toxicity of some essential oils and pure constituents to the ova, larva and adults of human ectoparasites indicating prospects of their application as anti-parasitic agents. The utilisation of essential oils as antiparasitic agents may overcome the problem of resistance exhibited by parasites to products currently in use. Essential oils that have shown prospects as pediculocides/ovicides include cinnamon bark (*Cinnamomum zeylanicum* Blume), lippia (*Lippia multiflora* Moldenke) and tea tree oils. The vapour phases of these oils have demonstrated higher activity than by direct contact of the oils on the lice, implying that the highly volatile constituents of the oils have stronger pediculocidal activity (Oladimeji *et al.*, 2000, 2005; Yang *et al.*, 2005).

Lippia oil was observed to be more highly effective than Delvap Super (a brand of dichlorvos) concentrate against body lice (*Pediculus humani corporis*) and head lice (*Pediculus humani capitis*). While a 10% solution of lippia oil in liquid paraffin exhibited similar activity as the Delvap Super® concentrate, dilutions of the latter were relatively inactive (Oladimeji *et al.*, 2000). Priestley *et al.* (2006) have reported (+)-terpinen-4-ol as being the most effective against body lice of a series of essential oil constituents studied.

Nerolidol, another essential oil constituent, was highly lethal to eggs of the lice but was ineffective against adult lice. Terpineol and α-pinene kill body lice (Weston *et al.*, 1997) while α- and β-pinene are known insecticides (Windholz, 1983). Lippia oil contains terpineol (2.9%), α-pinene (1%) and β-pinene (4%) which in part, may be responsible for its strong pediculocidal activity (Oladimeji *et al.*, 2000). Walton *et al.* (2004) found 5% tea tree oil highly more effective, killing mites in a shorter time than conventional drugs used in the treatment of scabies. Terpinen-4-ol, a constituent of the oil, at the concentration (2.1%) at which it is present in 5% tea tree oil was also effective though to a lesser extent than the whole oil. In a clinical trial study, Lippia oil (*Lippia multiflora* Moldenke) at 20% as an emulsion was more effective than 25% benzyl benzoate emulsion on human subjects suffering from scabies. The preparations, however, needed to be applied consecutively for 5 days to achieve complete cure (Oladimeji *et al.*, 2000). The antimicrobial activity of these two essential oils on microorganisms that cause secondary infections in scabies is an added advantage (Oladimeji *et al.*, 2004).

Leishmania amazonensis, a protozoon that causes cutaneous diseases, is susceptible to essential oils such as the eugenol chemotype ocimum oil, linalool-rich croton (*Croton cajucara* Benth.) oil and chenopodium (*Chenopodium ambrosioides* L.) oil as well as to pure eugenol (do Socorro *et al.*, 2003; Monzote *et al.*, 2006; Ueda-Nakamura *et al.*, 2006). Tea tree and eucalyptus oils have anti-viral activity against the herpes simplex virus while some essential oils are used anecdotally to clear plantar warts (Forbes and Schmid, 2006). Koch *et al.* (2008) studied the in-vitro antiviral activity of some essential oils against herpes simplex virus type 2 (HSV-2) as well as their mode of inhibitory effect. The essential oils, which included hyssop (*Hyssopus officinalis* L.), thyme (*Thymus vulgaris* L.), ginger (*Zingiber officinale* Roscoe) and chamomile (*Matricaria recutita* L.) oils, were virucidal and they affected HSV-2 mainly before adsorption to cells possibly by interacting with the viral envelope. Chamomile oil was highly effective and demonstrated prospects of a potential topical therapeutic virucidal agent for the treatment of herpes genitalis (Koch *et al.*, 2007). Burke *et al.* (2004) reported that a once-daily topical application of a 10% solution of Australian lemon myrtle (*Backhousia citriodora* F. Muell.) essential oil remarkably reduced lesions in children suffering from *Molluscum contagiosum*, which is a common viral illness of childhood.

Menthol, a constituent of some essential oils, is used in certain hair products as a hair growth stimulator. Although this compound is not a constituent of ocimum oil, the oil has been observed to stimulate hair growth on shaved animals and humans, and to prevent damage to hair and other skin structures caused by the administration of cyclophosphamide, a cancer chemotherapeutic agent (Orafidiya *et al.*, 2003, 2004a, 2004b). Essential oils such as thyme (*Thymus vulgaris* L.), rosemary (*Rosmarinus officinalis* L.), lavender (*Lavandula angustifolia* Mill.) and cedar wood (*Juniperus virginiana* L.), when used alone, mixed or in conjunction with electromagnetic pulses, have demonstrated the ability to improve alopecia (Bureau *et al.*, 2003).

Systemic studies on the anti-inflammatory activity of many essential oils have demonstrated their high potential as anti-inflammatory agents. However, there is still a paucity of studies on the anti-inflammatory activity of essential oils on the skin. Koh *et al.* (2002) reported that neat tea tree oil reduced mean wheal volume but not mean flare area when topically applied on histamine-induced wheal and flare. The oil also reduced erythema and flare caused by nickel-induced contact hypersensitivity in humans. Studies revealed terpinen-4-ol, but not 1,8-cineole or α-terpineol, as modulating the vasodilation and plasma extravasation associated with histamine-induced inflammation in humans (Khalil *et al.*, 2004). The leaf essential oil of *Lippia sidoides* Cham. exhibited anti-inflammatory properties by significantly reducing ear oedema induced by 12-otetradecanylphorbol 13-acetate (TPA) in mice (Monteiro *et al.*, 2007).

Topical application of products with insect repellent activity is one way of controlling the spread of parasitic diseases for which such insects are vectors. Ocimum oil at 20% is repellent for at least 2 h against blackflies that spread onchocerciasis; and the mosquitoes that spread malaria, filariasis, yellow fever, dengue and mosquito-borne encephalitides (Oyedele *et al.*, 2000; Usip *et al.*, 2006). Vanillin (10%) has been shown to significantly increase the mosquito repellency of the essential oil of *Zanthoxylum piperitum* (L.) DC (Choochote *et al.*, 2007). Gillij *et al.* (2008) while studying the mosquito repellency of some essential oils have suggested limonene and camphor as constituents that might be responsible for the repellent effects.

Toxicity of essential oils

Toxic manifestations of essential oils may be in the form of damage to internal organs and tissues or externally as allergic reactions, sensitisation or phototoxicity. The manifestation of systemic toxicity may not be due to direct oral administration of the causative essential oil, but may occur from inhalation of the vapour during topical application or through percutaneous absorption in topical preparations. Pulmonary and percutaneous absorption of limonene from sweet orange oil, cold expressed from *Citrus aurantium* var. *sinensis* L., Osbeck ex. Brazil, was reported to have occurred during aromatherapy by Fewel *et al.* (2007). In the pilot study, limonene was detected in blood within 10 minutes of commencing massage. Hayes and Markovic (2003) studied the percutaneous absorption of lemon myrtle (*Backhousia citriodora* F. Muell.) essential oil. Citral, consisting of isomers geranial and neral, was the only component of the oil that was found to have been absorbed through the skin throughout the 12-hour duration of the experiment. A formulated product of the oil also demonstrated absorption of citral only but elicited lesser damage to epidermal cells than the neat oil. Darben *et al.* (1998) reported a case of systemic eucalyptus oil toxicity following extensive application of a home remedy containing the oil on the body of a 6-year-old girl while treating urticaria. The girl presented with slurred speech, ataxia and muscle weakness progressing to unconsciousness. This toxicity would have arisen from percutaneous and possible nasal absorption of the toxic components of the eucalyptus oil. Gynaecomastia has been observed in three prepubertal boys using topical products that contained lavender and tea tree oils. The condition resolved shortly after the use of the products was discontinued. Studies carried out using human cells showed that the two oils had oestrogenic and antiandrogenic activities suggesting that lavender and tea tree oils might be responsible for the gynaecomastia observed in the boys (Henley *et al.*, 2007).

Orafidiya *et al.* (2004a) observed that ocimum oil demonstrated, in rats, the ability to prevent damage to hair and other skin structures caused by cyclophosphamide at skin sites other than where it was applied. The oil also enhanced hair growth at shaved sites on which it was not directly applied, implying percutaneous absorption of the oil into the circulatory system. Studies on the acute and subchronic toxicity of ocimum oil revealed a dose-dependent weakness, susceptibility to fatigue, sedative and sleep-inducing effects, suggesting that ocimum oil could have sedative and central nervous system depressant activities. Significant increases in the weights of the liver and brain were also observed (Orafidiya *et al.*, 2004c). These effects could be expected to also manifest through extensive topical use of ocimum oil. Weyers and Brodbeck (1989) have shown that 1,8-cineole, the principal component of eucalyptus oil, was bioavailable after topical application. The extent of percutaneous absorption was enhanced by the use of an occlusive dressing. However, topical application of eucalyptus oil preparations, when properly used, is well tolerated on the skin (Willms *et al.*, 2005). Peppermint oil (*Mentha piperita* L.) is absorbed through the skin just as it is absorbed in the gastrointestinal tract. Menthol, a constituent of peppermint oil has demonstrated skin-enhancing penetration of other agents (Nair, 2001).

There are many reports of adverse reactions to topically applied essential oils. The effects range from burning sensation to contact dermatitis. The European Council (2003), in the amendment to the European Cosmetics Directive, listed 26 fragrance ingredients whose concentrations in finished cosmetic products should not exceed 0.01% for leave-on products. Included in the lists are cinnamyl alcohol, citral, eugenol, geraniol, linalool, limonene, citronellol and farnesol.

Lavender oil is regarded as one of the mildest essential oils and it is mainly used as a perfume in cosmetics. In-vitro studies using endothelial cells and fibroblasts revealed that this oil is cytotoxic to human skin cells (Prashar *et al.*, 2004). The oil consists mainly of linalyl acetate (51%) and linalool (35%). When tested in their pure forms, linalool's activity was the same as that of the whole oil, while linalyl acetate demonstrated a cytotoxicity that was higher than that of the neat oil, suggesting that some components of lavender oil suppress activity of linalyl acetate in the whole oil. When lavender oil was applied directly to human skin in a skin patch test, contact allergy was observed. In this study, which was carried out over a period of 9 years, an increase in the number of subjects reacting positively to lavender oil was observed when the use of dried lavender flowers in pillows, drawers, cabinets or rooms became a new fashion in Japan (Sugiura *et al.*, 2000). The authors concluded that the increase in sensitivity to lavender oil was due to its aromatherapy administration rather than to the oil in cosmetic products. The sesquiterpene lactones, costunolide and dehydrocostuslactone, have been identified as the haptens responsible for the allergic contact dermatitis caused by costus (*Saussurea lappa* C.) essential oil which is used in perfumery. Cheminat *et al.* (1981) were able to remove these lactones from the oil by binding them to a polymer, aminoethyl-polystyrene. Tests carried out on guinea pigs showed that the animals could be sensitised to the untreated oil but not to the polymer-treated oil. Hence, the polymer could be used to render essential oils non-allergenic.

Tea tree oil causes low allergic contact dermatitis (Fritz *et al.*, 2001). Khanna *et al.* (2000) reported erythema multiform-like reaction that is secondary to allergic contact dermatitis caused by tea tree oil. Subsequent to this, adverse reactions such as linear immunoglobulin A disease and systemic hypersensitivity reactions were reported (Perrett *et al.*, 2003; Crawford *et al.*, 2004). Mozelsio *et al.* (2003) have reported the case of an immediate systemic hypersensitivity reaction in a 38-year-old man after topical application of tea tree oil. The man experienced immediate flushing, pruritus, throat constriction and light-headedness. High concentrations of tea tree oil, applied to the round winder of the ear for a relatively short time could be ototoxic to the high-frequency region of the cochlea (Zhang and Robertson, 2000). High doses of tea tree oil used in the treatment of dermatological conditions in dogs and cats resulted in depression, weakness, incoordination and muscle tremors (Villar *et al.*, 1994).

Peppermint oil is currently used in cosmetic formulations as a fragrance since its use as a flavouring agent is being discouraged. The oil has been found to be non-toxic, non-carcinogenic and to produce minimal skin reactions. However, pulegone, one of its constituents, is toxic and its safe concentration in the peppermint oil has been limited to $\leq 1\%$. This level could be achieved by controlling the time of harvest of the plant and the processing technique for the oil distillation (Nair, 2001).

There are some allergenic substances that do not elicit any obvious reaction at first exposure but would have sensitised the individual such that subsequent exposures manifest allergic reactions. As an example, the case of a patient with recurring eczema that was resistant to therapy was traced to her previous exposure to some essential oils (lavender, jasmine, etc.), which she had used for over a year in aroma lamps in her home and whose odours persisted even after she had discontinued the therapy. This can be regarded as a case of delayed manifestation of allergic reaction or sensitisation. For this patient, complete renewal of the interior of her flat was considered essential to the management of the allergy (Schaller and Korting, 1995).

In a study carried out by Rubel *et al.* (1998), volunteers who initially tested negative to patch testing of tea tree oil reacted strongly to subsequent applications of preparations containing the sesquiterpenoid fractions of the oil. Aromatherapists are highly susceptible to allergic reactions as they are exposed to a wide variety of essential oils, either directly on the hands while massaging or indirectly through inhalation of vapours of the oils. They are, therefore, more exposed to cross sensitisation from multiple essential oils. Bleasel *et al.* (2002) have reported the case of three aromatherapists and one chemist with interest in aromatherapy, who apart from presenting with hand dermatitis, also exhibited sensitisation to multiple essential oils. Workers exposed to essential oils in factories and plantation fields are equally susceptible to sensitisation effects. The allergic contact dermatitis experienced by myoga (*Zingiber mioga* [Thunb.] Roscoe) cultivators in Japan has been attributed mainly to R-(+)-limonene, one of its volatile constituents, while limonene oxide was found to be a much stronger skin sensitiser than myoga itself (Wei *et al.*, 2006). The main causes of allergic contact dermatitis observed among the staff of a perfume factory were two perfume oils and geraniol, benzaldehyde, cinnamic aldehyde, linalool, neroli oil, terpenes of lemon oil and orange oil which are ingredients of the perfumes (Schubert, 2006). Friedrich *et al.* (2007) assessed the sensitisation potential of 10 monoterpenes found in essential oils using rat popliteal lymph node assay (PLNA). The monoterpenes: citral, α-terpinene, β-myrcene, (−)-α-pinene, (−)-menthol, 1,8-cineole, (±) citronellal, (+)-limonene, (±) camphor and terpineol, however, proved to be non-sensitising.

Phototoxicity is a skin reaction caused by concurrent topical or systemic exposure to a susceptible substance and ultraviolet radiation or direct sunlight. The furocoumarin derivatives found in lemon oil (*Citrus limonum* Risso) and bitter-orange oil (*Citrus aurantium* L.), in particular oxypeucedanin and bergapten, are known to cause phototoxicity. Oxypeucedanin elicited photopigmentation on guinea pig skin without a preceding visible erythema (Naganuma *et al.*, 1985) while phototoxicity occurred in a subject who had applied bergamot (*Citrus bergamia* Risso et Poit.) oil on the body and had a session in a solarium (Weisenseel and Woitalla, 2005).

Poorly stored or oxidised essential oils have caused more allergic symptoms than fresh oil samples. They are also implicated in sensitisation and phototoxicity. The allergic reactions to oils rich in terpenes obtained from citrus (*Citrus* spp.), pine (*Pinus sylvestris* L.), juniper (*Juniperus communis* L.), black pepper (*Piper nigrum* L.), among others, have been attributed to the hydroperoxides found during storage. The peroxides, epoxides and endoperoxides, for example ascaridol and 1,2,4-trihydroxymenthane, formed during oxidation of tea tree oil were 3 times stronger in causing skin hypersensitivity than the fresh oil (Hausen *et al.*, 1999; Khanna *et al.*, 2000; Fritz *et al.*, 2001). Ascaridol was found for the first time in tea tree oil in the oxidised samples which were kept in open and closed bottles placed on window sills. Poor storage of the oil by consumers was considered responsible for the development of allergic contact dermatitis seen in persons self-treating with tea tree oil. Orange peel oil was previously thought to be carcinogenic because of D-limonene. However, studies have shown that oxidised compounds derived from D-limonene and other terpenes induced cancer (Homburger and Boger, 1968; Elegbede *et al.*, 1986). D-Limonene, on the other hand, is a chemopreventive agent against mammary, liver, lung and ultraviolet-induced skin cancer (Crowell, 1997; Brudnak, 2006).

A mild burning sensation whose intensity reduced with continuous application of 5% ocimum oil preparation was reported by subjects who were involved in the clinical trials for acne management (Orafidiya *et al.*, 2002). However, when the neat oil was applied directly on shaved skin of rats, the skin wrinkled extensively, giving an appearance of burns, and was subsequently shed. Neat ocimum oil also caused hardening of the skin of rabbits (Orafidiya *et al.*, 2004a).

Concurrent administration of essential oils with other drug substances may modify the therapeutic outcomes of the latter as some essential oils have been shown to affect the activity of human cytochrome P450 enzymes, which are major drug-metabolising enzymes in man. Chamomile (*Matricaria recutita* L.) essential oil has inhibited CYP1A2, CYP3A4, CYP2C9 and CYP2D6 to varying extents.

Chamazulene, *cis*-spiroether and *trans*-spiroether, constituents of the oil, were observed to be potent inhibitors of CYP1A2 (Ganzera *et al.*, 2006). Safrole caused potent competitive inhibition of CYP1A2 activity and non-competitive inhibition of CYP2A6 and CYP2E1 activities (Ueng *et al.*, 2005).

Conclusions

Essential oils have found application in the management and treatment of many skin disorders. However, for these potential therapeutic agents to be used as pharmaceutical preparations, more research efforts are required in the area of their formulation, clinical trials and toxicity studies.

References

Adesina SK (2005). *Effect of Formulation Variables on the Wound Healing Properties of the Leaf Essential Oil of* Ocimum Gratissimum *Linn. Lamiaceae*. PhD thesis. Department of Pharmaceutics, Obafemi Awolowo University, Ile-Ife, Nigeria.

Baiju N, Modak SM (2007). Broad-spectrum disinfectant composition containing a synergistic combination of cinnamon oil and citric acid. *Int J Essential Oil Ther* 1: 117–121.

Bassett IB, Pannowitz DL, Barnetson RS (1990). A comparative study of tea tree oil versus benzoyl peroxide in the treatment of acne. *Med J Aust* 153: 455–458.

Biju SS, Ahuja A, Khar RK, Chaudhry R (2005). Formulation and evaluation of an effective pH balanced topical antimicrobial product containing tea tree oil. *Pharmazie* 60(3): 208–211.

Bleasel N, Tate B, Rademaker M (2002). Allergic contact dermatitis following exposure to essential oils. *Aust J Dermatol* 43(3): 211–213.

Brudnak M (2006). Cancer-preventing properties of essential oil monoterpenes D-limonene and perilly alcohol. www.positivehealth.com/permit/Articles/cancer/bruds5 3.htm (accessed 20 Mar 2006).

Bureau JP, Ginouves P, Guilbaud J, Roux ME (2003). Essential oils and low-intensity electromagnetic pulses in the treatment of androgen-dependent alopecia. *Adv Ther* 20 (4): 220–229.

Burke BE, Baillie JE, Olson RD (2004). Essential oil of Australian lemon myrtle (*Backhousia citriodora*) in the treatment of *Molluscum contagiosum* in children. *Biomed Pharmacother* 58(4): 245–247.

Cheminat A, Stampf LL, Benezra C *et al.* (1981). Allergic contact dermatitis to costus: removal of haptens with polymers. *Acta Derm Venereol* 61(6): 525–529.

Choochote W, Chaithong U, Kamsuk K *et al.* (2007). Repellent activity of selected essential oils against *Aedes aegypti. Fitoterapia* 78(5): 259–364.

Crawford GH, Sciacca JR, James WD (2004). Tea tree oil: cutaneous effects of the extracted oil of *Melaleuca alternifolia. Dermatitis* 15(2): 59–66.

Crowell PL, (1997). Monoterpenes in breast cancer chemoprevention. *Breast Cancer Res Treatment* 46: 191–197.

Darben T, Cominos B, Lee CT, (1998). Topical eucalyptus oil poisoning. Australas *J Dermatol* 39(4): 265–267.

Elegbede JA, Maltzman TH, Verma AK *et al.* (1986). Mouse skin tumour promoting activity of orange peel oil and D-limonene: a re-evaluation. *Carcinogenesis* 7(12): 2047–2049.

European Council (2003). Amendment to the European Cosmetics Directive. *Offic J Eur Union* L66, 11 Mar, 26–35.

Fewell F, McVicar A, Gransby R, Morgan P (2007). Blood concentration and uptake of D-limonene during aromatherapy massage with sweet orange oil. A pilot study. *Int J Essential Oil Ther* 1: 97–102.

Forbes MA, Schmid MM (2006). Use of OTC essential oils to clear plantar warts. *Nurse Pract* 31(3): 53–55, 57.

Friedrich K, Delgado IF, Santos LMF *et al.* (2007). Assessment of sensitization potential of monoterpenes using the rat popliteal lymph node assay. *Food Chem Toxicol* 45(8): 1516–1522.

Fritz TM, Burg G, Krasovec M (2001). Allergic contact dermatitis to cosmetics containing *Melaleuca alternifolia* (tea tree oil). *Ann Dermatol Venereol* 128 (2): 123–126.

Ganzera M, Schneider P, Stuppner H (2006). Inhibitory effects of the essential oil of chamomile (*Matricaria recutita* L.) and its major constituents on human cytochrome P450 enzymes. *Life Sci* 78(8): 856–861.

Gillij YG, Gleiser RM, Zygadlo JA (2008). Mosquito repellent activity of essential oils of aromatic plants growing in Argentina. *Bioresource Technol* 99(7): 2507–2515.

Hammer KA, Carson CF, Riley TV (1999). Antimicrobial activity of essential oils and plant extracts. *J Appl Microbiol* 86: 985–990.

Hausen B, Reichling J, Harkenthal M (1999). Degradation products of monotopenes are the sensitizing agents in tea tree oil. *Am J Contact Derm* 10: 68–72.

Hayes AJ, Markovic B (2003). Toxicity of Australian essential oil *Backhousia citriodora* (lemon myrtle). Part 2. Absorption and histopathology following application to human skin. *Food Chem Toxicol* 10: 1409–1416.

Henley DV, Lipson N, Korach KS, Bloch CA (2007). Prepubertal gynecomastia linked to lavender and tea tree oils. *New Engl J Med* 356(5): 479–485.

Homburger F, Boger E (1968). The carcinogenicity of essential oils, flavors and spices: a review. *Cancer Res* 28: 2372–2374.

Inouye S, Uchida K, Abe S (2006). Vapour activity of 72 essential oils against a *Trichophyton mentagrophytes. J Infect Chemother* 12(4): 210–216.

Inouye S, Uchida K, Nishiyama Y *et al.* (2007). Combined effect of heat, essential oils and salt on fungicidal activity against *Trichophyton mentagrophytes* in a foot bath. *Nippon Ishinkin Gakkai Zasshi* 48(1): 27–36.

Khalil Z, Pearce AL, Satkunanatan N *et al.* (2004). Regulation of wheal and flare by tea tree oil: complimentary human and rodent studies. *J Invest Dermatol* 123: 683–690.

Khanna M, Qasem K, Sasseville D (2000). Allergic contact dermatitis to tea tree oil with erythema multiforme-like id reaction. *Am J Contact Derml* 11(4): 238–242.

Kishore N, Mishra AK, Chansouria JP (1993). Fungitoxicity of essential oils against dermatophytes. *Mycoses* 36 (5–6): 211–215.

Koch C, Reichling J, Schneele J, Schnitzler P (2008). Inhibitory effect of essential oils against herpes simplex virus type 2. *Phytomedicine* 15(1–2): 71–78.

Koh KJ, Pearce AL, Marshman G *et al.* (2002). Tea tree oil reduces histamine-induced skin inflammation. *Br J Dermatol* 147: 1212–1217.

Lertsatitthanakorn P, Taweechaisupapong S, Aromdee C *et al.* (2006). In vitro bioactivities of essential oils used for acne control. *Int J Aromather* 16(1): 43–49.

Messager SK, Hammer A, Carson CF, Rite TV (2005). Assessment of the antibacterial activity of tea tree oil using the European EN 1276 and EN 1499. *J Hosp Infect* 59: 220–228.

Monteiro MV, de Melo Leite AK, Bertini LM *et al.* (2007). Topical anti-inflammatory, gastroprotective and antioxidant effects of the essential oil of *Lippia sidoides* Cham. Leaves. *J Ethnopharmacol* 111(2): 378–382.

Monzelsio NB, Harris KE, McGrath KG, Grammer LC (2003). Immediate systemic hypersensitivity reaction associated with topical application of Australian tea tree oil. *Allerg Asthma Proc* 24: 73–75.

Monzote L, Montalvo AM, Almanonni S *et al.* (2006). Activity of the essential oil from Chenopodium ambrosiodes grown in Cuba against Leishmania amazonensis. *Chemotherapy* 52(3): 130–136.

Naganuma M, Hirose S, Nakayama Y *et al.* (1985). A study of the phototoxicity of lemon oil. *Arch Dermatol Res* 278(1): 31–36.

Nair B, (2001). Final report on the safety assessment of *Mentha piperita*, (Peppermint) oil, *Mentha piperita* (Peppermint) leaf extract, *Mentha piperita* (Peppermint) leaf, and *Mentha piperita* (Peppermint) leaf water. *Int J Toxicol* 20 (Suppl. 3): 61–73.

Oladimeji FA, Orafidiya OO, Ogunniyi TAB *et al.* (2000). Pediculocidal and scabicidal properties of *Lippia multiflora* essential oil. *J Ethnopharmacol* 72: 305–311.

Oladimeji FA, Orafidiya LO, Okeke IN (2004). Physical properties and antimicrobial activities of leaf essential oil of *Lippia multiflora* Moldenke. *Int J Aromather* 14: 162–168.

Oladimeji FA, Orafidiya OO, Ogunniyi TAB, Adewunmi TA, Onayemi O (2005). A comparative study of the scabicidal activities of formulations of essential oil of *Lippia multiflora* Moldenke and benzyl benzoate emulsion BP. *Int J Aromather* 15: 87–93.

Orafidiya LO, Agbani EO, Oyedele AO, Babalola OO, Onayemi O (2002). Preliminary clinical tests on topical preparations of *Ocimum gratissimum* Linn. leaf essential oil for the treatment of *Acne vulgaris*. *Clin Drug Invest* 22(5): 313–319.

Orafidiya LO, Agbani EO, Abereoje OA, Awe T, Abudu A, Fakoya FA (2003). An investigation into the would-healing properties of essential oil of *Ocimum gratissimum* Linn. *J Wound Care* 12(9): 331–334.

Orafidiya LO, Agbani EO, Adelusola KA *et al.* (2004a). A study on the effect of the leaf essential oil of *Ocimum gratissimum* Linn. on cyclophosphamide-induced hair loss. *Int J Aromather* 14: 119–128.

Orafidiya LO, Agbani EO, Oyedele AO *et al.* (2004b). The effect of aloe vera gel on the anti-acne properties of the essential oil of *Ocimum gratissimum* Linn leaf – a preliminary clinical investigation. *Int J Aromather* 14: 15–21.

Orafidiya LO, Agbani EO, Iwalewa EO *et al.* (2004c). Studies on the acute and sub-chronic toxicity of the essential oil of *Ocimum gratissimum* L. leaf. *Phytomedicine* 11: 71–76.

Orafidiya LO, Fakoya FA, Agbani EO, Iwalewa EO (2005). Vascular permeability-increasing effect of the leaf essential oil of *Ocimum gratissimum* Linn. as a mechanism for its wound healing property. *Afr J Trad Compliment Altern Med* 2(3): 253–258.

Oyedele AO, Orafidiya LO, Lamikanra A, Olaifa JI (2000). Volatility and mosquito repellency of *Hemizygia welwitschii* Rolfe oil and its formulations. *Insect Sci Appl* 20(2): 123–128.

Penfold AR, Grant R (1925). The germicidal values of some Australian essential oils and their pure constituents, together with those for some essential oil isolates, and synthetics. Part III. *J Roy Soc New South Wales* 59: 346–349.

Perrett CM, Evans AV, Russell-Jones R (2003). Tea tree oil dermatitis associated with linear IgA disease. *Clin Exp Dermatol* 28(2): 167–170.

Prashar A, Locke IC, Evans CS (2004). Cytotoxicity of lavender oil and its major components to human skin cells. *Cell Proliferation* 37(3): 221–229.

Priestley CM, Burgess IF, Williamson EM (2006). Lethality of essential oil constituents towards the human louse, *Pediculus humanus*, and eggs. *Fitoterapia* 77(4): 303–309.

Rubel DM, Freeman S, Southwell IA (1998). Tea tree oil allergy: what is the offending agent? Report of three cases of tea tree oil allergy and review of the literature. *Aust J Dermatol* 39(4): 244–247.

Schaller M, Korting HC (1995). Allergic airborne contract dermatitis from essential oils used in aromatherapy. *Clin Exp Dermatol* 20(2): 143–145.

Schubert H (2006). Skin diseases in workers at a perfume factory. *Contact Dermatitis* 55(2): 81–83.

Shahi SK, Shukla AC, Bajaj AK *et al.* (2000). Broad spectrum herbal therapy against superficial fungal infections. *Skin Pharmacol Appl Skin Physiol* 13(1): 60–64.

Sinico C, Alessandro De Logu A, Francesco Lai F *et al.* (2005). Liposomal incorporation of *Artemisia arborescens* L. essential oil and in vitro antiviral activity. *Eur J Pharm Biopharm* 59(1): 161–168.

do Socorro SRM, Mendonza-Filho RR, Bizzo HR *et al.* (2003). Anitleishmanial activity of a linalool-rich essential oil from *Croton cajucara. Antimicrob Agents Chemother* 47: 1895–1901.

Sugiura M, Hayakawa R, Kato Y *et al.* (2000). Results of patch testing with lavender oil in Japan. *Contact Dematitis* 43(3): 157–160.

Tyler VE, Brady LR, Robbers JE (1981). *Pharmacognosy*, 8th edn. Lea and Febiger, Philadelphia, pp. 103–143.

Ueda-Nakamura T, Mendonça-Filho RR, Morgado-Diaz JA *et al.* (2006). Antileishmanial activity of Eugenol-rich oil from *Ocimum gratissimum. Parasitol Int* 55(2): 99–105.

Ueng YF, Hsieh CH, Don MJ (2005). Inhibition of human cytochrome P45O enzymes by the natural hepatoxin safrole. *Food Chem Toxicol* 43(5): 707–712.

Usip LP, Opara KN, Ibanga SE, Atting IA (2006). Longitudinal evaluation of repellent activity of *Ocimum gratissimum* (Labiatae) volatile oil against *Simulium damnosum. Mem Inst Oswaldo Cruz* 101: 201–205.

Villar D, Knight MJ, Hansen SR, Buck WB (1994). Toxicity of melaleuca oil and related essential oils applied topically on dogs and cats. *Vet Hum Toxicol* 36(2): 139–142.

Walton SF, Mckinnon M, Pizzutto S *et al.* (2004). Acaricidal activity of *Melaleuca alternifolia* (tea tree) oil: *In vitro* sensitivity of *Sarcoptes scabiei* var hominis to terpinen-4-ol. *Arch Dermatol* 140: 563–566.

Warnke PH, Sherry E, Russo PAJ *et al.* (2005). Antibacterial essential oils reduce tumour smell and inflammation in cancer patients. *J Clin Oncol* 23 (7): 1588–1589.

Wei Q, Harada K, Ohmori S *et al.* (2006). Toxicity of the volatile constituents of Myoga utilizing acute dermal irritation assays and the guinea-pig maximization test. *J Occup Health* 48(6): 480–486.

Weisenseel P, Woitalla S (2005). Toxic mustard plaster dermatitis and phototoxic dermatitis after application of bergamot oil. *MMW Fortschr Med* 147: 53, 55.

Weston SE, Burgess I, Williamson EM (1997). Oils against headlice in 'Development in Pharmacognosy'. *Pharm J* 259: 482.

Weyers W, Brodbeck R (1989). Skin absorption of volatile oils. Pharmacokinetics. *Pharm Unserer Z* 18(3): 82–86.

Willms RU, Funk P, Walther C (2005). Local tolerability of two preparations with euclyptus oil and pine needle oil. *NNW Fortsch Med* 147 (Suppl. 3): 109–112.

Windholz M, (1983). *The Merck Index*. Rahway, USA, p. 761 (1073).

Yang YC, Lees HS, Clark JM *et al.* (2005). Ovicidal and adulticidal activities of *Cinnamomum zeylanicum* bark essential oil compounds and related compounds against *Pediculus humanus capitis* (Anoplura: Pediculicidae). *Int J Parasitol* 35(14): 1595–1600.

Zhang SY, Robertson D (2000). A study of tea tree oil ototoxicity. *Audiol Newootol* 5(2): 64–68.

26

Shelf-life of herbal remedies: challenges and approaches

DB Anantha Narayana and Rajendra M Dobriyal

Introduction

All products undergo changes, depending on the way that they are stored after they are manufactured, and herbal medicinal products (HMPs) are no exception; the World Health Organization has issued *Guidelines for Assessment of Herbal Remedies* (WHO, 1991), which suggest that all herbal remedies should also be assessed for their stability or shelf-life. However, none of the other guidelines issued by WHO elaborate this aspect, nor is there any guideline which advises on how this is to be done (WHO, 1994, 1998). A document issued by the US Food and Drug Administration (US FDA, 2004) requires submission of stability studies data for botanical drug applications, although no specific and detailed guidance on how such studies are to be performed is given in the document.

The European Medicine Agency (EMEA) has also dealt with this aspect and a few guidelines are understood to be in the draft stage (EMEA, 2006), although it is not expected that any specific guidance of how shelf-life of herbal preparations is to be assessed will be given in this document. In India regulatory requirements for traditional medicines, i.e. Ayurvedic, Unani and Siddha, do not make it mandatory for manufacturers to label the products with an expiry date or shelf-life period. However, in 2006, the government of India issued a draft notification in the *Gazette of India* providing for proposed shelf-lives to be marked on products of Ayurveda, Unani and Siddha systems, which is currently under scrutiny from academia and industry. It is noteworthy that in the *Ayurvedic Formulary of India*, expiry periods within which these products need to be used are specified.

The HMP formulations discussed in this chapter include dosage forms prepared with primarily plant-based raw materials, but may include one or more ingredients from minerals, metals, animal or marine origin. However, recently, formulation of single herb-based dosage forms has also been started and are included below.

The need for shelf-life marking of HMPs

Most of the regulatory bodies in the world do not mandate the printing of shelf-life or expiry date information for HMP formulations, although in recent years there has been a demand by consumers, and suggestions by others, that HMP formulations need to be labelled with an expiry date. However, it is a known fact that many regulators, by habit of reviewing conventional medicines dossiers, ask for such data for HMP formulations as well. These formulations are not based on single chemical entity compounds, and hence evaluation and discussions regarding their shelf-life can be compared easily on similar lines to food products. In such formulations it is extremely difficult to specify an expiry date (a date after which the potency of the actives would be lost or reduced to subpotent levels), so it is preferable to evaluate a 'best before' date. This is the date after which one or more properties of the formulations would have shown considerable changes/degradation, perceived by the consumers/patients and leading to doubts about the quality of the formulation and hence its efficacy. An attempt is made here to deal with evaluations for the 'best before' date.

Changing factors affecting shelf-life of HMP formulations

HMP medicines are used by consumers based on a recommendation/prescription from a traditional medicines practitioner (known by various names according to the culture), or based on informed self-medication in other cases, as for herbal dietary supplements. In the former, the traditional medicines doctor prepared these concoctions of formulations at their 'pharmacies', and dispensed in quantities for a week or so at a time, asking the patients to come for a review when the next dose is to be dispensed. In such circumstances, considerations for shelf-life were limited only to short time intervals and modern packaging technologies were not adopted.

However, in modern times, traditional medicines are manufactured in large batch sizes and are packaged and made available to practitioners as well as the public. Technologies are being adopted using modern equipment and processes so that large quantities can be processed, untouched by human hand, yet mimicking the processes prescribed in the traditional books. Many HMP formulations are known to use modern, safe, approved, pharmaceutical aids, i.e. excipients and adoption of modern dosage forms, e.g. tablets and capsules, to improve appeal and to provide unit dosages per serving. In such circumstances, considerations for shelf-life become necessary.

Various factors have an effect on the shelf-life of the formulations, related to manufacturing processes and environmental conditions. The initial quality of the material used is dealt with in Chapters 27 and 28 and it should be remembered that factors such as temperature, light, relative humidity/moisture and exposure to oxygen must be controlled for better shelf-life of the formulation.

Reference to various authentic Ayurvedic texts such as *Sharangdhar Samhita* (Vidyasagar, 1931) reveals that the aspect of shelf-life had been previously recognised. Some of the *Granthas* (Ayurvedic official texts) have given guidance regarding factors that make formulations degrade or become unfit for use and, in some cases, the period from the time from making the preparation to the end of its use is prescribed. This is continued in the *Ayurvedic Formulary of India* (Govt of India, 2003) where a period of 1 year is specified for a simple admixture of powdered herbs for oral or external usages.

Modern technological advances have made it possible to control and regulate various aspects of processing during production so as to minimise or even eliminate the ill-effects of factors affecting shelf-life. These include temperature and humidity in the processing and manufacturing areas, thereby consolidating stability of the formulation during processing and packing.

Advances in design and development of packaging technology have been achieved, so that the requisite barrier properties to build stability of the formulations can be provided, particularly with transportation and storage in mind.

The following factors have a direct bearing on the shelf-life of the formulations:

- heat (temperature during storage)
- moisture/humidity (inherent moisture and moisture absorbed during storage)
- exposure to light
- exposure to oxygen (air)
- exposure to microbes (storage in unhygienic packs/conditions and ingress of air into pack).

Formulations need to be carefully studied to select suitable packaging material so that the products are compatible with the materials and retain their original properties. Changes in colour, odour, physical structure, particle size, moisture, viscosity, taste, pH and other physicochemical parameters give evidence of shelf-life of the product.

The use of inert excipients such as stabilisers and preservatives also serves to improve and maintain the stability of the formulations.

Judicious adoption of modern technologies has made it possible for formulations to be given a 'best before' date much higher than those applicable to HMPs made by traditional methods.

Difficulties in conducting shelf-life studies in HMP formulations

Until any regulatory authority prescribes or issues widely accepted guidelines for shelf-life studies of HMP formulations, it is best to compare and find the closest categories of products comparable with them. HMPs are different from synthetic, chemical-based conventional medicines so adoption of guidelines used, e.g. ICH (2003), for such is to be avoided. These ICH guidelines largely work on studying kinetics of degradation of known/characterised compounds and their impurities/degradation compounds by adopting sophisticated analytical techniques indicating stability of individual compounds. Elaborate guidance is available regarding storage conditions including challenge conditions for different climatic zones in the world, for accelerated stability studies.

However, HMP formulations do not easily fit into such constraints as they are predominantly polyherbal and multi-component in nature. The closest category with which they can be compared is food products, as these are also of predominantly vegetal origin. In the case of HMP formulations, just as for foods and food products, the consumer can note degradation signs by apparent changes in appearance, colour, taste, smell, physical aspects and occasionally a combination of one or more of these properties.

However, many aspects of ICH guidelines can definitely be adopted while performing shelf-life studies on HMP formulations. Tables 26.1 and 26.2 show a comparison of physicochemical and quantitative assays for shelf-life studies for single chemical entities versus HMP formulations.

In the absence of ability to test the rate or extent of degradation of a known compound, it may be more appropriate to study other critical parameters in the case of HMP formulations.

Determination of critical parameters and critical points

To arrive at a point when a formulation can be considered to have 'gone off' and be not suitable for use, it is recommended that studies are conducted before shelf-life studies are initiated. These pre-shelf-life studies are aimed at identifying parameters that are critical to the particular formulation/dosage form and the point at which these parameters show changes, making it unfit for usage. This is done by intentionally exposing the formulation to conditions promoting their degradation and determining the critical parameter and critical point. In many cases a reasonable identification of the critical parameters can be made, while a set of experiments may be required to determine the critical point of such a parameter. A few examples are given below to elaborate this aspect.

Colour of the formulation: a change in colour, which would vary considerably from the normal colour of such formulation, raises doubts in the mind of the consumer about the stability of the product. The product may become darker or lighter when exposed to one or more factors such as heat, light and oxygen. It is desirable to confirm if such changes in colour are critical for the particular formulation. Samples of the same formulation may be exposed to higher temperatures, air or direct sun light and changes in colour can be observed. The minimum

Table 26.1 Comparison of analysability of physicochemical and quantitative assays for shelf-life studies

Test parameters	For synthetic chemical actives based products	For HMP formulations
Description	Can be measured in some cases where change occurs	Can be measured in most of the cases
Taste	Difficult to measure	Can be measured discerningly; is a test prescribed by traditional books[a]
Colour	May not change always	Changes in most of the cases
Smell	Difficult to measure	Obvious and can be measured
Consistency	Can be measured	Can be measured
pH	Can be measured	Can be measured
Quantitative assays	It is possible always	Rarely possible; even if possible only quantification of one of the markers may be possible[b]
Quantitative assay for degradation compounds or impurities	Always possible	Rarely possible, examples of such possibilities not seen in literature

[a]For medicated wine dosage forms (eg. *Asavas* and *Arishtas* of Ayurveda) the classical texts declare a product to be unfit for use if it becomes sour. Sour taste development is an indication of conversion of alcohol to acetic acid.

[b]Markers than can be analysed quantitatively may or may not be the bioactive compounds. Data related to dose–response relationship with reference to marker compounds and their percentages are not reported in literature commonly.

Table 26.2 Comparison of consumer perceptibility of physicochemical changes seen during storage/shelf-life of products

Test parameters	For synthetic chemical actives based products	For HMP formulations
Description	Consumer may not perceive	Generally perceivable
Taste	Difficult to measure	Easily perceivable and give great importance
Colour	The changes may not be consumer perceptible	Easily perceivable and give great importance
Smell	Difficult to measure	Easily perceivable and give great importance
Consistency	Can be perceived	Easily perceivable and give great importance
Microbial growth	Can be perceived	Easily perceivable and give great importance

change that can be allowed so as not to be perceived by the consumer as an indication of degradation will become the critical point of colour as a parameter. Changes in colour may be measured by a skilled person or instrumentally, e.g. a Levibound Tintometer, P-fund meter, use of standard colour shade cards or ultraviolet spectrophotometer.

Moisture: this is known to be absorbed by some herbal formulations, converting them to a coherent mass, reducing flowability and causing colour changes. Such absorption actually increases the degradation of the formulation rapidly. For some powdered dosage forms, moisture is a critical parameter and samples of such formulations should be intentionally exposed to high humidity and the moisture content measured at suitable time intervals until the product has absorbed enough water to make it unacceptable. For example *Churnas* (an Ayurvedic dosage form made of a coarsely powdered blend of herbs) has 3.5% moisture normally, but when their moisture increases to greater than 7–10%, they look different and degradation occurs rapidly. Determination of moisture in these experiments may be done by measuring loss on drying at 1050°C or by infrared moisture balance or by Karl Fischer's titration method, depending upon the availability of the facility. Methods given in any of the pharmacopoeias may be adopted for these studies (*British Pharmacopoeia* 2008; *Indian Pharmacopoeia* 1996; *USP National Formulary*, 2004).

Similarly other critical parameters and their critical points need to be determined. Table 26.3 shows a few of the critical points for various dosage forms of HMP formulations.

Once the critical parameters and the point at which they would become the benchmarks for use in the accelerated or the real-time studies are determined, relevant tests on products can be carried out.

Suggested evaluation methods

There are two clear objectives of the stability study.

- Is the quality of a product intact for the required period of time irrespective of whatever it is packed in? (Inherent phytochemical stability.)
- Is the selected packaging material capable of protecting the product for the required period of time? (Evaluation of the packaging material.)

Keeping in mind the different needs for shelf-life studies of HMP formulations, three approaches are suggested, depending on the nature of product, i.e. existing product, product in a new packaging or a new formulation.

Retrospective shelf-life studies

Any guideline should be applicable to both existing formulations and new formulations (products under development). In many case, manufacturers may have access to control samples/materials from old batches of existing products. Using such products, for which the manufacturer is confident that no intentional/accidental change has occurred in its composition and standards of practice, makes it possible to adopt a 'cross-sectional approach' to determine the shelf-life of the products. Such studies are referred to as retrospective shelf-life studies and are a form of real-time study.

Method

Samples of existing formulations in their current packaging may be collected from control samples or even from storage. At least three samples of each formulation should be collected from each station covering at least 6 months from their manufacturing dates. These samples may be tested for the critical parameters (see Table 26.3) and any other parameters that the manufacturer may feel necessary for that particular formulation. The results of these tests are compared with results from a freshly manufactured batch of the same formulation, or the specifications for those tests, for deciding the shelf-life.

The following aspects must be recorded in the data of such studies:

- name of formulation
- sample number and packing in which the sample is packed
- batch number, date of manufacture and time elapsed from manufacture (months/years)
- parameters/critical parameters analysed/studied
- specifications/requirements for each of the parameters/critical parameters
- actual results for each of the parameters/critical parameters
- inference of the results and calculation of shelf-life period to be assigned for the product.

Table 26.3 Recommended critical parameters for various dosage forms/formulation

Number	Dosage forms for herbal formulations	Critical parameters
1	Powdered herbs	Colour, odour, moisture
2	Pills and compressed tablets	Colour, moisture, DT, hardness
3	Calcined metallic preparations including those prepared using mercury and sulphur	Colour, moisture, flowability
4	Metallic preparations	Colour, moisture, flowability
5	Self-fermented, medicated wines	Taste, clarity, sedimentation, pH/acidity
6	Semi-solid pasty mass for oral administration	Colour, consistency, separation, smell and taste, appearance, pH, TPC, YMC
7	Preparations made with Guggulu resin	Colour, moisture, hardness
8	Calcined Iron ore based preparations	Appearance, colour, moisture, particle size, TPC, YMC
9	Preparations of herbalised ghee (clarified butter-based preparations)	Colour, consistency, acid value, peroxide value and smell
10	Medicated oils	Colour, consistency, acid value, peroxide value and smell
11	Distillates of herbs (essential oil distillates)	Colour, pH, content of volatile matter
12	Extracts (infusions/decoctions)	Appearance, colour, physical separation, pH, any specific marker(s)
13	Salts/salts left behind after herbs or fruits are incinerated to get ash like substances	Appearance, colour
14	Ointments for external application	Colour, physical separations, cracking, TPC, YMC
15	Liniments	Colour, physical separations, cracking
16	Concentrated extracts/dry or liquid extracts	Appearance, colour, physical separation, pH, any specific marker(s)
17	Products obtained by sublimation process	Colour, moisture, flowability
18	Fruit pulps fried with oil/ghee to get pasty mass	Colour, consistency, separation, smell and taste, appearance, pH, TPC, YMC
19	Aqueous decoction	Colour, sedimentation, pH, TSS, TPC, YMC
20	Drops for eye, nose and ear administration – may be oily or ghee based or water based	Colour, smell, clarity, pH (acidity and peroxide value where applicable), sterility
21	Granules for oral administration	Colour, odour, moisture, YMC
22	Inhalers	Weight
23	Compressed tablets with or without coating	Colour, moisture, DT, hardness, TPC, YMC
24	Hard or soft capsules	Moisture, DT, caking of contents, TPC, YMC

Table 26.3 *(continued)*

Number	Dosage forms for herbal formulations	Critical parameters
25	Modern gel formulations	Appearance, colour, physical separation, pH (content of volatile if present)
26	Liquid orals like syrups, suspensions	Colour, taste, pH, sedimentation/cracking, TPC, YMC

Note 1: Additional parameters may be selected for particular formulations.
Note 2: Wherever in the above formulation, knowledge of one or more actives and the method of determination of the same are available, the same may be selected as the critical parameters, e.g. menthol content, camphor content, antioxidant activity.
Note 3: Preservative efficacy tests are not included in these guidelines.
Note 4: It may not be necessary to do microbiological tests such as TPC, YMC at all 'stations of studies'. They may be analysed for TPC/YMC at initial and at selected stations as preservative efficacy studies are done normally at pre-formulations stage.

Prospective shelf-life studies for new formulations or for formulations in new packaging

An approach of adopting simple quality-assessment parameters, and the methods of testing these parameters as a means of evaluating shelf-life of HMP formulations has been developed by the present authors. This is directly relevant to what a consumer or a patient recognises as a change which shows that a particular HMP formulation is different from what it was expected to be, raising the doubts about the quality of the product. Some would expect HMP formulation also to be studied for their stability using typical pharmaceutical approaches for single chemical entity drugs, where not more than 10% deterioration of the active molecule occurs when it is stored at conditions that the manufacturers decide. This approach is not suggested nor recommended for HMP formulations for the following reasons.

- Formulations are generally polyherbal or herbomineral.
- Formulations, even if based on single herbs are multi-component in terms of chemical constituents.
- Active chemical molecules in the HMP formulations are inadequately known and markers, which are currently used, do not necessarily reflect a true correlation with biological activity.
- Assaying a single marker is against the principle of the holistic approach of therapy of HMP formulations, as it is difficult to pinpoint that the entire health benefit of HMPs is caused by one such compound identified.

As an alternative, it is suggested that the easiest and most practical method to evaluate shelf-life of HMP formulations is to decide requisite conditions and parameters during processing, and conditions during packing as well as a selection of intended packaging materials. The packs are then exposed to challenging conditions with a view to studying the behaviours of the formulations. One to three batches of samples of formulations manufactured using conditions that would be used during manufacturing should be taken for conducting the shelf-life studies. Properly closed, selected packs with one or more intended packaging materials should be also taken and exposed to controlled conditions of temperature, humidity, light and exposure to air. Samples from production batches may also be used for stability studies. If more than one packaging material (with different constructions) or packaging changes are to be studied, portions of the same batch of formulations would need to be packed in each packaging material or pack to get adequate numbers for study. ICH has divided the world into four different zones depending on the climatic conditions: temperature and humidity, so the conditions for storage for various zones as specified in ICH guidelines may be drawn up.

Examples of challenging conditions for storage of packs for accelerated studies include:

At 45°C ± 2°C.
At 40°C ± 2°C/75% ± 5% relative humidity.

For comparison purposes one set of samples is stored in a refrigerator (not in the freezer chamber).

Samples are to be evaluated on predetermined parameters at 0, 1, 2, 3 and 6 months.

Real-time studies

While the above would apply to studies done under accelerated conditions, manufacturers may also conduct real-time studies by keeping the packs of formulations at 30°C ± 2°C/65% ± 5% RH for long periods and evaluate them for predetermined parameters. For such real-time studies samples may be evaluated at 0, 3, 6, 12, 18 and 24 months.

Parameters to be evaluated

Parameters mentioned in Table 26.4 may be selected for the stability studies on varying formulations depending on the dosage forms, ingredients, stabilisers and preservatives present or absent. A thorough knowledge of the formulations would help

Table 26.4 Parameters to be assessed for stability studies of HMP formulations

1	Appearance
2	Colour
3	Odour
4	Taste
5	Particle size
6	Flowability
7	Viscosity
8	Clarity
9	pH
10	Moisture content
11	Sedimentation
12	Flocculation
13	Emulsion breakage
14	Friability
15	Hardness
16	Extractive values (in selected solvents)
17	Volatile matter content
18	Free fatty acids/acidity
19	Peroxide value
20	Microbiological parameters, namely total viable count (TPC) yeast and mould counts (YMC), coli form count and other pathogens
21	Comparative thin-layer chromatograph to compare the profiles
22	Assay – quantitative analysis of one or more analytical marker or biomarker
23	Specific parameters applicable to the formulation/dosage form

the identification of parameters that are likely to change or show changes caused by the ill effects of the factors affecting the stability of formulations.

Accelerated stability studies

The current guidelines for synthetic chemical-based drugs and formulations adopt accelerated stability studies as a common approach. Most of the regulatory requirements demand accelerated stability data of at least 6 or 9 months from the manufacturers as part of the registration dossier. This approach is valid and scientific, since synthetic drugs usually consist of a single, well-characterised chemical substance. Exposing them to high temperature and humidity and measuring the degraded compounds are not only analytically possible but also provide good information. No national or international regulatory agency has commented on the applicability of accelerated stability studies for HMP formulations. However, it is logical that industry would need to perform accelerated studies, to be able to decide a shelf-life and reduce the time to market. A cautious approach of an accelerated study protocol and studies up to 3–4 months under challenging conditions can still be adopted for HMP formulations. Such short studies would provide possible gross changes that may occur as a measure of good caution.

Documentation

Records of all the shelf-life studies need to be maintained. It is necessary to record the batch number of formulations, batch size, date of manufacturing, different packaging materials, packs taken up for studies, condition of exposure for studies, stations at which samples were analysed are recorded. Tests conducted at each time point for formulations and their packs and their actual results obtained are recorded for both formulations and packs. Wherever microbiological tests are to be done, a separate/unopened pack is used. Tests for parameters of assessment can be done from public test houses or other laboratories/research labs. At the end, such data may be tabulated so that conclusions and shelf-life may be assigned, based on data generated.

Additional approaches

The above strategy provides a basic framework for assessing, in a systematic way, the shelf-life of the HMP formulations. Wherever possible and practicable, additional techniques such as fingerprinting by TLC and/or HPTLC methods, or testing by HPLC may be done. Such techniques for the presence and absence of marker compounds, qualitatively or quantitatively, may be undertaken by those who wish to do shelf-life evaluation using such technologies. Manufacturers may add their own parameters and methods to further strengthen the guideline.

It is normal to accept that, when comparative HPTLC or HPLC testing is done of samples of HMP formulations from different stations, they should have a comparable chromatographic profile. The word 'comparable' here means 'similar', though in some cases appearance or absence of one or more additional spots/peaks in a TLC/HPTLC may be seen. In the absence of data, whether these changes in fact affect the bioactivity or the safety profile, it is difficult to make a reasoned conclusion, hence more scientific data need to be generated before prescribing chromatography testing as part of the stability studies requirement.

As an example, amla (*Emblica officinalis*), commonly called 'Indian gooseberry', is well known for its antioxidant and immunomodulatory activity and a few commercial dietary supplements are available. These products are either powder of dried fruits or an aqueous extract of the same. Amla is rich in tannins and polyphenols and ascorbic acid, gallic acid, ellagic acid and other polyphenolic compounds are seen in a TLC test. It is known that exposure of amla to higher temperature in the presence of moisture actually increases the gallic acid content and such samples actually show a higher antioxidant activity when tested by DPPH titrimetric methods. However, despite the changes seen in the chromatographic profile, the product has not shown any change in safety and efficacy historically. Hence adoption of ion chromatographic testing has to be done carefully.

Manufacturers may take another approach in monitoring TLC/HPTLC fingerprinting by including assays of markers and generation of data, by determining the extent of bioactivity as a means of stability testing. Bioactivity of the product against standard bacterial/fungal strains or in-vitro bioactivities, including those involving cell lines, also provides excellent stability data. In fact, studying biological activity data using validated in-vitro methods would be an ideal method, though its adoptability by large sections of the HMP industry is in doubt.

By determining the time required for formulations to degrade to a level of the critical points of the parameters selected under accelerated conditions, one can assess and extrapolate to ambient conditions for deciding the 'best before' dates for them. It is obvious that optimisation of packaging material with shelf-life requirements will need to be done to achieve the desired shelf-life at an affordable cost of packaging.

Communication with consumers

Consumers need to be told how to store and handle HMPs, as well as about their 'best before' dates. Such communications need to be done in a consumer-friendly form, so that it is well understood by the user. Information needs to be provided on the inner-most packaging material in contact with the pack and on all subsequent packaging materials. In a study conducted involving the storage conditions given on the well-regulated pharmaceutical products, the situation was contrary to this. The language and texts used by manufacturers on products surveyed showed a high level of 'consumer un-friendliness' and in some cases even the pharmacists who stored them in their pharmacies did not understand them correctly (Narayana *et al.*, 2002).

A small survey on labels of pharmaceutical formulations also reveals the following different texts, obviously meant for consumer benefit/education.

- Sealed for freshness
- Keep away from children
- Replace lid after each use tightly
- Store in cool place
- Store in cool and dry place
- Store in cool, dry place and away from moisture
- Store protected from sunlight
- For external use only
- Keep away from your eyes
- Use before . . . (please see bottom of pack) (Seen only on some packs; not very common.)
- Expiry date . . . (please see bottom of pack)
- Shake well before use.

We did not encounter any pack of HMP formulation requiring or directing the pack to be stored in chilled or frozen conditions.

Table 26.5 shows meanings of some of the statements generally printed on the labels.

Table 26.5 Meaning of the statements mentioned on the product packs regarding storage for the products

Text to be printed on the label/wrapper	What it means
'Do not store over 8°C'	To be stored in refrigerator (from +2°C to 8°C)
'Do not store over 30°C'	To be stored at room temperature (from +2°C to 30°C)
'Do not freeze'	To be stored in refrigerator (from +2°C to 8°C but not in the freezer chamber)
'Store in a cool place'	To be stored at room temperature (from +2°C to +30°C, away from exposure to direct sunlight)
'Protect from moisture'	To be stored in normal humidity at room temperature (RH <60%), product to be provided by the manufacturers in a moisture-resistant container
'Protect from light'	To be stored in light-resistant cupboards/drawers; product to be provided by the manufacturers in light-resistant containers

It is obvious that the consumers may not be able to decipher these directions properly as they cannot be expected to decide the temperatures that meet the terms 'cool' or 'cold'. Nor can they be expected to fully understand the terms such as 'keep away from moisture' or 'protect from sunlight'. Even if some consumers are able to do so, they are not equipped to achieve them by way of proper packaging, if manufacturers have not provided such packaging. The publication *Good Storage Practices for Pharmaceutical Substances* (WHO, 2003) has dealt with this aspect and provided fairly clear, consumer-friendly guidelines for labelling related to storage aspects of medicines. It puts the onus of providing proper packages to achieve storage for protection from moisture, as well as storage for protection from sunlight, on the manufacturer, who has to provide such products in packs which can achieve such storage.

Labelling

Packs of formulations need to be labelled in a manner that is easily understood by consumers as well as wholesale and retail personnel. Drawing from the above document from WHO, this would be broadly applicable to HMP formulations as well. The following statements are hence recommended for use on labels, wrappers and other printed packaging materials for HMP formulations also. In addition to the storage guides, it is necessary to specify the 'best before' date suitably. These dates would then mean that the HMP formulations are not recommended to be used after this date. The exact way this needs to be done can be by giving the 'month and year' as the use before dates or can also be given as ' . . . months from manufacturing for use'.

Conclusions

There is a strong case to be made for more systematic shelf-life studies to be carried out and also for more open publications of data made available by industrial companies. Such shelf studies would benefit from a cross-functional team of scientists expert in the chemistry of natural products, analytical science and biological science.

References

British Pharmacopoeia (2008). London: British Pharmacopeia Commission.

Delhi Pharmaceutical Trust (2002). *Good Storage Practices (GSPs) for Pharmaceutical Products at a Retail Pharmacy*. Delhi Pharmaceutical Trust, New Delhi.

Govt of India (2000). *Schedule T, Good Manufacturing Practices (GMPs) for Ayurvedic, Siddha and Unani Medicines, Amendment to Drugs & Cosmetics Rules – (1945)*. Ministry of Health & Family Welfare.

Govt of India (2001). *National Formulary of Unani Medicine*, Part III. Ministry of Health & Family Welfare, Govt. of India, New Delhi.

Govt of India (2003). *Ayurvedic Formulary of India*, Part-1, 2nd Edn. Ministry of Health & Family Welfare, Govt. of India, New Delhi.

Govt of India (2005). Draft Notification, GSR 691(E), *Gazette of India*. Govt. of India, New Delhi.

EMEA/CVMP/814 (2006). *Guidelines on Quality of Herbal Medicinal Products/Traditional Herbal Medicinal Products*. European Medicine Agency, London.

ICH (2003). *Stability Testing of New Drug Substances and Products, Q1A (R2)*. The International Conference on Harmonization of Technical Requirements for Registration of Pharmaceuticals for Human Use.

Indian Pharmacopoeia (1996). Vols I & II. Indian Pharmacopoeia Commission, Govt of India, New Delhi.

Narayana DBA, Mittal MP (2002). Storage of Medicines – Findings of the Survey of 100 retail outlets in Delhi. *IDMA Bull* 21. Indian Drugs Manufacturers Association, Mumbai.

Drugs & Cosmetic Rules (1945). Schedule P. Ministry of Health & Family Welfare, Govt of India.

US FDA (2004). *Guidelines for Industry: botanical drugs products*. CDER, Food & Drugs Administration, USA.

USP National Formulary (2004). United States Pharmacopoeia 27, National Formulary 22, Asian Edition. US Pharmacopoeia Consortium Inc.

Vidyasagar PS (1931). (Ed.). *Sharngdhar Samhita*. Chaukhambha Orientalia, Varanasi.

WHO (1991). *Guidelines for the Assessment of Herbal Remedies* (WHO/TRM/91.4). World Health Organization, Geneva.

WHO (1994). *Guidelines for Formulation of National Policy on Herbal Medicines*. Alexandria, World Health Organization Office for the Eastern Mediterranean.

WHO (1996). Good Manufacturing Practices: Guidelines on the Validation of Manufacturing Processes. In: WHO Expert Committee on Specifications for Pharmaceutical Preparations, 34th Report, Geneva, World Health Organizations, *Technical Report Series*, No. 863, 80–96.

WHO (1998). *Regulatory Situation of Herbal Medicines: A worldwide review*. (WHO/TRM/98.1). World Health Organization, Geneva.

WHO (2003). Guide to good storage practices for pharmaceuticals, Annexure 9. World Health Organization *Technical Report Series*, No. 908, Geneva.

Part 4

Evaluation of quality and safety

27

Authentication and quality assessment of botanicals and botanical products used in clinical research

Roy Upton

Introduction

The tremendous increase in interest in the use of herbal drugs over the past decade has led to an increased desire to subject these drugs to scientific evaluation, to determine their true potential as medicinal agents in modern healthcare. Numerous national and international organisations and initiatives such as those by the American Herbal Pharmacopoeia (AHP), European Pharmacopoeia (EP), European Scientific Cooperative on Phytotherapy (ESCOP), United States Food and Drug Administration (FDA), Office of Dietary Supplements (ODS), US Pharmacopoeia (USP), and World Health Organization (WHO) are working to ensure that herbal drugs are subjected to critical scientific review (see Table 27.1). Additionally, there are increased funding opportunities for the evaluation of herbal drugs (e.g. National Institutes of Health and National Center for Complementary and Alternative Medicine in the US).

Such trials require complete characterisation of the raw materials and finished product of the herbal drug being investigated to ensure its identity, purity, quality, consistency, and reproducibility (Table 27.2). Without such knowledge, the findings of any clinical trial will be subject to question as well as be irreproducible. Testing methodologies that are applied to medicinal plants include botanical, macroscopic, microscopic, chemical and molecular methods of testing, which provide analytical tools that can be used for full botanical product characterisation. Each testing methodology has advantages and disadvantages and has specific application for assessing a particular aspect of herbal product quality that will vary from herb to herb. Most often it is best to use both physical and chemical methods of assessment.

A key principle in choosing the appropriate tests is to ensure that the methodology has a sufficient degree of specificity for the desired analytical endpoint. Additionally, herbal product quality is neither dependent upon the presence of chemical

Table 27.1 Organisations and resources contributing to scientific knowledge on medicinal plants

American Herbal Pharmacopoeia: http://www.herbal-ahp.org
American Herbal Products Association: http://www.ahpa.org
AOAC International: http://www.aoac.org
Ayurvedic Pharmacopoeia: Government of India, Ministry of Health and Family Welfare Therapeutic Goods Administration (Australia): Questions & Answers for the Identification of Herbal Materials and Extracts: http://www.tga.gov.au/cm/idherbal.htm
Complementary Healthcare Council of Australia: Code of Practice for Ensuring Raw Material Quality and Safety: http://www.chc.org.au/lib/pdf/rawmat.pdf
Considerations for NCCAM Clinical Trial Grant Applications: http://nccam.nih.gov/research/policies/clinical-considerations.htm
European Scientific Cooperative on Phytomedicines (ESCOP): http://www.escop.com/
European Medicines Agency (EMEA): http://www.emea.eu.int/index/indexh1.htm
CPMP/QWP/2819/00 (EMEA/CVMP/814/00) Note for Guidance on Quality of Herbal Medicinal Products (CPMP/CVMP adopted July 01): http://www.emea.eu.int/pdfs/human/qwp/281900en.pdf
CPMP/QWP/2820/00 (EMEA/CVMP/815/00) Note for Guidance on Specifications: Test procedures and Acceptance Criteria for Herbal Drugs, Herbal Drug Preparations and Herbal Medicinal Products (CPMP/CVMP adopted July 01): http://www.emea.eu.int/pdfs/human/qwp/282000en.pdf
Health Canada Natural Health Products Regulations: http://www.hc-sc.gc.ca/hpfb-dgpsa/nhpd-dpsn/regs_cg2_tc_e.html
European Pharmacopoeia/ Directive for Quality of Medicines: http://www.pheur.org/site/page/_628.php
Ingredient Identity Testing records and Retention: http://www.cfsan.fda.gov/~dms/facgmp.html
International Code of Botanical Nomenclature (Saint Louis Code) 2000: http://www.bgbm.fu-berlin.de/iapt/nomenclature/code/SaintLouis/0000StLuistitle.htm
International Pharmacopoeias: e.g. Japan: http://jpdb.nihs.go.jp/jp14e/
Pharmacopoeia of the People's Republic of China: Ministry of Health & Welfare NSF International: http://www.nsf.org
Saskatchewan Herb and Spice Association and the National Herb and Spice Coalition: Good Practices for Plant Identification for the Herbal Industry: http://www.saskherbspice.org/Good%20Practices%20for%20plant%20identification.pdf
U.S. Food and Drug Administration: Current Good Manufacturing Practice in Manufacturing, Packing, or Holding Dietary Ingredients and Dietary Supplements: http://www.cfsan.fda.gov/~lrd/fr030313.html
U.S. Food and Drug Administration: Food, Drug & Cosmetic Act: http://www.fda.gov/opacom/laws/fdcact/fdctoc.htm
United States Pharmacopoeia: http://www.usp.org
World Health Organization: http://whqlibdoc.who.int/publications/2003/9241546271.pdf

marker compounds alone, as is often done in clinical investigations of herbal drugs, nor can herbal product quality be assessed by chemical means alone. Rather herbal quality is very much dependent upon growing, harvesting and processing conditions, the application of good manufacturing practices (GMP) in the manufacture of the actual product, and a host of other considerations. The need for a comprehensive approach to herbal assessment has not been a focus in the herbal trade in North America but has been given considerable attention in Europe, with many European Union countries being much more advanced and sophisticated in their approach to herbal medicine than the US.

Table 27.2 Botanical characterisation requirements of the National Center for Complementary and Alternative Medicine (NCCAM)

Plant identification	Identify to genus/species including botanical authority, reference to archived voucher including botanical expert who identified; harvest information, compliance with WHO or other guidelines for wild material
Supplier	Name and contact information for supplier
Adherence to independent standard	Compliance with pharmacopoeial monograph (e.g. AHP, EP, USP, WHO), justification for deviating from a monograph, or a description of suitable tests performed specific to the botanical study material; comparison against an authenticated reference material
Macroscopic description	Physical characteristics of plant part
Product specifications	Characterisation of extraction conditions, starting extract, and finished product: e.g. solvent used, herb to extract ratio, excipients and % excipients, markers for standardisation, chemical fingerprint to the extent allowed by current science including method, contaminant analysis, e.g. heavy metal, microbial; identification of process controls to assure consistency of product; stability, disintegration, dissolution, bioavailability (if known), assurance of batch to batch reproducibility, analytical guidelines for testing during course of study and information on matching placebo, if applicable; availability of retention samples for future testing if desired

Considerations for NCCAM Clinical Trial Grant Applications: http://nccam.nih.gov/research/policies/clinical-considerations.htm

Accepted standards for herbal products are collated in monographs in pharmacopoeias which identify, assess for purity and usually also give some quantitative standard for the drug in question (see Chapter 1). The tests described below deal primarily with techniques and approaches used for identity tests, i.e. verifying that the herbal material is what it is claimed to be.

Botanical drug versus drug from botanical

The unique differences of herbal drugs present unique challenges in establishing the identity, quality, and consistency of efficacy of herbal drugs – requirements of all medicinal compounds. The differentiation of conventional and herbal drugs can be minimally considered from regulatory, economic, and technical perspectives.

Internationally, most nations regulate herbal medicines as 'traditional medicines', applying an approval criteria that is much less onerous and expensive than the approval of conventional drugs. This is due to the long history of use of traditional medicines, the historical record of safety and efficacy, and the long-standing presence of herbal preparations in the public domain. This is in contrast to most conventional medications, which have not been in the public domain and for which little, or no historical data regarding safety or efficacy exist.

Economically, the cost of development and/or approval of traditional medicines is much less than for conventional drugs. There is also a greater degree of patent protection typically offered for the often novel compounds of modern pharmaceuticals rather than those in the public domain. The costs associated with drug approval differ from nation to nation and substance to substance. As a point of reference, in the US, the cost for conventional drug development has been estimated at a staggering US$802 million (DiMasi *et al.*, 2003) to US$1.7 billion per single drug (Crawford, 2004). As the US has no traditional medicines or natural health product regulatory model, no cost can be estimated for approval of a traditional herbal drug.

In the European Union (EU), unofficial estimates for the approval of a new active substance as of 2006 is €62 300. For approval of a known active substance, including an herbal drug, it is €17 700. Currently, the new EU traditional medicines regulations are too new for an accurate estimate of approval of a traditional drug. However, this has been estimated to be approximately €5000–10 000 (personal communication [2006] with Dr Willmar Ulrich, Director International Division, Schwabe Pharmaceuticals, Karlsruhe, Germany).

From a technical perspective, generally speaking, conventional drugs are well characterised, typically consisting of single ingredient preparations (e.g. morphine from the opium poppy) in which the composition, pharmacokinetics, pharmacology, dosage, safety, quality control requirements, etc., are well known. In contrast these parameters are seldom known for botanicals as the active compound(s) are often not known, multiple species of plants may be used as the same medicine (e.g. Radix Rheum), there is inherent natural variability in raw botanical materials that can only be partially controlled for, and different manufacturers will manufacture by different parameters resulting in varying constituent profiles and varying levels of efficacy.

Moreover, the majority of herbal practitioners worldwide utilise combinations of botanicals (consisting of 2–45 different botanicals), each with dozens or hundreds of constituents, the individual activity of which, from a Western biomedical perspective, has not been investigated, let alone the activity of the combination of compounds. While the safety and use of many traditionally used herbal preparations are well understood by traditional herbalists, such preparations defy conformity to testing and characterisation requirements applied to modern single-entity drugs.

It is equally important to note what does not constitute a traditional medicine. Multiple definitions for traditional medicines exist internationally (see Box 27.1). Generally speaking, crude plant materials and relatively crude herbal preparations, also often referred to as Galenic preparations, that have been used historically, and which do not contain chemically defined or isolated chemical compounds, may be classified as traditional medicines.

Box 27.1 World Health Organization definition of a traditional medicine

'Finished, labeled medicinal products that contain as active ingredients aerial or underground parts of plants, or other plant material, or combination thereof, whether in the crude state as plant preparations. Plant material also includes juices, gums, fatty oils, essential oils, and any other substances of this nature. Herbal medicines may contain excipients in addition to active ingredients.

Medicines containing plant material combined with chemically-defined active substances, including isolated constituents of plants, are not to be considered herbal medicines.'

Physical identification and quality assessment tests

Skilled physical assessment of a plant part is one of the most effective means for determining the identity and relative quality of a medicinal plant part and has been utilised for many centuries, e.g. by Dioscorides in classical Greek medicine (Riddle, 1985) and in Ayurvedic medicine (Kaviratna and Sharma, 1996). Coupled with appropriate chemical characterisation these two methodologies allow for a relatively complete characterisation of an herbal drug. The greatest limitation of physical assessment is its relative inappropriateness for evaluating material that has been extracted, as the structural characteristics of extracted botanicals are not present. The only physical assessment of herbal extracts that can be performed is an organoleptic analysis, which can provide indicators to identity and quality, but is less than definitive.

Botanical identification

Accurate identification of botanicals for use in herbal medicines is both a fundamental and regulatory requirement. Botanical identification is the primary means by which a plant is accurately identified and must be done by someone with the requisite skills, ideally a formally trained botanist. From earliest times until the mid-19th century much attention was given to plant identification, specifically so that adulterations could be avoided. The very early works suffered botanically because of the relative infancy of botany as a science, but the later works were drawn with exquisite detail, providing medical professionals with a relatively high degree of accuracy to ensure the identity of their materia medica.

Unfortunately, in the present medicinal herb trade, botanicals are seldom subjected to direct identification by a trained botanist but are gathered either by wildcrafters who, by experience, believe they are gathering the correct botanical, or are cultivated by farmers who purchase seeds from suppliers they believe to be reputable. In both cases documentation regarding an appropriate assessment is often lacking and therefore, not documentable. Additionally, medicinal plants are traded as plant parts after harvest and processing, often lacking the flowers, typically critical for making a definitive botanical identification. The lack of formal botanical identification can lead to adulteration, sometimes with dire consequences, since toxic herbs are sometimes substituted for those that are non-toxic (e.g. *Aristolochia fang ji* for *Stephania tetrandra*).

Identification of botanicals to be used medicinally should be made either in their native habitat when flowering or at the source of cultivation. Alternatively a representative of the plant population is identified by comparison with a botanical voucher (a pressing of the plant with characteristic identifiers). Vouchers should be properly archived in a herbarium in case future reference to the specimen must be made, such as if a question arose about the accuracy of the identification. Without a botanical documentation trail, the identity of the botanical used in a study or product will always be in question.

There are advantages and disadvantages of only using botany in the identification and quality assessment of medicinal plants. The primary advantage is that there is a plethora of botanical keys in floras clearly articulating the unique identifying characteristics of the plant species, so that a definitive identification to genus, species and subspecies can be made. Botany can only be applied in the medicinal plant trade for identification purposes and, unless the botanist is also trained in principles of commercial sourcing or traditional herbal practices, they may not know that a plant is ideally picked at a specific time of year, might have to be a certain age before being used or needs to be processed in a certain way. Botanists may not be familiar with changes with age in the cellular structures and organoleptic qualities.

Familiarity with these subtleties of herb quality is critically important if using botany as the primary identification tool for the subsequent physical and chemical characteristic of plant parts and should ideally be coupled with knowledge about proper harvesting and initial processing guidelines. There are some plant genera, such as *Crataegus* and *Salix* that can be extremely difficult for even trained botanists to identify to species definitively. In such cases, and especially when potentially toxic compounds or adulterants may be present, chemical testing for those compounds or chemical fingerprinting should be employed as a complementary verification.

Harvest and post-harvest conditions

In addition to appropriate botanical identification, botanicals must be harvested at the proper time. Herbalists historically adhered to such principles and many of these principles continue to be adhered to by professional herbal wildcrafters. However, where herbs are grown industrially, greater consideration is often given to commercial issues, such as time of increased biomass, or maximum yield of specific marker compounds, which may or may not relate to 'quality' or efficacy.

After optimal harvest times, post-harvest processing such as washing, drying, initial processing, and storage is most critical in ensuring the quality of a botanical drug. For example, the activity of valerian root (*Valeriana officinalis*) is predominantly found in the essential oil, partially associated with valerenic acid content, and contained within cells that are highly concentrated at the surface of the rhizome (Bos, 1997). If subjected to inappropriate handling these cells are damaged, thus exposing the valerenic acid to oxidation and therefore a decrease in essential oil yield. Valerenic acid is also subject to degradation at drying temperatures in excess of 45°C (Samuelsson, 1992; Bos, 1997). Therefore, post-harvest conditions for medicinal plants should be controlled for and documented as a quality control parameter. This is seldom done in the medicinal herb trade.

Macroscopic characterisation

After botanical identification, macroscopic assessment is an effective tool for determining identity of plant material. Macroscopic evaluation is an assessment of the plant material, either with the naked eye or with simple magnification such as with a hand lens or stereomicroscope. It typically includes gross morphological characteristics including colour, form, size, texture, and fracture (how the plant part breaks; usually associated with roots and barks) along with the plant's organoleptic characteristics (taste, aroma, quality). Similar species of plants can share similar morphological characteristics and so appropriate training is needed to acquire macroscopic identification skills.

Early texts, e.g. by Wallis and Greenish (UK), and Sayer and Youngken (US) provided a tremendous amount of information about these characteristics of medicinal plants which were in international trade, but it should be noted that many widely used contemporary herbal drugs were not included in these texts. Emphasis of macroscopy has been almost completely discarded in relatively modern texts of pharmacognosy (e.g. Tyler *et al.*, 1988) and its use in identification is now rare in North America where trade of powdered material is predominant, but important in other parts of the world, e.g. traditional Chinese herbs.

Macroscopic examination also allows for a relative qualitative assessment of adulterating species, filth, organic and non-organic contaminants, and material degradation is readily observed. This is in contrast to powders that do not allow for such an assessment. It should also be noted that when plants are retained in as whole a form as possible they generally retain their potency as less surface area is exposed to air, heat, and light.

Microscopic characterisation

Botanical microscopy was also once an integral part of pharmacognosy training and is currently in a rapid decline, not only because of the over-reliance on chemistry, but also because of the lack of skilled personnel familiar with the techniques. Microscopy of medicinal plants focused on the observation of the cellular structures, and their content, of plant material by use of a compound microscope.

Today, electron microscopy is also used, predominantly for investigative purposes, but it is not readily applied for analysis of medicinal plants in commercial trade. For a period of time in the late 1800s to middle 1900s microscopy was one of the most utilised techniques for the identification of plant parts and purity assessment and, when properly performed, can be used to identify plant parts to genus and species and detect adulterating matter such as other organic and non-organic matter, insect fragments, and in some cases, deteriorated materials.

In their relatively whole form, many plant parts possess a uniquely characteristic arrangement of cells that give the plant its unique identifiable characteristics. Once powdered, the arrangement of the cells, thus the plant part's unique characteristics, are lost and, in some cases, even diagnostic cell structures are destroyed (Houghton, 1998). Microscopy can be applied to powders but many similar plant parts will share the same cellular structures making identification of actual species difficult or impossible.

Advantages of microscopy are similar to macroscopy in that a proper identification can often be made if a botanical identification has not been performed; adulterants and foreign matter can be detected; though not as readily as with macroscopic examination; it is a cost-effective analytical tool; and the technique is relatively environmentally sound as only small amounts of chemical reagents are needed.

Disadvantages of microscopy include the inability to identify powders with definitiveness; less of an ability to perform a qualitative purity assessment as compared with macroscopic evaluation; a lack of appropriately trained personnel; and a general lack of appropriate keys and reference texts to which to refer.

Botanical reference standards

Physical assessment of botanicals is ideally performed using a botanical reference standard. A standard for the medicinal plant part of interest has its identity, purity and/or quality independently determined and may comprise whole, fragmented or powdered material. It should be as consistent as possible with material in commercial trade and, ideally, chemically characterised to reflect a minimum quality standard as established by appropriate pharmacopoeias, or as reflected in the historical or clinical literature.

Using such a standard, other commercial samples can be compared for consistency either physically or chemically and this can greatly increase the accuracy of a physical or chemical examination of a test sample. Many pharmacopoeias provide such standards for those botanicals for which pharmacopoeial monographs exist. Analysts using botanical reference standards should know the means by which identity, purity and/or quality of the reference standard were ascertained and whether or not the reference material can be used for both qualitative (identification) and quantitative (constituent concentration) purposes.

Chemical characterisation

Since the turn of the 19th century, chemical detection, identification, elucidation, isolation, and synthesis have dominated as an analytical technique in the development of modern medicines. Chemistry has also been extensively applied to medicinal plant characterisation, so that modern pharmacognosists are almost completely chemical in orientation and almost completely lacking in the physical skills so prevalent in earlier generations.

Chemical characterisation is an important technique in determining absolute concentrations of particular compounds, assessing relative consistency of products, and in some cases, determining plant identity and detecting adulterants. Many plants contain unique sets of compounds in characteristic ratios that can allow for the differentiation of even closely related species (e.g. *Echinacea*) (Bauer and Tittel, 1996) and even different plant parts of the same plant (e.g. *Panax quinquefolium*) (Ma *et al.*, 1998).

Chemistry is especially useful when specific active compounds of a plant are known or if a product is to be standardised to a particular compound for quality control purposes. Chemical analysis can be applied to determine optimum harvesting, drying, processing and extracting conditions, stability, and batch-to-batch consistency, and can provide a relatively objective tool for quality-control documentation. There are many different techniques that can be applied, ranging from simple colorimetric tests to sophisticated chromatography (see below). However, chemical analysis without physical assessment (botanical, macroscopic, or microscopic) has its limitations since alone it often will not be able to determine the identity of a plant so definitively as physical assessment. This is because there are some closely related species and different plant parts of the same plant that share remarkably similar chemical profiles, so they that cannot be easily differentiated.

Chemistry alone often cannot be used to make a qualitative assessment of a plant part, e.g an immature fruit can have a similar chemical profile as an appropriately ripe fruit (e.g. *Crataegus* berries). Organic and inorganic impurities cannot be readily detected chemically but they can physically. Chemical tests can also oftentimes be easily fooled by adding pure compounds to medicinal plants to increase the yield of a particular compound or group of compounds, e.g. *Ginkgo biloba* extract often has pure flavonoids (e.g. rutin and quercetin) added to increase flavonol glycoside concentration (Xie, 2002).

A key challenge in all types of chemical evaluation is in the interpretation of the analytical data. Plants and plant products can vary greatly in their constituent profile despite all the best efforts of growers and manufacturers to standardise all processes, so the absence or presence of key compounds and their varying levels or ratios may only tell part of the story of the medicinal efficacy of the plant.

Chemical analysis is very expensive relative to physical testing methodologies, and by its very nature, is not an environmentally sound technique, since it requires the use of highly toxic solvents and reagents. Use of such compounds, and the negative impact they have on the environment, are inconsistent with the philosophy of a large segment of the population who chooses natural medicines over synthetic. This is a point often not realised or considered in the medicinal plant trade. As noted, in most cases, the combination of both physical and chemical tests is ideal for the identity and qualitative assessment of medicinal plants.

Colorimetric tests

In the early development of chemical testing, colorimetric tests, where a reagent applied to a test material produces a consistent colour reaction, were commonly used. For example, Chinese star anise *Illicium verum* is often adulterated with Japanese star anise *I. anisatum*. When boiled in dilute potassium hydroxide solution, Chinese star anise produces a blood-red colour reaction while the adulterating Japanese star anise produces a yellowish-brown colour reaction (Youngken, 1930). The predicted colour reaction provides a confirmatory piece of evidence to determine identity. Colorimetric tests are generally very easy to perform and are cost-effective, but are usually specific to groups of compounds rather than individual species of plants so can be used as an indicator of identity but not for making a definitive identification.

Thin-layer chromatography and high-performance thin-layer chromatography

Thin-layer chromatography (TLC) assessment was among the earliest of chemical methods applied to medicinal plants. With it, characteristic chemical fingerprints can be developed that represent the identity and relative quality of a medicinal plant. As an analytical technique, TLC has been far overshadowed by other, more specific analytical methodologies, such as high-performance liquid chromatography (HPLC) with a prevailing perception of a superiority of specific methods over TLC. Many chemists remain unaware of the value of modern high-performance TLC (HPTLC) technologies in the assessment of medicinal plants. In recent years, increasing levels of sophistication have been applied to TLC, including higher-quality silica plates, automatic application and plate development equipment, the ability to perform quantitative analyses, and documentation systems with automated software interfaces.

The most important consideration regarding TLC or HPTLC as an analytical technique is to recognise the technique as another tool, with both advantages and disadvantages, available to the medicinal plant analyst. Many analysts believe TLC to be among the most valuable and versatile tool for chemical assessment of medicinal plants. The primary advantage of HPTLC is the relatively inexpensive cost in comparison with more specific analytical techniques. Another advantage is that much more chemical profiling information can be obtained from a single run using HPTLC than with many other methods, because of the ability to utilise a variety of detection methods which gives a multidimensional profile of a plant, compared with the typical single-dimensional chromatogram of HPLC. Additionally, up to 20 samples of the same or different botanicals can be assayed in a single analytical run, whereas with HPLC only one sample at a time can be assayed.

Disadvantages of HPTLC include those that exist with most chemical methods, i.e. that they will often not detect foreign organic or inorganic matter, cannot provide a non-chemical assessment of quality, and are relatively environmentally unsound because of the need for large amounts of chemical solvents and reagents. Additionally, while HPTLC can be used for the quantitation of specific compounds, other, more specific methods of quantitation such as HPLC are more accurate in this regard for quantitation, although in some cases, limits for detecting the presence of compounds may be more sensitive with HPTLC.

Quantitative analytical methods

Spectrophotometric and chromatographic (especially HPLC and gas chromatography [GC]) are the primary analytical tools for quantifying specific compounds in a substance. Spectrophotometric methods generally lack specificity and can be used for quantifying groups of similarly related structures such as proanthocyanidins in bilberry (*Vaccinium myrtillus*) or the hypericins (hypericin and pseudohypericin analysed collectively) in St John's wort.

Other spectrophotometric techniques such as Fourier transform infrared spectroscopy (FTIR) are also applied to medicinal plant analysis, since some botanical FTIR patterns will be characteristic, although in many others there is too much interference to give a distinguishing fingerprint. As the activity of many botanicals is often associated with groups of compounds, photometric analysis may provide a more representative picture of the composition of certain medicinal plants than more specific methods. They generally lack the specificity needed if analysis of an individual compound is required.

GC is specifically useful in the analysis of essential oil-rich materials and has a tremendous amount of analytical power to separate hundreds of closely related compounds when great specificity is required.

In the American and European herbal trade, individual active or marker compounds are typically tested for, often mimicking the Western conventional drug model. HPLC is the technique most often applied in the North American herb trade to quantify individual compounds. Both HPLC and GC can also be applied to quantify multiple compounds. In Asia, these techniques are as much applied with a focus of obtaining a characteristic chemical fingerprint or profile, as they are for quantitative purposes. This is in recognition of the fact that the activity of a medicinal plant is very seldom correlated with a single constituent. In addition, with chemical fingerprinting, attention is given to specific ratios that may help in differentiating closely related species or detecting adulterations. Such fingerprint analysis allows for broader assessment of identification and quality than the identification of a single marker compound, which cannot be used to determine identity and can only partially be used to assess quality.

Quantitative methods of analysis are best employed when there is a specific analyte of interest, such as an active or surrogate marker. HPLC and GC specifically can yield more accurate data regarding concentrations of compounds contained within a plant than non-specific methods and can be powerful tools for assessing consistency of a product. Their most significant disadvantage is that they seldom can be used to establish the identity of a plant ingredient definitively, although thay can help to determine the identity of the plant material. The equipment needed is also relatively expensive to purchase and run and can only analyse one sample at a time, so there is slow output compared with some of the other methods described. Lastly, there are very few, well-validated HPLC methods for medicinal plants. Different laboratories performing different analyses of exactly the same sample, using the same testing parameters, can produce widely different results.

Chemical reference standards

Chemical assessment of botanicals most often includes or requires the use of a pure chemical reference standard, such as hypericin for the analysis of St John's wort. Chemical reference standards are typically individual compounds that ideally have the highest degree of characterisation and purity as is practically possible. Chemical reference standards are available from commercial suppliers (e.g. Chromadex, US and Phytolab-Addipharma, Germany), from pharmacopoeial sources (e.g. American Herbal Pharmacopoeia or European Pharmacopoeia), or from government sources (e.g. National Institute for Standards Testing, US).

For the results of quantitative analyses to be considered valid, the purity of the reference standard(s) used must be accurately disclosed. Many commercial suppliers of reference standards do not accurately disclose either the purity of the standards or the manner in which purity was determined. Often, standards purity is determined using methods that are not optimal for purity assessment, such as TLC. Use of inaccurately characterised standards will yield varied quantitative values that will skew the results of testing. Those involved in the analysis of medicinal plants must ensure that the identity and purity of the chemical reference standards used are accurately disclosed.

Conclusions

Each of the analytical techniques described has advantages and disadvantages regarding their technical applicability, cost and environmental impact. In most cases, a combination of physical and chemical tests is needed for a complete identity and quality assessment of botanical drugs, which is a minimal requirement for all botanical products. Physical and chemical assessments typically require quality control personnel consisting of those with requisite training in botany, pharmacognosy, traditional herbal practices, microscopy and chemistry. The tests applied must have a great enough degree of specificity for the intended analytical endpoint.

In most cases, use of authenticated botanical and chemical reference standards is either required or can greatly increase the accuracy of both identification and qualitative assessment. Each of the methods discussed should be applied, as appropriate, to the assessment of herbal products, either if used as dietary supplements or medicines. There is a legal and ethical responsibility of manufacturers for ensuring the identity, purity, and relative quality of herbal products and the tools presented above can be used for these purposes.

Ultimately, well-characterised herbal medicine products must be subjected to appropriate preclinical and clinical testing to determine what analytes are most correlated with efficacy, which will then provide guidance as to the most appropriate analytical methods to be applied to individual medicinal plants.

References

Bauer R, Tittel G (1996). Quality assessment of herbal preparations as a precondition of pharmacological and clinical studies. *Phytomedicine* 2: 193–198.

Bos R (1997). *Analytical and Phytochemical Studies on Valerian and Valerian Based Preparations.* Rijksuniversiteit Groningen, Groningen, p. 184.

Crawford L (2004). Healthcare Institutional Investor Conference, Bank of America Securities. http://www.fda.gov/oc/speeches/2004/bascrty0707.html.

DiMasi JA, Hansen RW, Grabowski HG (2003). The price of innovation: new estimates of drug development costs. *J Health Econom* 22: 151–185.

Houghton PJ (1998). Establishing identification criteria for botanicals. *Drug Inform J* 32: 461–469.

Kaviratna AC, Sharma P (1996). *Caraka Samhita.* Volume 1. *Indian Med Sci Ser* 41: 286.

Ma YC, Luo M, Malley L *et al.* (1996). Distribution and proportion of major ginsenosides and quality control of ginseng products. *Chin J Med Chem* 6: 11–20.

Riddle JM (1985). *Dioscorides on Pharmacy and Medicine.* Austin: Univ Texas Pr., p. 298.

Samuelsson G (1992). *Drugs of Natural Origin: a textbook of pharmacognosy.* Swedish Pharm Pract, Stockholm.

Tyler V, Brady L, Robbers J (1988). *Pharmacognosy.* Lee & Febiger, Philadelphia.

Xie PS (2002). Overview on the quality control of traditional Chinese medicines. In: *First International Conference on the Modernization of Traditional Chinese Medicine.* Hong Kong Jockey Club, Hong Kong.

Youngken HW (1930). *A Textbook of Pharmacognosy.* Blakiston, Philadelphia.

28

Quality control of Chinese herbal drugs

Eva M Wenzig and Rudolf Bauer

Introduction

In recent decades, traditional Chinese medicine (TCM) has become very popular in Western countries. However, incidents such as the cases of nephropathy after consumption of adulterated Chinese herbs in Belgium have reinforced the requests for enhanced quality and safety control of these preparations.

Apart from the implementation of good agricultural practice (GAP), good sourcing practice (GSP) and good manufacturing practice (GMP) rules in cultivation, harvesting and processing, analytical methods have to be adapted to the special needs of TCM preparations. Great scientific effort has been made in the past few years to develop methods for correct authentication, detection of contaminants and quality assurance.

Authentication of Chinese medicinal herbs is crucial as, on the one hand, nomenclature is not always consistent and one common name can refer to different drugs in different geographical regions, but, on the other hand expensive and scarce drugs are sometimes substituted with cheaper ones. The most common authentication methods are macroscopic and microscopic analysis and chromatographic methods such as thin-layer chromatography (TLC), high-performance liquid chromatography (HPLC), gas chromatography (GC) and capillary electrophoresis (CE). More recently, DNA-related techniques have increasingly been used.

Many problems of contamination are similar to those concerning herbal drugs in Europe, e.g. microbial contamination, pesticide and heavy metal residues. A special problem occurring in TCM preparations is adulteration with synthetic drugs. These adulterations are most often detected by GC, HPLC and hyphenated techniques, but because of the big variety of possible adulterations, their reliable detection is critical.

For quality assurance, mainly chromatographic techniques such as TLC, HPLC, CE and GC are used and hyphenation with detection methods such as ultraviolet, diode array detection (DAD), mass spectrometry (MS) or evaporative light scattering detection (ELSD) are very common. Apart from analysis of markers and biomarkers, fingerprint analysis is increasingly applied, as it has been shown to be feasible for the analysis of very complex mixtures. For a meaningful fingerprint analyis, combination with chemometric methods has proven to be useful.

Background

Traditional Chinese medicine (TCM) has its origin at the beginning of civilisation in China. The first written documents dealing with the effort to cure diseases in China date from the Shang dynasty (2nd millennium BC). Over the centuries, the medical system developed in an empirical manner through observation of effects a treatment produced on specific ailments and on certain parts of the body (Siow *et al.*, 2005).

In contrast with other traditional medical systems, TCM has always been regarded as a science, and it has been taught at medical schools for more than 2000 years.

TCM herbs

In total, more than 6000 medicinal plants are known in herbal medicine in China. Approximately 300–500 of them are currently used regularly in TCM (Dobos *et al.*, 2005). Herbs contained in a prescription are mainly classified according to four categories:

- The major one is called 'chief' or emperor (*Zhing*), containing the bioactive components.
- The minor ones are classified as 'adjuvant' or 'minister' (*Chen*), providing support for the major herb or alleviating secondary disease symptoms.
- The helper-like herbs are known as 'assistant' (*Zhou*). They modulate the action of the emperor herb (enhance activity, alleviate secondary symptoms or counteract adverse effects of the prescription).
- The additive herbs or 'guides' are called *Shi* in Chinese. They direct the action of the other herbs towards specific parts of the body. Each property may be represented by several herbs in the mixture (Cheng, 2000). A TCM prescription usually consists of 2–10 herbs, in differing quantities.

The pharmacological classification of TCM herbs strongly differs from Western understanding: first, the physical properties of an herb such as colour or taste can be linked to the theory of Five Phases. Second, the herbs are classified according to four properties: cold, hot, warm and cool (*Su-Chi*). Furthermore a herb can be classified by direction of its action: ascending (*sheng*), descending (*jiang*), floating (*fu*) and sinking (*chen*). The direction is also connected to the *Su-Chi* and the *Woo-Wei* theory: Herbs with acrid and sweet taste and warm to hot properties are mostly ascending and floating in action, whereas herbs with bitter, sour and salty tastes and cool to cold properties are mostly sinking and descending in action (see also Chapter 4).

TCM in Western countries

In recent decades, the acceptance of TCM as a form of complementary and alternative medicine has strongly increased in Europe and North America. However, contrary to China, where the education of TCM physicians and pharmacists is standardised by law, clear legal regulations on this issue are still missing in most Western countries. The legal status of herbal TCM drugs which are sold in China as over-the-counter drugs in specialised pharmacies or as prescription medicines, differs from country to country in the West.

In the USA, TCM herbs are generally classified as dietary supplements and not as conventional drugs. They have to comply with the Dietary Supplement Health and Education Act (DSHEA), which regulates statements and claims on product labels and prohibits misbranding and adulteration of dietary supplements.

In Germany, all Chinese herbs which are considered as drugs have to be sold in pharmacies and fall under the same legislation as conventional drugs. Their pharmaceutical quality has to be guaranteed by pharmacists who rely on certificates from qualified laboratories that ensure identity, purity and quality of a batch; additional identity testing has to be performed in the respective pharmacy. The quality of ready-made formulas also has to be guaranteed (Dobos *et al.*, 2005).

In the United Kingdom, crude drugs derived from herbs are exempt from licensing by law. This means that crude TCM herbs do not have to meet UK standards of pharmaceutical quality in manufacturing or purity. Ready-made herbal TCM formulas are currently also not required to hold a market authorisation. However, the UK health authorities are interested in changing this situation, and thus the UK Medicines and Healthcare Products Regulatory Agency recently played a major role in initiating the new EU legislation designed to regulate the traditional herbal sector (Traditional Herbal Medicinal Products Directive, 2004/24/EC), which passed into law in November 2005. This directive regulates herbal products sold over-the-counter without intervention of health professionals. According to the new directive which must be fully implemented throughout the EU by 2011, safe traditional use over at least 30 years, 15 years of which within the EU, has to be demonstrated for these products. Furthermore, they have to be produced according to GMP, and indications should be limited to minor health disorders (Dobos *et al.*, 2005).

Quality issues in Chinese herbal drugs

Authentication issues

The problem of correct authentication starts with nomenclature: In China, a particular trivial name can refer to different plants or drugs, depending on the region. For example, *fangji* is the name for *Stephaniae tetrandrae radix*, which is mainly harvested in the north and is officially known as *hanfangji*. However, fangji roots from southern parts of China, known as *guanfangji*, are derived from *Aristolochiae radix*. Mixing up these drugs was associated with more than 100 cases of kidney intoxication in Belgium. A weight-loss regimen containing a Chinese herbal preparation in combination with orthodox drugs has been applied. Radix Aristolochiae (guanfangji), containing aristolochic acids – compounds known to be nephrotoxic and carcinogenic – had been admixed to the herbal preparation instead of Radix Stephaniae Tetrandrae (hanfangji). Aristolochic acids are present in plants of *Aristolochia*, *Bragantia* or *Asarum* species and are the most monitored toxic adulterants so far (Vanherweghem *et al.*, 1993; Nortier and Vanherweghem, 2002).

Similar problems can occur with the drugs *mutong* (*Akebia quinata* Decne), *chuanmutong* (*Clematis armandii* Franch.) and *guanmutong* (*Aristolochia manshuriensis* Kom.) (Lord *et al.*, 1999; Zhao *et al.*, 2006).

Problems might also arise due to the fact that the Chinese pharmacopoeia (PRC Pharmacopoeia Committee, 2005) allows more than one species as a source for certain herbs as they possess similar functions in treating certain diseases. For example, according to the 2005 Chinese pharmacopoeia, Flos Magnoliae can be derived from *Magnolia biondii* Pamp., *M. denudate* Desr. and *M. sprengeri* Pamp.

In addition to the substitutes allowed in the Chinese pharmacopoeia, locally distributed varieties or species are common in China. These substitutes have a long regional practice and history, but since they are derived from different plant sources, their chemical constituents and therapeutic effects may differ (Zhao *et al.*, 2006).

Adulteration, substitution and contamination issues

Species variability, cultivation conditions and harvest time have an influence on the quality of plant material. Besides, the quality of herbal drugs can be deteriorated by substitution, contamination or adulteration.

Substitution means the replacement of a drug by another species, while adulteration is the intentional addition of undeclared substances. Herbs can be adulterated by 'spiking' with marker compounds, to reach the targeted level, by addition of pharmaceutical drugs or other plant material, to increase perceived potency or by admixture of inexpensive substances such as starch or pre-extracted plant material in case of rare or precious drugs. Contamination is the accidental inclusion of undeclared substances such as microorganisms, heavy metals, pesticides, radioactivity or the wrong plant or plant part (McCutcheon, 2002; Techen *et al.*, 2004).

Contamination of herbal material can have several reasons. First of all it can come from the environmental conditions under which the herbs are grown. Even though a GAP system for the cultivation of Chinese herbs has been established, most Chinese herbs are not yet cultivated under controlled conditions, but are collected from their natural habitat or harvested from small cultivation bases (Gao *et al.*, 2002). It was reported that, until June 2004, only 13 TCM herbs were grown in agricultural sites complying with GAP (Siow, 2005). Because only 1% of the TCM plants produced in China are currently exported to Europe, for many Chinese farmers it is not profitable to implement new cultivation processes. This situation may cause inconsistent quality and contamination problems.

In addition, contamination with foreign plant and non-plant materials may also happen during drying, processing, transport, storage and manufacturing processes.

Some of these factors can be controlled by implementation of standard operating procedures (SOPs) according to GAP, good laboratory practices (GLP), GSP and GMP (Chan, 2003). Thus, the first step in quality assurance is finding reliable raw material suppliers who are applying GAP, GSP and GMP for raw material production. This will become easier in future, as the number of suppliers from China implementing these rules will definitely increase. Apart from that, attempts have been made to cultivate Chinese plants under controlled conditions in other countries, and in some, e.g. Germany, quite promising results have been achieved with this approach (Bomme *et al.*, 2005, 2006).

Adulteration, contamination or substitution with foreign or toxic plant material

Admixture of toxic herbs may occur erroneously because of incorrect identification or for economic reasons, when a cheaper herb is substituted to replace a safer, more expensive one. Especially popular or scarce herbs are sometimes sold in poor quality, and in some cases traders even supplied toxic, fake herbs (Chan, 2003).

For some crude drugs, certain processing steps are obligatory for a safe and correct use. This processing may be needed to reduce toxicity of the respective material. For example in case of Aconiti Radix (*fuzi*) the use of non- or improperly processed plant material can have fatal effects (Chan, 2003; Bauer and Wagner, 2004).

Adulteration with undeclared synthetic drugs

To achieve a quick relief of disease symptoms, preparations of traditional Chinese medicines are sometimes illegally adulterated with synthetic drugs. This can be hazardous to health and result in various side-effects or drug allergies (Song *et al.*, 2000).

An investigation of 2609 TCM preparations in Taiwan revealed that 23.7% of the preparations were adulterated with at least one undeclared conventional pharmacological compound (Huang *et al.*, 1997).

In a systematic review dealing with this issue, Ernst (2002b) identified 18 case reports, two case series and four analytical investigations concerning TCM preparations contaminated with synthetic drugs. In several cases serious or life-threatening symptoms were described, such as agranulocytosis, Cushing´s syndrome, coma, hypoglycaemia, somnolence, hypertension and massive gastrointestinal bleeding. In other cases the adulterants were only discovered by chance without causing any symptoms, or because the suspicion of adulteration was raised because of an extraordinary good clinical response to the preparation. Detected adulterants cover a wide range of pharmaceuticals and some of them are associated with severe side-effects, e.g. corticosteroids, phenylbutazone, glibenclamide, sildenafil and phenytoin.

The screening for undeclared synthetic drugs in Chinese herbs is very challenging, as the variety of possible adulterations is very large. Chromatographic techniques such as TLC, GC, HPLC and CE are the techniques used most frequently. Hyphenation with mass spectrometry has been shown to be very feasible for this kind of analysis.

For example, Liu *et al.* (2001) developed an HPLC-DAD screening method for undeclared therapeutic substances in Chinese proprietary medicine preparations. GC-MS was used for confirmation of results. The method was applied to 41 samples from 7 categories, 25 of which were anti-asthmatic preparations. In one of them, undeclared codeine was detected.

Au and coworkers (2000) selected 134 synthetic compounds commonly found as adulterants in Chinese preparations sold in the United States and screened more than 500 Chinese patent medicine samples for the presence of these compounds using GC-MS analysis. About 10% of the samples contained undeclared drugs and/or toxic levels of heavy metals, which had been detected by atomic absorption spectroscopy (AAS). The authors state that GC-MS screening has limitations because non-volatile, large molecules or inorganic compounds cannot be detected by this technique. Therefore, negative GC-MS results do not necessarily mean that the respective preparations are free from synthetic adulterations.

Tseng and Lin (2002) employed LC-MS-MS for the detection and quantification of sildenafil citrate in a Chinese dietary supplement which was claimed to enhance sexual activity. The authors found an average sildenafil citrate amount of 48.2 mg/capsule, which corresponds to the sildenafil dosage of Viagra.

Contamination with heavy metals

According to a review of Ernst and Coon (2001), numerous case reports and case series of heavy metal poisoning associated with the use of TCM have been published. Lead, in particular, has relatively often been described as the substance of contamination but mercury, cadmium, arsenic and thallium have also been detected in Chinese herbs. There are several reasons for these findings: first, some Chinese prescriptions intentionally contain heavy metals; for example, arsenic and mercury are sometimes added as a part of certain formulations (Au *et al.*, 2000). Second, heavy metals might be present because of accidental contamination during manufacture, for example, from grinding weights or lead-releasing containers or manufacture utensils. Finally, the herbs themselves accumulate heavy metals when grown in heavily polluted soil, and some plants even accumulate heavy metals, especially cadmium, from regular soil (Kabelitz, 1998; Ernst and Coon, 2001; Ernst, 2002a; Chizzola *et al.*, 2003).

For detection of heavy metals, techniques such as atomic absorption spectroscopy (AAS) or induced coupled plasma mass spectrometry (ICP-MS) can be used. ICP-MS is more sensitive and allows the synchronous analysis of heavy metals, which makes the method more cost-efficient (Kabelitz and Sievers, 2004).

Lin *et al.* (2006) made a new approach to the quality control of Chinese herbs with regard to inorganic trace elements by developing a fingerprint analysis of inorganic compounds for *Gan-Yu-Lin*, a Chinese formulation consisting of 10 herbs, using ICP-MS. According to the authors this kind of fingerprint can provide valuable additional information on the quality of herbal formulations.

The *European Pharmacopoeia* (2005) provides a general monograph on the determination of heavy metals in plant drugs and fatty oils by AAS, but no limits are stipulated yet. Recommended limits differ from country to country in Europe. These tolerance levels are not without controversy, and for some plant materials exceedings are inevitable. The cadmium tolerance level especially is often difficult to maintain (Kabelitz, 1998; Chizzola *et al.*, 2003). The German Pharmaceutical Manufacturers' Association recently made a proposal to set a cadmium limit of 1 mg/kg. This is based on results of an industrial database which pooled the heavy metal contents of 20 000 analysed herbal drug samples. Additionally, for cadmium-accumulating species (e.g. *Salix, Hypericum*), higher tolerance levels have been suggested which can be matched by 90% of the batches of the respective herbal drugs (Kabelitz, 1998; Kabelitz and Sievers, 2004).

Nevertheless, since medicinal plants are predominantly consumed by ill people, a reasonable limitation of heavy metal contaminants in medicinal plants and a harmonised regulation for heavy metal limits in herbal drugs is highly desirable.

Contamination with pesticides

In the past, most Chinese herbs were collected in the wild, and therefore pesticide treatment did not play an important role for TCM herbs (Leung *et al.*, 2005). Nowadays, however, many TCM plants are cultivated. The cultivation of TCM plants often takes years and requires the use of pesticides, to reduce pest damage. Improper use of pesticides not only pollutes soil and ground water, but also leads to accumulation of pesticides in plants. Pesticide residues may therefore be present in Chinese herbs and preparations thereof (Ling *et al.*, 1999).

Pesticide residues can cause various adverse effects in humans, ranging from acute symptoms such as skin rashes and asthma attacks to chronic diseases such as emphysema or cancer (Leung *et al.*, 2005). Owing to their long residual actions, the use of organochlorine pesticides such as DDT has been restricted or banned in many countries (Zuin and Vilegas, 2000; Sohn *et al.*, 2004). The use of pentachloronitrobenzene (PCNB, quintozene), lindane and DDT has been prohibited in the US and many other countries, and the use of hexachlorobenzene has been banned worldwide. For various pesticides, regulatory standards have been stipulated in many pharmacopoeias (Leung *et al.*, 2005), e.g. the 2005 European Pharmacopoeia sets limits for 34 pesticides and guidelines for the determination of limits for other pesticides are provided. In several developing countries however, legislation concerning pesticide residues in herbal drugs is lacking or largely ignored.

The determination of pesticide residues in plant material is difficult because of the complexity of the plant matrix and the large variety of pesticides. In general, the methodology of pesticide residue analysis includes three main steps: extraction (usually followed by a clean-up procedure), separation and detection of pesticides. If the plant material of interest is of unknown origin and several groups of pesticides might be present, it is necessary to use methods that measure total organic chlorine, phosphorus, arsenic or lead prior to a detailed analysis, to find out which group of pesticides is present. For detailed identification and quantification, most frequently GC or HPLC methods are used (Zuin and Vilegas, 2000).

Extraction and clean-up of pesticides is a crucial step in pesticide analysis of herbal drugs as the compounds have to be extracted from a complex matrix. Ling *et al.* (1999) propose supercritical fluid extraction (SFE) as it is rapid and only requires small solvent amounts. In their study, the authors developed an SFE method for the simultaneous extraction and clean-up of 13 organochlorine pesticides from Chinese herbal materials.

In the 2005 Chinese pharmacopoeia, a GC-ECD (gas chromatography-electron capture detector) method is described for the determination of organochlorine pesticides in Chinese materia medica, traditional Chinese patent medicines and simple preparations. The 2005 European Pharmacopoeia gives a GC method for determination of pesticides in plant materials; the clean-up procedure and detection method differ depending on the respective class of pesticides.

Leung *et al.* (2005) used GC-ECD for screening and GC-MS for quantitative determination of 20 organochlorine pesticides in four frequently used Chinese herbs, namely Radix Angelicae Sinensis, Radix Notoginseng, Radix Salviae Miltiorrhizae and Radix Ginseng. Ten representative batches of different provenances were analysed from each herb. In all drugs except Radix Angelicae Sinensis, varying levels of quintozene and hexachlorocyclohexane could be detected. In Radix Ginseng, hexachlorobenzene and lindane were also found. In Radix Notoginseng samples, even the banned pesticide DDT and its derivatives were identified.

Some attempts have also been made to remove pesticide residues present in harvested or processed materials. For example, Sohn *et al.* (2004) presented a method for the removal of pesticide residues from aqueous ginseng extract by two-phase partition between water and soybean oil. The authors describe the method as cost- and labour-efficient, however, avoiding pesticide residues, for example, by applying GAP rules, might be the better approach than their later removal. The GAP system for the cultivation of Chinese medicinal plants provides an SOP on controlling insect pest and plant diseases and on the utilisation of agricultural chemicals (Gao *et al.*, 2002). Implementation of this model to as many cultivation bases as possible should ameliorate the problem of pesticide accumulation in future.

Microbiological contamination

Although microbiological contamination of medicinal plants is an important quality issue, literature reports dealing with the microbiological contamination of Chinese herbal drugs are scarce.

In the 2005 Chinese pharmacopoeia, limits are given for preparations. The limits stipulated for bacteria, yeast and mould counts are dependent on the kind of preparation, on the presence of crude plant material in the preparation and on the intended application (for examples, see Table 28.1). The 2005 European Pharmacopoeia provides tolerance levels for the microbial load of medicinal plants, which depend on intended application and on preparation technique. Herbal products are mainly assigned to categories 3B, 4A and 4B (Table 28.1). The allowed microbial load is higher when the plant drug is intended to be treated with boiling water prior to use, as this leads to a decrease in microbial contamination. The criteria of the European Pharmacopoeia are not mandatory, but are used as a recommendation for target levels. The tolerance levels recommended by WHO are also dependent on the intended use of the material (WHO, 1998). The European Herbal Infusion Association (EHIA) recommends tolerance levels for herbal infusion raw materials, which are generally higher than those given by the European Pharmacopoeia (EHIA, 2005) (Table 28.1).

The limits recommended by these authorities are not without controversy, and in many cases it is rather difficult to comply with them. Especially organically produced materials are treated with natural fertilisers such as stinging-nettle broth which contains considerably higher microbial levels, and they are also preferred by many insects which often carry contaminants (Kneifel *et al.*, 2002). Another problem is insufficient drying of the material, which often leads to the growth of moulds.

A reduction of microbial load can mainly be reached by application of GAP to the processes of harvesting, drying, storing and packaging of herbal material. Antimicrobial treatment of harvested or processed drugs is very problematic as methods such as ethylene oxide treatment or irradiation are either forbidden or handled very restrictively in most countries. Steam treatment is currently the method of first choice, however it is expensive and can lead to degradation of plant constituents and quality (Kabelitz, 2001; Kabelitz and Sievers, 2004).

Contamination with mycotoxins

Mycotoxins are metabolites produced by toxigenic fungi, such as *Aspergillus*, *Penicillium* or *Fusarium* species and include aflatoxins, ochratoxins and zearalenone (Kabelitz and Sievers, 2004). Mycotoxins are heat-stable, so they are not destroyed by cooking or normal industrial processing. The presence of mycotoxins and mycotoxin-producing fungi has repeatedly been reported in medicinal plants and preparations derived from them.

Mycotoxins demonstrate a wide range of toxic effects including teratogenicity and carcinogenicity (Creppy, 2002) and mycotoxin limits for certain food products have been specified in EU food regulations for a long time. In these regulations limits are given for aflatoxin B1, aflatoxin M1 as well as for total aflatoxins (B1, B2, G1, G2) and for other mycotoxins such as ochratoxin A, fusarium toxins and patulin. In these regulations the maximum levels for several spices such as *Capsicum* ssp., *Piper* ssp. and *Zingiber officinale* Rosc. have been set to 5 µg/kg aflatoxin B1 and 10 µg/kg aflatoxin B1+B2+G1+G2 (EC No. 1881/2006, EC No. 1126/2007). In the 2005 European Pharmacopoeia, no mycotoxin limits are specified yet for herbal drugs or herbal medicinal products but a method for the determination of aflatoxins in certain herbal drugs is currently in preparation. Germany has stipulated maximum levels for herbal drugs (Table 28.2) (Aflatoxin Verbots V, 2000).

Mycotoxins can be detected by TLC, HPLC, GC-MS or ELISA techniques. WHO suggested an HPLC method for aflatoxin determination including precolumn derivatisation and fluorometric detection of the derivatives (WHO, 1998). Tasseneeyakul *et al.* (2004) used HPLC for the determination of aflatoxins in 28 Thai herbal medicinal products where extracts prepared from the samples were cleaned up by an immunoaffinity column, followed by post-column derivatisation with iodine and fluorescence detection. They could detect aflatoxins in five of the samples, with total aflatoxin levels ranging from 1.7 to 14.3 ng/g, which is below the current tolerance level stipulated in Thailand (20 ng/g). However, attention has to be paid when exporting these products in countries with lower tolerance levels, e.g. Europe.

Reports on mycotoxin contamination of Chinese herbal drugs are scarce. Ihrig *et al.* (2004) found aflatoxin B1 levels significantly above the German limit of 2 µg/kg aflatoxin B1 in Semen Biotae samples (2.4 and 22 µg/kg in two different samples). The used determination method (DIN EN 12955, 1999) includes HPLC immunoaffinity column cleanup and post-column derivatisation.

Methods used for authentication, quality control and standardisation of Chinese herbal drugs

Quality can only be produced; it cannot be transferred into a product by applying analytical methods to it. Nevertheless, methods of quality control have to be applied at different stages of production (Chan, 2003).

In general, the methods for identification and quality control of herbal medicines involve sensory

Table 28.1 Microbiological threshold levels tolerated by Ph Eur[a], PhPRP[d], WHO[c] and EHIA[b]

Authority	Category	Bacteria, yeast and mould count	Enterobacteria and certain other Gram-negative bacteria	*E. coli*	*Salmonella*	*Staph. aureus*
Ph. Eur.[a]	3B (oral preparations containing raw materials of natural origin for which antimicrobial treatment is not feasible and for which microbial contamination exceeding 10^3 viable counts/g or mL is accepted, with exception of category 4)	bacteria: $\leq 10^4$ aerobic CFU/g or mL moulds: $\leq 10^2$ aerobic CFU/g or mL	$\leq 10^2$ CFU/g or mL	absent in 1 g or 1 mL	absent in 10 g or 10 mL	absent in 1 g or 1 mL
	4A (crude herbal materials to which boiling water is added before use)	bacteria: $\leq 10^7$ aerobic CFU/g or mL moulds: $\leq 10^5$ aerobic CFU/g or mL	not specified	$\leq 10^2$ CFU/g or mL	not specified	not specified
	4B (crude herbal materials to which boiling water is not added before use)	Bacteria: $\leq 10^5$ aerobic CFU/g or mL Moulds: $\leq 10^4$ aerobic CFU/g or mL	$\leq 10^3$ CFU/g or mL	absent in 1 g or 1 mL	absent in 10 g or 10 mL	not specified
EHIA[b]	Herbal infusion raw materials	bacteria: $\leq 10^8$/aerobic CFU/g yeasts: $\leq 10^6$ CFU/g moulds: $\leq 10^6$ CFU/g	not specified	$\leq 10^4$/g	absent in 25 g	not specified
WHO[c]	Untreated plant material harvested under acceptable hygienic conditions and intended for further processing (including additional decontamination by a physical or chemical process)	moulds: $\leq 10^5$ CFU/g	not specified	$\leq 10^4$ CFU/g	not specified	not specified
	Pretreated plant materials (e.g. infusions with boiling water) or topically used preparations	bacteria: $\leq 10^7$ aerobic CFU/g yeasts and moulds: $\leq 10^4$ CFU/g	$\leq 10^4$ CFU/g	$\leq 10^2$ CFU/g	absent in 10 g	not specified
	Other plant materials for internal use	bacteria: $\leq 10^5$ aerobic CFU/g yeasts and moulds: $\leq 10^3$ CFU/g	$\leq 10^3$ CFU/g	≤ 10 CFU/g	absent in 10 g	not specified

Table 28.1 (*continued*)

PhPRP[d] (Examples)	Tablets	Without crude drug powder	bacteria: $\leq 10^3$ CFU/g or mL yeasts and moulds: $\leq 10^2$ CFU/g or mL	not specified	absent in 1 g or 1 mL	not specified	not specified
		With crude drug powder	bacteria: $\leq 10^4$ CFU/g or mL yeasts and moulds: ≤ 100 /g or mL	not specified	absent in 1 g or 1 mL	not specified	not specified
	Medicinal granules	Without crude drug powder	bacteria: $\leq 10^3$ CFU/g or mL yeasts and moulds: $\leq 10^2$ CFU/g or mL	not specified	absent in 1 g or 1 mL	not specified	not specified
		With crude drug powder	bacteria: $\leq 10^4$ CFU/g or mL yeasts and moulds: $\leq 10^2$ CFU/g	not specified	not specified	not specified	not specified
	Medicinal teas	Without sugar	bacteria $\leq 10^4$ /g or mL yeasts and moulds $\leq 10^2$ CFU/g or mL	not specified	not specified	not specified	not specified
		With sugar	bacteria: $\leq 10^3$ CFU/g or mL yeasts and moulds $\leq 10^2$ CFU/g or mL	not specified	not specified	not specified	not specified
Authority	**Category**		**Bacteria, yeast and mould count**	**Enterobacteria and certain other Gram-negative bacteria**	***E. coli***	***Salmonella***	***Staph. aureus***

[a]European Pharmacopoeia, 2005; [b]EHIA, 2005; [c]WHO, 1998; [d]Pharmacopoeia of the People's Republic of China (2005).

Table 28.2 Tolerance levels for aflatoxins in drugs according to the German regulations[a]

Aflatoxin	Tolerance level
M1	≤0.05 μg/kg
B1	≤2 μg/kg
B1, B2, G1, G2	≤4 μg/kg

[a]Aflatoxin Verbots V, 2000.

inspection (macroscopic and microscopic examination), molecular biological methods and analytical inspection comprising mainly chromatographic and spectroscopic techniques.

Macroscopic, microscopic and botanical authentication

For botanical identification, the intact plant material is examined, ideally during collection or harvest, while for macroscopic identification the morphological or organoleptic (sensory) characteristics of particular plant parts or fragments are studied. These techniques require high expertise, and often access to voucher specimens in working herbaria or to a photographic reference library if necessary (Techen *et al.*, 2004).

Microscopic examination allows the identification of crude plant material in the whole, fragmented or powdered stage. The method also requires high expertise, and sometimes it may not provide unequivocal authentication because of the fact that different medicinal materials, particularly from related species, often possess similar microscopic characteristics. Factors such as climate, harvesting period and storage conditions may also influence the microscopic structure of the material (Shaw *et al.*, 2002a; Bauer and Wagner, 2004).

Compared with other techniques, macroscopic and microscopic identification are very cost- and time-efficient. Therefore, these authentication methods play an important role in the monographs on herbs in many pharmacopoeias, including the Chinese and the European pharmacopoeias. The book *Microscopic Identification of Chinese Materia Medica*, edited by Zhao (2005) contains photographs of the microscopic characteristics of 126 commonly used Chinese materia medica, which are very helpful for microscopic authentication of these materials.

DNA-based techniques

DNA-based authentication comprises various techniques which are used for analysing DNA sequences and fingerprints. These techniques are employed in various fields such as taxonomy, physiology, embryology and genetics and have been successfully applied in the field of commercially important plants such as food crops and horticultural plants. The application of molecular methods to the authentication of Chinese medicinal materials was initiated in the mid-1990s (Shaw *et al.*, 2002b; Joshi *et al.*, 2004) when DNA-based techniques were used for differentiation of accessions collected at different geographic regions, differentiation of inter- and intraspecific variations, authentication of plants frequently substituted with species which are indistinguishable by macroscopic, microscopic or phytochemical methods, and for detection of adulterations. Attempts have also been made to identify DNA markers that can correlate DNA fingerprinting data with the quantity of phytochemical markers since this would allow the prediction of the concentration of active compounds and the marker-assisted selection of desirable chemotypes (Joshi *et al.*, 2004).

DNA markers are reliable for informative polymorphisms as the genetic composition is unique for each species and is not affected by age, physiological conditions and environmental factors. They are not tissue-specific and can be detected at any stage of organism development (Shaw *et al.*, 2002a; Chan, 2003). Only small sample amounts are needed for most methods. This makes DNA-based methods interesting for authentication of fragile, animal-derived and precious drugs. Despite these advantages, DNA-related techniques are not yet routinely used for authentication of TCM drugs as the methods are relatively expensive and as their application can be problematic in case of dried or processed materials (Zhao *et al.*, 2006).

Hybridisation-based methods

Hybridisation-based methods use cloned DNA elements or synthetic oligonucleotides as probes to hybridise DNA. The probes are labelled with radioisotopes or with conjugated enzymes which catalyse a colour reaction to detect hybridisation. DNA is either cleaved with restriction enzymes or first amplified by polymerase chain reaction (PCR), subsequently separated by gel electrophoresis and transferred to a solid support matrix (Shaw *et al.*, 2002a, Joshi *et al.*, 2004).

Restriction fragment length polymorphism (RFLP) is a technique in which organisms may be differentiated by analysis of patterns derived from cleavage of their DNA. It is a mostly hybridisation-based method used in paternity cases or criminal cases to determine the source of a DNA sample, but also widely applied in genome mapping, marker-aided breeding and phylogenetic studies. In this technique, restriction polymorphisms are detected by using a hybridisation probe. The quality of the assay is highly dependent on the choice of the DNA probe. Two types of DNA probes can be used, namely tandem repeats which occur as clusters among chromosomes and dispersed repeats which are scattered all over the chromosomes. Shorter repeating sequences (generally fewer than six base pairs) which are repeated from a few to many thousands of times, are abundant in the eukaryote genome. They are called microsatellites or single sequence repeat (SSR) (Shaw *et al.*, 2002a).

The major limitation of this method is its low sensitivity. It requires a large amount of high-quality genomic DNA, which is very difficult to obtain from processed herbal drugs. Also the stability and reproducibility are rather low because the quality of the assay highly depends on DNA quality and technical factors (Hon *et al.*, 2003).

For Chinese medicinal materials, PCR-RFLP is more suitable, as it requires a much lower amount of DNA. In this method a defined DNA sequence is first amplified by PCR and then selected restriction enzymes are employed to generate fragments unique to the respective species (Shaw *et al.*, 2002a).

Polymerase-chain-reaction-based methods

PCR enzymatically multiplies particular DNA sequences or loci of a template DNA with the help of arbitrary or specific oligonucleotide primers.

It is not easy to standardise PCR-based authentication procedures for medicinal plants. Reasons for variations are different DNA polymerases used, different buffer formulations as well as different equipment used. Variations can be reduced if the same commercial kits or polymerase mixtures are used in each lab performing the same test. Problems also occur when the plant material of interest contains compounds such as phenolics which can interact with the DNA and directly inhibit DNA polymerase or damage the structural integrity of DNA. The way a plant is harvested, stored and processed can also influence DNA quality (Techen *et al.*, 2004).

Various PCR-based techniques have been employed to authenticate and characterise medicinal plants; some of them do not require prior knowledge of the DNA sequence, for example AFLP, random amplified polymorphic DNA (RAPD), arbitrarily primed PCR (AP-PCR) and inter simple sequence repeat (ISSR); while for others, such as SSR, prior sequence information is required.

Amplified fragment length polymorphism

This fingerprinting technique is based on the detection of multiple DNA restriction fragments by means of PCR amplification and has the capacity to detect thousands of independent loci (Joshi *et al.*, 2004). Genomic DNA is digested by appropriate restriction enzymes (preferably a hexa-cutter or tetra-cutter), which cut DNA at defined sequence sites. A subset of the resultant fragments is then ligated to synthetic double-stranded adaptors (DNA segments) at each end and subsequently amplified using two specific adaptor-homologous primers. The amplified and labelled restriction fragments are separated on denaturating gels or by capillary electrophoresis. The complexity of the AFLP profiles depends on the primers and restriction enzymes chosen and on the level of sequence polymorphism between the tested DNA samples (Shaw *et al.*, 2002a).

The number of amplified bands of the preselected PCR is usually so high that a second round of PCR (selective PCR with fluorescent dyes) has to be performed to reduce the number of amplified products. This is done by using primers that possess 1–3 additional bases at the 3′ end. Several combinations have to be tested for optimisation. Digestion, ligation and two rounds of PCR make this method expensive and time-consuming. However, it is a very reliable and robust technology, and it has been widely applied in screening DNA markers linked to genetic traits, parentage analysis, forensic genotyping and population genetics (McGregor *et al.*, 2000; Techen *et al.*, 2004). However, the feasibility for the authentication of Chinese herbs might be limited, because high-quality DNA, especially high-molecular-weight DNA, is required, which might be a problem in the case of processed or dried medicinal materials (Ha *et al.*, 2002).

Arbitrarily primed PCR and random amplified polymorphic DNA

These methods have been simultaneously developed by two groups in 1990. Basically, instead of using region-specific PCR primers or adaptors, one single, arbitrarily chosen oligonucleotide is used as both the forward and reverse primer in a PCR reaction. This sequence consists of about 10 nucleotides in case of RAPD and about 20 nucleotides in case of AP-PCR. A product is produced when the primer binds on opposite strands, in the reverse orientation and within an amplifiable distance. PCR fragments are generated from different locations of the genome, because there are multiple sites within the genome for the primer to bind. Thus, multiple loci may be examined simultaneously. Using series of different primers allows the generation of a genetic fingerprint of a plant or a specific species (Shaw *et al.*, 2002a; Techen *et al.*, 2004).

RAPD analysis is a quick, rather easy and relatively cheap method; a major drawback is that reproducibility between laboratories has been shown to be low because the procedure is very sensitive to different PCR parameters, especially to slight variations in annealing temperature because of the low annealing temperatures required (McGregor *et al.*, 2000; Techen *et al.*, 2004). Nevertheless, RAPD and AP-PCR have extensively been used to study the genetic diversity of various Chinese medicinal plants, to discriminate different plant populations and to differentiate plant batches of different provenances (Shaw *et al.*, 2002a).

Zhang *et al.* (2001) successfully used an RAPD technique to distinguish *Lycium barbarum* L. from other closely related species of the same genus which are not listed for medical use in the 2005 Chinese pharmacopoeia.

Cheng (2002) employed an RAPD method for the identification of three plant species from an herbal mixture with one single primer. After screening 40 different primers, one was selected to simultaneously identify *Astragalus membranaceus* (Fisch.) Bge., *Atractylodes macrocephala* Koidz and *Ledebouriella seseloides* Wolff in the prescription. Ten samples purchased from different stores were evaluated and showed the three markers simultaneously, but the intensity of the *L. seseloides* marker varied among the samples. According to the authors, it remains to be investigated whether the admixture of closely related species can be detected with this method.

Fico *et al.* (2003) investigated different *Aconitum* species and subspecies using both RAPD and phytochemical analysis, and they found that the patterns of relatedness observed in the chemical profiles seem to correspond with the genetic profiles, suggesting that there may be a genetic basis for the chemical profiles observed.

Inter simple sequence repeat (ISSR)

ISSR makes use of anchored primers to amplify simple sequence repeats. The primers are not totally arbitrary but are composed of repeated di-, tri-, tetra- or pentanucleotid motifs which are scattered throughout the eukaryote genome. As in RAPD analysis, a product is achieved when the same repeat is present in the two DNA strands within an amplifiable distance. Specificity and reproducibility can be enhanced by addition of a different base at 3′ or 5′. Because longer primers are used, the method is more reliable and less sensitive to annealing temperature than RAPD analysis; however, the annealing temperature has to be optimised for each primer and species DNA. Compared with AFLP and SSR analysis, the method is rather quick, straightforward and economic (McGregor *et al.*, 2000; Techen *et al.*, 2004).

Simple sequence repeat (SSR)

For this technique, prior sequence information is required. SSR markers or microsatellites (also termed simple sequence length polymorphism [SSLP] or sequence-tagged microsatellite site [STMS]) are tandem repeats scattered throughout the genome. They can be amplified using primers that flank these regions. The technique has been successfully used to construct detailed genetic maps of several organisms and to study genetic variation within populations of the same species (Shaw *et al.*, 2002a). As the markers are usually species-specific, their development is rather costly, but once they have been developed the method becomes quite inexpensive (McGregor *et al.*, 2000).

Hon *et al.* (2003) compared the advantages and limitations of some PCR-based techniques, namely RAPD, and AP-PCR, PCR-RFLP and microsatellite marker techniques, and of a hybridisation-based technique, namely DNA fingerprinting with low-cost (rapid reassociating fraction) DNA probes, using ginseng as an example. They conclude that microsatellite marker techniques are most suitable for the authentication of ginseng samples, because unambiguous identification of botanical identity and origin was possible. The authors point out that the main limitations of this technique are the high costs and labour-intensive search for informative loci. However, it is superior to other methods in terms of information content, accuracy, sensitivity, reliability and reproducibility. Moreover, the method can be fully automated, which makes it interesting for large-scale, high-throughput authentication.

Sequencing-based markers and microarray techniques

Concerning these techniques, DNA sequences from the nuclear and chloroplast genome are used for identification of plants at several taxonomic levels. Certain sequences such as the 5S rDNA spacer and the internal transcribed spacer (ITS) regions between the 16S and 26S rDNA are highly variable and can thus be used for authentication at species level. Sequences such as nuclear 18S or plastidal rbcL, ndhF or matK however, are conserved among species and therefore suitable for discrimination at genus or family level (Shaw *et al.*, 2002a, 2002b; Joshi *et al.*, 2004; Techen *et al.*, 2004). DNA sequence-based techniques have widely been used for authentication of Chinese herbs.

For example, Zhao *et al.* (2003) amplified and sequenced the 5S rRNA spacer domains of three different *Angelica* species, namely *A. sinensis* (Oliv.) Diels (*Danggui*) and its potential substitutes *A. acutiloba* (Sieb. Et Zucc.) Kitag., which is mainly found in Japan as well as *A. gigas* Nakai, which mainly occurs in Korea. The authors demonstrated that the diversity of the spacer regions can be used for genetic differentiation of the three species. Additionally, HPLC analyses were performed, to study the chemical profile of the three species and of different provenances.

In a similar study, Xia *et al.* (2005) performed a DNA sequence analysis and a chemical fingerprint analysis of five *Curcuma* species, namely *C. wenyujin* Y.H. Chen et C. Ling, *C. phaeaocaulis* Val. and *C. kwangsiensis* S.G. Lee et C.F. Liang, which are used as Rhizoma Curcumae, and *C. longa* L. and *C. chuanyujin* C.K. Hsieh et H. Zhang, which are frequently found as adulterants of Rhizoma Curcumae. Sequence analysis of the 5S-rRNA spacer domains revealed that the three species officinal as Rhizoma Curcumae are closely related, whereas the other two species show significant DNA differences. The same result was obtained by cluster analysis of the respective HPLC fingerprints.

Microarray-based methods work by hybridisation of RNA or DNA to complementary DNA molecules bound at specific locations on the array. Hybridisation can be detected by labelling with hybridisation indicators or by other changes resulting from the binding event. With microarrays, thousands of sequences can simultaneously be detected quickly, sensitively and selectively. As different species possess different genomes, each species will produce a specific array pattern (Shaw *et al.*, 2002b).

Carles *et al.* (2001) have been working on the development of a DNA microarray technique for the identification of Chinese medicinal plants, and presented a DNA micorarray which is feasible for the authentication of 20 different toxic Chinese herbs (Carles *et al.*, 2005). Species-specific oligonucleotide probes were derived from the 5S rRNA gene, but also from the leucine tRNA gene of the respective plants.

In summary, DNA-based authentication methods have several advantages which make them suitable for the identification of Chinese herbs:

- the techniques are independent from the physical form of the material
- only a low amount of material is required
- DNA-based markers represent the most basic signature of an organism and are therefore much less affected by environmental influences than phenotypic markers.

On the other hand, some limitations have to be considered:

- some of the methods are strongly dependent on DNA quality, which might be a problem in the case of dried or processed materials
- certain plant compounds or fungal contamination may also influence DNA extraction or PCR reaction.

To establish a marker for identification of a particular species, DNA analysis of closely related species and/or varieties as well as common contaminants and adulterants is necessary, a very expensive and time-consuming process (Joshi *et al.*, 2004).

The DNA-based investigation of herbal samples for unknown contaminants is at present extremely difficult and costly because of the broad spectrum of possible admixtures. More comprehensive databases of DNA fingerprints and DNA sequences comprising a wide range of plant species would therefore be required (Techen *et al.*, 2004).

The application of DNA-related techniques in the quality control of herbs is also limited by the fact that the DNA fingerprint of a plant is the same for the whole plant, while the content of biomarker or marker compounds is often strongly dependent on the plant part. Moreover, DNA fingerprinting might allow correct authentication of a plant but at present, it does not give information about the concentration of active constituents or marker compounds. This means that a combination of DNA-related and phytochemical techniques is necessary for quality control applications (Joshi *et al.*, 2004). Some attempts have been made to match the results of DNA-related techniques to chemical profiles of Chinese herbs (Fico *et al.*, 2003; Xia *et al.*, 2005), but it is too early to draw general conclusions on the feasibility of this approach.

Finally, DNA-based techniques generally cannot be used for preparations containing herbal extracts, even though the successful authentication of herbal starting materials based on DNA extracted from small amounts of plant cells which are still present in herbal extracts and tinctures has been recently reported (Novak *et al.*, 2007). However, more experience is required to evaluate the general feasibility of such a technique.

To summarise, DNA-related techniques are a valuable complement, but not a replacement for macroscopic, microscopic and phytochemical methods.

Immunochemical methods

Antibodies are very powerful identification tools. A single difference in the amino acid sequence may change the epitope of a protein which is recognised by an antibody (Shaw *et al.*, 2002a). Antibodies can also be raised against conjugates of proteins and naturally occurring plant constituents. These antibodies can then be used for qualitative and quantitative determination of the respective compounds.

As an example, Fukuda *et al.* (2000) produced a monoclonal antibody against ginsenoside Rg1, which only showed very low cross-reactivity with structurally closely related compounds and is therefore feasible for the determination of ginsenoside Rg1 in crude plant extracts without any pretreatment.

Lu and coworkers (2003) developed a quantitative ELISA using monoclonal antibodies for the detection of paeoniflorin and albiflorin in crude drugs and preparations of *Paeonia lactiflora* Pallas. The results of quantitative determination showed good agreement with results obtained by HPLC analysis. The ELISA kit was about 100 times more sensitive than the HPLC method.

Immunochemical analyses are highly reproducible and show high selectivity and sensitivity. Diagnostic kits can be developed for rapid testing. They can be used for raw materials as well as for processed drugs and extracts. However, development of immunochemical methods is extremely elaborate and time consuming.

Chromatographic techniques

Chromatographic techniques are the most versatile tools for the analysis of Chinese herbs. They can be employed for identification and authentication as well as for determination of various adulterants and contaminants and for standardisation purposes. In contrary to macroscopic, microscopic and many molecular biological methods they are not restricted to the raw herb, but can also be applied to pharmaceutical preparations.

There are two approaches in the use of chromatographic methods for quality-control purposes:

- analysis based on marker or biomarker compounds
- chromatographic fingerprint analysis.

A marker compound can be any constituent characterising a plant of interest; biomarkers are bioactive plant constituents, representing a plant's pharmacological activity (Techen *et al.*, 2004). Conventional research and quality control of herbal medicines focus on the analysis of one or several bioactive or characteristic lead compounds (Bauer, 1998). This approach is widely used in industry and also in many pharmacopoeial monographs.

If the bioactive compound is known, the preparation can be standardised on this compound in terms of a normalisation. This means that the content of the active principle can be adjusted by addition of inert material or by blending with a highly concentrated batch. In case of several bioactive constituents, standardisation is more complicated, because the ratios of active constituents can vary from batch to batch. The material has to be standardised by blending with batches of higher or lower quality. In case the active principles of an herb are unknown, characteristic marker compounds must be used for quality control. However, normalisation on these marker compounds is not recommendable as they might not be related to therapeutic activity (Bauer, 1998; McCutcheon, 2002). For this reason the 2005 European Pharmacopoeia discriminates between standardised extracts (standardisation to a certain content of known active compounds is achieved by mixing with inert material or by blending with other extract batches), quantified extracts (not all active compounds known; standardisation to a defined range of active markers is achieved by blending of extract batches) and other extracts, which are mainly defined by their production process (starting material, solvent, extraction conditions).

In many TCM herbs standardisation referring to one lead compound is difficult, as reference compounds are often not available. In addition the complexity of many herbal medicines makes this kind of analysis during pharmaceutical quality control rather tedious. In this case fingerprint analysis might be a more appropriate method for quality control (Bauer, 1998; Li *et al.*, 2004a; Yang *et al.*, 2005). To additionally represent bioactivity by the chromatographic fingerprint, the suggestion has been made to match the fingerprint profile of an herbal preparation to the results of biological assays or clinical studies (Yuan and Lin, 2000).

The concept of chromatographic fingerprinting for herbal materials is also appreciated by some authorities: The US Food and Drug Administration (FDA) proposed to accept the technique for the identification of herbal materials (FDA, 2000) and the World Health Organization (WHO) has also shown interest (WHO, 2000). Furthermore, in China, the State Drug Administration (SFDA) decided that registration of injections made of Chinese medicines requires chromatographic fingerprints characterising the products (Wong *et al.*, 2002).

A chromatographic fingerprint is a chromatogram representing the chemical characteristics of an herbal material. (HP)TLC, GC, HPLC, CE, high-speed countercurrent chromatography and some hyphenated techniques have already been used for the development of chromatographic fingerprints (Fan *et al.*, 2006). Hyphenated techniques have been shown to be very useful because of the additional spectral information, which allows elimination of instrumental interferences and correction of retention time shifts and leads to better selectivity and measurement precision (Liang *et al.*, 2004).

Thin-layer chromatography

The advantages of using TLC for quality control of herbal drugs are its simplicity, versatility, high velocity, specificity, sensitivity and simple sample preparation. With the help of image analysis and digital technologies developed in computer science, the evaluation of similarity between different samples is possible. Various pharmacopoeias such as the 2005 Chinese pharmacopoeia as well as the series *Chinese Drug Monographs and Analysis* (Wagner *et al.*, 2006) use TLC to provide characteristic fingerprints of Chinese herbs (for example see Figure 28.1).

TLC is widely used for a first screening and semi-quantitiative evaluation and very often combined with other chromatographic methods.

As an example, Blatter and Reich (2004) developed two improved HPTLC methods for the quality

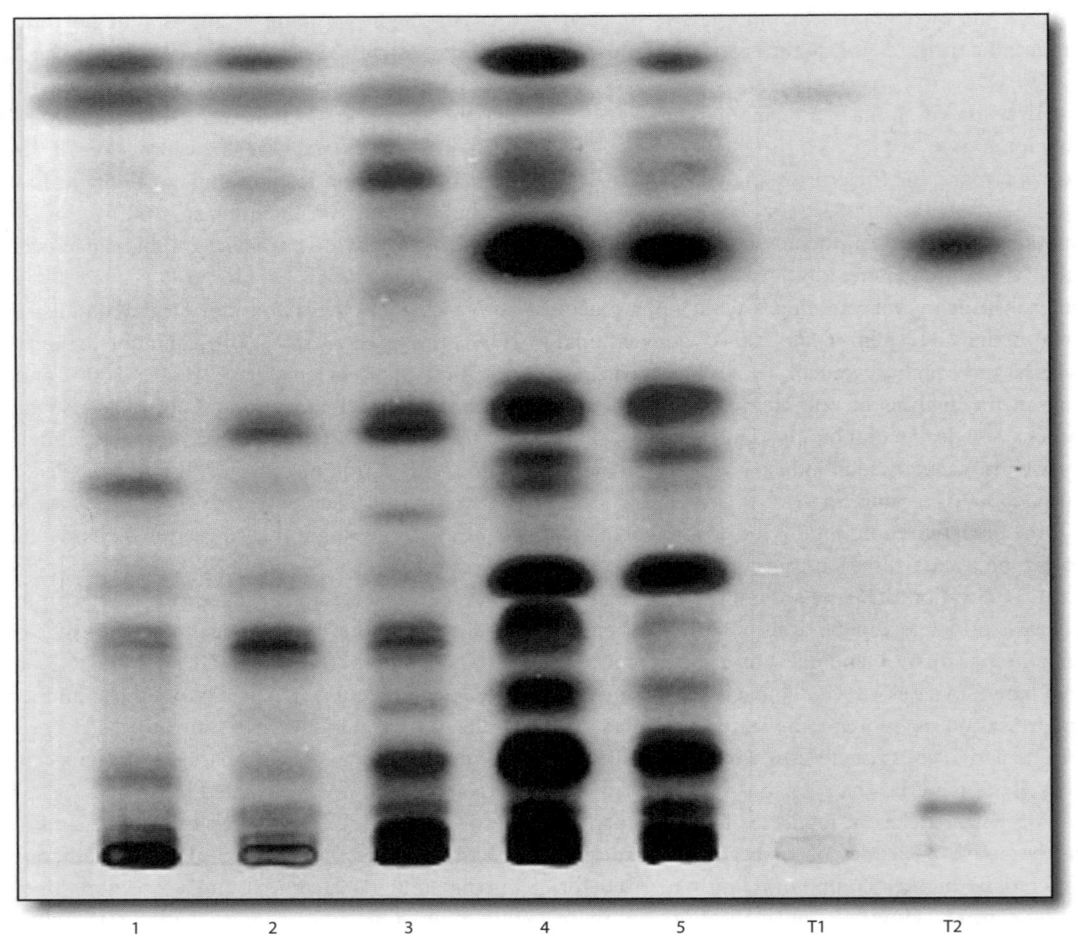

Figure 28.1 Thin-layer chromatogram of different *Atractylodes* species and reference compounds (Silica, n-hexane/ethylacetate 95:5; detection: anisaldehyde-sulphuric acid reagent, VIS) (reprinted from Resch *et al.*, 1999). Samples: 1 = *Atractylodes macrocephala* rhizomes (TCM-hospital Kötzting, Germany); 2 = *A. japonica* rhizomes (Botanical Garden of the University of Düsseldorf); 3 = *A. koreana* rhizomes (Kang Weon Province, Korea); 4 = *A. lancea* rhizomes (TCM-hospital Kötzting, Germany); 5 = *A. chinensis* rhizomes (Kunming); reference compounds: T1 = atractylon; T2 = atractylodin I.

control of *Stephania tetrandra* S. Moore. The first method allowed unambiguous identification of the herb as well as quantitative determination of the main alkaloid tetrandrin using scanning densitometry at 210 nm. The second method was developed to detect adulteration of the drug with drugs containing aristolochic acid. The method allowed the detection of 1 ppm aristolochic acid after derivatisation with tin(II) chloride.

Zhao *et al.* (2005) developed a densitometric HPTLC method, which allows the simultaneous qualitative and quantitative determination of emodin, resveratrol and polydatin, the main bioactive constituents of *Polygonum cuspidatum* Willd. ex Spreng.

Di *et al.* (2003) used HPTLC with automated multiple development (AMD), a technique which allows gradient elution in TLC, for fingerprint profiling of carbohydrates from the fruiting bodies of various *linghzi* (*Ganoderma*) species. The method consisted of an optimised acid hydrolysis of the carbohydrates extracted with water from linghzi followed by AMD separation and post-chromatographic derivatisation with 4-aminobenzoic acid and densitometric detection. Although some species could be successfully differentiated, the authors had problems with the differentiation of closely related species because of the similarity of the profiles obtained.

HPLC and hyphenated techniques

Over the past decades, HPLC has been widely applied for the analysis of herbal medicines because of its high separation capacity. It can be employed to analyse almost all constituents of herbal products provided that an optimised procedure is developed which involves optimisation of mobile and stationary phase (Li *et al.*, 2005). Another advantage of this technique is the possibility of coupling it to various detection techniques such as ultraviolet diode array detection (DAD), mass spectrometry (MS) or even nuclear magnetic resonance (NMR). These hyphenated techniques can provide information about the structure of the compounds present in a chromatogram. In addition, some hyphenated methods provide higher sensitivity compared with conventional approaches.

HPLC-DAD

HPLC-DAD is by far the most common hyphenated instrument, and for most TCM manufacturers it is a practical and meaningful technique for efficient quality control. DAD can be used for identification of chromatogram peaks, simultaneous determination, peak purity control, chromatographic discrepancy correction and fingerprint generation (Yan *et al.*, 2005a). The technique is also widely applied for identification and quality control of Chinese herbs in various pharmacopoeial monographs, as well as in the series *Chinese Drug Monographs and Analysis* (Wagner *et al.*, 2006). Only a few examples are mentioned below.

He *et al.* (2005) analysed methanolic extracts of 44 samples of cassia bark (*Cinnamomum* spp.) and related materials from different regions as well as four types of commercial commodities (debarked cortex, *qi-bian-gui*, bark and twigs) by HPLC with respect to four marker compounds. The chromatographic fingerprint and the content of marker compounds varied considerably depending on species and commercial commodity. Thus, authentication and quality assessment of genuine cassia bark (*C. cassia* Presl.) was possible with this method.

Zschocke *et al.* (2005) developed an HPLC-DAD method for the analysis of *Ligusticum chuanxiong* Hort. For the unequivocal direct identification of the main constituents of the hexane extract, namely the phtalides senkyunolide A, butylphtalide, neocnidilide and Z-ligustilide, the authors used HPLC-NMR and HPLC-MS, which made isolation of these compounds unnecessary. Having confirmed the structures, HPLC-DAD proved to be a feasible tool for analysis of the extract because, owing to their different chromophores, the DAD spectra of the compounds were very characteristic (Figure 28.2).

Yang *et al.* (2005) developed a fingerprint-based, quality-control method for *Hypericum japonicum* Thunb. (*tianjihuang*) using HPLC-DAD. Hydroethanolic extracts of 56 authentic samples were compared and similarity was mathematically assessed using a software recommended by the SFDA. They showed that the similarity of fingerprints was very strongly dependent on the geographic origin of the respective herbs. Within the provenances, time-dependent changes in secondary metabolite profiles were found, providing information for optimum harvest time.

Fan *et al.* (2006) propose multiple chromatographic fingerprinting which involves more than one fingerprint and represents the whole chemical characteristics of the analyte as a strategy for quality control of complex herbal medicines. They demonstrated their approach by developing and validating a binary HPLC fingerprint method for Danshen Dropping Pill, a popular Chinese formulation, which is composed of *Salvia miltiorrhiza* Bunge (*danshen*) and *Panax notoginseng* (Burk.) F.H. Chen (*sanqi*). Two fingerprint chromatograms were produced, one for the depsides and one for the saponins present in the preparation. A data fusion-based method was employed to evaluate the similarity of multiple chromatographic fingerprints, and principal component analysis (PCA) was used for the detection of frauds.

Yan *et al.* (2005a) propose two-dimensional fingerprint analysis, to fully utilise DAD information. As an example, they used *Qinkailing* injection, a very complex preparation containing eight medical materials. They achieved the 2D-fingerprint by PCA of the HPLC-DAD data and successfully applied it to classify various Qinkailing samples.

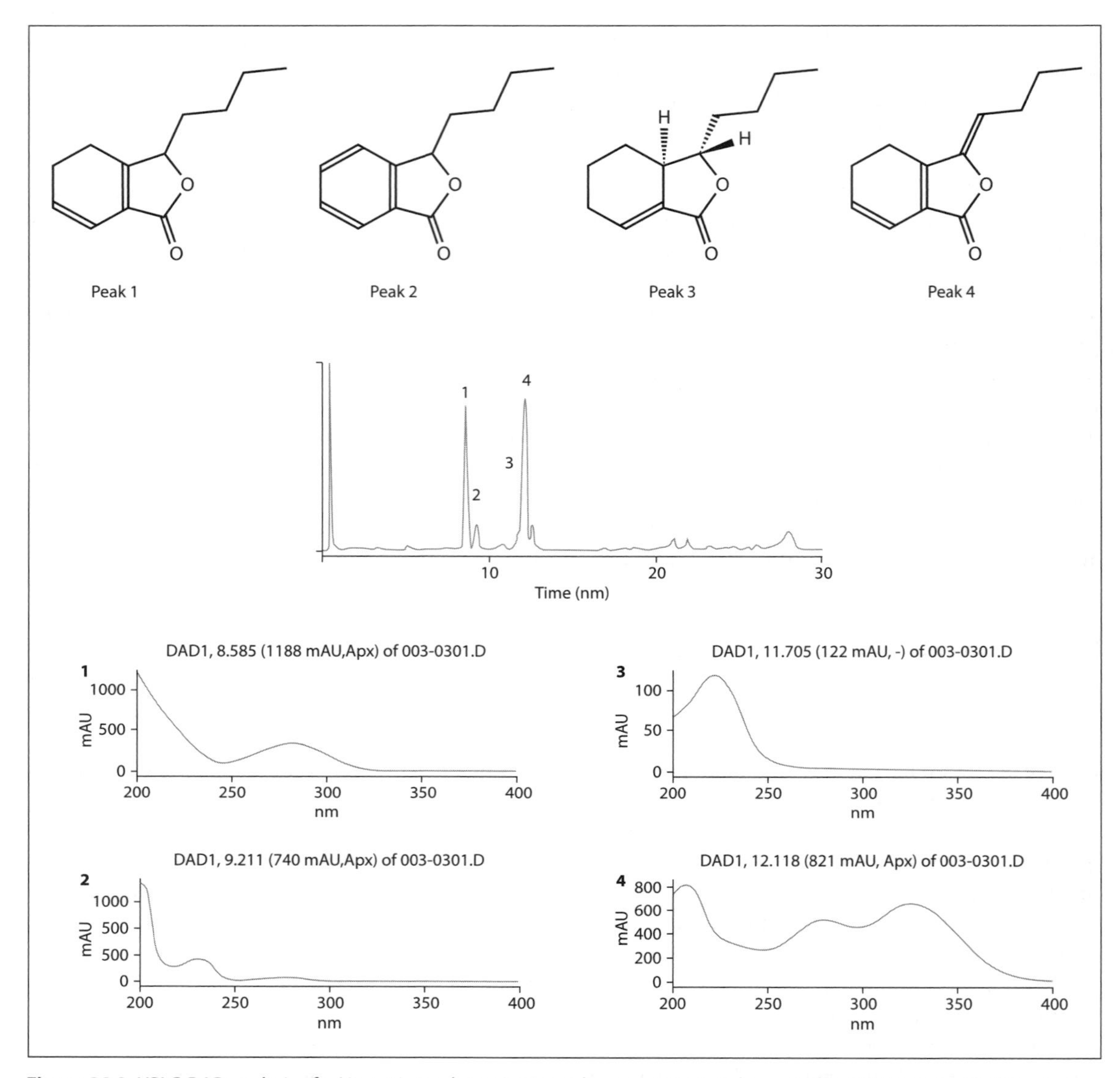

Figure 28.2 HPLC-DAD analysis of a *Lingusticum chuanxiong* root hexane extract. Column: LiChroCART 125-4 with LiChroSpher 100 RP-18 (5 μm), Merck; precolumn: LiChroCART 4-4 with LiChroSpher 100 RP-18 (5 μm), Merck. Mobile phase: A = distilled water, B = acetonitrile; gradient: 40–55% B, linear in 15 min, 55–95% B, linear in 18 min, 95% B, isocratic for 2 min; flow: 1 ml/min; column temperature: 40 °C; UV-detection: 210 nm. Peak 1: senkyunolide A, peak 2: butylphtalide, peak 3: neocnidilide, peak 4: Z-ligustilide. (From Zschocke *et al.*, with permission from Springer Science and Business Media.)

HPLC-MS and HPLC-DAD-MS

The importance of LC-MS has strongly increased in Chinese medicinal product research, because with this technique a wide variety of plant constituents ranging from small molecules to macromolecules such as peptides, proteins, carbohydrates and nucleic acids can be characterised. Apart from quantitative analysis, applications have been expanding rapidly into the area of structural elucidation and characterisation of active compounds (Cai *et al.*, 2002).

Coupling liquid chromatography with mass spectrometry has become possible with the atmospheric pressure ionisation methods, electrospray ionisation (ESI) and atmospheric pressure ionisation (APCI)

(Wang *et al.*, 2003). Other ion sources frequently applied in natural product analysis are thermospray ionisation and matrix-assisted laser desorption ionisation (MALDI) (Wolfender *et al.*, 1998; Wang *et al.*, 2003).

Tandem mass spectrometry (MS-MS) is highly feasible for detection of target compounds in complex matrices. The advantages of this technique are its selectivity, high sensitivity and fast screening capabilities. Among the various mass filters, quadrupole mass filters show excellent properties in terms of quantitative analysis, while ion trap MS has been widely used for structural identification. LC-MS with ion trap mass analysis offers the possibility of multiple-stage tandem mass spectrometry (MS^n), as the ion trap produces fragment product ions through multiple generations. This is a powerful tool for the unambiguous identification of plant constituents (Cai *et al.*, 2002).

Continuous MALDI sources, configured with time of flight-mass spectrometers (TOF-MS), which are extensively used in protein, nucleotide and sequence analysis, have also already been used for the analysis of medicinal herbs (Wang *et al.*, 2003). This technique is especially useful for determination of polar plant constituents (Cai *et al.*, 2002).

The main challenge of the application of LC-MS to the analysis of herbal extracts consists in finding an ionisation method suitable for the large variety of compounds present in a crude plant extract. Even though many interfaces are available, no single one allows universal detection of all constituents (Wolfender *et al.*, 1998). Optimum ionisation conditions are structure-dependent, for example, most phenolic acids can only be ionised in the negative ion mode. Thus, analysis of an unknown sample requires the application of different conditions, e.g. different interfaces, to ionise all constituents of interest. The application of other spectroscopic techniques might be necessary in addition. LC-DAD-MS has been used very frequently for the analysis of plant extracts, because it provides on-line ultraviolet and MS information for each peak in a chromatogram, which often allows direct identification (He, 2000). Only a few examples are mentioned below, to illustrate the usefulness of this technique for the quality control of Chinese herbs.

Lin *et al.* (2005) used an LC-UV-ESI-MS combination for the determination of 12 constituents, most of them isoflavones and their glycosides, in Puerariae Radix 70% methanolic extracts. Parameters such as eluent composition, HPLC column and ion source were optimised, to achieve highly resolved separation and reliable identification of the compounds.

Zschocke *et al.* (1998) developed TLC, HPLC and LC-MS methods for the differentiation of *Angelica sinensis* (Oliv.) Diels from its related umbelliferous drugs *A. pubescens* Maxim. *f. biserrata* Shan et Yuan, *A. dahurica* (Fisch. Ex Hoffm.) Benth et Hook, *Ligusticum chuanxiong* Hort., *L. porteri* Coulter and Rose and *Levisticum officinale* Koch. The authors found that HPLC analysis was best suited for differentiation between the four drugs *Levisticum officinale*, *Ligusticum chuanxiong*, *L. porteri* and *Angelica sinensis* as mainly quantitiative differences of their main constituents were found. LC-MS analysis of *A. sinensis* and *L. officinale* was not found to be advantageous with respect to differentiation of the two drugs. Nevertheless, the method provided the possibility to identify thermolabile ligustilide dimers in the APCI mode.

Cai *et al.* (2005) determined the phenolic constituents of an 80% methanolic *Rosa chinensis* Jacq. extract by LC-ESI-MS. Additionally, the authors used MALDI-QIT-TOF-MS, a hybrid mass spectrometer equipped with a MALDI source and a quadrupole ion trap followed by time-of-flight analysis, to verify the obtained results and to tentatively identify two ellagitannins which could not be identified by LC-ESIMS analysis. This could be done without any further purification of the crude extract. In total, the authors identified 36 phenolics in the extract.

Chen *et al.* (2004) used a comprehensive two-dimensional LC-DAD-APCIMS system for the separation and identification of Rhizoma Chuanxiong constituents. In a comprehensive two-dimensional system, all analytes from the first dimension separation are acted upon equally as fractions and analysed on the second dimension column. The authors used a CN column for first and an ODS column for second dimension separation. Molecular-weight information achieved from the MS detector adds a third dimension to the system because overlapping peaks can be identified without chromatographic resolution. From a methanolic extract, more than 52 compounds were separated in less than 215 min and 11 of them could be identified simultaneously. According to the authors, this comprehensive two-dimensional approach is highly feasible for separation and identification of complex traditional Chinese medicines because of its high peak capacity, sensitivity and powerful resolution potential.

LC-MS technique is also frequently applied for the detection of undesired or toxic compounds in Chinese herbal preparations. For example, Wong *et al.* (2002) used an LC-MS-MS method for qualitative and quantitative analysis of toxic constituents in materials such as Radix Aconiti Lateralis, Radix Sophorae Tonkiniensis, Semen Strychni and Venenum Bufonis. The presence of the respective constituents was verified by their mass spectra, and quantitative determination was performed using multiple reaction monitoring (MRM).

Ioset *et al.* (2002) developed an LC/DAD-UV/MS method for the detection and quantification of aristolochic acid I in herbal samples. The limit of detection was 2 ng for ultraviolet and for MS in the selective ion monitoring (SIM) mode and 15 ng in the MS full scan mode. Additionally, a TLC prescreening for aristolochic acid I was developed. The authors applied these methods to Chinese phytomedicines and dietary supplements used as slimming regimens (Ioset *et al.*, 2003).

Huang *et al.* (2005) developed a similar method for the determination and quantification of aristolochic acids I and II in Chinese medical preparations which were suspected to contain aristolochic acids based on previous TLC analysis. Quantification was performed using the very sensitive MRM method (detection limits: 2 ng/mL for aristolochic acid I, 2.8 ng/mL for aristolochic acid II).

Adams *et al.* (2006) developed an LC-MS method for the determination of trace amounts of atropine in *Lycium barbarum* L. berries (*Gouquizi*), which are widely used in China as medicine and functional food. LC-MS analyses were conducted using a quadrupole MS as well as an ion trap operated in the SRM (selected reaction monitoring) mode. Traces of atropine with maximum 19 ppb of dry weight were found in all eight analysed batches. The authors conclude that these amounts are not hazardous to health even at high consumption levels. Concerning MS conditions the authors conclude that the ion-trap method offers better selectivity in complex mixtures because of the quantification of specific fragmentation reactions in the SRM mode, whereas the quadrupole system provides higher sensitivity, less variation and therefore lower limits of quantitation.

HPLC-ELSD

In recent years, evaporative light scattering detection (ELSD) has been increasingly used. In contrast to the hyphenated techniques mentioned above, HPLC-ELSD does not provide additional structural information, but it allows the determination of compounds lacking a chromophore without derivatisation. Since this technique shows good applicability to complex mixtures, it seems to offer a useful alternative to conventional detection methods. HPLC-ELSD has already been employed for determination of various non-chromophoric compounds such as saponins, terpenes, steroids and carbohydrates, but it might also be used as a quasi-universal detector for determining all constituents of a preparation.

Wenkui and Fitzloff (2001) used HPLC-ELSD for the determination of astragaloside IV in Radix Astragali methanolic extracts. The compound is difficult to analyse by HPLC-UV because of its poor ultraviolet absorption.

Chai *et al.* (2005) determined seven triterpenoid saponins in Flos Lonicerae (*Jinyinhua*) hydroethanolic extracts. According to the 2005 Chinese pharmacopoeia, this herb can be derived from four sources, namely *L. japonica* Thunb., *L. hypoglauca* Miq., *L. dasystyla* Rehder and *L. confusa* DC. As the saponin profile alone did not allow the clear distinction of botanical origin, the authors suggest combination with conventional identification methods.

Yan *et al.* (2005b) employed the technique for the simultaneous determination of the major bioactive compounds in Qingkailing injection, namely adenosine, geniposide, chlorogenic acid, baicalin, ursodeoxycholic acid, cholic acid and hyodeoxycholic acid. Because of the poor ultraviolet absorption of some of these compounds, HPLC-DAD analysis cannot be performed, making HPLC-ELSD a useful alternative.

Gas chromatography and hyphenated techniques

As many bioactive constituents of herbal medicines are volatile, GC analysis can often be used for authentication and quality control. By the use of GC-MS, reliable information on the identity of compounds is available and it has very good separation power, which allows generation of fingerprints of high quality. Furthermore, by mass spectrometry and the use of mass spectral databases, the qualitative and quantitative composition of the volatile compounds can be analysed. A disadvantage of this technique is the fact that polar and non-volatile compounds (and adulterations) are not detectable (Liang *et al.*, 2004). To improve the chromatographic resolution of complex mixtures, chemometric methods are often applied.

Guo and coworkers (2004) used this approach to develop a GC fingerprint of *Artemisia capillaris* Thunb. volatile oil. They applied subwindow factor analysis (SFA), to resolve clusters of overlapping peaks. They obtained 75 resolved peaks and identified 43 of them using an MS database. To compare the received fingerprint chromatogram to chromatograms of other samples, an orthogonal projection method was adopted to identify each component directly in the sample chromatograms. Using this technique, tedious similarity search for each single peak and also subjective assumption to the analytical results can be avoided. After comparison of samples from four different sources, 51 common components were identified. It was also shown that differentiation from *Artemisia sacrorum* Ledeb., a common substitute of the drug, is possible with the developed method.

Li *et al.* (2003) used GC-MS combined with chemometric resolution methods to compare the volatile fractions from *Schisandra chinensis* (Turcz.) Baill. obtained by six different extraction methods. SFA was applied to confirm the equality of identical chemical components in different volatile fractions by their mass spectra.

Recently, comprehensive two-dimensional gas chromatography (GC × GC) has been described as an appropriate tool to achieve highly resolved chromatograms from very complex mixtures: GC × GC couples two columns with different separation mechanisms via a modulator, which traps, focuses and reinjects the slices into the second column. The advantages of this technique are enhanced sensitivity, superior resolution and group separation that facilitate the identification of unknown compounds (Shellie *et al.*, 2002; Wu *et al.*, 2004). The retention times on the two columns are plotted in a two-dimensional way. Using this plot, it is easy to compare different samples with regard to presence and absence of chromatographic peaks. Improved resolution of sample components and isolation of analyte signals from the chemical background additionally improves the quality of mass spectra. Additional information can be obtained when using bubble plots with the centre of the bubble representing the 1D and 2D coordinate, and the area of the bubble representing the size of a chromatographic peak. Resolution of individual components is best represented when a 3D surface plot or a 2D contour/colour plot of the 2D separation space is used (Shellie *et al.*, 2003).

Shellie *et al.* (2003) applied two-dimensional gas chromatography with flame ionisation detection (GC × GC) and with quadrupole mass spectrometry detection (GC × GCqMS) to the analysis of the semi-volatile oils of three ginseng species, namely *Panax ginseng* C.A. Mey., *P. notoginseng* (Burk.) F.H. Chen and *P. quinquefolium* L. They performed chromatogram matching by correlating GC × GC-qMS with GC × GC (FID) results. This method allows FID to be used for quantitation of MS-identified peaks, as peak areas can be more accurately determined using FID.

Wu *et al.* (2004) used GC × GC, hyphenated with a TOFMS instead of a quadrupole MS, for the qualitative analysis of *Pogostemon cablin* (Blanco) Benth. volatile oil. They compared this technique to GC-MS and impressively demonstrated the enhanced sensitivity and superior resolution of GC × GC as compared with one-dimensional GC. Under the same operation conditions, GC-chromatograms displayed only 79 peaks, while about 800 peaks were resolved with GC × GC (Figure 28.3).

Electrophoretic methods and hyphenated techniques

As a micro-column separation technique, capillary electrophoresis (CE) has been shown to be effective and convenient in various fields, including the analysis of herbal medicines (Li *et al.*, 2005). The advantages of CE are that only small sample amounts are required and that samples can be rapidly analysed with very good separation efficiency. Additionally,

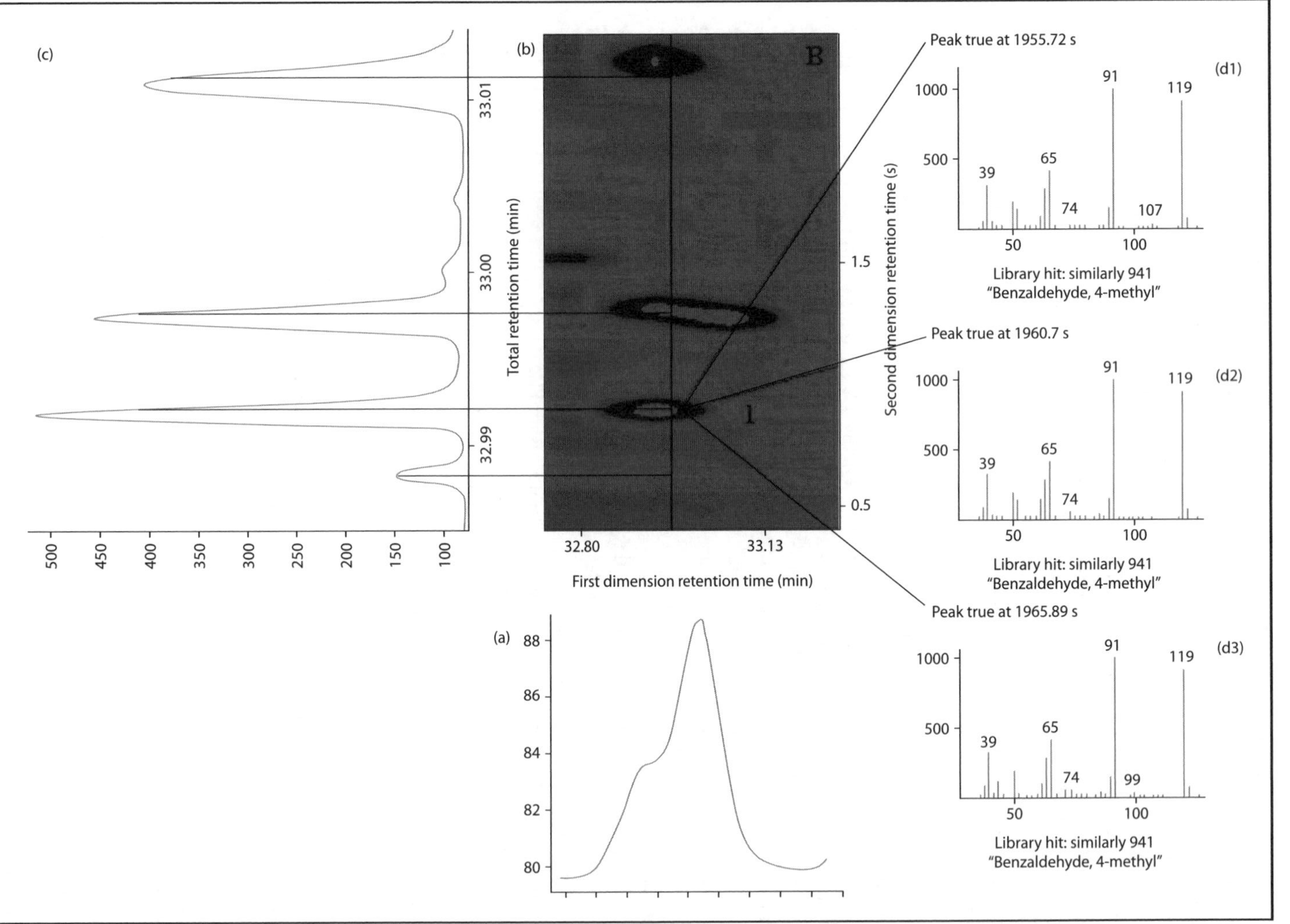

Figure 28.3 Detailed comparison of 1D-GC with GC × GC chromatograms of *Pogostemon cablin* (Blanco) Benth. volatile oil (same injection amount, split ratio and the same velocity of carrier gas). (a) Detail of 1D-GC chromatogram; (b) detail of GC × GC contour plot; (c) detail of GC × GC chromatogram. The vertical line at 32.96 min indicates the second-dimension chromatogram that is shown in (c). In (b), peak 1 was modulated three times by GC × GC, therefore, identified three times by TOF MS, the spectra D1, D2, D3 were corresponding deconvoluted mass spectrum. Column: 1D-GC, SOLGELWAX (60 m × 0.25 mm i.d. × 0.25 μm); GC × GC, first: SOLGELWAX (60 m × 0.25 mm i.d. × 0.25 μm), second: cyclodex-B (3 m × 0.1 mm i.d. × 0.1 μm). The modulation time of GC × GC was 5 s. The Chemstation acquired data at 100 Hz for both 1D GC and GC × GC. (Reprinted from Wu *et al.*, with permission from Elsevier.)

the capillaries reach equilibrium more easily than HPLC columns and the problem of column contamination is avoided (Liang *et al.*, 2004; Li *et al.*, 2005).

The techniques most widely used are capillary zone electrophoresis (CZE), capillary gel electrophoresis (CGE) and capillary isoelectric focusing (cIEF) (Liang *et al.*, 2004). Techniques such as micellar electrokinetic chromatography (MEKC), microemulsion electrokinetic chromatography (MEEKC) and non-aqueous capillary electrophoresis (NACE) have also repeatedly been employed in the analysis of herbal extracts (Li *et al.*, 2005).

CZE is a useful method for the separation of charged natural products, especially for polyphenolic compounds such as flavonoids, coumarins and organic acids (Li *et al.*, 2005). For example, Jiang *et al.* (2005) developed a CZE method for the separation and quantitative determination of chalcones from *Carthamus tinctorius* L. preparations. Yue *et al.* (2004) analysed flavonoids in *Hippophae rhamnoides* L. preparations by CZE.

As it allows good separation of both charged and electrically neutral analytes, MEKC offers wider application possibilities than CZE. Neutral compounds can be separated because of their different partition between the micelle and aqueous phase. Separation is based on a combination of electrophoretic and chromatographic mechanisms (Li *et al.*, 2005). This method has been widely used for the analysis of herbal preparations. As a recent example, Yu *et al.* (2006) developed a MEKC method for the determination and quantitative analysis of paeonol and paeoniflorin, two bioactive compounds of Cortex Moutan, the dry root bark of *Paeonia suffruticosa* Andr. The compounds could also be determined in a granulate preparation of the drug. Müller *et al.* (2004) used MEKC for the qualitative and quantitative analysis of biologically active constituents of Herba Verbenae (*Verbena officinalis* L.), a herb that is used in European as well as in Chinese medicine. With the optimised MEKC method, five markers belonging to three different classes of compounds (iridoids, phenylethanoids and flavonoids) could be baseline separated within 25 minutes.

MEEKC is a relatively new technique, which is characterised by the use of buffers containing surfactant-coated oil droplets for electrokinetic separations. In comparison with MEKC, the simultaneous separation of compounds with a wide solubility range is enhanced (Zhai *et al.*, 2006).

Zhai *et al.* (2006) developed an MEEKC method for the separation and quantitative analysis of six aristolochic acid derivatives. With the optimised experimental conditions, baseline separation within 16 minutes was achieved (Figure 28.4). When the method was applied to methanolic extracts of five different samples derived from *Aristolochia* species, the contents of four of the aristolochic acids were successfully determined with satisfactory recovery, sensitivity and reproducibility.

Non-aqueous CE (NACE) is based on the use of electrolyte solutions prepared from pure organic solvents. Compared with aqueous CE, it offers a number of interesting characteristics such as alteration of selectivity, reduced electrophoretic current and improved MS compatibility as well as enhanced solubility and stability of hydrophobic compounds. The fact that the physical and chemical properties of organic solvents and water differ greatly allows a simple selective manipulation of separation performance (Qi *et al.*, 2005). The technique has been repeatedly used for the separation and identification of Chinese herb constituents. For example, Li *et al.* (2004c) could separate the three toxic *Aconitum* alkaloids aconitine, hypaconitine and mesaconitine within 6 minutes using an NACE method. The method was successfully applied to determine these compounds in the Chinese drugs *Chuanwu* (dry root of *Aconitum carmichaeli* Debx.) and *Caowu* (dry root of *A. kusnezoffii* Reichb.).

Qi *et al.* (2005) determined bioactive flavone derivatives such as eupatilin, artenoflavone and hispidulin in ethanolic extracts of different Chinese herbs using an NACE technique.

In recent decades, hyphenated CE instruments such as CE-DAD, CE-MS and CE-NMR have been developed. This approach combines efficient CE separation with specific and sensitive detection methods, and additionally helps to overcome to a certain extent problems of artefact formation because of separation buffer chemistry or hidden instrumental constraints (Liang *et al.*, 2004).

Feng *et al.* (2003) used CE-MS to analyse the alkaloids present in *Wutou* (Radix Aconiti Praeparata) and *Maqianzi* (the seed of *Strychnos pierreana* A.W. Hill) before and after detoxicant

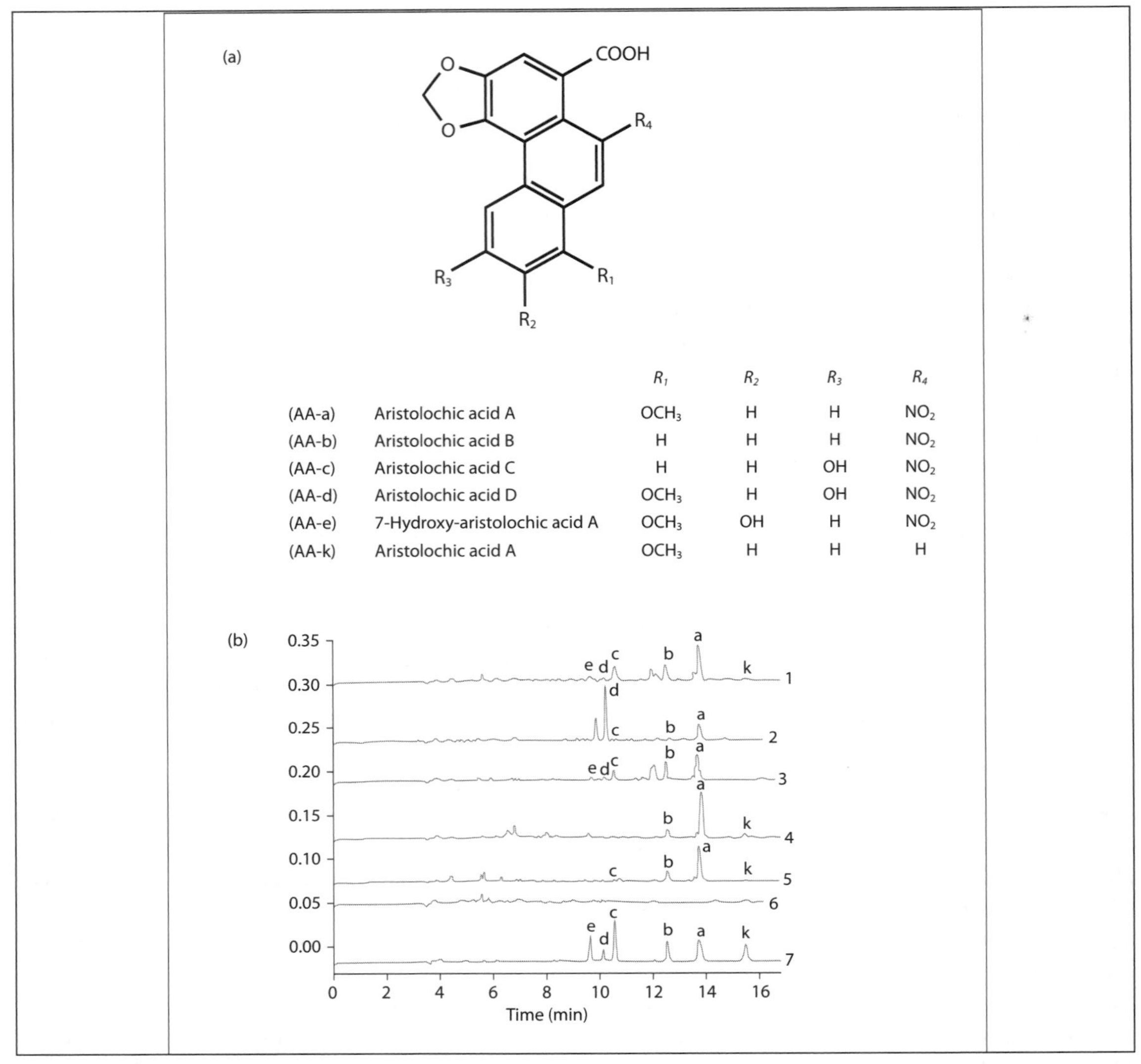

Figure 28.4 MEEKC method for the separation and quantitation of aristolochic acid derivatives. (a) Analysed aristolochic acid derivatives. (b) Representative electropherograms: Herba Aristolochiae (1), Fructus Aristolochiae (2), Radix Aristolochiae (3), Radix Aristolochiae Fangchi (4), Caulis Aristolochiae Manshuriensis (5), Herba Asari (6) and standards (7). (Reprinted from Zhai *et al.* (2006) with permission from Elsevier.)

processing of the materials. As good separation of the Maqianzi alkaloids was obtained, they could be measured in the total ion current mode. For the aconite alkaloids and their degradation products however, no satisfactory CE separation was achieved, so determination was only possible in the selective ion-monitoring mode.

Hyphenation of CE with less common detection methods such as laser-induced fluorescence detection (Hsieh *et al.*, 2006) or electrochemical detection at a carbon-fibre microdisk electrode (Zhou *et al.*, 2006) has recently been successfully used for sensitive determination of aristolochic acids.

The method developed by Zhou *et al.* (2006) has also been successfully applied to provide fingerprints of the methanolic extracts of different *Aristolochia* species, showing that CE is also feasible for fingerprint development.

Application and evaluation of chromatographic fingerprint data in quality control of herbal drugs

Despite the widespread acceptance of chromatographic fingerprint techniques for quality control, the establishment of a characteristic fingerprint chromatogram for the quality control of herbal medicines remains a critical task (Wong *et al.*, 2004). The ability to obtain a good chromatographic fingerprint representing phytoequivalence of an herb depends on several factors such as extraction method, measurement instruments and measurement conditions. These factors have to be optimised, to achieve meaningful fingerprints. After having solved these problems the question arises how to evaluate the information provided by a chromatographic fingerprint reasonably and efficiently (Liang *et al.*, 2004).

The chromatographic profile should be featured by the fundamental attributions of 'integrity' and 'fuzziness', or 'sameness' and 'differences' which chemically represent the investigated herbal product. This means that by the use of chromatographic fingerprints the accurate authentication and identification of herbal medicines should be possible ('integrity'), even though the amount and/or concentration of the characteristic constituents vary from batch to batch ('fuzziness') or, that chromatographic fingerprints should be able to successfully demonstrate the 'sameness' and 'differences' between various samples (Liang *et al.*, 2004). Chemometric methods have been shown to be a helpful tool in the generation and evaluation of chromatographic fingerprints.

Calculation of information content

A chromatographic fingerprint of an herbal product is a multivariate system and its information content can be calculated by means of various approaches.

For local approaches, signal intensity, retention time, peak area and/or peak height of each independent peak without overlapping, but not the whole chromatographic curve, are taken into consideration. This makes the identification of each single peak and the estimation of the noise and/or error level of a fingerprint necessary, and in case of overlapping peaks, calculation of information content becomes very complex (Gong *et al.*, 2003; Liang *et al.*, 2004).

Gong *et al.* (2003) used a more global approach, namely information theory, to select the fingerprint with maximum information content from several different chromatograms. In this method, a chromatographic fingerprint is regarded as a continuous signal determined by its chromatographic shape. They applied this method to different chromatographic fingerprints of *Ginkgo biloba* L. and Rhizoma Chuanxiong, and selected the fingerprint with the highest information content, which corresponds to an optimum separation degree and a uniform concentration distribution of all constituents.

Correction of retention time shifts

Chromatographic retention time shifts are a frequent problem in fingerprint analysis. They occur for several reasons, such as successive degradation of the stationary phase, minor changes in the composition of the mobile phase, detector and other instrumental shifts, column overloading or interactions between analytes. These shifts have to be corrected prior to evaluation of similarity and difference between chromatograms since they might lead to erroneous results (Li *et al.*, 2004d; Liang *et al.*, 2004). There are several approaches for peak synchronisation. A very useful method is the addition of an internal standard (Liang *et al.*, 2004). Mathematical retention time correction can be performed by using methods such as local least squares analysis (LLS) or spectral correlative chromatography (SCC) (Li *et al.*, 2004b; 2004d).

In LLS, the correction of shifts is applied to fingerprint clusters in a piecewise manner, which makes the LLS-corrected fingerprints comparable in compositional distribution (Li *et al.*, 2004b). The idea of SCC is that the same chemical component should possess the same spectrum no matter when it is eluted through diverse chromatographic columns. This means that for this technique also spectral data are required. With the help of this method, it is also possible to determine the presence or absence of compounds of interest among different fingerprint chromatograms (Li *et al.*, 2004d; Liang *et al.*, 2004).

Similarity evaluation of fingerprints

As mentioned above, SCC can be employed to demonstrate similarities and dissimilarities of chromatographic fingerprints and to detect frauds (Li *et al.*, 2004d), but the method requires two-way data.

A simple method for the evaluation of similarity is the calculation of correlation coefficient or congruence coefficient. The SFDA suggested to judge herbal chromatographic fingerprints by their similarities which come from the calculation of the correlation coefficient and/or cosine value of vectorial angle of original data (Yang *et al.*, 2005). Yang *et al.* (2005) used the evaluation software recommended by the SFDA for data analysis when evaluating HPLC-DAD-generated fingerprints of 56 *Hypericum japonicum* Thunb. (*tianjihunang*) samples from six Chinese provinces for similarity. The authors used the correlation coefficient for similarity calculation, with a reference fingerprint representing the median of all chromatograms. The chromatogram with the highest correlation coefficient was selected as an authentic reference fingerprint.

Principal-component analysis (PCA) is also frequently used for comparison of chromatographic fingerprints and detection of outliers. PCA is a common method to reduce multivariate data sets to their lowest dimensionality (Johnson *et al.*, 2003). In PCA the original multivariate data are projected on a set of orthogonal axes defining a subspace of the original multivariate data space that maximally describes the variation contained within that multivariate data. The axes are known as principal components. They are arranged in descending order of the amount of variation in the original data they explain. Each principal component has an associated loadings and scores vector (Johnson *et al.*, 2003). By extraction of useful information from object data, PCA is able to construct a theoretical model that has prerequisites or limited validity of principal components. When a fingerprint shows unexpected properties diverging from those of major good fingerprints or features not fitting in the theoretical major good fingerprint model, it is excluded from the model and diagnosed to be different (Li *et al.*, 2004b).

Li *et al.* (2004b) performed a series of PCAs on the LLS-corrected HPLC-fingerprints of 33 *Erigeron breviscarpus* samples. They found that direct PCA of the LLS-corrected fingerprints without any further data transformation led to indefinite or unclear classification, and identification of unexpected fingerprints was very difficult with this method. For this reason, data pretreatment prior to PCA was necessary. Normalisation and standard normal variate (SNV) transformation led to an improved classification of fingerprints, the latter technique performing best (Figure 28.5).

Chemometric resolution of two-way data

Data obtained by hyphenated instruments are generally called two-way or two-dimensional data. They are very beneficial for the analysis of complex mixtures such as Chinese medical preparations because of the additional spectral information they provide. However, some problems have to be solved when using these techniques: On one hand, the spectra are often influenced by the background and overlapping peaks, which makes similarity-matching using spectral databases difficult. On the other hand, peak overlapping leads to a loss of analytical information. Several chemometric resolution techniques for two-dimensional data have been developed in the last decade to solve these problems (Li *et al.*, 2003). The resolution methods can be divided into iterative methods such as iterative transformation factor analysis (ITTFA), orthogonal projection approach (OPA) and elementary matrix transformation (IMEMT), and non-iterative methods, which can be regarded as evolving methods. Examples for this approach are evolving factor analysis (EFA), window factor analysis (WFA), heuristic evolving latent projections (HELP), subwindow factor analysis (SFA) and evolving window orthogonal projection (EWOP) (Guo *et al.*, 2003).

Guo and coworkers (2003) applied an iterative method, namely OPA, and a non-iterative method, namely EWOP, to the chemometric resolution of GC-MS chromatograms of *Notopterygium incisum* Ting ex H.T. Chang. In general, when separation performance is good, an iterative method is applied for resolution, and in case of bad separation performance, rather a non-iterative method is applied. The authors could separate 98 constituents in the essential oil of the plant, and 65 of them, accounting for 92.13% of the volatile oil, could be identified.

Examples for the application of SFA have already been described in detail in Chapter 3 (Li *et al.*, 2003; Guo *et al.*, 2004).

Spectroscopic techniques

Near-infrared spectroscopy

NIR spectroscopy is rapid, non-destructive, simple to use in routine operation and, since no sample

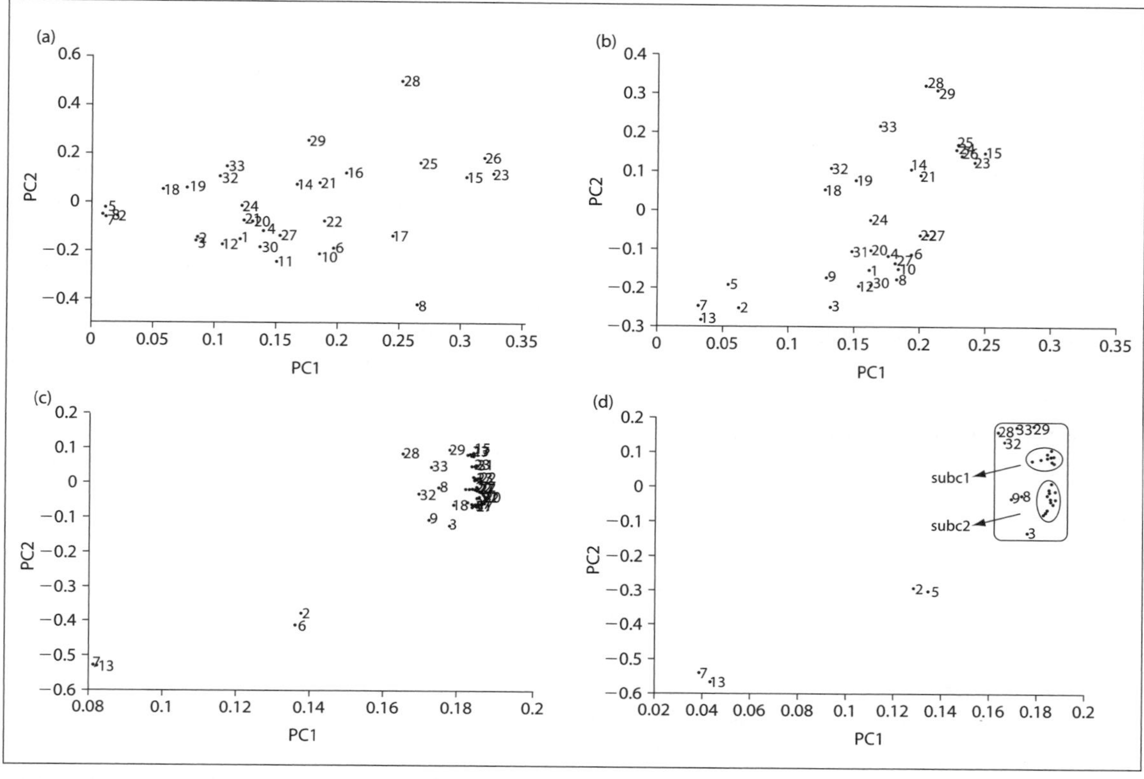

Figure 28.5 Principal component projection plot of PC1 to PC2 of the LLS-corrected fingerprints of 33 herbal samples of *Erigeron breviscarpus* with and without data transformation. (a) Representation of 33 herbal fingerprints of *E. breviscarpus* samples on PC1 and PC2 (96% variance explained) with no data transformation after LLS correction; (b) on PC1 and PC2 (94% variance explained) after LLS correction and closure to 1; (c) on PC1 and PC2 (92% variance explained) after LLS correction and normalisation; (d) on PC1 and PC2 (89% variance explained) after LLS correction and SNV. (Reprinted from Li *et al.* (2004b) with permission from Elsevier.)

preparation is required, it is also interesting for the quality control of Chinese medical herbs (Chen and Sørensen, 2000; Fuzzati, 2004).

The major drawback is that for quantitative analysis the instrument has to be calibrated with a set of 20–50 samples with known analyte concentration obtained by suitable reference methods. The calibrations also have to be checked regularly by comparison with reference methods, to assure the compliance between calibration set and analysed samples (Chen and Sørensen, 2000; Fuzzati, 2004). Calibration models are produced using multiple linear regression (MLR), partial least squares (PLS) or principal component regression (PCR). Data pretreatment using mathematical transformation of the NIR spectra can be applied to enhance spectral features and/or to remove or reduce unwanted sources of variation during calibration model development (Fuzzati, 2004).

Chen and Sørensen (2000) used NIR spectroscopy for the determination of glycyrrhizin in Radix Glycyrrhizae and of ginsenosides in Radix Notoginseng. The samples could be successfully classified into low-, medium- and high-quality materials.

Woo *et al.* (2005) developed a NIR spectroscopy method for the discrimination between Chinese and Korean Angelicae Gigantis Radix. Samples of both origins were collected from various cultivation areas during a period of more than one year, and soft independent modelling of class anology (SIMCA) was used to build a calibration model for classification. Samples could be successfully discriminated by using the characteristic band of decursin which provided the most significant difference between the two provenances.

Wang *et al.* (2007) used NIR spectroscopy for the classification of *Glycyrrhiza uralensis* Fisch. batches and for the prediction of their glycyrrhizin content. The authors could demonstrate that NIR spectroscopy combined with PCA or SIMCA algorithm is suitable for the classification of liquorice samples according to their geographical origins, growing conditions and plant parts. Additionally they applied a combination of NIR spectroscopy and a partial least square analysis using HPLC data as a reference for the prediction of glycyrrhizic acid levels in the samples.

Nuclear magnetic resonance spectroscopy

Apart from its frequent application in structure elucidation, NMR spectroscopy has recently become an interesting tool for metabolomic analyses. The term 'metabolome' describes the sum of metabolic constituents, observable as chemical profile or fingerprint of the metabolites in whole organisms or parts of them. [^{1}H]NMR spectroscopy in combination with PCA has been successfully utilised to differentiate plants based on their metabolomes. Especially high-resolution NMR and two-dimensional NMR techniques have been shown to be feasible for the analysis of highly complex plant extracts (Yang *et al.*, 2006).

Yang *et al.* (2006) applied [^{1}H]NMR and *J*-resolved spectroscopic methods in combination with PCA to the metabolomic fingerprinting of three different commercial ginseng preparations and four kinds of ginseng roots. *J*-resolved two-dimensional spectra lead to a considerable increase of signal resolution within a short time, and moreover, by projection to a spectral axis, all protons appear as singlets, simplifying the spectra of complex mixtures. From the results obtained, the authors conclude that the presented method is promising for the quality control of other herbal medicinal products.

Conclusions

The application of Chinese herbs in Western countries has dramatically increased during recent decades. However, the legal basis for this kind of medicine only exists in rudimentary form, and harmonisation between countries is still missing. In some countries such as Germany, Chinese herbs are regarded as drugs, in others such as the US, they are classified as dietary supplements.

Incidents with Chinese preparations containing hazardous or toxic constituents, such as the toxic effects caused by herbs containing aristolochic acid, led to a serious discussion about the safety of TCM preparations. To minimise the risk of such incidents, it is necessary to ensure that quality and safety of TCM preparations meet Western standards. To a certain extent, this can be achieved by the application of good agricultural, sourcing and manufacturing practices to the production process and by the development of quality-control methods that give consideration to the special properties of Chinese herbal preparations.

Many safety issues do not substantially differ from the problems concerning herbal drugs in Europe, e.g. microbial contamination, pesticide and heavy metal residues. The fact that GAP rules are not yet fully implemented in many Chinese cultivation bases might, however, aggravate these problems in Chinese drugs. Adulteration with undeclared synthetic drugs is a problem more frequently occurring in Chinese herbal preparations than in Western ones, and it is difficult to handle, as the variety of possible adulterations is very large.

Special attention has to be paid to the correct authentication of the plant material. Compared with Western medicinal plants, this is more critical in Chinese plants for several reasons: on the one hand, nomenclature is not always consistent and one name can refer to different drugs in different geographical regions; on the other hand, expensive and scarce drugs are sometimes substituted by cheaper ones. For such cases, appropriate authentication markers are needed. The most common authentication methods are macroscopic and microscopic analysis and chromatographic methods such as TLC, HPLC, GC, CE and hyphenated techniques. In recent years, DNA-related techniques have increasingly been used. It is apparent that no single method exists that allows 100% authentication; instead, a combination of techniques is needed.

Appropriate quality of herbal materials also has to be ensured, as is the case for Western herbal materials. However, in TCM, herbal mixtures consisting of up to 10 plants are common, which makes quality assurance an extremely challenging task. Apart from standardisation based on markers and biomarkers, fingerprint analysis using hyphenated chromatographic techniques seems to be a promising approach for quality assurance of complex herbal preparations. This concept is also favoured by authorities such as the WHO, the FDA and the Chinese State Drug Administration. However, the development of a meaningful fingerprint as well as the evaluation of similarity is not an easy task and often chemometric methods have to be applied to transform complex chromatographic data into meaningful quality information.

In summary, great scientific efforts have been made to provide appropriate methods that allow quality assurance of Chinese herbal drugs. However, for global safe use of TCM preparations in the future, harmonised legislation for TCM in general and for safety and quality requirements of TCM herbs in Western countries is needed.

References

Adams M, Wiedenmann M, Tittel G, Bauer R (2006). HPLC-MS trace analysis of atropine in *Lycium barbarum* berries. *Phytochem Anal* 17: 279–283.

Aflatoxin VerbotsV (2000). *Verordnung u-umlautber das Verbot der Verwendung von mit Aflatoxinen kontaminierten Stoffen bei der Herstellung von Arzneimitteln*. 19.7.2000, BGBI I, p. 1081 (1505).

Au AM, Ko R, Boo FO *et al.* (2000). Screening methods for drugs and heavy metals in Chinese patent medicines. *Bull Environ Contam Toxicol* 65: 112–119.

Bauer R (1998). Quality criteria and standardization of phytopharmaceuticals: Can acceptable drug standards be achieved? *Drug Inform J* 32: 101–110.

Bauer R (2001). Traditionelle Chinesische Medizin. In: *Arzneimittel der komplementa-umlautren Medizin*, Eds. Müller-Jahncke W-D, Borchardt A. Govi-Verlag, Stuttgart, Germany, pp. 184–210.

Bauer R, Wagner H (2004). Analytik von TCM-Drogen. *Dtsch Apoth Ztg* 144: 5007–5011.

Blatter A, Reich E (2004). Qualitative and quantitative HPTLC methods for quality control of *Stephania tetrandra*. *J Liq Chromatogr Relat Technol* 27: 2087–2100.

Bomme U, Bauer R, Heubl G (2005). Erste Ergebnisse zur botanischen Identifizierung sowie zum Ertrags- und Inhaltsstoffverhalten verschiedener Saatgutherkünfte von *Angelica dahurica* und *Saposhnikovia divaricata*. *Z Arznei Gewu-umlautrzpflanzen* 10: 28–36.

Bomme U, Heubl G, Bauer R (2006). Erste Ergebnisse der Untersuchungen zur botanischen Charakterisierung sowie zum Ertragsverhalten und Inhaltsstoffspektrum verschiedener Herkünfte von *Prunella vulgaris* L., *Leonurus japonicus* Houtt. und *Sigesbeckia pubescens* Makino. *Z Arznei Gewu-umlautrzpflanzen* 11: 81–91.

Cai Z, Lee FSC, Wang XR *et al.* (2002). A capsule review of recent studies on the application of mass spectrometry in the analysis of Chinese medicinal herbs. *J Mass Spectrom* 37: 1013–1024.

Cai Y-Z, Xing J, Sun M *et al.* (2005). Phenolic antioxidants (hydrolyzable tannins, flavonols, and anthocyanins) identified by LC-ESI-MS and MALDI-QIT-TOF MS from *Rosa chinensis* flowers. *J Agric Food Chem* 53: 9940–9948.

Chai X-Y, Li S-L, Li P (2005). Quality evaluation of Flos Lonicerae through simultaneous determination of seven saponins by HPLC with ELSD. *J Chromatogr A* 1070: 43–48.

Chan K (2003). Some aspects of toxic contaminants in herbal medicines. *Chemosphere* 52: 1361–1371.

Carles M, Lee T, Moganti S *et al.* (2001). Chips and Qi: microcomponent-based analysis in traditional Chinese medicine. *Fresenius J Anal Chem* 371: 190–194.

Carles M, Cheung MKL, Moganti S *et al.* (2005). A DNA microarray for the authentication of toxic traditional Chinese medicinal plants. *Planta Med* 71: 580–584.

Chen Y, Sørensen LK (2000). Determination of marker constituents in Radix Glycyrrhizae and Radix Notoginseng by near infrared spectroscopy. *Fresenius J Anal Chem* 367: 491–496.

Chen X, Kong L, Su L *et al.* (2004). Separation and identification of compounds in *Rhizoma chuanxiong* by comprehensive two-dimensional liquid chromatography coupled to mass spectrometry. *J Chromatogr A* 1040: 169–178.

Cheng J-T (2000). Review: drug therapy in Chinese traditional medicine. *J Clin Pharmacol* 40: 445–450.

Cheng KT (2002). Authentication of the components from a mixture of herbal materials. In: *Authenication of Chinese Medicinal Materials by DNA Technology*, Eds. Shaw PC, Wang J, But PPH. World Scientific Publishing Co. Pte. Ltd., Singapore, pp. 69–84.

Chizzola R, Michitsch H, Franz C (2003). Monitoring of metallic micronutrients and heavy metals in herbs, spices and medicinal plants from Austria. *Eur Food Res Technol* 216: 407–411.

Creppy EE (2002). Update of survey, regulation and toxic effects of mycotoxins in Europe. *Toxicol Lett* 127: 19–28.

Di X, Chan KKC, Leung HW *et al.* (2003). Fingerprint profiling of acid hydrolyzates of polysaccharides extracted from the fruiting bodies and spores of Lingzhi by high-performance thin-layer chromatography. *J Chromatogr A* 1018: 85–95.

European Committee for Standardization (1999). *Foodstuffs – Determination of Aflatoxin B1, B2, G1 and G2 in Cereals, Shell-Fruits and Derived Products – High*

Performance Liquid Chromatographic Method with Post Column Derivatization and Immunoaffinity Column Clean up. DIN EN 12955.

Dobos GJ, Cohen MH, McIntyre M *et al.* (2005). Are national quality standards for traditional Chinese herbal medicine sufficient? Current governmental regulations for traditional Chinese herbal medicine in Eastern and Western countries. *Complement Ther Med* 13: 183–190.

(EC) No. 1881/2006 (2006). Commission regulation (EC) No. 1881/2006 of 19 December 2006 setting maximum levels for certain contaminants in foodstuffs. *Offic J Eur Union* L364/5–L364/24.

(EC) No. 1126/2007 (2007). Commission regulation (EC) No. 1126/2007 of 28 December 2007 amending Regulation (EC) No 1881/2006 setting maximum levels for certain contaminants in foodstuffs as regards Fusarium toxins in maize and maize products. *Offic J Eur Union* L255/14–L255/17.

EHIA (2005). *Guidelines for good agricultural and hygiene practices for raw materials used for herbal infusions (GAHP)*. http://www.ehia-online.org/documents/gahp_edition_2005.pdf, p. 18 (accessed 17 Apr 2007).

Ernst E (2002a). Toxic heavy metals and undeclared drugs in Asian herbal medicines. *Trends Pharmacol Sci* 23: 136–139.

Ernst E (2002b). Adulteration of Chinese herbal medicines with synthetic drugs: a systematic review. *J Intern Med* 252: 107–113.

Ernst E, Coon JT (2001). Heavy metals in traditional Chinese medicines: A systematic review. *Clin Pharmacol Ther* 70: 497–504.

European Pharmacopoeia. *Europäisches Arzneibuch* (2005). Ausgabe, Verlag Österreich Gmbh.

Fan X-H, Cheng Y-Y, Ye Z-L *et al.*(2006). Multiple chromatographic fingerprinting and its application to the quality control of herbal medicines. *Anal Chim Acta* 555: 217–224.

FDA *Guidance for Industry Botanical Drug Products* (2000). US Department of Health and Human Services, Food and Drug Administration, Center for Drug Evaluation and Research (CDER), Rockville, MD, USA.

Feng H-T, Yuan L-L, Li SFY (2003). Analysis of Chinese medicine preparations by capillary electorphoresis-mass spectrometry. *J Chromatogr A* 1014: 83–91.

Fico G, Spada A, Braca A *et al.* (2003). RAPD analysis and flavonoid composition of Aconitum as an aid for taxonomic discrimination. *Biochem System Ecol* 31: 293–301.

Fukuda N, Tanaka H, Shoyama Y (2000). Formation of monoclonal antibody against a major ginseng component, ginsenoside Rg1 and its characterization. *Cytotechnology* 34: 197–204.

Fuzzati N (2004). Analysis methods of ginsenosides. *J Chromatogr B* 81: 119–133.

Gao W, Duan H, Huang L (2002). Good agricultural practice (GAP) and sustainable resource utilization of Chinese Materia Medica. *J Plant Biotechnol* 4: 103–107.

Gong F, Liang Y-Z, Xie P-S, Chau F-T (2003). Information theory applied to chromatographic fingerprint of herbal medicine for quality control. *J Chromatogr A* 1002: 25–40.

Guo F-Q, Liang Y-Z, Xu C-J, Huang L-F (2003). Determination of the volatile chemical constituents of *Notopterygium incisum* by gas chromatography-mass spectrometry and iterative or non-iterative chemometrics resolution methods. *J Chromatogr A* 1016: 99–110.

Guo F-Q, Liang Y-Z, Xu C-J, Huang L-F, Li X-N (2004). Comparison of the volatile constituents from *Artemisia capillaris* from different locations by gas chromatography-mass spectrometry and projection method. *J Chromatogr A* 1054: 73–79.

Ha W-Y, Yau FC-F, Shaw P-C, Wang J (2002). Differentiation of *Panax ginseng* from *P. quinquefolius* by amplified fragment length polymorphism. In: *Authentication of Chinese Medicinal Materials by DNA Technology,* Eds. Shaw PC, Wang J, But PPH. World Scientific Publishing Co. Pte. Ltd., Singapore, pp. 109–124.

He X-G (2000). On-line identification of phytochemical constituents in botanical extracts by combined high-performance liquid chromatographic–diode array detection–mass spectrometric techniques. *J Chromatogr A* 880: 203–233.

He ZD, Qiao CF, Han QB *et al.* (2005). Authentication and quantitative analysis on the chemical profile of Cassia bark (Cortex Cinnamomi) by high-pressure liquid chromatography. *J Agric Food Chem* 53: 2424–2428.

Hon CC, Chow YC, Zeng FY, Leung FCC (2003). Genetic authentication of ginseng and other traditional Chinese medicine. *Acta Pharmacol Sin* 24: 841–846.

Hsieh SC, Huang MF, Lin BS, Chang HT (2006). Determination of aristolochic acid in Chinese herbal medicine by capillary electrophoresis with laser-induced fluorescence detection. *J Chromatogr A* 1105: 127–134.

Huang WF, Wen KC, Hsiao ML, Hsiao ML (1997). Adulteration by synthetic therapeutic substances of traditional medicines in Taiwan. *J Clin Pharmacol* 37: 334–350.

Huang CY, Tseng MC, Lin JH (2005). Analyzing aristolochic acids in Chinese herbal preparations using LC/MS/MS. *J Food Drug Anal* 13: 125–131.

Ihrig M, Kaunzinger A, Baumann J *et al.* (2004). Qualitätsmängel bei TCM-Drogen. *Pharm Z* 149: 3776–3783.

Ioset J-R, Raoelison GE, Hostettmann K (2002). An LC/DAD-UV/MS method for the rapid detection of aristolochic acid in plant preparations. *Planta Med* 68: 856–858.

Ioset J-R, Raoelison GE, Hostettmann K (2003). Detection of aristolochic acid in Chinese phytomedicines and dietary supplements used as slimming regimens. *Food Chem Toxicol* 41: 29–36.

Jiang T-F, Lv Z-H, Wang Y-H (2005). Separation and determination of chalcones from *Carthamus tinctorius* L. and its medicinal preparation by capillary zone electrophoresis. *J Sep Sci* 28: 1244–1247.

Johnson KJ, Wright BW, Jarman KH *et al.* (2003). High-speed peak matching algorithm for retention time alignment of gas chromatographic data for chemometric analysis. *J Chromatogr A* 996: 141–155.

Joshi K, Chavan P, Warude D, Patwardhan B (2004). Molecular markers in herbal drug technology. *Curr Sci* 87: 159–165.

Kabelitz L (1998). Heavy metals in herbal drugs. *Eur J Herbal Med (Phytother)* 4: 1–9.

Kabelitz L (2001). Zur mikrobiologischen Qualität von Arznei- und Gewürzdrogen. Sind die bisherigen Anforderungen sachgerecht? *Z Arznei- und Gewuumlautrzpflanz* 6: 174–175.

Kabelitz L, Sievers H (2004). Contaminants of medicinal and food herbs with a view to EU regulations. *Innov Food Technol* 2004: 25–27.

Kneifel W, Czech E, Kopp B (2002). Microbial contamination of medicinal plants – a review. *Planta Med* 68: 5–15.

Leung KS-Y, Chan K, Chan C-L, Lu G-H (2005). Systematic evaluation of organochlorine pesticide residues in Chinese Materia Medica. *Phytother Res* 19: 514–518.

Li X-N, Cui H, Song Y-Q *et al.* (2003). Analysis of volatile fractions of *Schisandra chinensis* (Turcz.) Baill. using GC-MS and chemometric resolution. *Phytochem Anal* 14: 22–33.

Li B-Y, Hu Y, Liang Y-Z *et al.* (2004a). Spectral correlative chromatography and its application to analysis of chromatographic fingerprints of herbal medicines. *J Sep Sci* 27: 581–588.

Li B-Y, Hu Y, Liang Y-Z (2004b). Quality evaluation of fingerprints of herbal medicine with chromatographic data. *Anal Chim Acta* 514: 69–77.

Li Y, Qi S, Chen X, Hu Z, (2004c). Separation and determination of aconitine alkaloids in traditional Chinese herbs by nonaqueous capillary electrophoresis. *Electrophoresis* 25: 3003–3009.

Li B-Y, Hu Y, Liang Y-Z (2004d). Spectral correlative chromatography and its application to analysis of chromatographic fingerprints of herbal medicines. *J Sep Sci* 27: 581–588.

Li W, Chen Z, Liao Y, Liu H (2005). Separation methods for toxic components in traditional Chinese medicines. *Anal Sci* 21: 1019–1029.

Liang Y-Z, Xie P, Chan K (2004). Quality control of herbal medicines. *J Chromatogr B* 812: 53–70.

Lin C-C, Wu C-I, Sheu S-J (2005). Determination of 12 pueraria components by high-performance liquid chromatography-mass spectrometry. *J Sep Sci* 28: 1785–1795.

Lin I-H, Lee M-C, Chuang W-C (2006). Application of LC/MS and ICP/MS for establishing the fingerprint spectrum of the traditional Chinese medicinal preparation Gan-Lu-Yin. *J Sep Sci* 29: 172–179.

Ling Y-C, Teng H-C, Cartwright C (1999). Supercritical fluid extraction and clean-up of organochlorine pesticides in Chinese herbal medicine. *J Chromatogr A* 835: 145–157.

Lord GM, Tagore R, Cook T, Gower P, Pusey CD (1999). Nephropathy caused by Chinese herbs in the UK. *Lancet* 354: 481–482.

Lu Z, Morinaga O, Tanaka H, Shoyama Y (2003). A quantitative ELISA using monoclonal antibody to survey paeoniflorin and albiflorin in crude drugs and traditional Chinese herbal medicines. *Biol Pharm Bull* 26: 862–866.

McCutcheon A (2002). *An Exploration of Current Issues in Botanical Quality: a discussion paper*, 2002. Natural Health Products Directorate, Health Products and Food Branch, Canada.

McGregor CE, Lambert CA, Greyling MM *et al.* (2000). A comparative assessment of DNA fingerprinting techniques (RAPD, ISSR, AFLP and SSR) in tetraploid potato (*Solanum tuberosum* L.) germplasm. *Euphytica* 113: 135–144.

Nortier JL, Vanherweghem JL (2002). Renal interstitial fibrosis and urothelial carcinoma associated with the use of a Chinese herb (*Aristolochia fangchi*). *Toxicology* 181–182: 577–580.

Novak J, Grausgruber-Gröger S, Lukas B (2007). DNA-based authentication of plant extracts. *Food Res Int* 40: 388–392.

PRC Pharmacopoeia Committee (2005). *Pharmacopoeia of People's Republic of China*. People's Health Publishers, Beijing.

Qi S, Li Y, Wu S, Chen X, Hu Z (2005). Novel nonaqueous capillary electrophoresis separation and determination of bioactive flavone derivatives in Chinese herbs. *J Sep Sci* 28: 2180–2186.

Resch M, Wagner H, Bauer R, Xiao PG, Chen JM (1999). Rhizoma Atractylodis macrocephalae – Baizhu. In: *Chinese Drug Monographs and Analysis*, Eds. Wagner H, Bauer R, Peigen X *et al.* Vol. 2 (10) Verlag für Ganzheitliche Medizin, Dr. Erich Wühr GmbH, Kötzting, Germany.

Shaw PC, Ngan FN, But PPH, Wang J (2002a). Molecular markers in Chinese medicinal materials. In: *Authenication of Chinese Medicinal Materials by DNA Technology*, Eds. Shaw PC, Wang J, But PPH. World Scientific Publishing Co. Pte. Ltd., Singapore, pp. 1–24.

Shaw PC, Wang J, But PPH *et al.* (2002b). Outlook. In: *Authenication of Chinese Medicinal Materials by DNA Technology*, Eds. Shaw PC, Wang J, But PPH. World Scientific Publishing Co. Pte. Ltd., Singapore, pp. 212–224.

Shellie R, Mondello L, Marriott P, Dugo G (2002). Characterisation of lavender essential oils by using gas chromatography–mass spectrometry with correlation of linear retention indices and comparison with comprehensive two-dimensional gas chromatography. *J Chromatogr A* 970: 225–234.

Shellie RA, Marriott PJ, Huie CW (2003). Comprehensive two-dimensional gas chromatography (GCxGC) and GCxGC-quadrupole MS analysis of Asian and American ginseng. *J Sep Sci* 26: 1185–1192.

Siow YL, Gong Y, Au-Yeung KKW *et al.* (2005). Emerging issues in traditional Chinese medicine. *Can J Physiol Pharmacol* 83: 321–334.

Sohn S-H, Kim S-K, Kang H-G, Wee J-J (2004). Two-phase partition chromatography using soybean oil eliminates pesticide residues in aqueous ginseng extract. *J Chromatogr A* 1042: 163–168.

Song Y, Cheng H-L, Her G-R, Wen K-C (2000). Analysis of synthetic drugs in Chinese medicine by high performance liquid chromatography/mass spectrometry with in-source collision induced dissociation. *J Chin Chem Soc* 47: 475–480.

Techen N, Crockett SL, Khan IA, Scheffler BE (2004). Authentication of medicinal plants using molecular biology techniques to compliment conventional methods. *Curr Med Chem* 11: 1391–1401.

Tseng M-C, Lin J-H (2002). Determination of sildenafil citrate adulterated in a dietary supplement capsule by LC/MS/MS. *J Food Drug Anal* 10: 112–119.

Vanherweghem J-L, Depierreux M, Tielemans C *et al.* (1993). Rapidly progressive interstitial renal fibrosis in young women: Association with slimming regimen including Chinese herbs. *Lancet* 341: 387–391.

Wagner H, Bauer R, Peigen (Eds.). (2006). *Chinese Drug Monographs and Analysis* Verlag für Ganzheitliche Medizin, Dr. Erich Wühr GmbH, Kötzting, Germany.

Wang X, Kapoor V, Smythe GA (2003). Extraction and chromatographic-mass spectrometric analysis of the active principles from selected Chinese herbs and other medicinal plants. *Am J Chin Med* 31: 927–944.

Wang L, Lee FSC, Wang (2007). Near-infrared spectroscopy for classification of licorice (*Glycyrrhizia uralensis* Fisch) and prediction of the glycyrrhizic acid (GA) content. *Lebensm Wiss Technol* 40: 83–88.

Wenkui L, Fitzloff JF (2001). Determination of astragaloside IV in radix astragali (*Astragalus membranaceaus* var. *monghulicus*) using high-performance liquid chromatography with evaporative light-scattering detection. *J Chromatogr Sci* 39: 459–462.

Wolfender J-L, Rodriguez S, Hostettmann K (1998). Liquid chromatography coupled to mass spectrometry and nuclear magnetic resonance spectroscopy for the screening of plant constituents. *J Chromatogr A* 794: 299–316.

Wong S-K, Tsui S-K, Kwan S-Y (2002). Analysis of proprietary Chinese medicines for the presence of toxic ingredients by LC/MS/MS. *J Pharm Biomed Anal* 30: 161–170.

Wong S-K, Tsui S-K, Kwan S-Y, Su X-L, Lin R-C, Tang L-M, Chen X-J (2004). Establishment of characteristic fingerprint chromatogram for the identification of Chinese herbal medicines. *J Food Drug Anal* 12: 110–114.

WHO (1998). *Quality Control Methods for Medicinal Plant Materials.* World Health Organization, Geneva, Switzerland.

WHO (2000). *General Guidelines for Methodologies on Research and Evaluation of Traditional Medicine.* World Health Organization, Geneva, Switzerland.

Woo Y-A, Kim HJ, Ze K-R, Chung H (2005). Near-infrared (NIR) spectroscopy for the non-destructive and fast determination of geographical origin of Angelicae gigantis Radix. *J Pharm Biomed Anal* 36: 955–959.

Wu J, Lu X, Tang W *et al.* (2004). Application of comprehensive two-dimensional gas chromatography-time-of-flight mass spectrometry in the analysis of volatile oil of traditional Chinese medicines. *J Chromatogr A* 1034: 199–205.

Xia Q, Zhao KJ, Huang ZG *et al.* (2005). Molecular genetic and chemical assessment of Rhizoma Curcumae in China. *J Agric Food Chem* 53: 6016–6026.

Yan S-K, Xin W-F, Luo G-A *et al.* (2005a). Simultaneous determination of major bioactive components in Qingkailing injection by high-performance liquid chromatography with evaporative light scattering detection. *Chem Pharm Bull* 53: 1392–1395.

Yan S-K, Xin W-F, Luo GA (2005b). An approach to develop two-dimensional fingerprint for the quality control of *Qingkailing* injection by high-performance liquid chromatography with diode array detection. *J Chromatogr A* 1090: 90–97.

Yang L-W, Wu D-H, Tang W *et al.* (2005). Fingerprint quality control of Tianjihuang by high-performance liquid chromatography-photodiode array detection. *J Chromatogr A* 1070: 35–42.

Yang SY, Kim HK, Lefeber AWM *et al.* (2006). Application of two-dimensional nuclear magnetic resonance spectroscopy to quality control of ginseng commerical products. *Planta Med* 72: 364–369.

Yuan R, Lin Y (2000). Traditional Chinese medicine: an approach to scientific proof and clinical validation. *Pharmacol Ther* 86: 191–198.

Yue M-E, Jiang T-F, Shi P-Y (2004). Fast determination of flavonoids in *Hippophae rhamnoides* and its medicinal preparation by capillary zone electrophoresis using dimethyl-β-cyclodextrin as modifier. *Talanta* 62: 695–699.

Zhai Z-D, Luo X-P, Shi Y-P (2006). Separation and determination of aristolochic acids in herbal medicines by microemulsion electrokinetic chromatography. *Anal Chim Acta* 561: 119–125.

Zhang YB, Leung HW, Yeung HW, Wong RNS (2001). Differentiation of *Lycium barbarum* from its related *Lycium* species using random amplified polymorphic DNA. *Planta Med* 67: 379–381.

Zhao KJ, Dong TTX, Tu PF, Song ZH, Lo CK, Tsim KWK (2003). Molecular genetic and chemical assessment of Radix *Angelica* (Danggui) in China. *J Agric Food Chem* 51: 2576–2583.

Zhao R-.Z, Liu S, Zhou L-L (2005). Rapid quantitative HPTLC analysis, on one plate, of emodin, resveratrol, and polydatin in the Chinese herb *Polygonum cuspidatum*. *Chromatographia* 61: 311–314.

Zhao Z (Ed.) (2005). *An Illustrated Microscopic Identification of Chinese Materia Medica.* International Society for Chinese Medicine, Hong Kong.

Zhao Z, Hu Y, Liang Z *et al.* (2006). Authentication is fundamental for standardization of Chinese medicines. *Planta Med* 72: 865–874.

Zhou X, Zheng C, Sun J, You T (2006). Analysis of nephrotoxic and carcinogenic aristolochic acids in *Aristolochia* plants by capillary electrophoresis with electrochemical detection at a carbon fiber microdisk electrode. *J Chromatogr A* 1109: 152–159.

Zschocke S, Liu J-H, Stuppner H, Bauer R (1998). Comparative study of roots of *Angelica sinensis* and related umbelliferous drugs by thin layer chromatography, high-performance liquid chromatography and liquid chromatography-mass spectrometry. *Phytochem Anal* 9: 283–290.

Zschocke S, Klaiber I, Bauer R, Vogler B (2005). HPLC-coupled spectroscopic techniques (UV, MS, NMR) for the structure elucidation of phtalides in *Ligusticum chuanxiong*. *Mol Divers* 9: 33–39.

Zuin VG, Vilegas HY (2000). Pesticide residues in medicinal plants and phytomedicines. *Phytother Res* 14: 73–88.

29

Clinical trials as signposts to efficacy

Alexander G Panossian and Georg C Wikman

Introduction

The medicinal uses of plants are classified in WHO monographs according to the level of supporting data (World Health Organization, 1999, 2002). To be included in the highest category, the medicinal indications must be well-established in a number of countries and validated by clinical studies, the results of which have been disseminated through open publication in the international scientific literature. Medicinal uses that are well known in some countries and are incorporated into official pharmacopoeias, national monographs or in traditional systems of medicine, are included in a second category. Well-established indications with a plausible pharmacological basis supported by dated scientific studies requiring confirmation using more up-to-date techniques, are also included in this category. The lowest category includes those uses described in unofficial pharmacopoeias, other similar literature, and in folk medicine. Typically, it is not possible to assess the validity of these claims owing to the absence of supporting experimental or clinical data. The possible use of such remedies should be carefully considered in the light of more appropriate therapeutic alternatives.

Medicinal plants that have been traditionally employed in many countries, perhaps even for centuries, still require clinical evaluation of their efficacy and safety and comparison with the current standard treatment(s). In this context, the clinical trial provides a good example of the need for contemporary society to justify its choice of medication on the basis of the objectivity perceived to be inherent in quantitative and statistical data.

Types of clinical trials

Clinical trials are arranged on several categories.

Phase I

These trials examine clinical pharmacology and toxicity. The studies are usually performed on 20–80 healthy, human volunteers. The objectives of these studies are related to:

- estimation of suitable *single* dosage causing no serious side-effects
- drug bioavailability and metabolism

- determination of most suitable repeated dose schedule for use in Phase II.

Phase II

These trials are the initial clinical studies of efficacy and safety of a drug. They are pilot, small-scale studies on 100–200 patients requiring close monitoring of each patient. The aims of Phase II trials are:

- to estimate the efficiency of the dosing regimen determined in Phase I
- to verify the safety of the treatment.

Phase III

These multicentre trials are the full-scale evaluation of treatment, aimed to compare the study drug with the standard treatment(s) for the same condition in large trials involving a significant number of patients.

Phase IV

After approval for marketing, monitoring for adverse effects and additional large-scale, long-term studies of morbidity and mortality are essential.

Since the middle of the 20th century, the clinical trial has become firmly established as a standard procedure in the evaluation of new drugs. The key features of such a trial include the involvement of a control group whose members do not receive the experimental treatment, the allocation of subjects to the experimental group or to the control group in a fully randomised manner, and the use of blind or masked assessment so that neither the researchers nor the subjects are aware of which group they are in during the period of study.

In general, clinical trials may be classified as controlled, randomised, double-blind studies, open trials, or as well-documented observations of therapeutic applications. While clinical trials may take a variety of different forms, they are all *prospective* in that the observations are made over a period of time following application of the treatment. Perhaps the most common design for a clinical trial is the fixed sample size, parallel group design with random allocation of subjects to groups.

However, a different strategy may be required when there is considerable variability in the initial disease state of the subjects or in their response to therapy. Under these circumstances, large numbers of subjects may need to be included in the trial, to estimate the magnitude of any difference between treatments reliably. In such cases a more precise comparison of treatments might be achieved using a crossover design in which each subject receives more than one treatment. An example of this type of trial is the simple 2×2 crossover study in which one group of subjects receives treatment A followed by treatment B while another group receives these treatments in the reverse order. Clearly such a design is only suitable for use with chronic conditions in which the objective is limited to the study of a patient's response to relatively short periods of therapy (Everitt and Pickles, 2004).

Possible designs of controlled clinical trials can be described as follows (Deeks *et al.*, 2003).

Experimental designs

A study in which the investigator has control over at least some study conditions, particularly decisions concerning the allocation of participants to different intervention groups.

Randomised, controlled trial

Participants are randomly allocated to intervention or control groups and followed up over time to assess any differences in outcome rates. Randomisation with allocation concealment ensures that on average known and unknown determinants of outcome are evenly distributed between groups.

Quasi-randomised trial

Participants are allocated to intervention or control groups by the investigator, but the method of allocation falls short of genuine randomisation and allocation concealment (e.g. allocated by date of birth, hospital record number, etc.).

Non-randomised trial/quasi-experimental study

The investigator has control over the allocation of participants to groups, but does not attempt randomisation (e.g. patient or physician preference). Differs from a 'cohort study' in that the intention is experimental rather than observational.

Observational designs

The following categories are used for the various studies where the effect of a treatment on health outcomes is carried out.

Controlled before-and-after study

A follow-up study of participants who have received an intervention and those who have not, measuring the outcome variable both at baseline and after the intervention period, comparing either final values if the groups are comparable at baseline, or change scores. It can also be considered an experimental design if the investigator has control over, or can deliberately manipulate, the introduction of the intervention.

Concurrent cohort study

A follow-up study that compares outcomes between participants who have received an intervention and those who have not. Participants are studied during the same (concurrent) period either prospectively or, more commonly, retrospectively.

Historical cohort study

A variation on the traditional cohort study where the outcome from a new intervention is established for participants studied in one period and compared with those who did not receive the intervention in a previous period, i.e. participants are not studied concurrently.

Case–control study

Participants with and without a given outcome are identified (cases and controls respectively) and exposure to a given intervention(s) between the two groups compared.

Before-and-after study

Comparison of outcomes from study participants before and after an intervention is introduced. The before and after measurements may be made in the same participants, or in different samples. It can also be considered an experimental design if the investigator has control over, or can deliberately manipulate, the introduction of the intervention.

Cross-sectional study

Examination of the relationship between disease and other variables of interest as they exist in a defined population at one particular time point.

Case series

Description of a number of cases of an intervention and outcome (no comparison with a control group).

Regulation of herbal preparations and quality of clinical trials

Herbal preparations can be categorised according to the quality and level of the data (efficacy and safety) supporting the medicinal indications and/or uses claimed. In EC countries, for example, herbal preparations are categorised as:

- *herbal medicinal products* with a well-established use, a recognised efficacy and an acceptable level of safety
- *traditional herbal medicines*
- *dietary supplements* (EMEA/HMPWG/104613/2005, 2006; Directive 2001/83/EC, 2001).

In the United States, botanicals can be used as drugs or dietary supplements, while in Russia they may be employed as drugs or biologically active additives. An important consequence of this type of legal classification is that the claims that can be made for each category of herbal preparation are highly restricted.

In the US, the Food and Drug Administration (FDA) regulates dietary supplements as foods, and not as drugs. The FDA does not pre-approve dietary supplements on their safety and efficacy (unlike drugs) and requires that every supplement be labelled a dietary supplement (Kurtzweil, 1998). A dietary supplement sold or promoted on its label or in labelling as a treatment, prevention or cure for a specific disease or condition would be considered an unapproved – and thus illegal – drug.

By law, manufacturers may make three types of claims for their dietary supplement products: health claims, structure/function claims, and nutrient content claims. Some of these claims describe:

- the link between a food substance and disease or a health-related condition
- the intended benefits of using the product
- the amount of a nutrient or dietary substance in a product.

A disclaimer – 'This statement has not been evaluated by the FDA. This product is not intended to diagnose, treat, cure, or prevent any disease' is required by law when a manufacturer makes a structure/function claim on a dietary supplement label. In general, these claims describe the role of a nutrient or dietary ingredient intended to affect the structure or function of the body. In the European Union (EU), the Food Supplements Directive (Directive 2002/46/EC, 2002) requires that supplements be demonstrated to be safe, both in quantity and quality.

Herbal preparations have a limited range of indication on labelling. The indication fields for traditional medicinal products contain the additional statements 'traditionally used' and they are: 'for strengthening . . .', 'for improvement of the general condition . . .', 'adjuvant treatment of the organic function of . . .', 'prevention of . . .', 'mildly acting medicinal product for . . .' (Directive 2004/24/EC, 2004).

In the EC, claims made for 'herbal medicinal products with well-established medicinal use, recognised efficacy' and 'acceptable level of safety' (EMEA/HMPWG/104613/2005, 2006) must be supported by an adequate level of evidence before marketing approval can be granted to the product (EMEA/CPMP/HMPWG/1156/03, 2004).

Major claims: level I; grade A

- 'For the treatment, cure or management of any serious disease or disorder.'
- 'For the prevention of any serious disease or disorder' should be reserved for products with high level of evidence only.

Medium claims: level IIa, IIb, III; grade B

For products with a medium level of evidence, the following claims may be acceptable:

- reduction of the risk of a disease/disorder
- reduction in frequency of a discrete event
- aids/assists in the management of a named symptom/disease/disorder
- relief of symptoms of a named disease or disorder.

Minor claims: level IV, grade C

For products with a general level of evidence, the following claims may be acceptable:

- relief or management of symptoms of a minor, self-limiting disease/disorder that does not require medical intervention for diagnosis or monitoring
- description of a pharmacological action related to management of symptoms of a minor, self-limiting disease/disorder that does not require medical intervention for diagnosis or, if general evidence is submitted to support such claims, additional supporting evidence, e.g. pharmacological data, may be also necessary.

According to WHO, 'well-established medicinal use', and 'recognised efficacy' implies a 'long history of medical use' which may be defined, depending on the history of a given country (or community), as not less than several decades. Well-established use implies that a sufficient number of patients were treated by the concerned product or by a product essentially similar to the concerned product.

In the case of well-established herbal medicinal products, the requirements for proof of efficacy and the documentation required to support the indicated claims depend on the nature and the level of the indication. For treatment of minor disorders a lower level of evidence may be adequate, especially when the extent of long-term use, the experience with that particular herbal medicinal product and supportive pharmacological data were taken into account. The level of evidence and the grading of recommendations corresponds to the nature of the disease that is treated.

In the assessment of well-established herbal medicinal products, all bibliographic documents on clinical trials have to be taken into consideration. Old reports are judged for their credibility. Various type of documents are used: controlled clinical trials, other clinical trials, cohort or longitudinal studies, observational (non-interventional) studies, case–control studies, other collections of single cases allowing a scientific evaluation, scientifically documented medical experience, for example, scientific literature and expertise from scientific medical associations. These bibliographic records are assessed, to establish if they can demonstrate a sufficient level of safety and efficacy (EMEA/HMPWG/104613/2005).

When studying clinical safety and efficacy using bibliographic references, the following are evaluated:

- number of patients
- specific diagnosis
- preparation used
- dosage
- duration of administration
- criteria for evaluation (e.g. improvement of symptoms)
- applicable statistical analysis.

The following factors increase the relevance and credibility of published data:

- multiple studies conducted by different investigators and/or independent literature reports where the findings across studies/reports are consistent
- high level of detail in the published reports, including clear and adequate descriptions of statistical plans, analytic methods (prospectively determined), and study endpoints, and a full accounting of all enrolled patients
- clearly appropriate endpoints that can be objectively assessed and are not dependent on investigator judgement (e.g. overall mortality, blood pressure, or microbial eradication). Such endpoints are more readily interpreted than more subjective endpoints such as relief of symptoms
- robust results achieved by protocol-specified analyses that yield a consistent conclusion of efficacy and do not require selected post-hoc analyses, such as covariate adjustment, subsetting, or reduced data sets (e.g. analysis of only responders or compliant patients, or of an 'eligible' or 'evaluable' subset)
- conduct of studies by groups with properly documented operating procedures and a history of implementing such procedures effectively (EMEA/HMPWG/104613/2005).

Reviews of the literature identify the current level of evidence of the safe and effective use of a herbal medicinal product. WHO recommends following definitions of the types of evidence (Table 29.1) and the grading of recommendations (Table 29.2).

The description of the traditional use of a preparation with no accompanying clinical or experimental data would not be considered sufficient

Table 29.1 Levels of evidence

Level	Type of evidence
Ia	Evidence obtained from meta-analysis of randomised, controlled trials
Ib	Evidence obtained from at least one randomised, controlled trial
IIa	Evidence obtained from at least one well-designed, controlled study without randomisation
IIb	Evidence obtained from at least one other type of well-designed, quasi-experimental study
III	Evidence obtained from well-designed, non-experimental, descriptive studies, such as comparative studies, correlation studies and case–control studies
IV	Evidence obtained from expert committee reports or opinions and/or clinical experience of respected authorities

Table 29.2 Grading of recommendations

Grade	Recommendation
A (Evidence levels Ia, Ib)	Requires at least one randomised, controlled trial as part of the body of literature of overall good quality and consistency addressing the specific recommendation
B (Evidence levels IIa, IIb, III)	Requires availability of well-conducted, clinical studies but no randomised clinical trials on the topic of recommendation
C (Evidence level IV)	Requires evidence from expert committee reports or opinions and/or clinical experience of respected authorities. Indicates absence of directly applicable studies of good quality

evidence of efficacy. However, most medicines, the indications of which could be described as well established, are typically supported by numerous clinical studies (EMEA/HMPWG/104613/2005).

The highest level of evidence (Ia) is the *Evidence obtained from meta-analysis of randomised controlled trials*. Meta-analysis is a statistical method for combining the results from two or more independent studies. It is used when it is felt that the studies are similar enough to make combining the results a sensible thing to do. Judging the advisability of combining drugs requires clinical common sense and an assessment of the quality of the studies carried out on each drug separately. Meta-analysis is a two-stage process. First the data for each study are summarised, and then those summaries are statistically combined. All widely used methods of meta-analysis are of this type (Altman *et al.*, 2002).

While, for a whole variety of reasons, some clinical trials may not provide accurate information concerning the efficacy or safety of a studied drug, those that have been conducted according to GCP standards should offer an acceptable standard of reliability.

In 1996, ICH-consolidated guidelines were developed with consideration of the current good clinical practices (GCPs) of the EU, Japan and the US, as well as those of Australia, Canada, the Nordic countries and the World Health Organization.

GCP is an international ethical and scientific quality standard for designing, conducting, recording and reporting trials that involve the participation of human subjects. Compliance with this standard provides public assurance that the rights, safety and wellbeing of trial subjects are protected, consistent with the principles that have their origin in the Declaration of Helsinki, and that the clinical trial data are credible.

The objective of the ICH GCP guidance was to provide a unified standard for the EU, Japan and the US to facilitate the mutual acceptance of clinical data by the regulatory authorities in these jurisdictions.

The principles of ICH GCP are:

- Clinical trials should be conducted in accordance with the ethical principles that have their origin in the Declaration of Helsinki (World Medical Association, 2000), and that are consistent with GCP and the applicable regulatory requirement(s).
- Before a trial is initiated, foreseeable risks and inconveniences should be weighed against the anticipated benefit for the individual trial subject and society. A trial should be initiated and continued only if the anticipated benefits justify the risks.
- The rights, safety and wellbeing of the trial subjects are the most important considerations and should prevail over interests of science and society.
- The available non-clinical and clinical information on an investigational product should be adequate to support the proposed clinical trial.
- Clinical trials should be scientifically sound, and described in a clear, detailed protocol.
- A trial should be conducted in compliance with the protocol that has received prior institutional review board (IRB)/independent ethics committee (IEC) approval/favourable opinion.

- The medical care given to, and medical decisions made on behalf of, subjects should always be the responsibility of a qualified physician or, when appropriate, of a qualified dentist.
- Each individual involved in conducting a trial should be qualified by education, training, and experience to perform his or her respective task(s).
- Freely given informed consent should be obtained from every subject prior to clinical trial participation.
- All clinical trial information should be recorded, handled and stored in a way that allows its accurate reporting, interpretation and verification.
- The confidentiality of records that could identify subjects should be protected, respecting the privacy and confidentiality rules in accordance with the applicable regulatory requirement(s).
- Investigational products should be manufactured, handled and stored in accordance with applicable good manufacturing practice (GMP). They should be used in accordance with the approved protocol.
- Systems with procedures that assure the quality of every aspect of the trial should be implemented.

The use of reliable data in support of medical and public health decisions is essential, particularly when it concerns clinical trials of herbal preparations.

While it is practically impossible to ascertain whether certain clinical trials performed before the 1980s complied fully with the principles of GCP, it is possible to evaluate the quality of the reports to some extent.

There are three methods to assess the quality of clinical trials: individual markers, checklists, and scales. Scales have the theoretical advantage over the other methods in that they provide quantitative estimates of quality that could be replicated easily and incorporated formally into the peer review process and into systematic reviews. Most frequently Jadad's scale is used for assessments of quality of clinical trials (Jadad *et al.*, 1996). The instrument contained the three questions related directly to measure the likelihood of bias in research reports:

- Was the study described as randomised (this includes the use of words such as randomly, random, and randomisation)?
- Was the study described as double blind?
- Was there a description of withdrawals and dropouts?

Points awarded for items 1 and 2 depended on the quality of the description of the methods to generate the sequence of randomisation and/or the quality of the description of the method of double blinding. If the trial had been described as randomised and/or double blind, but there was no description of the methods used to generate the sequence of randomisation or the double-blind conditions, one point was awarded in each case. If the method of generating the sequence of randomisation and/or blinding had been described, one additional point was given to each item if the method was appropriate.

A method to generate randomisation sequences was regarded as adequate if it allowed each study participant to have the same chance of receiving each intervention, and if the investigators could not predict which intervention was next. Methods of allocation using date of birth, date of admission, hospital numbers, or alternation should be not regarded as appropriate. A study must be regarded as double blind if the word 'double blind' is used. Double blinding was considered appropriate if it was stated or implied that neither the person doing the assessment nor the study participant could identify the intervention being assessed or if in the absence of such a statement the use of active placebos, identical placebos or dummies is mentioned. Conversely, if the method of generating the sequence of randomisation and/or blinding was described but not appropriate, the relevant item was given zero points. The third item, withdrawals and dropouts, was awarded zero points for a negative answer and one point for a positive. For a positive answer, the number of withdrawals and dropouts and the reasons had to be stated in each of the comparison groups. If there were no withdrawals, it should have been stated in the report (Jadad *et al.*, 1996).

In the absence of randomised, controlled trials (RCTs), healthcare practitioners and policymakers rely on non-randomised studies to provide evidence of the effectiveness of healthcare interventions. However, there is controversy over the validity of non-randomised evidence, related to the existence and magnitude of selection bias. Systematic evaluation of non-randomised intervention studies (Deeks *et al.*, 2003) showed that results of non-randomised studies sometimes, but not always, differ from results of randomised studies of the same intervention. Non-randomised studies may still give seriously misleading results when treated and control groups appear similar in key prognostic factors. Standard methods of case-mix adjustment do not guarantee removal of bias. Residual confounding may be high even when good prognostic data are available, and in some situations adjusted results may appear more biased than unadjusted results. Although many quality-assessment tools exist and have been used for appraising non-randomised studies, most omit key quality domains.

Healthcare policies based upon non-randomised studies or systematic reviews of non-randomised studies may need re-evaluation if the uncertainty in the true evidence base was not fully appreciated when policies were made. The inability of case-mix adjustment methods to compensate for selection bias and our inability to identify non-randomised studies that are free of selection bias indicate that non-randomised studies should only be undertaken when RCTs are infeasible or unethical. Recommendations for further research include:

- applying the resampling methodology in other clinical areas to ascertain whether the biases described are typical
- developing or refining existing quality-assessment tools for non-randomised studies
- investigating how quality assessments of non-randomised studies can be incorporated into reviews and the implications of individual quality features for interpretation of a review's results
- examination of the reasons for the apparent failure of case-mix adjustment methods
- further evaluation of the role of the propensity score (Deeks *et al.*, 2003).

The value of evidence concerning the effectiveness of healthcare interventions derived from studies involving non-randomised designs is somewhat controversial. Advocates for quasi-experimental and observational (QEO) studies argue that evidence from randomised, controlled trials (RCTs) is often difficult or impossible to obtain, or is inadequate to answer the question of interest. Advocates for RCTs point out that QEO studies are more susceptible to bias and refer to published comparisons that suggest QEO estimates tend to find a greater benefit than RCT estimates. However, comparisons from the literature are often cited selectively, may be unsystematic and may have failed to distinguish between different explanations for any discrepancies observed.

QEO study estimates of effectiveness may be valid if important confounding factors are controlled for. The small size of discrepancies for high-quality comparisons also implies that psychological factors (e.g. treatment preferences or willingness to be randomised) had a negligible effect on outcome. However, the authors caution against generalising their findings to other contexts, for three main reasons:

- Few papers were reviewed, and the findings may depend on the specific interventions evaluated.
- Most high-quality comparisons studied RCT and QEO study populations that met the same eligibility criteria, which may have reduced the importance of controlling for confounding.
- The literature reviewed is likely to have been subject to some form of publication bias.

Authors of papers appeared to have strong a priori views about the usefulness of evidence from QEO studies, and the findings of papers appeared to support these views (MacLehose *et al.*, 2000).

Clinical trials of selected medicinal plants

Table 29.3 summarises the results of clinical trials of selected medicinal plants that are included in WHO and ESCOP monographs (World Health Organisation, 1999, 2002; ESCOP Monographs, 2003).

Table 29.3

Plant name and part used	Dosage forms	Diagnosis/indications/use	Pharmacological effect related to indication/use
Absinthii Herba, *Arememisia absinthium* L., Wormwood	Infusions or decocts, dry alcoholic extract suspended in water	Hepatopathy, anorexia, dyspeptic complaints	Increases gastrointestinal secretions
Agni Casti Fructus, *Vitex agnus* castus L., Chaste tree fruit	Extracts	Premenstrual syndrome (mastodinia, mastalgia) and menstrual cycle disorders (polymenorrhoea, amenorrhoea, olygomenorrhoea)	Reduction of frequency and severity of premenstrual symptoms and cholesterol lowering, fibrinolitic and antihypertensive effects, vasodilatation of precapillary arterioles, improve of elastic property of the aorta
Allii Sativi Bulbus, *Allium sativum* L., Garlic	Fresh bulbs, dried powder, volatile oil, oil macerates, juice, aqueous or alcoholic extracts, aged garlic extracts, tablets, capsules, powder	Atherosclerosis, hyperlipidemia; age-dependent changes in blood vessels	
Allii Cepae Bulbus, *Allium cepa* L., Onion	Fresh juice, 5% and 50 % EtOH extracts. Dried bulbus	Atherosclerosis, age-dependent changes in blood vessels, loss of appetite	Antibacterial, antifungal effect, inhibition of platelet aggregation, cholesterol lowering, fibrinolitic and antihypergycaemic effect
Aloe Capensis, *Aloe vera* (L.) Burm.f.	Powdered, dried juice and preparations thereof for oral use	For short-term use in cases of occasional constipation	Laxative effect
Altheaeae Radix	Crude drug, and galenic preparation thereof	Dry cough, irritation of the oral, pharyngeal or gastric mucosa	Mucous protective effect from local irritation. Anti-tussive, anti-inflammatory, immuno-modulatory effects
Andrographidis Herba	Crude drug, capsules, tablets and pills	Prophylaxis and symptomatic treatment of upper respiratory infections, such us common cold, uncomplicated sinusitis, bronchitis, pharingotonsilitis, lower urinary tract infections, acute diarrhoea	Antiviral, immunostimulatory, anti-inflammatory, antipyretic, antihepatotoxic activity.
Anisi Fructus	Crude drug for infusions	Dyspeptic complaints such as mild spasmolytic gastrointestinal complaints, bloating, flatulence. Catarrh of upper respiratory tract	Secretolitic, antispasmolitic and secretomotor effects
Angelicae Sinensis Radix	Powdered crude drug and fluid extracts	Menopausal symptoms	Premenstrual pain relief effect
Arnicae Flos	Ointments, creams, gels or compresses made with 5–25% tinctures, extracts, dicuted extracts or decoctions of dried flowers	Treatment of bruises, sprains and inflammation caused by insect bites, gingivitis and aphthous ulcers, symptomatic treatment of rheumatic complaints, chronic venous insufficiency	Anti-inflammatory, antimicrobial, cytotoxic and tumour-inhibiting effects

Table 29.3 (*continued*)

Plant name and part used	Dosage forms	Diagnosis/indications/use	Pharmacological effect related to indication/use
Astragali Radix, *Astragalus membranaceus* (Firch.) Bunge	Crude plant material, extracts	Common cold	Immunostimulant
Betulae Folium	Crude plant material for infusion, tincture, fresh juice	Irrigation of urinary tract, especially in cases of inflammation and renal gravel, and as an adjuvant in the treatment of bacterial infections of the urinary tract	Diuretic effect
Bruceae Fructus, *Brucea javanica* (l) Merr.	Seeds for decoction, or capsules	Amoebic dysentery	Amoebicidal and antibacterial activity
Bupleuri Radix, *Bupleurum falcatum* L.	Decoction	Common cold, malaria, influenza, pneumonia/fever	Antipyretic activity
Calendulae Flos	Infusion for topical use, extracts, tinctures and ointments	Symptomatic treatment of minor inflammations of the skin and mucosa as an aid to the healing of minor wounds	Immunomodulatory, antibacterial, antiviral, anti-inflammatory and wound healing activity
Cheledoni Herba	Tea infusion, standardised extracts, tinctures	Symptomatic treatment of mild to moderate spasms of the upper gastrointestinal tract; minor gall bladder disorders; dyspeptic complaints such as bloating and flatulence	Antispasmodic, choleretic and anti-inflammatory effects
Centellae Herba, *Centella asiatica* (L.) Urban	Dried drug for infusion, galenic preparations for oral administration, powder or extract for topical application	Treatment of wounds, burns, and ulcerous skin ailments. Prevention of keloid and hypertrophic scars. Stomach and duodenal ulcer	Stimulation of collagen and mucopolysaccharide synthesis in foreskin fibroblasts, inhibition of the inflammatory phase of hypertrophic scars and keloids. Reduction of stress-induced gastric ulceration by stimulation of GABA
Chamomillae Flos, *Chamomilla recutita* (L) Rauschert	Extracts, tinctures and other galenicals	1. Treatment of digestive ailments such as dyspepsia, epigastric bloating, impaired digestion, flatulence 2. Insomnia 3. Inflammations of the skin and mucosa (skin cracks, bruses, frostbite, insect bites), including irritations and infections of the mouth and gums, and haemorrhoids	Anti-inflammatory
Cimicifugae Racemosae Rhizoma	Crude drug, extracts	Treatment of climacteric symptoms such as hot flushes, profuse sweating, sleeping disorders and nervous irritability	Oestrogenic activity, a decrease in serum luteinising hormone and climacteric symptoms Anti-depressive effect
Coptidis Rhizoma, Coptis chinensis Franch	Crude plant material, powder, and decoction	Cholera and non-cholera diarrhoea	Antibacterial activity, antisecretory effect in enterotoxigenic *E. coli*-induced diarrhoea

(*continued overleaf*)

Table 29.3 *(continued)*

Plant name and part used	Dosage forms	Diagnosis/indications/use	Pharmacological effect related to indication/use
Crategi Folium cum Flore	Crude drug for infusion and extracts	Treatment of congestive heart failure stage II	Increases myocardial performance, improves myocardial circulatory perfusion and tolerance in cases of oxygen deficiency, antiarrythmic Inotropic, chronotropic, antihypertensive effects, effect on coronary blood flow Vasodilatatory, potassium channel agonist
Curcumae Longae Rhizoma Curcuma longa L.	Crude plant material, powder in galenic preparations	Treatment of acid, flatulent and atonic dyspepsia	Anti-inflammatory, inhibition of gastric secretion, stimulation of gastic wall mucus and increase in the mucin content in gastric juice
Cynarae Folium	Dried leaf aqueous dry extract or infusion	Adjuvant to a low-fat diet in the treatment of mild to moderate hyperlipidaemia. Digestive complaints (e.g. stomach ache, nausea, vomiting, feeling of fullness) and hepatobiliary disturbances	Choliretic, hypolipidaemic, thermogenic, antidispeptic, hepatoprotective effect
Echinaceae Pallidae Radix	Hydroethanolic extracts	Adjuvant therapy and prophylaxis of recurrent infections of the upper respiratory tract (common cold)	Immunomodulatory and antioxidant effects
Echinaceae Purpureae Herba	Powdered aerial part, pressed juice and galenic preparations thereof for internal and external use	Supportive therapy for colds, the respiratory tract and urinary infections. External used include promotion of wound healing	Immunomodulatory and antiviral effects
Echinaceae Purpureae Radix	Crude plant material, powder in galenic preparations	Supportive therapy for colds, the respiratory tract and urinary infections	Stimulation of the immune system
Eleutherococci Radix	Powdered crude drug or extracts in capsules, tablets, teas, syrup, fluid extracts	As a prophylactic and restorative tonic for enhancement of mental and physical capacities in cases of weakness, exhaustion and tiredness, and during convalescence	Adaptogenic and antistress activity, immunomodulating, antioxidant, antiviral, hepatoprotective and endocrine effects
Ephedrae Herba	Powdered plant material, extracts and other galenicals	Nasal congestion due to hay fever, allergic rhinitis, acute coryza, common cold and sinusitis. Bronchodilatator in the treatment of bronchial asthma	Sympathomimetic effect, stimulation of α-adrenoreceptors when applied topically to nasal and pharyngeal mucosal surface. Stimulation of β-adrenoreceptors in lung
Eucalypti Aetheroleum	Essential oil in solid, semisolid or liquid preparations and galenical preparations	Symptomatic treatment of common cold, reducing in nasal congestion	Stimulation of nasal cold receptors, Antimicrobial, anti-inflammatory activity

Table 29.3 *(continued)*

Plant name and part used	Dosage forms	Diagnosis/indications/use	Pharmacological effect related to indication/use
Filipendulae Ulmariae Herba	Local allocation of an ointment containing decoction	Cervical dysplasia	Anticancerogenic effect
Frangulae Cortex	Finely cut and powdered crude drug, powder, dried extract, liquid and solid preparations	Short-term treatment of occasional constipation. As a single dose for total intestinal evacuation	Laxative effect
Gentianae Radix	Decoction, macerate and tincture	Anorexia, dyspeptic complaints (heartburn, vomiting, nausea, constipations, flatulance), inflammatory conditions of gastrointestinal tract	Stimulation of secretion of gastric juice and bile. Improvement in dyspeptic symptoms
Ginkgo Folium	Coated tablets and solutions prepared from standardised extracts	Symptomatic treatment of mild to moderate cerebrovascular insufficiency (demential syndromes) with the following symptoms: memory deficit, disturbance of concentrations, depressive emotional conditions, dizziness, tinnitus, headache. Peripherial occlusive disease and post-phlebitis syndrome. Treatment of inner ear disorders	Multiple effects: to improve global and local blood flow and microcirculation, to protect against hypoxia, to improve rheology, including inhibition of platelet aggregation, to improve metabolism and to reduce capillary permeability
Ginseng Radix	Crude plant material, capsules and tablets of powdered drugs, extracts, tonic drinks, wines, and lozenges	A prophylactic and restorative agent for enhancement of mental and physical capacities, in cases of weakness, exhaustions, tiredness and loss of concentrations, and during convalescence	Multiple activities producing an adaptogenic effect
Glycyrrhizae Radix	Crude plant material, dried extract, liquid extract	Peptic and duodenal ulcers	Anti-inflammatory, cytoprotective effect due on the gastric mucosa to inhibition of 15-hydroxy-prostaglandin dehydrogenase and Δ13-PG reductase
Hamamelidis Folium et Cortex	Dried leaves and bark for decoctions, steam distillate, ointment and suppositories. Fresh leaves and twigs are used for preparation of a steam distillate	Topically for minor skin lesions, bruises and sprains, local inflammation of the skin and mucous membranes, haemorrhoids and varicose veins	Astrigent and venotonic activities. Antibacterial and anti-inflammatory activity
Hamamelidis Aqua	Water solutions and semi-solid preparations	Atopic dermatitis, atopic eczema, treatment of bruises, skin irritation, sunburn, insect bites. Minor inflammatory conditions of the skin and mucosa. Episiotomy pain	Anti-inflammatory and analgesic effect
Hamamelidis Cortex	Ointment containing fluid extract	First-degree haemorrhoids	Anti-inflammatory. Improvement in symptoms (pruritus, bleeding, burning sensation and pain)

(continued overleaf)

Table 29.3 (*continued*)

Plant name and part used	Dosage forms	Diagnosis/indications/use	Pharmacological effect related to indication/use
Hamamelidis Folium	Cream containing fluid extract	Atopic neurodermitis	Anti-inflammatory and analgesic effect
Harpagophyti Radix	Hydro-ethanolic extracts	Arthrosis and arthritis, relief of low back pain	Anti-inflammatory and analgesic effects
Hederae Helicis Folium	Hydro-ethanolic dry extracts in oral liquids	Cough associated with hypersecretion of viscous mucus. As adjuvant treatment of bronchial diseases	Spasmolitic and anti-inflammatory effects
Hippocastani Semen	Crude drug and extracts	Internally, for the treatment of symptoms of chronic venous insufficiency, including pain, feeling of heaviness in the legs, nocturnal calf-muscle spasms, itching and oedema. Externally, for the symptomatic treatment of chronic venous insufficiency, sprains and bruises	Anti-inflammatory and vasoactive effects
Hiperici Herba	Dried crude drug for decoction, powdered drug or extracts in capsules, tablets, tinctures and drops. Topical preparations include the oil, infusions, compresses, gels and ointments	Symptomatic treatment of mild and moderate depressive episodes	Antidepressant activity
Lichen Islandicus	Decoction, pastilles containing aqueous extract	Dry cough; irritation or inflammation of the oral and pharyngeal mucosa	Antibacterial, antiviral, immunomodulatory and antiproliferative activities
Lini Semen	Seeds, powdered and soaked in water	Constipation, irritable bowel syndrome, diverticular disease, gastritis and enteritis. Painful skin inflammations – externally	Laxative effect, effect on gastrointestinal complaints. Oestrogenic effect, effects on blood glucose and lipid level
Matricariae Flos	External use: hydroalcoholic extracts in solid and semisolid preparations (ointment, cream, etc.), infusions, extracts. Internal use: Infusions, dry and fluid extracts	Gastrointestinal complaints (gastritis, flatulence or minor spasms of the stomach), dermatoses, haemorrhoids, wounds healing. UV-induced erythema	Anti-inflammatory, antispasmodic, wound healing effects
Meliloti Herba	Hydroalcoholic extract taken orally or applied topically	Symptomatic treatment problems related to varicose veins, lymphoedema and mastalgia	Myotropis action, anti-inflammatory
Melaleucae Alternafpliae Aethroleum	Essential oil	Topical application for symptomatic treatment of common skin disorders such as acne, tinea pedis, bromidrosis, furunculosis and mycotic onychia, and of vaginitis due to *Thrichomonas vaginalis* or *Candida albicans*, cystitis and cervicitis	Antimicrobial activity

Table 29.3 *(continued)*

Plant name and part used	Dosage forms	Diagnosis/indications/use	Pharmacological effect related to indication/use
Melissae Folium	Comminuted crude drug, powder, tea bags, dried and fluid extracts for infusions and other galenical preparations	Externally, for symptomatic treatment of herpes labialis	Antiviral activity
Menthae Piperitae Aethroleum	Internal use: essential oil (in lozenges or enteric-coated capsules) for digestive disorders and irritable bowel syndrome External use: essential oil in dilute, semisolid or oily preparations	Internally for symptomatic treatment of irritable bowel syndrome and digestive disorders such as flatulence and gastritis	Antimicrobal and antispasmodic activity
Menthae Piperitae Aetheroleum	Aqueous preparations, enteric-coated capsules	Irritable bowel syndrome, symptomatic treatment in common cold, tension-type headache	Spasmolytic effect, analgesic effect, secretolytic in the bronchi, and decongestant in the nose
Myrrha	Solutions, volatile oil	Schistosomiasis and fascioliasis	Anthelmintic antiparasitic effect
Myrtilli Fructus	Dry fruit, decoction	Peripheral vascular diseases (limb varicose syndrome, chronic venous insufficiency), ophthalmic disorders (tapetoretinal degeneration, refractory defects, etc.)	Antioxidant, vasoprotective, anti-inflammatory, antiatherogenic and ophthalmic activity
Ocimi Sancti Folium	Crude drug and preparations thereof	Diabetes	Hypoglycaemic activity
Oenotherae Biennis Oleum	Fixed oil, neat or in capsule form	Internally for symptomatic treatment of atopic eczema, diabetic neuropathy, mastalgia and rheumatoid arthritis	Anti-inflammatory, inhibition of nerve conduction velocity, inhibition of platelet aggregation. Inhibition of clinical symptoms in atopic eczema, mastalgia, diabetic neuropathy, menopausal flashing, rheumatoid arthritis
Orthosiphonis Folium	Infusions	Irrigation of urinary tract – inflammation and bacterial infections: uratic diathesis, cholicystitis and cholangitis	Diuretic and choleretic activity
Passiflorae Herba	Infusions, tincture	Tenseness, restlessness and irritability with difficulty in falling asleep, anxiety, opiate addictions	Sedative effect, inhibition of GABA receptors
Piperis Methystici Rhizoma, Kava kava	Comminuted crude drug and extracts for oral use	Short-term symptomatic treatment of mild states of anxiety or insomnia, due to nervousness, stress or tension	Behavioural and neuroprotective effect
Plantaginis Ovatae Semen	Seeds, powder and granules	Chronic and temporary constipation due to illness or pregnancy, duodenal ulcer and diverticulitis. Irritable bowel syndrome. Softening of stool of those with haemorrhoids	Laxative, increases the volume of the faeces by absorbing water, which stimulates peristalsis. Antidiarrhoeal effect due to increase in the viscosity of the intestinal contents

(continued overleaf)

Table 29.3 *(continued)*

Plant name and part used	Dosage forms	Diagnosis/indications/use	Pharmacological effect related to indication/use
Plantaginis Lanceolatae Folium/Herba	Extract	Catarrhs of the respiratory tract – acute bronchitis	Anti-inflammatory, immunostimulant and spasmolitic activity
Plantaginis Ovatae Testa	Crude drug	Idiopatic constipation, diarrhoea. Mild to moderate hypercholisterolaemia	Laxative, antidiarrhoeal and cholesterol-lowering effects
Polygalae Radix	Extract	Productive cough, catarrh, chronic bronchitis	Expectorant effect – reduction of expectorant fluid viscosity
Pruni Africanae Cortex	Lipophilic extract of the crude drug	Treatment of lower urinary tract symptoms of benign prostatic hyperplasia stages I and II	Inhibition of cell proliferation, anti-inflammatory activity, improvements in the clinical symptoms of nocturia, daytime polyuria, dysuria, hesitancy and urgency of micturition. Enhancing of the secretory activity of the prostate and seminal vesicles, testosterone-antagonistic activity. Inhibition of oestrogen binding
Rauwolfiae Radix	Crude drug and powder	Mild essential hypertension	Hypotensive effect
Rhamni Purshianae Cortex	Finely cut crude drug powder, dried extracts, liquid and solid preparations	Short-term treatment of occasional constipation	Laxative effect
Rhei Radix and Rhizoma	Dried plant material and standardised preparations	Short-term treatment of occasional constipation	Stimulates and irritates the gastrointestinal tract due to stimulation of colonic motility, and increasing the parecellular permeability across the colonic mucosa
Rusci Rhizoma	Solid or liquid extracts	Supportive therapy for symptoms of chronic venous insufficiency (tired and heavy legs, tingling and swilling), varicoses. Haemorrhoids	Vasoprotection and vasoconstriction, effect on permeability and lymphatic vessels
Salicis Cortex	Hydroalcoholic and water extracts	Relief of exacerbation of chronic low back pain. Symptomatic relief of mild osteoarthritis and rheumatic complaints	Anti-inflammatory and antipyretic effects
Salviae Officinalis Folium	Aqueous extracts	Hyperhidrosis	Reduction in sweat secretion
Sambuci Flos	Crude drug for decoctions and infusions	Diaphoretic activity for the treatment of fever	Increases the response of the sweat glands to heat stimuli and increase diaphoresis
Senegae Radix	Chopped crude drug for decoctions and extracts	Cough due to bronchitis and catarrh of the upper respiratory tract	Expectorant activity

Table 29.3 *(continued)*

Plant name and part used	Dosage forms	Diagnosis/indications/use	Pharmacological effect related to indication/use
Sennae Folium	Dried plant material, powder, oral infusion, and standardised extracts	Short-term treatment of occasional constipation	Stimulation of peristaltic contraction and inhibition of local contraction, resulting in an accelerated colonic transit, thereby reducing fluid absorption. Stimulation of mucus and active chloride secretion
Sennae Fructus	Crude plant material, powder, oral infusion, and standardised extracts	Short-term treatment of occasional constipations	The same as above
Serenoae Repentis Fructus	Crude drug, lipophilic extracts and preparations thereof	Treatment of lower urinary tract symptoms (nocturia, polyuria, dysuria, urinary retention) secondary to BPH stages I and II, in cases when diagnosis of prostate cancer is negative	Anti-inflammatory, antigonadotropic effects
Silybi Mariae Fructus	Standardised extracts, crude drug for decoction	Supportive treatment of acute or chronic hepatitis and cirrhosis induced by alcohol, drugs or toxins	Antioxidant, antihepatotoxic, anti-inflammatory activity
Solidaginis Virguariae Herba	Infusions	Irrigation of the urinary tract – inflammation and renal gravel. Adjuvant treatment of bacterial infections of the urinary tract	Anti-inflammatory, diuretic, spasmolitic effects
Tanaceti Parthenii Herba	Crude drug for decoction; powdered drug or extracts in capsules, tablets, tinctures and drops	Prevention of migraine	Anti-inflammatory activity, inhibition of platelet aggregation and inhibition of serotonin binding
Thymi Herba	Dried herb for infusion, extract and tincture	Uncomplicated respiratory tract infections, bronchial catarrh and bronchitis	Spasmolitic, antimicrobial, anti-inflammatory effects
Trigonellae Foenugraeci Semen	Powdered seeds	Adjuvant therapy in diabetes mellitus: type II diabetes (non-insulin-dependent). As an adjunct in the treatment of mild to moderate hypercholesterolaemia	Hypoglycaemic and hypocholesterolaemic effects
Urticae Radix	Crude drug for infusion; hydroalcoholic extracts	Symptomatic treatment of lower urinary tract disorders (nocturia, polyuria, dysuria, urinary retention) secondary to BPH stages I and II, in cases when diagnosis of prostate cancer is negative	Effects on benign prostatic hyperplasia: sex hormone-binding globulin, prostate growth, enzymatic activity (5-α-reductase) and aromatase
Urticae Folium and Herba	Hydroalcoholic extracts, infusions	Adjuvant treatment of arthritis, arthroses and/or rheumatic conditions	Anti-inflammatory, analgesic effects
Uvae Ursi Folium	Crude drug for infusion or cold macerates, hydroalcoholic extracts and solid forms for oral administration	Internally, mild urinary antiseptic for moderate inflammation of urinary tract and bladder	Antibacterial activity

(continued overleaf)

Table 29.3 *(continued)*

Plant name and part used	Dosage forms	Diagnosis/indications/use	Pharmacological effect related to indication/use
Valerianae Radix	Internal use as the expressed juice, tincture, extracts and other galenic preparations. External use as a bath additive	Mild sedative and sleep-promoting agent. For the treatment of states of nervous excitation and anxiety-induced sleep disturbances	Sedative effect, depression of CNS activity by stimulation of GABA synthesis in synaptosomes. Spasmolytic effect due to relaxation of smooth muscle, apparently by modulating Ca^{2+} entry into the cell
Zingiberis Rhizoma	Dried powder, extract, tablets and tincture	Nausea, vomiting associated with motion sickness, postoperative nausea, pregnancy, and sea sickness	Antinausea and antiemetic activity due to increasing gastric motility and acids. Anti-inflammatory effect

Some peculiarities in the evaluation of the efficacy of medicinal plants

A very important problem in evaluation of efficacy of herbal medicinal products is the complex chemical composition of plant extracts, containing as a rule several active compounds. Their content in the extracts is dependent on many factors, such as geographic region, soil and climate where it was growing, harvesting season, day time, drying, storage conditions, processing method, etc. Consequently the content of active and inactive compounds varies from batch to batch, but must be standardised in the final product, to have reproducible results in clinical trials. Meanwhile, the contribution of each ingredient in efficacy of the product can have an importance, because of its possible effects on:

- the stability of the product during the storage
- the absorbance of the active ingredients into the blood, their distribution and bioavailability
- possible interactions with other ingredients in the organism.

As a result, synergistic, when the cumulative effects of two active ingredients is more than just their sum, or antagonistic interactions of active and inactive ingredients can take place (Williamson, 2001). Therefore, results of clinical trials of a standardised extract produced by one manufacturer, cannot be extended to the similar extracts of the same plant produced by other manufacturers, even if the chemical content of the active ingredients is the same.

Assuming that the product was produced in accordance with GMP standards, this implies reproducible from batch to batch chemical composition not only of active but of all other ingredients of plant extract. An even more complicated situation is with combinations of various plants extracts.

Finally, to come to a conclusion regarding the efficacy of a medicinal plant based on results of various clinical trials, the bioequivalence of studied drugs has to be taken into account. If they are not bioequivalent, the results of meta-analysis cannot be considered as trustworthy. It should be mentioned that many contradictory results concerning efficacy or safety of plant extracts are caused by lack of any data related to their chemical and bioequivalence.

Some plant extracts contain many active compounds acting via different mechanisms and unique interactions collectively have very high efficacy. Thus, treatment of cerebral insufficiency in humans with *Gingko biloba* extracts has been shown to improve global and local blood flow and microcirculation (Költringer *et al.*, 1989; Jung *et al.*, 1990), to protect against hypoxia (Schaffler and Reeh, 1985), to improve rheology, including inhibition of platelet aggregation (Witte, 1989; Artmann and Schikarski, 1993), to prevent damage to membranes by free radicals (Kleijnen and Knipschild, 1992), to improve metabolism and to reduce capillary permeability (Lagrue *et al.*, 1986). Moreover, the same extract is used for the treatment of other conditions, such as peripherial occlusive disease, post-phlebitis syndrome and inner ear disorders.

A characteristic feature of many medicinal plants is that they are usually used for treatment of many disorders. What is really efficient, and what is not? That is the key question for practitioners while they search for the most efficient drug for the treatment of a particular disorder – as a rule there is a very large choice of various plants, but very scarce information about their comparative efficacy.

References

Altman DG, Deeks JJ (2006). Meta-analysis, Simpson's paradox, and the number needed to treat BMC. *Med Res Methodol* 2: 1–5.

Artmann GM, Schikarski C (1993). *Ginkgo biloba* extract (EGb761) protects red blood cells from oxidative damage. *Clin Hemorheol* 13: 529–539.

Deeks JJ, Dinnes J, D'Amico R *et al.* (2003). International Stroke Trial Collaborative Group; European Carotid Surgery Trial Collaborative Group. Evaluating non-randomised intervention studies. *Health Technol Assess* 7: iii–x, 1–173.

Directive 2001/83/EC (2001). European Parliament and of the Council of 6 Nov 2001. On the Community code relating to medicinal products for human use. *Offic J Eur Union* 311: 67–128.

Directive 2002/46/EC (2002). European Parliament and of the Council of 10 June 2002 on the approximation of the laws of the Member States relating to food supplements. *Offic J Eur Union* 183: 51–57.

Directive 2004/24/EC (2004). European Parliament and of the Council of 31 March 2004 amending, as regards traditional herbal medicinal products, Directive 2001/83/EC on the Community code relating to medicinal products for human use. *Official Journal of European Union:* L 136, 85–90.

EMEA/CPMP/HMPWG/1156/03 (2004). *Final concept paper on the implementation of different levels of scientific evidence in core-data for herbal drugs.* London, 3 Mar 2004.

EMEA/HMPWG/104613/2005 (2006). *Guideline on the assessment of clinical safety and efficacy in the preparation of community herbal monographs for well-established and of community herbal monographs/entries to the community list for traditional; herbal medicinal products/substances/preparations.* London, 7 Sep 2006.

ESCOP monographs (2003). The Scientific Foundation for Herbal Medicinal Products, 2nd ed. Thieme, Stuttgart, 556.

Everitt BS, Pickles A (2004). *Statistical Aspects of the Design and Analysis of Clinical Trials (Revised Edition).* World Scientific Publishing Co., London, pp. 340.

Jadad AR, Moore RA, Carroll D *et al.* (1996). Assessing the quality of reports of randomized clinical trials: is blinding necessary? *Control Clin Trials* 17: 1–12.

Jung F, Mrowietz C, Kiesewetter H, Wenzel E (1990). Effect of *Ginkgo biloba* on fluidity of blood and peripheral microcirculation in volunteers. *Arzneimittelforschung* 40: 589–593.

Kleijnen J, Knipschild P (1992). *Ginkgo biloba* for cerebral insufficiency. *Br J Clin Pharmacol* 34: 352–358.

Ko-umlautltringer P, Eber O, Klima G *et al.* (1989). Microcirculation in parenteral *Ginkgo biloba* extract therapy. *Wien Klin Wochenschr* 101: 198–200.

Kurtzweil P (1998). An FDA guide to dietary supplements. *FDA Consumer Magazine* Sep–Oct 1998. http://www.fda.gov/fdac/features/1998/598_guid.html; http://www.cfsan.fda.gov/~dms/supplmnt.html.

Lagrue G, Behar A, Kazandjian M, Rahbar K (1986). Idiopathic cyclic edema. The role of capillary hyperpermeability and its correction by *Ginkgo biloba* extract. *Presse Med* 15: 1550–1553.

MacLehose RR, Reeves BC, Harvey IM *et al.* (2000). A systematic review of comparisons of effect sizes derived from randomised and non-randomised studies. *Health Technol Assess* 4: 1–154.

Schaffler K, Reeh PW (1985). Doppelblindstudie zur hypoxieprotektiven Wirkung eines standardisierten *Ginkgo biloba* – Präparates nach Mehrfachverabrcichung an gesunden Probanden. *Arzneimittelforschung* 35: 1283–1286.

Williamson E (2001). Synergy and other interactions in phytomedicins. *Phytomedicine* 8: 401–409.

Witte S (1989). Therapeutical aspects of *Ginkgo biloba* flavone glucosides in the context of increased blood viscosity. *Clin Hemorheol* 9: 323–326.

World Health Organization. (1999). *WHO Monographs on Selected Medicinal Plants.*Volume 1: WHO: Geneva, 295pp.

World Health Organization (2002). *WHO Monographs on Selected Medicinal Plants.*Volume 2: WHO: Geneva, 358 pp.

World Medical Association (2000). *Declaration of Helsinki. Ethical principles for medical research involving human subjects.* 18th WMA General Assembly Helsinki, Finland, June 1964; 52nd WMA General Assembly Edinburgh, Scotland, Oct 2000.

30

Toxicological evaluation of herbal medicines: approaches and perspectives

Stanley O Aniagu

Introduction

The use of medicinal plants dates back to prehistoric times. From time immemorial, humans have always recognised the great value of various herbs, plants and plant products.

Hence it is not surprising that there are a wide variety of these herbs and herbal products still in use. In addition to their use in industrialised nations, herbal prescriptions are commonly employed in developing countries for the treatment of various diseases, this practice being an alternative way to compensate for some perceived deficiencies in orthodox pharmacotherapy (Sofowora, 1989). Unfortunately, there is limited scientific evidence regarding safety and efficacy to back up the continued therapeutic application of these natural remedies. The rationale for the utilisation of herbal medicines has rested largely on long-term clinical experience (Zhu, 2002). However, with the upsurge in the use of these remedies coupled with the increasing demands made by regulatory bodies (e.g. the US Food and Drug Administration (FDA); the Committee on Safety of Medicines in the UK, the National Agency for Food and Drug Administration and Control), it has now become imperative to provide adequate clinical and toxicological data to support their continued folkloric applications.

This chapter introduces a rational approach for the toxicological assessment of herbal medicines. In particular, attention is drawn to the Organisation for Economic Co-operation and Development (OECD) test guidelines on toxicity studies in experimental animals, since this represents a harmonised approach in the application of toxicological study protocols. No doubt the reader will benefit from having a closer look at these guidance documents in addition to consulting other guidelines as may be set out by the relevant authorities in each country. Efforts aimed at establishing the no-observed adverse effect levels (NOAEL), tolerable daily intakes (TDI) and margins of safety (MOS) for each herbal medicine should be actively encouraged. In fact, these are the major challenges for toxicologists and risk assessors in various regulatory agencies.

What are herbal medicines?

Herbal medicines consist of products used in therapies that utilise plants, plant extracts or other plant remedies in the treatment of diseases, and can rightly be regarded as the oldest known form of medicine. Through serendipity, careful observation of animals or by trial and error, our ancestors found the most effective curative remedies for their ailments. But with the advent and rapid progress in scientific knowledge, we can now identify the exact chemical constituents of these plants, and therefore can rationalise the pharmacological bases of their healing powers. One of the most remarkable things about herbal medicine is that it takes a more holistic approach in the treatment of diseases. Herbalists are either naturally gifted or are trained in comparable diagnostic skills as orthodox doctors but in their own case, they look for the underlying cause(s) of the ailment. In the world of herbal medicine, symptomatic treatment or suppression of symptoms is insufficient to achieve total cure since diseases can only occur when there is a perturbation or imbalance in one of the body systems. That is why herbalists use different plants or plant remedies to restore the balance of the body first and foremost, enabling the body to muster its own natural healing powers. Herbal preparations in the form of tablets, powders, capsules, fluid extracts, syrups, tinctures, creams and ointments promote health as a positive state and can be employed in a wide range of conditions including malaria, arthritis, insomnia, stress, headaches and migraines, tonsillitis and influenza; allergic responses such as hay fever and asthma; skin problems such as acne, dermatitis and eczema; digestive disorders such as peptic ulcers and irritable bowel syndrome; circulatory diseases such as angina, high blood pressure, varicose veins; and gynaecological disorders such as premenstrual syndrome.

Perspectives on toxicity of herbal medicines

One of the major issues with herbal medicines is the fact that there is still insufficient scientific evidence to back up their safety and efficacy. This may in part be due to the relative difficulty of evaluating a complete mixture of herbal medicines using the conventional battery of pharmacological and toxicological assays. However, we must bear in mind that herbal medicines work on a holistic basis and herbalists use either whole plant extracts or parts of the whole plant (e.g. leaf, root, bark, fruit) and these contain hundreds (maybe thousands) of different chemical entities.

Of course, many orthodox medicines and pharmaceuticals in use today are based on the principle of single-chemical isolation from plants or large-scale synthesis of these chemicals in the laboratory. But from the point of view of herbal medicine, it is not a good idea to try to isolate one active chemical compound for therapeutic purposes because, more often than not, these single chemical entities elicit unwanted or adverse effects when used alone. On the contrary, herbalists believe that the active constituents in a plant are rightly balanced within the plant and any possible untoward or toxic effects of one component would be neutralised by the presence of complementary constituents.

For instance, synthetic diuretics such as furosemide seriously deplete potassium levels in the body prompting co-medication with potassium supplements or alternative prescriptions containing potassium-sparing diuretics. In contrast, dandelion leaves have potent diuretic effects, yet contain potassium to replace the ions lost during treatment naturally (Bradley, 1992). That is why it is important to note that the toxic effect produced by the active principle(s) isolated from a plant may be totally different from the effects produced by the whole plant extract.

However, being herbal does not mean a remedy is innocuous, since there are several published reports on the potential toxic effects of herbal medicines in the population (Vora and Mansoor, 2005; Schoepfer *et al.*, 2007). These may have several causes.

Contamination of herbal medicines

A worrisome trend on the toxic effects of herbal medicines and dietary supplements is related to reports on the hepatotoxicity, nephrotoxicity, neurotoxicity, haematological, mutagenic and cardiovascular toxicities of some herbs. Hepatoxicity seems to be the most common observation and effects can range from mild elevations of liver enzymes to fulminant liver failure. However, the reported toxicities of herbal products could be complicated because of the presence of confounding factors such as contamination with pesticides, herbicides, naturally occurring toxins, microbes or adulteration with orthodox medicines (El-Nahhal, 2004). Some so-called herbal products and dietary supplements actually contain other synthetic compounds, which are less well characterised. Hence it is the duty of regulatory agencies and lawmakers to impose strict labelling conditions for all herbal medicinal products, especially for products with the potential for significant toxicity. The labels should contain a frank declaration of the composition of these products and will aid in the evaluation and reporting of any adverse effects or interactions.

In-vivo versus in-vitro toxicity studies

There is much debate about the replacement of experimental animals with in-vitro toxicology models (for instance, see Funds for the Replacement of Animals in Medical Experiments [FRAME] website: http://www.frame.org.uk/). The objectives of FRAME are linked to the three Rs – *r*efinement, *r*eduction and *r*eplacement. It is possible that a wide range of in-vitro techniques, using both transformed and unmodified human and rodent cells, could serve as useful media in various toxicity assays. These in-vitro assays can play a big role in flagging or pointing out possible toxicological endpoints, with subsequent animal studies following on a lower scale (reduction). However, the complete replacement of whole animal studies with in-vitro techniques may never be a realistic option since there are marked differences in the behaviour of similar cells under in-vivo and in-vitro conditions. The most realistic target is to refine the procedures for animal experiments such that:

- The minimum number of animals required to establish the desired toxicological endpoints could be used.
- Little or no suffering is inflicted on the animals used for in-vivo studies.

Approaches to integrated safety assessment of herbal medicines

Toxicology as hazard-identification stage of safety assessment

There is no doubt that toxicological studies provide an appropriate platform for hazard identification. Most regulatory agencies rely on the results of in-vivo toxicity studies conducted according to standard protocols (e.g. OECD, FDA or WHO test guidelines) for risk assessment purposes. The type, nature and extent of effect obtained during toxicity studies can help in adequately classifying herbal medicines as non-toxic, moderately toxic or severely toxic on selected body systems. The following are dealt with in this chapter:

- acute, subacute and sub-chronic toxicity studies
- combined chronic toxicity and carcinogenicity studies
- developmental and reproductive toxicity studies
- genotoxicity and neurotoxicity assays.

Table 30.1 summarises the various types of toxicity studies.

Acute toxicity studies

This describes the toxic effects elicited by any substance or mixture of substances when administered in single (or in rare cases, multiple) doses to experimental animals over a period not exceeding 24 h. It is useful in providing preliminary identification of target organs of toxicity and, occasionally, revealing delayed effects. Acute toxicity studies may also aid in the selection of starting doses for Phase 1 human studies or dose-ranges for subsequent repeat-dose studies. In addition, acute toxicity studies are invaluable in cases of acute overdosing in humans. The test compound should be administered (up to the maximum feasible dose) to animals to identify doses causing no adverse effect and doses causing major life-threatening toxicities. Ideally, the acute toxicity studies in animals should be conducted using the route intended for human administration (orally in most cases).

Table 30.1 Summary of the various types of toxicity studies and test systems required

Toxicity type	Duration	OECD test guidance	Routes	Test system
Acute	≤14 days	420/423/425	Oral/inhalation	Rat (female)
Subacute	14–28 days	407	Oral/diet/drinking water	Rat
Subchronic	30–90 days	408	Oral/diet/drinking water	Rat
Chronic	≥ 6 months	452	Oral/diet/drinking water	Rat
Combined chronic and carcinogenicity	18 months to 2.5 years	453	Oral/dermal/inhalation	Rat/mice/hamster
Carcinogenicity	2 years	451	Oral/dermal/inhalation	Rat/mouse/hamster
Genotoxicity	Variable	473–486	In vitro/in vivo	Variable
Developmental and reproductive	Variable	414/415/416	Oral	Rat, dog
Neurotoxicity	Variable	424	Oral/dermal/inhalation	Rat

Preliminary considerations

Test material

The test material should be clearly defined (e.g. part of plant or herb used, what sort of extract – freeze-dried aqueous, organic; extraction method; percentage yield, etc.). If test substances are stored in the fridge or freezer, they should be allowed to attain room temperature (22 ± 3°C) prior to dosing. To avoid causing excessive pain or tissue damage in the animals, preparations with irritant or caustic properties are not recommended. Results of any other in-vivo or in-vitro toxicity tests on herb or toxicological data on a compound structurally related to those found in the plant will be invaluable in the selection of the most appropriate starting doses.

Selection of animals

The choice of animals to be used would depend on the regulatory requirement in each country and any prior sensitivity issues with the herb in question. Young, healthy, adult rats of either sex could be used (age range 8–12 weeks). The OECD, however, recommends nulliparous and non-pregnant female rats for acute toxicity testing (OECD, 1998). This is because in certain instances where there are sensitivity differences between male and female rats, females are usually more sensitive than males in picking up subtle effects.

Before the test, animals should be randomised and assigned to the required number of test groups. The weight variation in animals or between groups used in a test should not exceed ±20% of the mean weight. Feeding should be done ad libitum with standard feed and the test animals should have free access to drinking water. If test substance is to be given orally, an overnight food starvation is recommended. In addition, the animals should be maintained under standard conditions of humidity (30–70%), temperature (22 ± 3°C) and 12 h light/darkness cycle and should be acclimatised to the environment for a week prior to commencement of the studies.

It is advisable to follow both the standard good laboratory practice (GLP) regulations of the OECD and WHO (OECD, 1982; WHO, 1990) and the *Guide for the Care and Use of Laboratory Animals* (NIH, 1985). In general, studies should be designed so that the maximum amount of information is obtained from the smallest number of animals. Moreover, calculating lethality parameters such as LD_{50}, as done previously using large numbers of animals, is no longer required.

Preparation and administration of test doses

The maximum volume of freshly prepared herbal medicine that can be administered at once in rodents is usually 1 mL/100 g of body weight (although in some cases 2 mL/100 g has been used). For vehicles other than water, the toxicological characteristics of the vehicle should be known. The preparation should be administered in a single dose by gavage using a stomach tube or a suitable intubation cannula. In the unusual circumstance that a single dose is not possible, the dose may be given in smaller fractions over a period not exceeding 24 hours. After the substance has been administered, food may be withheld for a further 3–4 h in rats or 1–2 h in mice.

Observations and data monitoring

Animals should be observed individually after dosing at least once during the first 30 min, periodically during the first 24 h (with special attention given during the first 4 h), and daily thereafter, for a total of 14 days. The times at which signs of toxicity appear and disappear are important, especially if there is a tendency for toxic signs to be delayed. Systematic observations for each animal should include changes in skin and fur, eyes and mucous membranes, respiratory, circulatory, autonomic and central nervous systems; somatomotor activity and behaviour pattern including cases of convulsions, salivation, diarrhoea, lethargy, sedation and coma. Gross necropsies should be performed and recorded for each animal including those sacrificed moribund, found dead, or terminated at day 14. It may be necessary to perform histopathological examination of organs showing evidence of gross pathology in animals surviving for 24 h or more after the initial dosing.

Data collection and test reporting

Individual animal and group data should be summarised in tabular form and the test report must include the following information, as appropriate:

- test substance (physical nature, purity, and physico-chemical properties)
- test animals (number, age, and sex of animals)
- housing conditions, diet, etc.
- test conditions including dosing volumes and time of dosing
- details of food and water quality
- the rationale for the selection of the starting dose
- tabulation of response data and dose level for each animal
- tabulation of body weight and body weight changes
- individual weights of animals at the day of dosing, in weekly intervals thereafter, and at the time of death or sacrifice
- date and time of death if prior to scheduled sacrifice
- time course of onset of signs of toxicity, and whether these were reversible for each animal
- necropsy and histopathological findings for each animal, if available (OECD, 1998).

Methods

Previous methods of acute toxicity testing were based on the techniques proposed by Miller and Tainter (1944), Litchfield and Wilcoxon (1949) and Lorke (1983). These traditional methods for assessing acute toxicity relied on deaths of animals as endpoints, thus giving an LD_{50} value for each substance investigated. However newer and better techniques are now set out in the OECD test guidance documents no. 420 (fixed dose procedure), no. 423 (acute toxic class method) and no. 425 (up and down procedure). The following is a brief summary of the currently recommended methods for acute toxicity testing. For more detailed information on the application of these techniques, the reader should consult the relevant OECD documents and other references at the end of this chapter.

Fixed-dose procedure

As the name suggests, this technique relies on the observation of clear signs of toxicity at one of a series of fixed-dose levels, thus avoiding death as an endpoint. The procedure has been validated in a series of studies (Stallard and Whitehead, 1995) using mathematical models and has been shown to be reproducible in addition to allowing a substance to be ranked according to the globally harmonised system (GHS) for the classification of chemicals and mixtures, which cause acute toxicity (OECD, 1998). Basically, after an initial sighting study, groups of animals of a single sex are dosed in a stepwise procedure using the fixed doses of 5, 50, 300 and 2000 mg/kg. The initial dose level is selected on the basis of a sighting study and is expected to produce evident toxicity. In the absence of any data on the toxicity of the substance, starting doses should be 300 mg/kg. A minimum of 24 h is allowed between the dosing of each animal, after which all treated animals should be observed for at least 14 days for clinical signs and conditions associated with pain, suffering and impending death. Further groups of animals may be dosed at higher or lower fixed doses, depending on the presence or absence of signs of toxicity or mortality. This procedure continues until the dose causing evident toxicity or no more than one death is identified, or when no effects are seen at the highest dose or when deaths occur at the lowest dose. A total of five female rats (including one from the sighting study) will normally be used for each dose level investigated. Treatment of more animals at the next dose should be delayed for 3–4 days until one is confident of survival of the previously dosed animals.

Acute toxic class method

The acute toxic class (ATC) method (Roll *et al.*, 1986) is a reproducible, step-wise procedure based on biometric evaluations (Diener *et al.*, 1995; Diener and Schlede, 1999) with adequately separated, fixed doses of a substance to allow for GHS ranking and classification. Three female rats are used per step and depending on the mortality and/or the moribund status of the animals, a total of two to four steps may be necessary to allow judgement on the acute toxicity of the test substance.

The procedure uses very few animals and ranks substances in a similar manner to test guidelines 420 and 425. Four predefined doses of 5, 50, 300 and 2000 mg/kg body weight are used and the starting oral dose should most likely produce mortality in some of the dosed animals. Although the method is not intended for the calculation of a precise LD_{50}, it does allow for the determination of defined exposure ranges where lethality is expected, since death of a proportion of the animals is still the major endpoint of this test.

If one dose level causes a mortality lower than 100% and another dose level results in lethality higher than 0%, then an LD_{50} can be determined. Depending on the results obtained at one dose level, actions taken may be:

- no further testing needed
- dosing three additional animals at the same dose
- dosing three additional animals at the next higher or the next lower dose level.

A limit test should be conducted when available information suggests that mortality is unlikely at the highest starting dose level (2000 mg/kg body weight) but otherwise, for animal welfare reasons, starting doses of 300 mg/kg body weight are recommended. The time interval between treatment groups is determined by the onset, duration and severity of toxic signs but usually this is about 3–4 days to account for any delayed toxicity.

Up-and-down-procedure

The FDP allows for the estimation of LD_{50} and confidence intervals in addition to observation of signs of toxicity (ASTM, 1987). Substances are subsequently ranked and classified according to the GHS method. Computer simulations have shown that starting doses in the region of 175 mg/kg and using a dose progression of factor 3.2 (corresponding to half-log units) between doses will produce the best results. The main test consists of a single, ordered dose progression in which animals are dosed, one at a time, at a minimum of 48-h intervals. The first animal receives a dose a step below the level of the best estimate of the LD_{50}. If the animal survives, the dose for the next animal is increased 3.2 times the original dose; if it dies, the dose for the next animal is decreased by a similar factor. Using the default progression factor, doses would be selected from the sequence 1.75, 5.5, 17.5, 55, 175, 550, 1750, 2000 or 5000 mg/kg for specific regulatory needs.

The testing stops when one of the following stopping criteria first is met:

- three consecutive animals survive at the upper band
- five reversals occur in any six consecutive animals tested
- at least four animals have followed the first reversal and the specified likelihood-ratios exceed the critical value (OECD, 1998).

For most applications, testing will be completed with only four animals after initial reversal in animal outcome. The LD_{50} is calculated using the maximum likelihood method (SAS Institute Inc., 1990), except in some cases where the geometric mean of doses for the animals in the current nominal sample is used as a rough estimate of the LD_{50}. All deaths, whether immediate or delayed or humane kills, are incorporated for the purpose of the maximum likelihood analyses.

Preliminary considerations for repeat-dose studies

Repeat dose studies include 28-day, 90-day, 6-month and other studies lasting for a year or more. The determination of oral toxicity profiles of herbal medicines using repeat doses may be accomplished after initial acute toxicity testing. This study provides information on the possible health hazards that may occur over a specified period of time. The method should give an indication of herbs which have neurological, immunological or reproductive toxicity. It is critical to have in place the right experimental design before the commencement of these studies.

Selection of animal species

Selection of animal species and housing conditions are similar to the acute toxicity studies. The preferred rodent species is the rat, although other rodent species may be used. Animals may be housed individually, or be caged in small groups of the same sex; for group caging, no more than five animals should be housed per cage. At least ten animals (five female and five male) should be used at each dose level. If interim kills are planned, the number should be increased by the number of animals scheduled to be killed before the completion of the study. Consideration should be given to an additional satellite group of ten animals (five per sex) in the control and in the top dose group for observation of reversibility, persistence, or delayed occurrence of toxic effects, for at least 14 days after treatment.

Selection of dose levels

By regulatory requirement, at least three test groups and a control group should be used. But if from assessment of other available data, no effects are expected at 1000 mg/kg body weight per day, then a limit test may be performed at this dose level. There are many factors which come into play in the choice of dose levels for repeat dose toxicity studies, including intra- and interspecies variation, differences in metabolic and toxicokinetic profiles between rodents and humans, etc. But generally, the lowest dose is usually a simple multiple of the therapeutic dose whereas the highest dose is normally chosen to be a nearly toxic dose. However, the highest dose level should not cause a body weight decrease greater than 10–12% relative to concurrent control values and in a dietary study should not exceed 5% of the total diet because of potential nutritional imbalances caused at higher levels or produce severe toxic, pharmacological or physiological effects. The median dose lies somewhere between these two extremes (possibly a geometric mean of the two). If LD_{50} values are available, the recommended doses should be 0.1%, 1% and 10% of the oral acute toxicity LD_{50} values. Alternatively, two- to fourfold intervals are frequently optimal for setting the descending dose levels. Ideally, the lowest and median dose levels should be selected with a view to demonstrating any dose–response relationships while the lowest dose is expected to cause no observable adverse effects (i.e. NOAEL).

Preparation and administration of doses

The test compound should be administered by gavage or via the diet or drinking water. The animals are dosed with the test substance daily 7 days each week for the required duration. Substances administered via diet or drinking water should be monitored to ensure that the quantities of herbs involved do not interfere with normal nutritional status or cause water imbalance.

Clinical and functional observation battery

General clinical observations should be made at least once a day but recordings for morbidity and mortality should be done at least twice daily. Observed signs should include:

- changes in skin, fur, eyes, mucous membranes, occurrence of secretions and excretions and autonomic activity (e.g. lachrymation, piloerection, pupil size, unusual respiratory pattern)
- changes in gait, posture and response to handling as well as the presence of clonic or tonic movements
- stereotypies (e.g. excessive grooming, repetitive circling) or bizarre behaviour (e.g. self-mutilation).

In the fourth exposure week, sensory reactivity to stimuli of different types (e.g. auditory, visual and proprioceptive stimuli, assessment of grip strength

(Meyer *et al.*, 1979) and motor activity assessment (Crofton *et al.*, 1991)) should be conducted. The availability of data on functional observations from a repeat dose study may enhance the ability to select dose levels for a subsequent sub-chronic study.

Body weight, food and water consumption

The body weight of each animal should be assessed using a sensitive balance during the acclimatisation period, once before commencement of dosing, at least once weekly during the dosing period and once on the terminal day. Measurements of food and water consumption should be made daily or at least weekly.

Absolute and relative organ weights

At the end of the dosing period, all the animals should be killed humanely and the different organs such as the heart, liver, lungs, brain, spleen, kidneys, uteri, testes should be carefully dissected out and weighed in grams (absolute organ weight). The relative organ weight of each animal should then be calculated as follows:

relative organ weight = absolute organ weight/ terminal body weight × 100.

Haematology

The following haematological examinations should be performed at the end of the treatment period:

- haematocrit
- haemoglobin concentration
- erythrocyte count
- total and differential leucocyte counts
- platelet count
- erythrocyte morphology
- mean corpuscular volume
- mean corpuscular haemoglobin
- mean corpuscular haemoglobin concentration
- a measure of blood-clotting potential.

Chemical pathology (clinical biochemistry)

All animals should be investigated for major toxic effects in tissues such as the liver, kidney and heart using clinical chemistry measurements. Overnight fasting of the animals prior to blood sampling is recommended. Plasma or serum analyses should include:

- sodium
- potassium
- glucose
- total cholesterol
- urea
- creatinine
- total proteins and albumin
- at least two enzymes indicative of hepatocellular effects (such as alanine aminotransferase, aspartate aminotransferase, alkaline phosphatase, γ-glutamyl transpeptidase, lactate dehydrogenase and sorbitol dehydrogenase)
- factors related to metabolic profiles (e.g. calcium, phosphate, fasting triglycerides, specific hormones, methaemoglobin and cholinesterase).

In the last week of study, urinalysis could be performed to determine appearance, volume, osmolality, specific gravity, pH, protein, glucose and blood cells.

Gross necropsy and histopathology

A full, detailed, gross necropsy should be conducted for all animals. The wet weights of the liver, kidneys, adrenals, testes, epididymes, thymus, spleen, brain and heart of all surviving animals should be measured soon after dissection. Thereafter preservation of the following tissues in the most appropriate fixation medium (e.g. formol saline) should be carried out:

- all gross lesions
- brain (e.g. cerebrum, cerebellum)
- spinal cord
- stomach
- small and large intestines
- liver
- kidneys
- adrenals
- spleen
- heart
- thymus
- thyroid
- trachea and lungs
- gonads
- accessory sex organs (e.g. uterus, prostate)
- urinary bladder
- lymph nodes
- peripheral nerve and bone marrow sections.

Full histopathology should be carried out on all gross lesions and also on the preserved organs and tissues of all animals in the control and high-dose groups.

Toxicokinetics and metabolism data

Toxicokinetics (absorption, distribution, metabolism and elimination) can be very useful in the evaluation and interpretation of subchronic and chronic exposure studies (Paynter, 1984). For each herb in particular information can be obtained on:

- rate of absorption
- pattern of distribution in tissues, organs and fluid compartments
- reversible binding to tissue sites and plasma proteins
- pattern and rates of metabolism and excretion profiles.

However, the toxicokinetic evaluation of herbal medicines may pose difficult problems since the chemical constituents in most plants may be in the region of hundreds or thousands (e.g. alkaloids, glycosides, flavonoids, quinines, tannins, polyphenols, sugars). In any case, if the chemical composition of a plant is well known, then it may suffice to do a toxicokinetic profiling of the major active constituents.

Data analyses and test reporting

This is similar to reporting of acute toxicity testing, with the inclusion of additional toxicity parameters, e.g.

- nature, severity and duration of clinical observations (reversibility or otherwise)
- sensory activity, grip strength and motor activity assessments
- haematological tests with relevant baseline values
- clinical biochemistry tests plus baseline values
- terminal body and organ weight data
- necropsy findings
- a detailed description of all histopathological findings
- toxicokinetic data if available
- statistical analyses in addition to discussion of results and appropriate conclusions.

Subacute toxicity studies

An example of a subacute toxicity study is the repeat-dose, 28-day, oral toxicity study in rodents. This study provides information on the possible health hazards likely to arise from repeated exposure over a relatively limited period of time and comprises the basic repeat-dose toxicity study that may be used for herbal medicines, for which a 90-day study is not warranted. Test parameters to be monitored are similar to those outlined previously.

Subchronic toxicity studies

Subchronic toxicity studies are short-term, repeat-dose studies carried out as a follow-up to the 28-day, subacute toxicity studies. A short-term study has been defined (WHO, 1990) as 'having a duration lasting up to 10% of the animal's lifespan, 90 days in rats and mice, or 1 year in dogs'. The main purpose of subchronic testing is to identify any target organs and to establish dose levels for chronic exposure studies.

The 90-day study provides information on major toxic effects, target organs and the possibility of accumulation, and can provide an estimate of a no-observed-adverse-effect level of exposure, which can be used in selecting dose levels for chronic studies and for establishing safety criteria for humans. The herb should be orally administered daily in graduated doses to three groups of experimental animals and a concurrent control group for a period of 90 days. At least 20 animals (10 female and 10 male) are recommended at each dose level but, if interim kills are planned, the number should be increased accordingly. An additional satellite group of 10 animals (five per sex) in the control and in the top dose group may be included for observation of reversibility or persistence of any toxic effects post treatment. Toxicological parameters to be monitored are similar to those outlined earlier except that interim haematological and clinical chemistry evaluations may be performed at selected times.

Combined chronic toxicity and carcinogenicity studies

These long-term observations are defined as studies lasting for the greater part of the lifespan of the test animals, usually 18 months in mice and 2 years in rats (WHO, 1990). Typically the rat weanlings or post-weanlings have been used for a combined chronic toxicity/carcinogenicity assessment. Ideally, the design and conduct of the test should allow for the detection of neoplastic effects and a determination of carcinogenic potential as well as general toxicity, including neurological, physiological, biochemical, and haematological effects and exposure-related morphological effects. Preliminary studies providing data on acute, subchronic and toxicokinetic responses should have been carried out to permit an appropriate choice of animal species and strain (selected strains should not have a high spontaneous background tumour incidence). Dosing of the rodents should begin as soon as possible after weaning and acclimatisation, and preferably before the animals are 6 weeks old.

Experimental design and dosing

For a thorough biological and statistical evaluation, each dose level and concurrent control group should have at least 50 animals of each sex. A high-dose satellite group for evaluation of pathology other than neoplasia should contain 20 animals of each sex, while the satellite control group would contain 10 animals of each sex. If interim sacrifice is planned, the initial number should be increased accordingly. Based on the results of previous subchronic toxicity studies, at least three dose levels should be used in addition to the concurrent control group. The highest dose level should elicit signs of minimal toxicity without substantially altering the normal lifespan caused by effects other than tumours. The lowest dose should not interfere with the normal growth, development and longevity of the animal; and it must not otherwise cause any indication of toxicity (low dose is usually 10% or more of the high dose). For chronic toxicity testing, additional treated and concurrent control satellite groups are included in the study. The highest dose for satellite animals should be chosen so as to produce frank toxicity, to elucidate a toxicological profile of the test substance. Frequency of exposure is usually daily but may vary according to the route chosen – oral, dermal or inhalation. At interim periods of 3 months, 6 months and at every 6-month interval, urinalysis, haematological and biochemical examinations and should be performed. A complete gross and histopathological examination should be done on all animals including those that died during the experiment or were killed in moribund conditions.

Developmental and reproductive toxicity studies

The guidelines and procedures for developmental and reproductive toxicity studies are well documented in Korach (1998) as well as the OECD guidelines 414–416. Briefly, these studies are designed to provide general information on critical endpoints relating to potential toxic effects on reproductive parameters, including effects on mating behaviour (both sexes), fertility (both sexes), blastocyst implantation, gonadal function, oestrous cycling, conception, parturition, lactation, weaning, neonatal mortality, fetal development and survival. These studies could be one-generation (OECD 415), two-generation (OECD 416) or three-generation tests.

Important endpoints to assess within each generation include:

- time after pairing to mating
- mating behaviour
- percentage of females pregnant
- number of pregnancies going to full term
- litter size
- number of live births
- number of stillborns
- pup viability and weight at parturition, and postnatal days 4, 7, 14 and 21 days of age
- fertility index
- gestation index
- viability index
- lactation index
- gross necropsy and histopathology on selected parents.

Developmental toxicity studies (also called teratology studies) are designed to look at a wide spectrum of possible in utero outcomes for the conceptus, including death, malformations, functional deficits and developmental delays in fetuses. Exposure during sensitive periods may alter normal development resulting in immediate effects, or may subsequently compromise normal physiological or behavioural functioning. The following assessments are usually carried out:

- number of live litters
- sex ratio of fetuses
- fetal/litter weights
- number and percentage of fetuses/litter with malformations
- number and percentage of fetuses/litter with variations
- types of malformations and variations.

Genotoxicity and neurotoxicity studies

These are designed to determine whether test chemicals can perturb genetic material to cause gene or chromosomal mutations. A large number of assay systems, especially in-vitro systems, have been devised to detect the genotoxic or mutagenic potential of agents. These tests include:

- bacterial reversal mutations tests (e.g. Ames test)
- tests in mammalian sytems (e.g. chromosomal aberration tests, erythrocyte micronucleus test, sister chromatid exchange assay, unscheduled DNA synthesis)
- in-vitro gene mutation assays in yeast
- dominant lethal test in rodents and the mouse spot test.

Newer assays, which could provide additional information, include the Comet assay (DNA damage and repair), mutations in transgenic animals, fluorescent in-situ hybridisation and cell transformations.

In addition to genotoxicity tests, current thinking has also focused on epigenetic mechanisms of toxicity. In this regard, future evaluations could include effects on DNA methylation, histone acetylation, chromatin remodelling and transcription factors, which all act in concert to influence gene expression.

Neurotoxicity studies are aimed at identifying if the nervous system is permanently or reversibly affected by the treatment and to understand the underlying mechanisms involved. The following parameters are usually evaluated in addition to aforementioned clinical observations:

- functional tests (e.g. auditory, visual)
- ophthalmological examinations
- limb grip strength
- motor activity
- incidence of specific neurobehavioural, neuropathological, neurochemical or electrophysiological abnormalities.

If other toxicology data indicate potential neurotoxic effects, the inclusion of more specialised tests of sensory and motor function or learning could be considered.

Interpretation of toxicology data

The importance of choosing the right doses and toxicological endpoints cannot be overemphasised. The use of high doses, which overwhelm normal metabolic and detoxification pathways, or which cause tissue necrosis, could give rise to misleading conclusions. Moreover, responses produced by herbs in humans and experimental animals may differ markedly and could be physiological, pharmacological, toxic or adaptive (e.g. liver enzyme induction leading to hyperplasia). Hence, not all observed responses within a study would represent toxicity per se.

In terms of data analyses, there may be limitations associated with the use of statistics in toxicology (Gad and Weil, 1986, 1989; Waner, 1992). The key issues include the relationship between statistical and biological significance and the fact that lack of statistical significance does not necessarily prove safety. Findings should be considered on the basis of both statistical significance and likely biological variability. A non-statistically significant finding may have biological significance when considered in the light of predictable toxicological or pharmacological action of the test material or when combined with results from other studies. It is also essential to separate artefactual deaths from toxicity-induced deaths. The former includes deaths through age, acute or chronic infections, negligent handling or accidents. Deaths, which are clustered at a specific time period may reflect a spontaneous epidemic outbreak of limited duration.

Body weight changes are usually related to food intake, and analysis of one without an analysis of the other is of limited value (Weil and McCollister, 1963; Roubicek *et al.*, 1964; Heywood, 1981). Weight decrement may not always be related to toxicity per se (Seefeld and Petersen, 1984). The incorporation of herbal medicines into the diet may either increase or reduce palatability or may have no effect on appetite.

In clinical chemistry measurements, it is critical to consider the most relevant enzymes for analyses. For instance, in the assessment of hepatocellular function, alanine amino transaminase provides a more sensitive marker of hepatocellular damage than aspartate amino transaminase and within limits can provide a quantitative assessment of the degree of hepatocellular damage (Al-Mamary *et al.*, 2002). Creatine phosphokinase is mainly located in skeletal and heart muscle and is the most appropriate enzyme to detect muscle damage. For hepatobiliary function, alkaline phosphatase, γ-glutamyl transferase and total bilirubin are the most relevant measurements.

It is always important to ascertain whether changes in biochemical or haematological parameters are linked to changes in organ weight, gross pathology or histopathology. Age-related changes in animals may have over-riding influences on haematological, biochemical, toxicokinetic or histopathological parameters (Grice and Burek, 1983; Mohr *et al.*, 1994, 1996). Hence it is essential in all cases to differentiate between age-related and treatment-induced lesions with respect to the observed physiological, pharmacological and toxic responses. Overall, the evaluation and interpretation of test results should be correlated with more specific, sensitive, and reliable histopathological findings. The reader should consult Bush (1991) for a good review of factors that can complicate the interpretation of findings in toxicity studies.

Conclusions

After hazard identification through a battery of toxicity tests, the next step in safety assessment is to determine the exposure levels of the herbal medicine (i.e. how much of these herbs can an individual consume in a given period of time). The subsequent risk assessment is defined by the relationship between hazard and exposure (i.e. risk = hazard × exposure).

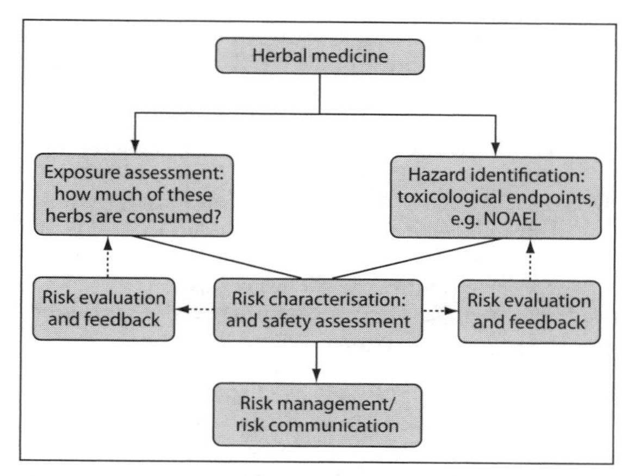

Figure 30.1 A simplified approach for the integrated risk assessment of herbal medicines.

In this case, a direct comparison is made between the NOAEL and exposure levels, giving a ratio referred to as the margin of safety (MOS). The MOS should be sufficiently large to such a degree that there is high enough confidence that the doses of herbal medicines taken will not cause adverse human health effects. A tolerable daily intake should also be defined for each herbal medicine. Following the risk-characterisation phase, a risk-management decision needs to be made as to whether the risk is acceptable or not. If unacceptable, suitable controls should be put in place to minimise the risk and this should be communicated appropriately (Figure 30.1).

References

Al-Mamary M, Al-Habori M, Al-Aghbari *et al.* (2002). Investigation into the toxicological effects of *Catha edulis* leaves: a short-term study in animals. *Phytother Res* 16: 127–132.

ASTM (1987). *E 1163–87, Standard Test Method for Estimating Acute Oral Toxicity in Rats.* American Society for Testing and Materials, Philadelphia PA, USA.

Bradley PR (Ed). (1992). *British Herbal Compendium*, vol. 1. Bournemouth: British Herbal Medicine Association; pp. 73–74.

Bush BM (1991). *Interpretation of Laboratory Results for Small Animal Clinicians.* Blackwell Scientific Publications, London.

Crofton KM, Howard JL, Moser VC *et al.* (1991). Interlaboratory comparison of motor activity experiments: implication for neurotoxicological assessments. *Neurotoxicol Teratol* 13: 599–609.

Diener W, Mischke U, Kayser D, Schlede E (1995). The biometric evaluation of the OECD modified version of the acute-toxic-class method (oral). *Arch Toxicol* 69: 729–734.

Diener W, Schlede E (1999). Acute toxicity class methods: alternatives to LD/LC_{50} tests. *ALTEX* 16: 129–134.

El-Nahhal Y (2004). Contamination and safety status of plant and food in Arab countries. *J Appl Sci* 4: 411–417.

FRAME: Funds for the replacement of animals in medical experiments. http://www.frame.org.uk/.

Gad SC, Weil CS (1986). *Statistics and Experimental Design for Toxicologists*. Telford Press, NJ.

Gad SC, Weil CS (1989). Statistics for toxicologists. In: Hayes AW. (Ed). *Principles and Methods of Toxicology*, 3rd edn. Raven Press, New York. Chapter 7, pp. 221–274.

Grice HC, Burek JD (1983). Age associated (geriatric) pathology: Its impact on long term toxicity studies. In: *Current Issues in Toxicology*. Springer Verlag, New York.

Korach KS (Ed) (1998). *Reproductive and Developmental Toxicology*. Marcel Dekker, New York.

Heywood R (1981). Target organ toxicity. *Toxicol Lett* 8: 349–358.

Litchfield JT, Wilcoxon FJ (1949). A simplified method of evaluating dose-effect experiments. *J Pharmacol Exp Ther* 96: 99–113.

Lorke D (1983). A new approach to practical acute toxicity testing. *Arch Toxicol* 54: 275–287.

Meyer OA, Tilson HA, Byrd WC, Riley MT (1979). A method for the routine assessment of fore- and hindlimb grip strength of rats and mice. *Neurobehav Toxicol* 1: 233–236.

Miller LC, Tainter ML (1944). Estimation of ED50 and its error by means of log-probit graph paper. *Proc Soc Exp Biol Med* 57: 261–269.

Mohr U, Dungworth DL, Capen CC (Eds) (1994). *Pathobiology of the Aging Rat*, Vol 2. ILSI Press, Washington, DC.

Mohr U, Dungworth DL, Ward J *et al.* (Eds) (1996). *Pathobiology of the Aging Mouse*, Vols 1 and 2. ILSI Press, Washington, DC.

NIH (1985). *Guide for Care and Use of Laboratory Animals*. Publication # 85-23. (1985, revised) DHHS. NIH Publication. Bethesda, Maryland, USA.

OECD (1982). *Good Laboratory Practice in the Testing of Chemicals*. Organisation for Economic Cooperation and Development, Paris, p. 62.

OECD (1981). Test Guideline 453. Combined chronic toxicity/carcinogenicity studies. In: *OECD Guidelines for the Testing of Chemicals*. Organisation for Economic Cooperation and Development, Paris.

OECD (1995). Test Guideline 407. *Repeated Dose 28-day Oral Toxicity Study in Rodents. In: OECD Guidelines for the Testing of Chemicals*. Organisation for Economic Cooperation and Development, Paris.

OECD (1998). Test Guideline 408. *Repeated Dose 90-day Oral Toxicity Study in Non-rodents. In: OECD Guidelines for the Testing of Chemicals*. Organisation for Economic Cooperation & Development, Paris.

OECD (1998). *OECD Guidelines for the Testing of Chemicals. Section 4: Health Effects. Vol. 2*, 10th Addendum, Oct 1998. Organisation for Economic Cooperation and Development, Paris.

OECD (2001). Test Guideline 414. Prenatal development toxicity study. In: *OECD Guidelines for the Testing of Chemicals*. Organisation for Economic Cooperation and Development, Paris.

OECD (2001). Test Guideline 420. Acute oral toxicity – fixed dose procedure (FDP). In: *OECD Guidelines for the Testing of Chemicals*. Organisation for Economic Cooperation and Development, Paris.

OECD (2006). Test Guideline 425. *Acute Oral Toxicity – Up and Down Procedure (UDP*. In: *OECD Guidelines for the Testing of Chemicals*. Organisation for Economic Cooperation and Development, Paris.

Paynter OE (1984). *Oncogenic Potential: Guidance for Analysis and Evaluation of Long Term Rodent Studies. Evaluation Procedure #1000.1*. Office of Pesticide and Toxic Substances, EPA, Washington, D.C.

Roll R, Höfer-Bosse TH, Kayser D (1986). New perspectives in acute toxicity testing of chemicals. *Toxicol Lett* (Suppl.) 31: 86.

Roubicek CB, Pahnish OF, Taylor RL (1964). Growth of rats at two temperatures. *Growth* 28: 157–164.

SAS Institute Inc. (1990). *SAS/STAT User's Guide*. Version 6, Fourth Ed. Cary, NC, USA.

Schoepfer AM, Engel A, Fattinger K *et al.* (2007). Herbal does not mean innocuous: Ten cases of severe hepatotoxicity associated with dietary supplements from Herbalife (R) products. *J Hepatol* 47 (4): 521–526.

Seefeld MD, Peterson RE (1984). Digestible energy and efficiency of feed utilisation in rats treated with 2,3,7,8-tetrachlorodibenzo-p-dioxin. *Toxicol Appl Pharmacol* 74: 214–222.

Sofowora EA (1989). *Medicinal Plants and Traditional Medicine in Africa*, 2nd edn. Spectrum Books Ltd., Ibadan, Nigeria.

Stallard N, Whitehead A (1995). Reducing numbers in the fixed-dose procedure. *Hum Exp Toxicol* 14: 315–323.

Vora CK, Mansoor GA (2005). Herbs and alternative therapies: relevance to hypertension and cardiovascular diseases. *Curr Hypertension Rep* 7: 275–280.

Waner T (1992). Current statistical approaches to clinical pathology data from toxicological studies. *Toxicolol Pathol* 20 (3), Part 2.

Weil SC, McCollister DD (1963). Relationship between short- and long-term feeding studies in designing an effective toxicity test. *Agric Food Chem* 11: 486–491.

WHO (1990). *Principles for the Toxicological Assessment of Pesticide Residues in Food*, Environmental Health Criteria 104. IPCS/WHO, Geneva.

Zhu M, Lew KT, Leung P (2002). Protective effects of plant formula on ethanol-induced gastric lesions in rats. *Phytother Res* 16: 276–280.

31

Safety evaluation of herbal medicines

S Bart A Halkes, Jenneke A Wijbenga, Edwin van den Worm, Burt H Kroes, Cees J Beukelman and Albert JJ van den Berg

Introduction

Following the advances in biomedical sciences in the 20th century, the use of herbal medicinal products (HMPs) strongly declined. However, in recent years a revival in the interest of herbal medicines has been observed (see Chapter 1). The main reason for the renewed interest seems to be the general belief that natural products are harmless or, at least, have fewer side-effects than synthetic drugs. Going along with the needs of consumers, pharmaceutical industries have started marketing an increasing number of (new) HMPs. A survey in The Netherlands in 1998, for instance, yielded a list of over 1500 products containing almost 800 different plant species (Commissie Toetsing Fytotherapeutica, 1999).

As a result of this growing popularity of HMPs, the necessity for the assessment of quality, safety, and efficacy of these products is increasingly felt. In particular, the evaluation of safety aspects should have priority since the above-mentioned assumption that HMPs only have beneficial effects has proven to be incorrect. Reports on toxic effects and/or adverse events associated with, amongst others, accidental or deliberate contamination or adulteration/substitution of plant material, the use of toxic plant (constituents), hypersensitivity reactions and herb–drug interactions have been regularly published (see, for example, Sharff and Bayer, 1982; Kumana *et al.*, 1983; De Smet, 1992; Fugh-Berman and Ernst, 2001; Cosyns, 2003; Palanisamy *et al.*, 2003; Cusack and Buckley, 2005; Izzo, 2005). Nevertheless, the number of these accounts still represents only a small proportion of the total amount of adverse drug reactions in the database of the World Health Organization (WHO) (Barnes, 1998).

This chapter gives a brief overview of the points to consider in relation to the safe use of HMPs. Approaches to deal with the evaluation of potential health risks of medicinal plants will also be described. In this respect, the combined application of analytical techniques and bioassays to obtain phytochemical markers to predict toxicity as well as a methodology to assess the clinical relevance of herb–drug interactions will be given as illustrative examples.

Health risks related to HMPs

Health risks associated with the use of HMPs may have multiple causes, but in general three categories can be distinguished. Two of these categories relate to the HMP itself. The first can be designated as extrinsic or non-plant-associated (Halkes, 2000); toxic effects or adverse reactions originating from accidental or deliberate contamination or adulteration/substitution of the plant material described on the label or from poor quality control.

The second category is more intrinsic or plant-associated in nature (Halkes, 2000). In this category, the plant material – as active ingredient in the HMP – produces health risks, for example, because it contains toxic constituents, or constituents that are known to affect the bioavailability and pharmacokinetic and/or pharmacodynamic interaction of other (plant) compounds or drugs, or it has been subjected to specific manufacturing processes resulting in highly concentrated or otherwise non-conventional extracts. The third category are 'consumer-dependent' causative factors, i.e. health risks associated with users or patients who show, for instance, hypersensitivity reactions or belong to a specific population which is much more prone to toxic effects and/or adverse events (De Smet, 2004). Each of these aspects will be discussed separately in the following sections.

Contaminations and adulterations/substitutions

A critical evaluation of the available reports in which toxicity of and/or adverse drug reactions to HMPs have been described shows that the detrimental effects in many cases were due to contamination or adulteration/substitution of the plant material. The risks associated with the use of such contaminated or adulterated products have been extensively reviewed (De Smet, 1992; De Smet, 2004). Therefore, this aspect of herbal safety will only be briefly commented upon here since they are discussed in Chapter 27. Contaminants and adulterants are often the result of ignorance or incompetence but cases of deliberate substitution by cheaper or more common plant species and conventional drugs are not uncommon.

Toxic plants and/or constituents

It has long been recognised that certain plants or plant constituents are (extremely) toxic and that their use can provide serious health risks. Amongst these plants are *Aconitum napellus* L., *Croton tiglium* L. (fatty oil from the seeds), *Digitalis* species, *Ricinus communis* L., and plants containing aristolochic acid or pyrrolizidine alkaloids (Sharff and Bayer, 1982; Kumana *et al.*, 1983; Roth *et al.*, 1984; Cosyns, 2003). The application of these plants as herbal medicines is generally obsolete and is legally restricted in many countries. However, despite the legislatorial exclusion of some notorious toxic plant species, the use of other potentially harmful herbs still persists, as may be concluded from a Dutch survey (Commissie Toetsing Fytotherapeutica, 1999) which confirmed previous observations from the German HMP market (Thesen, 1988).

Aristolochic-acid-induced nephrotoxicity

From the point of view of safety, the availability and use of potentially noxious plants, and HMPs is an obvious cause for concern. A striking example in this respect comes from Belgium where in 1992 a number of women using a Chinese herbal mixture to lose weight developed severe end-stage renal disease caused by interstitial nephritis and uroepithelial malignancies (Vanherweghem *et al.*, 1993; Depierreux *et al.*, 1994; Cosyns, 2003). To inhibit appetite, these women were intended to be treated with *Stephania tetranda* S. Moore and *Magnolia officinalis* Rehder and E.H. Wilson. However, root extracts of *S. tetranda* (in Chinese: *fangji*) were exchanged for or contaminated with roots of *Aristolochia fangchi* Y.C. Wu ex L.D. Chow and S.M. Hwang (Chinese name: *guang fangji*) (Vanhaelen *et al.*, 1994). *Aristolochia* species contain aristolochic acids, nephrotoxins and carcinogens which have been shown in both animal and human studies to induce tumours in the urinary tract (Thiele *et al.*, 1967; Mengs *et al.*, 1982, 1988). Aristolochic acids – in particular the nitrophenanthrene carboxylic acids aristolochic acid I and II – form DNA adducts after metabolic activation

(Arlt *et al.*, 2002). Such adducts were identified in the kidneys and urethric tissue of the Belgian patients (Schmeiser *et al.*, 1996). DNA damage by aristolochic acid may also lead to destructive fibrotic processes in the kidney (Lebeau *et al.*, 2001). This example highlights the need for adequate quality control and proper identification of ingredients in HMPs as this could have prevented this dramatic case, in particular since HMPs containing aristolochic acid are still marketed (Martena *et al.*, 2007).

Plants and/or constituents affecting bioavailability and pharmacokinetics

Several plants or plant constituents are renowned for their ability to affect bioavailability and pharmacokinetics of coadministered drugs. The most well-known and by far the best-investigated example in this respect is St John's wort (*Hypericum perforatum* L.). Numerous clinical studies and case reports have documented that St John's wort preparations lower serum concentrations of concomitantly used drugs and in this way – when serum concentrations are reduced to suboptimal or even below therapeutically effective levels – may pose health risks (for more details, see below). *Hypericum* extracts contain many (bioactive) constituents, including hyperforin, hypericin, flavonoids, and polyphenols. Of these compounds, hyperforin markedly induces cytochrome-P450 (CYP) 3A4 expression via activation of the pregnane receptor (Moore *et al.*, 2000). Since this isoenzyme is involved in the hepatic metabolism of a wide array of drugs, these findings provide a molecular mechanism for the interaction between St John's wort and these drugs.

Besides St John's wort, many other plant constituents have been shown to alter bioavailability and pharmacokinetics. Thus, the major alkaloid component in *Piper* species, piperine, has been reported to increase serum concentrations of drugs, such as the bronchodilator theophylline and the beta-blocker propranolol (Bano *et al.*, 1991) after oral administration in humans. This enhancement of systemic availability by piperine is most probably related to the inhibition of glucuronidation in the liver and the small intestine (Atal *et al.*, 1985; Singh *et al.*, 1986). Other plant constituents that may influence the biopharmaceutical parameters of a HMP include saponins and essential oil constituents; the former being able to increase the water solubility of non-polar compounds (Nakayama *et al.*, 1986; Schöpke and Bartlakowski, 1997) and the latter improving percutaneous absorption (Hori *et al.*, 1991; Williams and Barry, 1991). Plants containing this kind of constituents may constitute distinct safety problems. Especially when they are used in complex or combined preparations, the ability of such compounds to influence the bioavailability and pharmacokinetics of additional ingredients may significantly alter the toxicological profile of these products. A specific group of HMPs that should be considered in this respect are Ayurvedic preparations, since extracts of *Piper* species are part of most formulations used in this Indian traditional medical system.

Highly concentrated or otherwise non-conventional extracts

In the past decade, an increasing number of HMPs have been marketed which contain highly concentrated, enriched, partially purified extracts or extracts that have been prepared with non-conventional solvents. The profile of constituents present in such preparations substantially differs from traditionally used extracts (decoctions, percolates, macerates, tinctures, etc.), both in qualitative and quantitative aspects. Accordingly, the toxicological characteristics of such products may also significantly differ from traditional preparations. Safety data obtained for the latter, therefore, cannot provide an accurate and reliable insight into the actual dangers of extracts that have been subjected to specialised manufacturing processes. As a consequence, unexpected intoxications resulting from the use of products containing these highly concentrated or otherwise non-conventional extracts may emerge. This can be illustrated by recent case reports on hepatotoxic effects of kava (*Piper methysticum* G. Forst). Traditional extracts of kava – infusions of ground roots in cold water – have been consumed in the South Pacific for ages, apparently without serious side-effects (Steiner, 2000; Moulds and Malani, 2003).

When the use of kava for the treatment of anxiety and nervous disorders became popular in the Western world, concentrated alcohol and acetonic extracts replaced the traditional beverages. From

1990 to 2002, 39 patients were identified who had developed hepatic necrosis or cholestatic hepatitis following the use of these commercial products (Stickel *et al.*, 2003). Eight of these patients required liver transplantation and in total three lives were lost (Stickel *et al.*, 2003). Although the risk–benefit ratio of kava extracts still is considered to be good in comparison with that of other drugs used to treat anxiety, these casualties resulted in withdrawal of market authorisation and a ban on sales in many countries (Clouatre, 2004).

Initially, it was speculated that both immunoallergic and idiosyncratic reactions might underly the liver damage (Stickel *et al.*, 2003). However, several, more recent publications also suggest that differences in concentration and ratio of plant constituents in commercial preparations versus traditional kava beverages may play a role in hepatotoxicity. Thus, the concentration of kava-lactones in extracts prepared with organic solvents is significantly higher than that of aqueous extracts (Stickel *et al.*, 2003; Whitton *et al.*, 2003; Côté *et al.*, 2004) and has been linked to a more potent inhibition of the drug-metabolising potential of the liver (Côté *et al.*, 2004). Along with this, the kava-lactone to gluthathione ratio is negatively affected when extracts are prepared according to commercial methods which may result in glutathione depletion in the liver and subsequent saturation of its enzymatic detoxification pathways (Whitton *et al.*, 2003).

Finally, the use of non-polar extraction solvents has been associated with an increased hepatocellular toxicity, an effect that was due to preferential extraction of the hydroxychalcone flavokavain B from kava roots (Jhoo *et al.*, 2006). Likewise, introduction of a modified extraction procedure leading to St John's wort products with a higher hyperforin content has been associated with an increased number of herb–drug interactions (see also below) (Madabushi *et al.*, 2006).

Consumer-dependent toxic effects and/or adverse events

Toxic effects and/or adverse events are not always dependent on the HMP itself but may also be due to consumer-related factors, such as age, renal and hepatic functioning, hypersensitivity reactions, nutritional state or disease-related physiological disturbances (Huxtable, 1990; De Smet, 2004). Furthermore, otherwise perfectly well-tolerated HMPs may cause health problems under specific circumstances. In particular, long-term users, consumers of large amounts or many different HMPs simultaneously, and people who use prescribed drugs concomitantly (herb–drug interactions; see below) may be prone to detrimental effects, but also pregnant and lactating women or patients undergoing surgery are at risk (Huxtable, 1990; De Smet, 2004).

HMPs during pregnancy and lactation

Ever since the early sixties, when the world was shocked by the dramatic effects of thalidomide on the unborn child, there is consensus that the use of drugs during the first phases of pregnancy should in general be avoided. Only drugs that can be classified as pregnancy-category A and lactation-category I according to the Swedish classification can be considered safe for use by pregnant women (Sannerstedt *et al.*, 1980; Berglund *et al.*, 1984).

Similar precautions should be taken when HMPs are used during pregnancy and lactation since genotoxic, arbortifacient, uterine stimulatory, and emmenagogue effects have been reported for many herbs (Ernst, 2002). At present, only a few herbs have been clinically tested for safety and efficacy during pregnancy. Ginger (*Zingiber officinale* Roscoe.), as a herbal remedy for pregnancy-associated nausea and vomiting, is one of these exceptions, since its efficacy is proven in several randomised clinical trials and the incidence of birth defects, miscarriages or deformities in ginger-treated women is not higher than in the normal population (Boone and Shields, 2005; Borrelli *et al.*, 2005). However, for the vast majority of HMPs sufficient data on safety during pregnancy and lactation is lacking. Until this information is available, pregnant women should limit the use of HMPs or only do so after consultation of a general practitioner and/or gynaecologist.

Methods to evaluate the safety of herbal medicines

From a scientific point of view, it does not come as a surprise that health risks are associated with the use of HMPs since drug targets, e.g. receptors, enzymes or DNA, do not discriminate between the origin of molecules, whether these are derived from the plant kingdom or have been synthesised. Therefore, safety of a HMP is not dependent on its naturalness but on its chemical fingerprint and its ability to interact with physiological substrates of the human body (De Smet, 1995). Both of these aspects need to be considered in the safety evaluation of HMPs. This requires a multidisciplinary approach, involving analytical techniques and methodologies common to botany, pharmacology, pharmacotherapy, toxicology and epidemiology. Distinct features of HMPs which set these products apart from synthetic drugs – their complexity and available knowledge from traditional use – should, however, also be taken into account during safety evaluation.

Quality control

Quality control is dealt with in Chapter 28 so is mentioned here only to emphasise its important link with safety. Increased resolution chromatographic systems and sensitivity of detection methods have made it possible to detect and identify plant constituents in ever-decreasing concentrations (Hostettmann *et al.*, 1997; Kerns *et al.*, 1998; Vogler *et al.*, 1998).

Quality assurance is not only important to prevent the detrimental effects that contaminated or adulterated/substituted preparations may inflict on general health, or at least minimising these risks to occur, but also for another reason. Thus, it is inherent to the production process, as a result of differences in growing and harvesting conditions, that the chemical profile of the plant material used to prepare HMPs is not constant. This is valid both for the concentration of (biologically active) markers (Repčák *et al.*, 1998; Vogel *et al.*, 1999; Beekwilder *et al.*, 2006) but also for the levels of potentially noxious plant constituents (Table 31.1). Efforts to guarantee a constant quality – for instance, by standardisation to fixed (low) concentrations of active and/or toxic metabolites – as well as methods to quantify this are therefore necessary as they are a prerequisite for obtaining reproducible data on efficacy and safety and the reliable assessment of benefit-to-risk ratios.

Nevertheless, phytochemical standardisation alone may not be completely satisfactory, since HMPs that are comparable in content and/or pattern of one or more constituents still have been shown to vary in biological activity and bioavailability (Rininger *et al.*, 2000a,b; Kressmann *et al.*, 2002). In this respect, use of bioassays has been advocated as an instrument to better predict therapeutic efficacy (McLaughlin *et al.*, 1998; Rininger *et al.*, 2000a). By

Table 31.1 The concentration of (potentially) noxious constituents in HMPs depends on the plant variety, growing and harvesting conditions, and the plant part used. Standardisation to fixed (low) concentrations of these metabolites may help to obtain reproducible data on safety and to establish a positive benefit-to-risk ratio (Halkes, 2000)

The content of β-asarone, which showed carcinogenic activity in several in vivo studies, is dependent on the number of chromosomes in *Acorus calamus*; commercial products prepared from an American diploid variety contain no traceable amounts of β-asarone whereas those of European (triploid) and Indian (tetraploid) varieties yield low and high concentrations respectively of this compound (Stahl and Keller, 1981)
Roots of *Symphytum asperum* have higher levels of alkaloids in comparison to the aerial parts (Roitman, 1981)
Ginkgolic acids are detectable in both the leaves and seed covers of *Ginkgo biloba* but relative concentrations in the leaves are so low that allergic responses, especially dermatitis, can be excluded (Wagner *et al.*, 1989)
The pyrrolizidine alkaloid content in the leaves of different *Senecio* spp. varies widely, depending on the time of year or developmental stage at which the plant was collected (Johnson *et al.*, 1985)
Similar results were obtained with regard to the seasonal variation in the amounts of the neurotoxin 4′-O-methylpyridoxine in *Ginkgo biloba* leaves and seeds (Arenz *et al.*, 1996)
The concentration of alkaloids in *Senecio* spp. was found to be affected by the area in which the plants are collected (Johnson *et al.*, 1985)

analogy, toxicological testing in combination with quality control may serve to identify safety/toxicological markers more adequately. Thus, inhibitory activity of kava extracts towards various cytochrome-P450 isoenzymes (CYP 3A4, CYP 1A2, CYP 2C9, and CYP 2C19) was found to be dependent on kavalactone composition (Côté *et al.*, 2004). Likewise, the mutagenic potential of commercial ethanolic plant extracts could be correlated with their quercetin content (Schimmer *et al.*, 1988). Another example of combined application of analytical techniques and bioassays to identify phytochemical markers to predict potential toxic effects of herbal extracts is highlighted below.

Gallic acid content in tannic acid samples as a predictive marker for toxicity

Hydrolysable tannins are present in many different (medicinal) plants and have been included in many older editions of pharmacopoeias and are specifically referred to as Acidum Tannicum or tannic acid (Halkes *et al.*, 2001a). Tannic acid became the standard in local treatment of burn wounds in the first half of the 20th century when most clinicians agreed upon its effectiveness, but nowadays its use is generally considered to be obsolete, mainly because of early reports on hepatotoxicity (Hupkens *et al.*, 1995; Halkes *et al.*, 2001a).

Using analytical techniques in combination with a bioassay, we were able to establish that the toxic effects observed in patients with burns were not related to tannic acid itself but rather were, at least in part, caused by degradation products present in preparations used in early clinical trials and toxicity studies. A haemoglobin precipitation test was used as a model to study the protein-binding capacity, using tannic acids from different commercial sources. A highly purified tannic acid extensively used in the food and pharmaceutical industry was found to be most potent in this respect but other tannic acid samples, however, showed considerably less activity or were even unable to precipitate haemoglobin in the dosage range tested (Halkes *et al.*, 2001b).

Qualitative and quantitative analysis of these tannic acids demonstrated that the ability to bind proteins was inversely proportional to the content of free gallic acid, one of the constituents found after hydrolytic degradation of tannic acid (Figure 31.1a; Halkes *et al.*, 2001b). In subsequent experiments it was proven that gallic acid, even when present in such low concentrations of approximately 1–2%, (completely) blocked haemoglobin precipitation (Figure 31.1b) and that highly purified tannic acid with a gallic acid content below 0.1% did not elicit signs of hepatotoxicity (Halkes *et al.*, 2002). On the basis of these experiments, it was concluded that the free gallic acid concentration in tannic acid products is a predictive marker for safety. Too-high levels of gallic acid, by attenuating protein precipitation in the burn wound, may on the one hand hamper the fixation of endogenous toxins produced in the skin after thermal injury, thereby constituting a potential hazard to the liver as has been seen in several clinical trials (Halkes *et al.*, 2001a). On the other hand, inhibition of protein binding may also have caused an increase in the bodily uptake of topically applied tannic acids, thereby elevating the plasma concentrations to potentially toxic levels which might explain the adverse effects observed in several animal experiments (Halkes *et al.*, 2001a).

Safety assessment of traditionally used HMPs

In contrast to new chemical entities, many medicinal herbs have a long history of use and this may have generated a significant amount of published toxicological information including scientifically accepted monographs, clinical experience and epidemiological studies, as well as data from post-marketing surveillance programmes. This information may be used as a basis for a simplified registration procedure and may serve as a substitute for animal experiments and reduce the number of clinical trials in humans (Anonymous, 2004b; Committee on Herbal Medicinal Products, 2006).

Although prescribers and consumers of traditional HMPs will be able to recognise and report on major acute adverse events, such as dermatological reactions, nausea, and disturbances of the gastrointestinal tract, it has proven to be difficult to associate other more subtle symptoms of toxicity or long-term detrimental effects with the use of a particular herb and these may therefore have easily been missed. Consequently, data on traditional use are unlikely to provide information on chronic

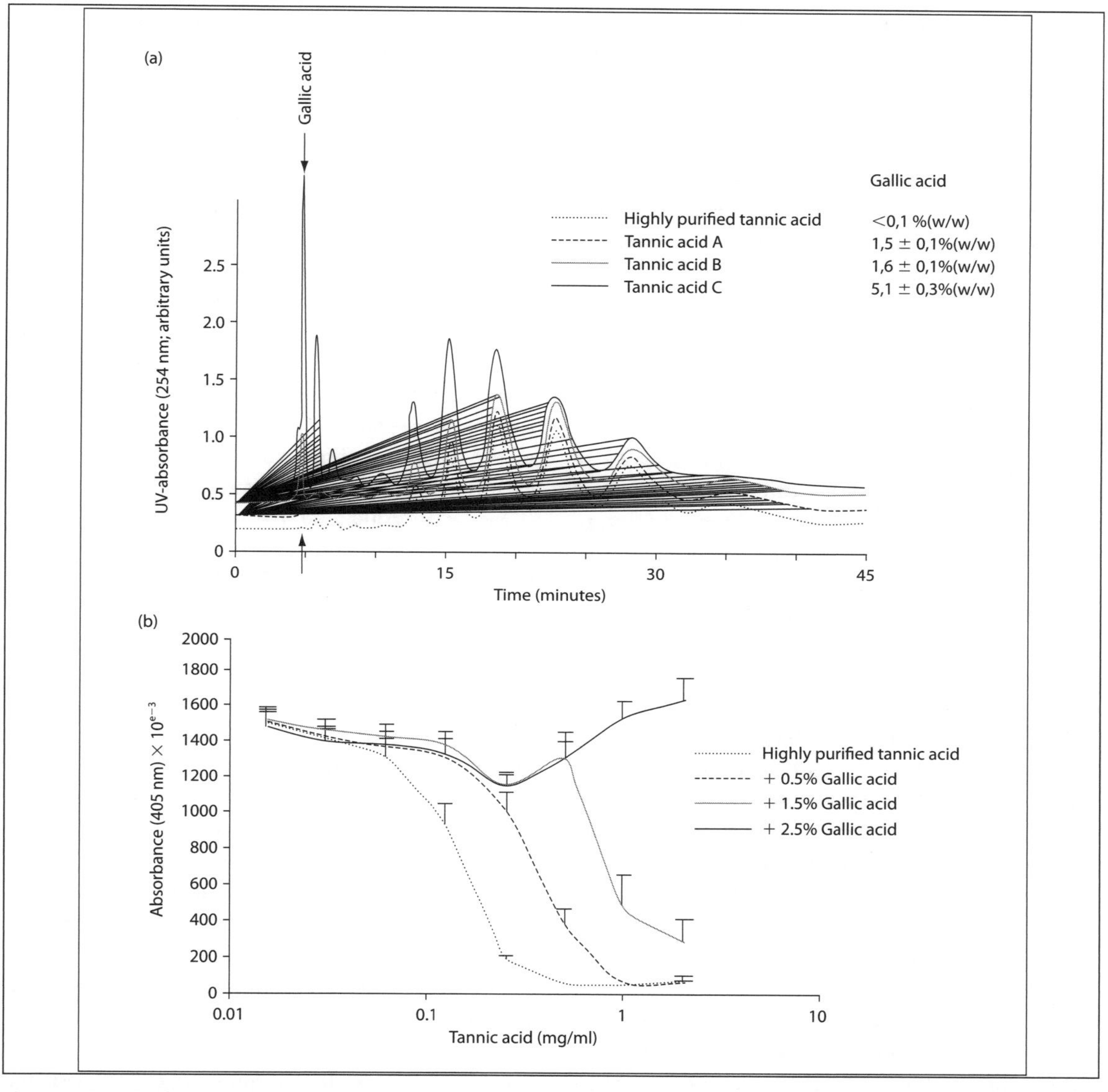

Figure 31.1 Use of analytical techniques in combination with bioassays to identify predictive markers for toxicity. (a) High-performance liquid chromatography profiles from some commercial tannic acids. High-molecular-weight polygalloyl-glucose esters elute between 12 and 40 min. The degradation-product gallic acid has a retention time of 4.7 minutes; (b) haemoglobin precipitation – measured as a decrease in absorbance at 405 nm – of tannic acids is markedly inhibited by the presence of low concentrations of gallic acid.

toxicity, carcinogenic, mutagenic, and/or teratogenic effects. Legislatory bodies have acknowledged this problem and have given the right to national and European authorities to demand such supplementary safety testing when bibliographic evidence is deemed to be insufficient to prove safety before marketing authorisation as a traditional HMP is issued (Anonymous, 2004b, 2006a).

Methods to establish safety of non-traditional HMPs

Safety evaluation of non-traditional HMPs requires a multidisciplinary approach involving a wide variety of data, including the chemical profile of (toxic) constituents present in the plant material, results from in-vitro or in-vivo pharmacological and toxicological studies, as well as information on toxic effects and adverse events observed in clinical trials or obtained from post-marketing surveillance databases. In particular, the human data are best suited to establish potential health risks and should take precedence in determining safety. When the number and rigour of the human studies is deemed sufficient by expert judgement, non-clinical testing may not even be required (Bast *et al.*, 2002).

Chemical profile of (toxic) constituents

Qualitative and quantitative determination of the (toxic) constituents present in a plant extract or HMP is fundamental to the evaluation of safety (see above). Quality control should guarantee levels of known, relevant toxins to be within acceptable limits which may be defined on the one hand by hazard characterisation of the substance(s) involved and on the other hand by their possible contribution to therapeutic efficacy. In this respect, products derived from *Valeriana officinalis* L. may serve as an example. Valepotriates present in this herb have been shown to possess in-vitro cytotoxic and mutagenic activity, most probably attributable to their alkylating properties (Bos *et al.*, 1997). However, reasonable doubt may be raised as to whether the toxic effects of valepotriates are of relevance in humans, since they are quite unstable and little is resorbed from the intestinal tract in unchanged form (Wagner and Jurcic, 1980). Thus, hazards associated with the presence of valepotriates may be graded as low. Nevertheless, since it is questionable whether the presence of valepotriates contributes to the beneficial effects of valerian preparations in the treatment of sleep disorders (Bos *et al.*, 1997), limits of these constituents may be set at the absolute minimum.

This applies even more so in the case of plants containing constituents which have been implicated in more severe toxic effects such as pyrrolizidine alkaloids or aristolochic acids. However, in other instances complete reduction of the levels of a potentially toxic component is not always possible. This is in particular true when a HMP contains constituents which are both pharmacologically active or detrimental, depending on the dosage; removal of these constituents will also render the product ineffective. It may then be useful to set specific limits, e.g. as done in the 2005 *European Pharmacopoeia* for the content of hydroxyanthracene derivatives in standardised *Aloe* dry extracts (Anon., 2004a).

Even if no known toxins are present, identification of (minor) constituents in a HMP may be of use during safety evaluation since it may provide input for a recently developed pragmatic risk assessment tool, the threshold of toxicological concern (Kroes *et al.*, 2004, 2005). This concept refers to the establishment of a level of exposure for all kind of substances below which there would be no appreciable risk to human health. The threshold of toxicological concern principle proposes that such levels can be identified – also in the absence of full-range toxicity data – on the basis of the molecular structure of the (plant) constituent and the known toxicity of chemicals that share similar structural characteristics (Kroes *et al.*, 2004, 2005).

Experimental, pharmacological and toxicological data

Where insufficient data are available or reasonable doubt exists as to whether or not a specific HMP can be safely used – e.g. when information on traditional use is lacking or (potentially) noxious constituents are present – complementary evidence should be supplied to prove the harmlessness of such a preparation. In this regard, like all new chemical entities that are being filed for a marketing authorisation, HMPs should satisfy the requirements for the acceptance of safe use as laid down by, for example, the European Union (Anon., 2001). Usually, this will require thorough research into the extracts or products in question; knowledge about the acute, subacute and chronic toxicity, potentially harmful effects on reproduction including embryo/fetal and perinatal toxicity, mutagenic and carcinogenic activity, tolerance, pharmacokinetic parameters, etc., should be established to minimise the health risks of these products (Anon., 1995, 1997, 2001). Based on the results of these toxicity tests, risks associated with the use of a HMP can be characterised and a safe dosage or acceptable daily intake established. In general, the safe dosage is determined based on the highest no observed adverse effect level (NOAEL) or the lowest observed adverse effect level (LOAEL) obtained from in-vivo experiments or human studies, which are divided by a safety or uncertainty factor (Bast *et al.*, 2002).

Human studies

Systematic studies in healthy volunteers or patients, whether these are clinical trials or case reports, may – in addition to providing evidence for efficacy – also be used to determine potential health risks (Anonymous, 2001). Clinical trials have their limitations in this respect, so the health risks of a HMP in daily practice can better be examined in population-based studies such as epidemiological and/or pharmacovigilance studies. Although confounding variables can influence the results, these studies may indicate unusual adverse events but, for instance, also herb–drug interactions. Implementation of HMPs in (inter)national post-marketing schemes, as has been done now for several years in the WHO Collaborating Centre for International Drug Monitoring (Barnes, 1998), may provide such evidence. However, since most herbal preparations are not authorised as medicines and consumers do not report to their healthcare professionals in this respect (Cuzzolin *et al.*, 2006), existing post-marketing systems may not adequately monitor reports on adverse events in these cases. Post-marketing surveillance studies specifically focusing on herbal preparations which have not been authorised as medicines and allowing for direct submission of consumer comments should therefore be developed (Bast *et al.*, 2002).

Direct evidence of toxic effects and/or adverse events from human studies is the most important source of information to establish health risks associated with the use of HMPs. Nevertheless, critical appraisal of these data is necessary during the process of safety evaluation. In particular, weighing of the clinical relevance of reported detrimental effects is essential as will be illustrated in the next section.

Assessment of the clinical relevance of herb–drug interactions: St John's wort as an example

A great number of possible herb–drug interactions can be found in scientific literature, e.g. a survey in 2001 yielded 250 plant species or genera being mentioned in connection with herb–drug interactions (Wijbenga *et al.*, 2004a). However, there is much variation in the level of evidence underlying these reports and, interactions are often merely assumed on the basis of (claimed) pharmacotherapeutic activity of the herb or its constituents. Sometimes, data from in-vitro or animal studies do suggest potential herb–drug interactions but it remains questionable whether these findings can be extrapolated to humans. Only in a limited number of cases are reports of herb–drug interactions substantiated by clinical trials and/or case reports (Wijbenga *et al.*, 2004a).

To be of use in daily practice, clinically relevant herb–drug interactions need to be distinguished from non-significant and putative ones, since too many warnings of unclear clinical significance will only increase the likelihood that healthcare professionals will ignore herb–drug interaction alerts. At present, the available literature mainly comprises of enumerations of herb–drug interactions (Izzo and Ernst, 2001; Bressler, 2005a,b; Hu *et al.*, 2005; Izzo, 2005; Van den Bout-Van den Beukel *et al.*, 2006). Although a non-validated scoring system to rate the probability of herb–drug interactions has been described (Fugh-Berman and Ernst, 2001), the clinical relevance of herb–drug interactions has, to our knowledge, not yet been systematically assessed. However, a structured procedure for the assessment of drug–drug interactions has been successfully adopted and included in computerised drug-interaction surveillance systems (Van Roon *et al.*, 2005), which has also been proven suitable to assess herb–drug interactions (Wijbenga *et al.*, 2004b,c,d,e,f; De Smet, 2006). Central to this algorithm to assess the clinical relevance of the interaction are two parameters: the evidence supporting the reported interaction, and the severity of the adverse event resulting from the interaction. In short, evidence is graded from 0 to 4; in-vitro and/or animal studies are graded 0; case reports are graded 1 or 2 – depending on the quality of documentation; clinical studies are graded 3 when they concern surrogate endpoints, or 4 when they concern clinically relevant endpoints. When only abstracts or posters from scientific meetings are available, they are graded 1 or (if the study is not published within three years) as 0. Severity is graded from A to F in order of increasing seriousness.

Although no strict limits can be defined, effects can broadly be categorised A or B when adverse events have not (yet) been observed or are considered minor (for instance lowered plasma levels in healthy volunteers, headache), C or D when moderately severe adverse events are observed or when there is an increased risk of serious but non-lethal disease, and E or F in cases of serious adverse events or increased risk of failure of life-saving therapies. The National Cancer Institute's Common Toxicity Criteria provides a useful six-step scale for gradually dividing adverse reactions of drugs (Van Roon *et al.*, 2005).

Of all medicinal herbs, St John's wort (*Hypericum perforatum*) has been most frequently mentioned in literature in connection with herb–drug interactions, so will be used as an example. Close to a hundred case reports and clinical studies could be identified in which herb–drug interactions were associated with the use of St John's wort (Table 31.2; updated from Wijbenga *et al.*, 2004c). Of these, the ones that undoubtedly had the greatest impact were those case reports and clinical trials reporting decreased cyclosporine blood levels resulting in a weakened immunosuppressant activity, in some cases even to such extent that rejection episodes in patients with organ transplants were observed. Both the level of evidence and severity of the adverse events can in this case be rated as high.

Cyclosporine is a substrate of both the cytochrome-P450 isoenzyme CYP3A4 and P-glycoprotein and St John's wort induces both of these enzymes, which can be seen within 2 weeks of starting its use (Dürr *et al.*, 2000). Other substrates of CYP3A4 and/or P-glycoprotein that have been reported in case reports and/or clinical studies to be influenced in patients who concomitantly use St John's wort, are digoxin, irinotecan, methadone, nevirapine, oral contraceptives, sildenafil and tacrolimus. Except for sildenafil, the level of evidence and/or severity point to a high clinical relevance (see Table 31.2).

In clinical studies with healthy volunteers, other substrates of CYP3A4 and/or P-glycoprotein have also been stated to be affected by St John's wort. The clinical relevance for patients in need of these therapies is not as strong, but still can be considered relatively high (see Table 31.2). Against expectations, no changes in pharmacokinetic parameters of the CYP3A4 substrates alprazolam and carbamazepine were observed in two studies with healthy volunteers (Burstein *et al.*, 2000; Markowitz *et al.*, 2000). Likely explanations for these discrepancies are the short period of use of St John's wort in the study with alprazolam and auto-induction of CYP3A4 in the study with carbamazepine.

An effect of St John's wort on other CYP-isoenzymes has also been suggested. For instance, several accounts of increased drug clearance and reduction of the international normalised ratio (INR) during simultaneous use of phenprocoumon or warfarin and St John's wort have been published (see Table 31.2). Since both phenprocoumon and warfarin are mainly metabolised by CYP2C9, this would imply an inducing effect of St John's wort on this isoenzyme. However, in clinical studies using the CYP2C9–substrate tolbutamide, induction of this isoenzyme by St John's wort could not be confirmed, possibly because the induction of other CYP-isoenzymes such as CYP3A4 was substantial enough to cause the observed effects. Nevertheless, taking into account the evidence and severity of the clinical effect, the interaction between St John's wort and phenprocoumon or warfarin can be considered as clinically relevant.

Initial indications of induction of CYP2C19 are not fully substantiated and the clinical relevance of these (potential) interactions is as yet unclear. For instance, clinical studies with theophylline and the CYP1A2–probe caffeine are not in agreement with the hypothesis arising from one case report that St John's wort might affect the metabolism of theophylline (see Table 31.2). Finally, no effect on the induction of CYP2D6 has been found in clinical studies using debrisoquin or dextromethorphan (see Table 31.2).

Aside from pharmacokinetic interactions such as those mentioned above, pharmacodynamic interactions might also be elicited by St John's wort. Case reports have linked it with symptoms of the serotonin syndrome when used in combination with a variety of drugs, e.g. fenfluramine, sertraline and venlafaxine. Manic symptoms have been observed when St John's wort was added to, or exchanged by the patient for other psychoactive drugs and an episode of delirium was reported when loperamide, valerian and St John's wort were used concomitantly. Although the implications may in some cases have been serious, the level of evidence for these pharmacodynamic interactions is still limited (see Table 31.2).

Table 31.2 Case reports and clinical studies of St John's wort-associated drug interactions with an assessment of their clinical relevance (modified and updated (June 2006) from Wijbenga *et al.*, 2004c)

Prescribed drug	St John's wort preparation	Reported effect	Reference relevance	Clinical
Blood-glucose-lowering drugs				
Rosiglitazone	Unknown	Increased clearance	Hruska *et al.*, 2005	1A
Tolbutamide	Esbericum capsules	No change	Arold *et al.*, 2005	3A
Tolbutamide	Capsules from Sundown Herbals	No change	Wang *et al.*, 2001	3A
Cardiovascular drugs				
Digoxin	St John's wort herbal tea	Digoxin poisoning after cessation of St John's wort	Andelic, 2003	1D
Digoxin	Esbericum capsules	No change	Arold *et al.*, 2005	3A
Digoxin	LI 160 extract	Decreased AUC	Dürr *et al.*, 2000	3A
Digoxin	Jarsin 300 (LI 160 extract)	Decreased AUC, C_{max} and trough concentrations	Johne *et al.*, 1999	3A
Digoxin	Powder from Kneipp-Werke hyperforin-rich; powder from Kneipp-Werke low in hyperforin; Jarsin 300 tablets (LI 160 extract); Johanniskrautöl-Kapseln S (oil extract); Sidroga Johanniskraut tea; Kneipp Johanniskrautsaft plant juice; Remotiv tablets (ZE 117 extract)	Decreased AUC, C_{max} and trough concentrations (hyperforin-rich powder; Jarsin 300) tablets; no change (powder low in hyperforin; Johanniskrautöl-Kapseln S; tea; juice; Remotiv tablets)	Mueller *et al.*, 2004	3A
Nifedipine	unknown	Reduced plasma concentration	Smith *et al.*, 2001	0C
Phenprocoumon	Unknown	Decreased INR	Bon *et al.*, 1999	1C
Phenprocoumon	LI 160 extract	Decreased AUC free phenprocoumon	Maurer *et al.*, 1999	0A
Pravastatin	TruNature caplets	No change	Sugimoto *et al.*, 2001	3A
Simvastatin	TruNature caplets	Decreased plasma concentration	Sugimoto *et al.*, 2001	3A
Verapamil	Movina tablets	Decreased plasma concentrations	Tannergren *et al.*, 2004	3A
Warfarin	Bioglan tablets	Increased clearance; decreased INR	Jiang *et al.*, 2004	4C
Warfarin	Unknown	Decreased INR	Yue *et al.*, 2000	1D
Drugs for the central nervous system				
Alprazolam	Esbericum capsules	No change	Arold *et al.*, 2005	3A
Alprazolam	Solaray capsules	No change	Markowitz *et al.*, 2000	3A
Alprazolam	Kira tablets (LI 160)	Increased clearance	Markowitz *et al.*, 2003	3A
Amitriptyline	Jarsin 300 (LI 160 extract)	Decreased AUC of amitriptyline and metabolites	Roots *et al.*, 2000; Johne *et al.*, 2002	3C

(*continued overleaf*)

Table 31.2 (*continued*)

Prescribed drug	St John's wort preparation	Reported effect	Reference relevance	Clinical
Bupropion; nortriptyline	Unknown	Manic symptoms	Moses and Mallinger, 2000	1D
Buspirone	Hypericum 2000 Plus	Symptoms suggestive of serotonin syndrome	Dannawi, 2002	1D
Buspirone; fluoxetine	Unknown	Hypomanic symptoms	Spinella and Eaton, 2001	1D
Carbamazepine	Tablets from Hypericum Buyers Club	No change	Burstein *et al.*, 2000	3A
Clonazepam; lithium; olanzapine	Unknown	Manic symptoms	Moses and Mallinger, 2000	1D
Fenfluramine	Unknown	Symptoms suggestive of serotonin syndrome	Beckman *et al.*, 2000	1B
Midazolam	Jarsin 300 dragees (LI 160)	Increased clearance	Dresser *et al.*, 2003	3A
Midazolam	Product from Wild Oats Markets	Increased metabolism	Gurley *et al.*, 2002	3A
Midazolam	Extract from Rexall-Sundown Pharmaceuticals	Increased clearance	Gorski *et al.*, 2002; Hall *et al.*, 2003	3A
Midazolam	Capsules from Sundown Herbals	Decreased AUC	Wang *et al.*, 2001	3A
Nefazodone	Unknown	Symptoms suggestive of serotonin syndrome	Lantz *et al.*, 1999	1B
Paroxetine	Unknown	Symptoms suggestive of serotonin syndrome	Beckman *et al.*, 2000	1B
Paroxetine	Unknown	Symptoms suggestive of serotonin syndrome	Gordon, 1998	1D
Paroxetine	Unknown	Symptoms suggestive of serotonin syndrome	Waksman *et al.*, 2000	0D
Quazepam	Caplets from TruNature	Decreased plasma concentration	Kawaguchi *et al.*, 2004	3A
Sertraline	Unknown	Symptoms suggestive of serotonin syndrome	Lantz *et al.*, 1999	1B
Sertraline; testosterone	Unknown	Manic symptoms	Barbenel *et al.*, 2000	1E
Trazodone	Unknown	Symptoms suggestive of serotonin syndrome	Fugh-Berman, 2000; Miller, 2001	1B
Venlafaxine	St John's wort mother tincture	Symptoms suggestive of serotonin syndrome	Prost *et al.*, 2000	1B
Drugs against HIV				
Indinavir	Tablets from Hypericum Buyers Club	Reduced AUC	Piscitelli *et al.*, 2000	3A
Nevirapine	Unknown	Increased clearance	De Maat *et al.*, 2001	1E

Table 31.2 (*continued*)

Prescribed drug	St John's wort preparation	Reported effect	Reference relevance	Clinical
Immunosuppressants				
Cyclosporine	Unknown	Subtherapeutic drug levels	Ahmed *et al.*, 2001	1E
Cyclosporine	Herbal tea mixture	Subtherapeutic drug levels	Alscher and Klotz, 2003	1E
Cyclosporine	Your Life tablets; St John's wort tablets	Subtherapeutic drug levels; chronic transplant rejection	Barone *et al.*, 2000; Barone *et al.*, 2001; Turton-Weeks *et al.*, 2001	1F
Cyclosporine	Jarsin 300TM tablets	Subtherapeutic drug levels	Bauer *et al.*, 2003	4E
Cyclosporine	Neuroplant	Subtherapeutic drug levels	Beer and Ostermann, 2001	1E
Cyclosporine	Unknown	Subtherapeutic drug levels; transplant rejection	Bon *et al.*, 1999	1E
Cyclosporine	Unknown	Subtherapeutic drug levels; transplant rejection	Breidenbach *et al.*, 2000a,b	1E
Cyclosporine	Jarsin 300 dragees (LI 160)	Increased clearance	Dresser *et al.*, 2003	3A
Cyclosporine	Unknown	Subtherapeutic drug levels; transplant rejection	Karliova *et al.*, 2000	2E
Cyclosporine	Jarsin 300	Subtherapeutic drug levels	Mai et al., 2000	2E
Cyclosporine	Jarsin 300; Jarsin 300 after supercritical carbon dioxide extraction to remove hyperforin	Subtherapeutic drug levels (Jarsin 300); no change (CO_2-extracted Jarsin 300)	Mai *et al.*, 2004	4E
Cyclosporine	Unknown	Subtherapeutic drug levels	Mandelbaum *et al.*, 2000	2E
Cyclosporine	Unknown	Subtherapeutic drug levels	Moschella and Jaber, 2001	2E
Cyclosporine	Unknown	Subtherapeutic drug levels	Rey and Walter, 1998	1E
Cyclosporine	Jarsin (LI 160 extract)	Subtherapeutic drug levels; transplant rejection	Ruschitzka *et al.*, 2000	1E
Mycophenolic acid	Jarsin 300 tablets	No change	Mai *et al.*, 2003	4A
Tacrolimus	Neuroplant	Subtherapeutic drug levels; decreased creatinine in serum	Bolley *et al.*, 2002	1E
Tacrolimus	Tablets from Lichtwer Pharma	Increased clearance	Hebert *et al.*, 2004	3A
Tacrolimus	Jarsin 300 tablets	Subtherapeutic drug levels	Mai *et al.*, 2003	4E
Oncolytics				
Imatinib	Kira (LI 160)	Increased clearance	Frye *et al.*, 2004	3A

(*continued overleaf*)

Table 31.2 (*continued*)

Prescribed drug	St John's wort preparation	Reported effect	Reference relevance	Clinical
Imatinib	Product from HBC	Reduced AUC	Smith *et al.*, 2004a,b	3A
Irinotecan	Tablets from Bio Nutrition Health Products	Decreased plasma levels of active metabolite SN-38; lower degree of myelosuppression	Mathijssen *et al.*, 2002	4E
Miscellaneous				
Anaesthetic drugs	Unknown	Delayed emergence	Crowe and McKeating, 2002	1B
Caffeine	Esbericum capsules	No change	Arold *et al.*, 2005	3A
Caffeine	Unknown	No change	Gewertz *et al.*, 1999	0A
Caffeine	Product from Wild Oats Markets	No change	Gurley *et al.*, 2002	3A
Caffeine	Capsules from Sundown Herbals	No change	Wang *et al.*, 2001	3A
Caffeine	Jarsin 300	No change	Wenk *et al.*, 2004	3A
Chlorzoxazone	Product from Wild Oats Markets	Increased metabolism	Gurley *et al.*, 2002	3A
Debrisoquin	Product from Wild Oats Markets	No change	Gurley *et al.*, 2002	3A
Dextromethorphan	Unknown	No change	Ereshefsky *et al.*, 1999	0A
Dextromethorphan	Solaray capsules	No change	Markowitz *et al.*, 2000	3A
Dextromethorphan	Kira tablets (LI 160)	No change	Markowitz *et al.*, 2003	3A
Dextromethorphan	Tablets from Hypericum Buyers Club	No change	Roby *et al.*, 2001	3A
Dextromethorphan	Capsules with extract from Sundown Herbals	No change	Wang *et al.*, 2001	3A
Dextromethorphan	Jarsin 300	No change	Wenk *et al.*, 2004	3A
Fexofenadine	Jarsin 300 dragee (LI 160)	Increased clearance	Dresser *et al.*, 2003	3A
Fexofenadine	Sundown capsules	Decreased plasma concentration	Wang *et al.*, 2002	3A
Loperamide; valerian	Unknown	Delirium	Khawaja *et al.*, 1999	1D
Methadone	Jarsin	Decreased drug concentration; withdrawal symptoms	Eich-Höchli et al., 2003	4C
Omeprazole	Tablets from Hypericum Buyers Club	Decreased plasma concentration	Wang et al., 2004, see also discussion in Xie *et al.*, 2005	3A
Oral contraceptive	Unknown	Breakthrough bleeding	Bon *et al.*, 1999	1C
Oral contraceptive	Extract from Rexall-Sundown Pharmaceuticals	Increased clearance; increased breakthrough bleeding	Gorski *et al.*, 2002; Hall *et al.*, 2003	4C
Oral contraceptive	Unknown	Breakthrough bleeding; unintended pregnancy	Henderson *et al.*, 2002	1F

Table 31.2 (*continued*)

Prescribed drug	St John's wort preparation	Reported effect	Reference relevance	Clinical
Oral contraceptive	Capsules from Hypericum Buyers Club	Reduced dose exposure; increased breakthrough bleeding	Murphy *et al.*, 2005	4C
Oral contraceptive	Jarsin tablets (LI 160 extract)	Decreased AUC 3-ketodesogestrel; increased intracyclic bleeding	Pfrunder *et al.*, 2003	4C
Oral contraceptive	LI 160 extract	Breakthrough bleeding	Ra-umlauttz *et al.*, 2001	1C
Oral contraceptive	Helarium 425; unknown	Unexpected pregnancy	Schwarz *et al.*, 2003	1F
Oral contraceptive	Remotiv (Ze 117 extract)	No change	Will-Shahab *et al.*, 2001	0A
Oral contraceptive	Unknown	Breakthrough bleeding	Yue *et al.*, 2000	1C
Sildenafil	Unknown	Lack of effect	Chen *et al.*, 2001	1C
Theophylline	TruNature caplets	No change	Morimoto *et al.*, 2004	3A
Theophylline	Unknown	Subtherapeutic drug level	Nebel *et al.*, 1999	1B
Voriconazole	Jarsin (LI 160 extract)	Increased clearance	Rengelshausen et al., 2005	3A

Finally, when considering herb–drug interactions, it is important to keep in mind that individual preparations of any one herb may significantly vary in composition and, consequently, in the effect they bring about. In the case of St John's wort, for instance, the occurrence of interactions with cyclosporine, digoxin or oral contraceptives has been associated with the presence of hyperforin (Will-Shahab *et al.*, 2001; Mai *et al.*, 2004; Mueller *et al.*, 2004; Arold *et al.*, 2005; Madabushi *et al.*, 2006). This, again, emphasises the indispensability of adequate quality control in the process of safety evaluation.

Conclusions

The consumer should be provided with reliable and safe HMPs, so it is essential to assess the health risks associated with these preparations. An objective scientific attitude should be adopted in this respect, i.e. it should neither be assumed that all HMPs are harmless nor should the use of botanicals be unconditionally rejected as dangerous nonsense. Like all drugs, this kind of products should be adequately controlled for pharmaceutical quality, to prevent contamination, substitution or adulteration of the plant material and to determine concentrations of (potentially) toxic constituents.

Quality control is also of importance to guarantee batch-to-batch consistency, which is essential for the effective and safe use of HMPs. Proper evaluation of existing data on traditional use, and pharmaco(toxico)logical and clinical research as well as post-marketing monitoring with an adequate system of pharmacovigilance, may further enhance the rational use of herbs and minimise (potential) health risks.

Information acquired should be disseminated to healthcare professionals and consumers in such a way that they are better aware of the hazards that inappropriate use of HMPs may incur. In this respect, the indirect health risks associated with the use of HMPs, particularly where a well-proven conventional approach is reduced, retarded or replaced by unsatisfactorily proven treatments – as well as the dangers of free and uncontrolled availability of herbal remedies via the Internet should also be pointed out to the public (De Smet, 1995, 2004). Nevertheless, despite all efforts to provide safe HMPs, unexpected negative effects, such as a rare idiosyncratic reaction, can never be prevented completely; HMPs in this respect are not different from synthetic drugs. Proper safety evaluation may, however, minimise the chance of such adverse events occurring.

Acknowledgement

Parts of the work described here were financially supported by Stichting Achmea Slachtoffer en Samenleving, the Dutch Burn Foundation, and the Dutch Ministry of Health, Welfare, and Sport (project 1075459).

References

Ahmed SM, Banner NR, Dubrey SW (2001). Low cyclosporin A level due to Saint John's wort in heart transplantation patients. *J Heart Lung Transplant* 20: 795.

Alscher DM, Klotz U (2003). Drug interaction of herbal tea containing St. John's wort with cyclosporine. *Transpl Int* 16: 543–544.

Andelic S (2003). [Bigeminy – the result of interaction between digoxin and St. John's wort]. *Vojnosanit pregl* 60: 361–364 (PubMed abstract).

Anon. (1995). *CPMP/ICH/141/95: Guidance on specific aspects of regulatory genotoxicity tests for pharmaceuticals S2A.* Step 4 version dated 19 Jul 1995. International Conference on Harmonization of Technical Requirements for Registration of Pharmaceuticals for Human Use.

Anon. (1997). *CPMP/ICH/174/95: Genotoxicity: a standard battery for genotoxicity testing of pharmaceuticals S2B.* Step 4 version dated 16 Jul 1997. International Conference on Harmonization of Technical Requirements for Registration of Pharmaceuticals for Human Use.

Anon. (2001). Directive 2001/83/EC of the European Parliament and of the Council of 6 November 2001, on the Community code relating to medicinal products for human use. *Off J Eur Union* 311: 67–128.

Anon. (2004a). Aloes dry extract, standardised, Aloes extractum siccum normatum. In: *European Pharmacopoiea*, 5th edn, volume 2. Strasbourg: Directorate for the Quality of Medicines, Council of Europe, 949.

Anon. (2004b). Directive 2004/24/EC of the European Parliament and of the Council of 31 March 2004, amending, as regards traditional herbal medicinal products, Directive 2001/83/EC on the Community code relating to medicinal products for human use. *Off J Eur Union* 136: 85–90.

Arenz A, Klein M, Fiehe K *et al.* (1996). Occurrence of neurotoxic 4′-O-methylpyridoxine in *Ginkgo biloba* leaves, *Ginkgo* medications and Japanese *Ginkgo* food. *Planta Med* 62: 548–551.

Arlt VM, Stiborova M, Schmeisser HH (2002). Aristolochic acid as a probable human cancer hazard in herbal remedies: a review. *Mutagenesis* 17: 265–277.

Arold G, Donath F, Maurer A *et al.* (2005). No relevant interaction with alprazolam, caffeine, tolbutamide, and digoxin by treatment with a low-hyperforin SJW extract. *Planta Med* 71: 331–337.

Assessment of Herbal Medicinal Products in The Netherlands. Assen: Stichting Toetsing. *Fytotherapeutica* 14–20.

Atal CK, Dubey RK, Singh J (1985). Biochemical basis of enhanced drug bioavailability by piperine: evidence that piperine is a potent inhibitor of drug metabolism. *J Pharmacol Exp Ther* 232: 258–262.

Bano G, Raina RK, Zutshi U *et al.* (1991). Effect of piperine on bioavailability and pharmacokinetics of propanolol and theophylline in healthy volunteers. *Eur J Clin Pharmacol* 41: 615–617.

Barbenel DM, Yusufi B, O'Shea D *et al.* (2000). Mania in a patient receiving testosterone replacement post-orchidectomy taking SJW and sertraline. *J Psychopharmacol* 14: 84–86.

Barnes J (1998). Herbal safety high on European phytotherapy agenda. *Inpharma* 1164: 20–21.

Barone GW, Gurley BJ, Ketel BL *et al.* (2001). Herbal supplements: A potential for drug interactions in transplant recipients. *Transplantation* 71: 239–241.

Barone GW, Gurley BJ, Ketel BL *et al.* (2000). Drug interaction between SJW and cyclosporine. *Ann Pharmacother* 34: 1013–1016.

Bast A, Chandler RF, Choy PC *et al.* (2002). Botanical health products, positioning and requirements for effective and safe use. *Environ Toxicol Pharmacol* 12: 195–211.

Bauer S, Stoörmer E, Johne A *et al.* (2003). Alterations in cyclosporin A pharmacokinetics and metabolism during treatment with SJW in renal transplant patients. *Br J Clin Pharmacol* 55: 203–211.

Beckman SE, Sommi RW, Switzer J (2000). Consumer use of St. John's wort: A survey on effectiveness, safety and tolerability. *Pharmacotherapy* 20: 568–574.

Beekwilder J, Jonker H, Meesters P *et al.* (2006). Antioxidants in raspberry: on-line analysis links antioxidant activity to a diversity of individual metabolites. *J Agric Food Chem* 53: 3313–3320.

Beer AM, Ostermann T (2001). Johanniskraut: Interaktion mit Cyclosporin gefährdet Nierentransplantat und erhöht die täglichen Medikationskosten. *Med Klin* 96: 480–484.

Berglund F, Flodh H, Lundborg P *et al.* (1984). Drug use during pregnancy and breast-feeding. A classification system for drug information. *Acta Obstet Gynecol Scand* 126 (supp.): 1–55.

Bolley R, Zu-umlautlke C, Kammerl M *et al.* (2002). Tacrolimus-induced nephrotoxicity unmasked by induction of the CYP3A4 system with St John's wort. *Transplantation* 73: 1009.

Bon S, Hartmann K, Kuhn M (1999). Johanniskraut: ein Enzyminduktor? *Schweiz Apoth Ztg* 16: 535–536.

Boone SA, Shields KM (2005). Treating pregnancy-related nausea and vomiting with ginger. *Ann Pharmacother* 39: 1710–1713.

Borrelli F, Capasso R, Aviello G *et al.* (2005). Effectiveness and safety of ginger in the treatment of pregnancy-induced nausea and vomiting. *Obstet Gynecol* 105: 849–856.

Bos R, Woerdenbag HJ, De Smet PAGM *et al.* (1997). *Valeriana* species. In: De Smet PAGM, Keller K, Hänsel R, Chandler RF, Eds. *Adverse Effects of Herbal Drugs*, Vol. 3. Berlin: Springer-Verlag, pp. 165–180.

Breidenbach T, Hoffmann MW, Becker T *et al.* (2000a). Drug interaction of St John's wort with ciclosporin. *Lancet* 355: 1912.

Breidenbach T, Kliem V, Burg M *et al.* (2000b). Profound drop of cyclosporin A whole blood trough levels caused by St John's wort (*Hypericum perforatum*). *Transplantation* 69: 2229–2230.

Bressler R (2005a). Herb–drug interactions. St. John's wort, prescription medications. *Geriatrics* 60: 21–23.

Bressler R (2005b). Herb–drug interactions: interactions between *Ginkgo biloba* and prescription medications. *Geriatrics* 60: 30–33.

Burstein AH, Horton RL, Dunn T *et al.* (2000). Lack of effect of St John's wort on carbamazepine pharmacokinetics in healthy volunteers. *Clin Pharmacol Ther* 68: 605–612.

Chen MC, Huang SM, Mozersky R *et al.* (2001). *Drug interactions involving St John's wort – data from FDA's adverse reaction reporting system.* Presented at the American Association of Pharmaceutical Scientists Annual Meeting; 2001 Oct 21–25; Denver, Colorado.

Clouatre DL (2004). Kava kava: examining new reports on toxicity. *Toxicol Lett* 150: 85–96.

Commissie Toetsing Fytotherapeutica (1999). *Inventarisatie en Proeftoetsing van Plantaardige Medicinale Bereidingen in Nederland* [A Survey and Trial].

Committee on Herbal Medicinal Products (2006). *EMEA/HMPC/32116/2005: Guideline on non-clinical documentation for herbal medicinal products in applications for marketing authorisation (bibliographical and mixed applications) and in applications for simplified registration.* Draft of 11 Jan 2006. Committee on Herbal Medicinal Products, European Medicines Agency.

Cosyns JP (2003). Aristolochic acid and 'Chinese herbs nephropathology': a review of the evidence to date. *Drug Saf* 26: 33–48.

Côté CS, Kor C, Cohen J *et al.* (2004). Composition and biologicial activity of traditional and commercial kava extracts. *Biochem Biophys Res Comm* 322: 147–152.

Crowe S, McKeating K (2002). Delayed emergence and St. John's wort. *Anesthesiology* 96: 1025–1027.

Cusack C, Buckley C (2005). Compositae dermatitis in a herbal medicine enthusiast. *Contact Dermatitis* 53: 120–121.

Cuzzolin L, Zaffani S, Benoni G (2006). Safety implications regarding use of phytomedicines. *Eur J Clin Pharmacol* 62: 37–42.

Dannawi M (2002). Possible serotonin syndrome after combination of buspirone and St John's Wort. *J Psychopharmacol* 16: 401.

De Maat MMR, Hoetelmans RMW, Mathot RAA *et al.* (2001). Drug interaction between St John's wort and nevirapine. *AIDS* 15: 420.

Depierreux M, Van Damme B, Vanden Houte K *et al.* (1994). Pathologic aspects of a newly described nephropathy related to the prolonged use of Chinese herbs. *Am J Kidney Dis* 24: 172–180.

De Smet PAGM (1992). Toxicological outlook on the quality assurance of herbal remedies. In: De Smet PAGM, Keller K, Hänsel R, Chandler RF, Eds. *Adverse Effects of Herbal Drugs*. Vol. 1. Berlin: Springer-Verlag, 1–72.

De Smet PAGM (1995). Health risks of herbal remedies. *Drug Saf* 13: 81–93.

De Smet PAGM (2004). Health risks of herbal remedies: an update. *Clin Pharmacol Ther* 76: 1–17.

De Smet PAGM (2006). Clinical risk management of herb–drug interactions. *Br J Clin Pharmacol* 63: 258–267.

Dresser GK, Schwarz UI, Wilkinson GR *et al.* (2003). Coordinate induction of both cytochrome P4503A and MDR1 by St John's wort in healthy subjects. *Clin Pharmacol Ther* 73: 41–50.

Dürr D, Stieger B, Kullak-Ublick GA *et al.* (2000). St John's Wort induces intestinal P-glycoprotein/MDR1 and intestinal and hepatic CYP3A4. *Clin Pharmacol Ther* 68: 598–604.

Eich-Höchli D, Oppliger R, Golay KP *et al.* (2003). Methadone maintenance treatment and St. John's wort; a case report. *Pharmacopsychiatry* 36: 35–37.

Ereshefsky B, Gewertz N, Lam YWF *et al.* (1999). Determination of SJW differential metabolism at CYP2D6 and CYP3A4 using dextromethorphan probe methodology. *Proceedings of the NCDEU 38th annual meeting*: poster 130.

Ernst E (2002). Herbal medicinal products during pregnancy: are they safe? *Br J Obstet Gynecol* 109: 227–235.

Frye RF, Fitzgerald SM, Lagattuta TF *et al.* (2004). Effect of St John's wort on imatinib mesylate pharmacokinetics. *Clin Pharmacol Ther* 76: 323–329.

Fugh-Berman A (2000). Herb–drug interactions. *Lancet* 355: 134–138.

Fugh-Berman A, Ernst E (2001). Herb–drug interactions: review and assessment of report reliability. *Br J Clin Pharmacol* 52: 587–595.

Gewertz N, Ereshefsky B, Lam YWF *et al.* (1999). Determination of the differential effects of St. John's wort on the CYP1A2 and NAT2 metabolic pathways using cafeine probe methodology (abstract). *Proceedings of the NCDEU 38th annual meeting*, P131.

Gordon JB (1998). SSRI's and St. John's wort: possible toxicity? *Am Fam Physician* 57: 950–953.

Gorski JC, Hamman MA, Wang Z *et al.* (2002). The effect of St. John's wort on the efficacy of oral contraception. *Clin Pharmacol Ther* 71: P25.

Gurley BJ, Gardner SF, Hubbard MA *et al.* (2002). Cytochrome P450 phenotypic ratios for predicting herb–drug interactions in humans. *Clin Pharmacol Ther* 72: 276–287.

Halkes SBA (2000). Safety issues in phytotherapy. In: Ernst E, Ed. *Herbal Medicine: a Concise Overview for Professionals*. Oxford: Butterworth-Heinemann, pp. 82–99.

Halkes SBA, Van den Berg AJJ, Hoekstra MJ *et al.* (2001a). The use of tannic acid in the local treatment of burn wounds: intriguing old and new perspectives. *Wounds* 13: 144–158.

Halkes SBA, Van den Berg AJJ, Hoekstra MJ *et al.* (2001b). Treatment of burns: new perspectives for highly purified tannic acids? *Burns* 27: 299–300.

Halkes SBA, Van den Berg AJJ, Hoekstra MJ *et al.* (2002). Transaminase and alkaline phosphatase activity in the serum of burn patients treated with highly purified tannic acids. *Burns* 28: 449–453.

Hall SD, Wang Z, Huang SM *et al.* (2003). The interaction between St John's wort and an oral contraceptive. *Clin Pharmacol Ther* 74: 525–535.

Hebert MF, Park JM, Chen YL *et al.* (2004). Effects of St. John's wort (*Hypericum perforatum*) on tacrolimus pharmacokinetics in healthy volunteers. *J Clin Pharmacol* 44: 89–94.

Henderson L, Yue QY, Bergquist C *et al.* (2002). St John's wort (*Hypericum perforatum*): drug interactions and clinical outcomes. *Br J Clin Pharmacol* 54: 349–356.

Hori M, Satoh S, Maibach HI *et al.* (1991). Enhancement of propranolol hydrochloride and diazepam skin absorption in vitro: effect of enhancer lipophilicity. *J Pharm Sci* 80: 32–35.

Hostettmann K, Wolfender JL, Rodriguez S (1997). Rapid detection and subsequent isolation of bioactive constituents of crude plant extracts. *Planta Med* 63: 2–10.

Hruska MW, Cheong JA, Langaee TY *et al.* (2005). Effect of St. John's wort administration on CYP2C8 mediated rosiglitazone metabolism. *Clin Pharmacol Ther* 77: P35.

Hu Z, Yang X, Ho PC *et al.* (2005). Herb–drug interactions: a literature review. *Drugs* 65: 1239–1282.

Hupkens P, Boxma H, Dokter J (1995). Tannic acid as a topical agent in burns: historical considerations and implications for new developments. *Burns* 21: 57–61.

Huxtable RJ (1990). The harmful potential of herbal and other plant products. *Drug Saf* 5 (supp. 1): 126–136.

Izzo AA (2005). Herb–drug interactions: an overview of the clinical evidence. *Fundam Clin Pharmacol* 19: 1–16.

Izzo AA, Ernst E (2001). Interactions between herbal medicines and prescribed drugs: a systematic review. *Drugs* 61: 2163–2175.

Jhoo JW, Freeman JP, Heinze TM *et al.* (2006). In vitro cytotoxicity of nonpolar constituents from different parts of kava plant (*Piper methysticum*). *J Agric Food Chem* 54: 3157–3162.

Jiang X, Williams KM, Liauw WS *et al.* (2004). Effect of St John's wort and ginseng on the pharmacokinetics and pharmacodynamics of warfarin in healthy subjects. *Br J Clin Pharmacol* 57: 592–599.

Johne A, Brockmoller J, Bauer S *et al.* (1999). Pharmacokinetic interaction of digoxin with an herbal extract from St John's wort (*Hypericum perforatum*). *Clin Pharmacol Ther* 66: 338–345.

Johne A, Schmider J, Brockmoller J *et al.* (2002). Decreased plasma levels of amitriptyline and its metabolites on comedication with an extract from St. John's wort (*Hypericum perforatum*). *J Clin Psychopharmacol* 22: 46–54.

Johnson AE, Molyneux RJ, Merrill GB (1985). Chemistry of toxic range plants. Variation in pyrrolizidine alkaloid content of *Senecio*, *Amsinckia*, and *Crotalaria* species. *J Agric Food Chem* 33: 50–55.

Karliova M, Treichel U, Malago M *et al.* (2000). Interaction of *Hypericum perforatum* (St. John's wort) with cyclosporin A metabolism in a patient after liver transplantation. *J Hepatol* 33: 853–855.

Kawaguchi A, Ohmori M, Tsuruoka S *et al.* (2004). Drug interaction between St John's Wort and quazepam. *Br J Clin Pharmacol* 58: 403–410.

Kerns EH, Volk KJ, Whitney JL *et al.* (1998). Chemical identification of botanical components using liquid chromatography/mass spectrometry. *Drug Inf J* 32: 471–485.

Khawaja IS, Marotta RF, Lippmann S (1999). Herbal medicines as a factor in delirium. *Psychiatr Serv* 50: 969–970.

Kramer MS, Leventhal JM, Hutchinon T *et al.* (1979). An algorithm for the operational assessment of adverse drug reactions. I. Background, description, and instructions for use. *JAMA* 242: 623–632.

Kressmann S, Biber A, Wonnemann M *et al.* (2002). Influence of pharmaceutical quality on the bioavailability of active components from *Ginkgo biloba* preparations. *J Pharm Pharmacol* 54: 1507–1514.

Kroes R, Kleiner J, Renwick AG (2005). The treshold of toxicological concern concept in risk assessment. *Toxicol Sci* 86: 226–230.

Kroes R, Renwick AG, Cheeseman M *et al.* (2004). Structure-based thresholds of toxicological concern (TTC): guidance for application to substances present at low levels in the diet. *Food Chem Toxicol* 42: 65–83.

Kumana CR, Ng M, Lin HJ *et al.* (1983). Hepatic veno-occlusive disease due to toxic alkaloid in herbal tea. *Lancet* 2(8363): 1360–1361.

Lantz MS, Buchalter E, Giambanco V (1999). St. John's wort and antidepressant drug interactions in the elderly. *J Geriatr Psychiatry Neurol* 12: 7–10.

Lebeau C, Arlt VM, Schmeisser HH *et al.* (2001). Aristolochic acid impedes endocytosis and induces DNA adducts in proximal tubule cells. *Kidney Int* 60: 1332–1342.

Madabushi R, Frank B, Drewelow B *et al.* (2006). Hyperforin in St. John's wort drug interactions. *Eur J Clin Pharmacol* 62: 225–233.

Mai I, Bauer S, Perloff ES *et al.* (2004). Hyperforin content determines the magnitude of the St John's wort-cyclosporine drug interaction. *Clin Pharmacol Ther* 76: 330–340.

Mai I, Kruger H, Budde K *et al.* (2000). Hazardous pharmacokinetic interaction of Saint John's wort

(*Hypericum perforatum*) with the immunosuppressant cyclosporin. *Int J Clin Pharmacol Ther* 38: 500–502.

Mai I, Sto-umlautrmer E, Bauer S *et al.* (2003). Impact of St John's wort treatment on the pharmacokinetics of tacrolimus and mycophenolic acid in renal transplant patients. *Nephrol Dial Transplant* 18: 819–822.

Mandelbaum A, Pertzborn F, Martin-Facklam M *et al.* (2000). Unexplained decrease of cyclosporin trough levels in a compliant renal transplant patient. *Nephrol Dial Transplant* 15: 1473–1474.

Markowitz JS, DeVane CL, Boulton DW *et al.* (2000). Effect of St John's wort (*Hypericum perforatum*) on cytochrome P450 2D6 and 3A4 activity in healthy volunteers. *Life Sci* 66: 133–139.

Markowitz JS, Donovan JL, DeVane CL *et al.* (2003). Effect of St John's wort on drug metabolism by induction of cytochrome P450 3A4 enzyme. *JAMA* 290: 1500–1504.

Martena MJ, Van der Wielen JCA, Van der Laak LFJ *et al.* (2007). Enforcement of the ban on aristolochic acids in Chinese traditional herbal preparations on the Dutch market. *Anal Bioanal Chem* DOI 10.1007/s00216–007–1310–3.

Mathijssen RHJ, Verweij J, De Bruijn P *et al.* (2002). Effects of St. John's wort on irinotecan metabolism. *J Natl Cancer Inst* 94: 1247–1249.

Maurer A, Johne A, Bauer S (1999). Interaction of St John's wort extract with phenprocoumon. *Eur J Clin Pharmacol* 55: A22.

McLaughlin JL, Rogers LL, Anderson JE (1998). The use of biological assays to evaluate botanicals. *Drug Inf J* 32: 513–524.

Mengs U (1988). Tumour induction in mice following exposure to aristolochic acid. *Arch Toxicol* 61: 504–505.

Mengs U, Lange W, Poch JA (1982). The carcinogenic action of aristolochic acid in rats. *Arch Toxicol* 51: 107–119.

Miller LG (2001). Drug interactions known or potentially associated with St. John's wort. *J Herbal Pharmacother* 1: 51–64.

Moore LB, Goodwin B, Jones SA *et al.* (2000). St John's wort induces hepatic drug metabolism through activation of the pregnane receptor. *Proc Natl Acad Sci USA* 97: 7500–7502.

Morimoto T, Kotegawa T, Tsutsumi K *et al.* (2004). Effects of St. John's wort on the pharmacokinetics of theophylline in healthy volunteers. *J Clin Pharmacol* 44: 95–101.

Moschella C, Jaber BL (2001). Interaction between cyclosporin and *Hypericum perforatum* (St. John's wort) after organ transplantation. *Am J Kidney Dis* 38: 1105–1107.

Moses EL, Mallinger AG (2000). St John's wort: three cases of possible mania induction. *J Clin Psychopharmacol* 20: 115–117.

Moulds FW, Malani J (2003). Kava: herbal panacea or liver poison? *Med J Aust* 178: 451–453.

Mueller SC, Uehleke B, Woehling H *et al.* (2004). Effect of St John's wort dose and preparations on the pharmacokinetics of digoxin. *Clin Pharmacol Ther* 75: 546–557.

Murphy PA, Kern SE, Stanczyk FZ *et al.* (2005). Interaction of St. John's Wort with oral contraceptives: effects on the pharmacokinetics of norethindrone and ethinyl estradiol, ovarian activity and breakthrough bleeding. *Contraception* 71: 402–408.

Nakayama K, Fujino H, Kasai R *et al.* (1986). Solubilizing properties of saponins from *Sapindus mukurossi* Gaertn. *Chem Pharm Bull* 34: 3279–3283.

National Cancer Institute (1999). *Common toxicity criteria*, v2.0 [online]. http://ctep.cancer.gov/reporting/ctc.html (accessed 23 Jun 2006).

Nebel A, Schneider BJ, Baker RK *et al.* (1999). Potential metabolic interaction between St. John's wort and theophylline. *Ann Pharmacother* 33: 502.

Palanisamy A, Haller C, Olson KR (2003). Photosensitivity reaction in a woman using an herbal supplement containing ginseng, goldenseal, and bee pollen. *J Toxicol Clin Toxicol* 41: 865–867.

Pfrunder A, Schiesser M, Gerber S *et al.* (2003). Interaction of St John's wort with low-dose oral contraceptive therapy: a randomized controlled trial. *Br J Clin Pharmacol* 56: 683–690.

Piscitelli SC, Burstein AH, Chaitt D *et al.* (2000). Indinavir concentrations and St John's wort. *Lancet* 355(9203): 547–548.

Prost N, Tichadou L, Rodor F *et al.* (2000). Interaction millepertuis–venlafaxine. *Presse Med* 29: 1285–1286.

Ra-umlauttz AE, von Moos M, Drewe J (2001). Johanniskraut: ein Phytopharmakon mit potentiell gefährlichen Interaktionen. *Praxis* 90: 843–849.

Rengelshausen J, Banfield M, Riedel KD *et al.* (2005). Opposite effects of short-term and long-term St John's wort intake on voriconazole pharmacokinetics. *Clin Pharmacol Ther* 78: 25–33.

Repčák M, Eliašovŏ A, Ruščančinová A (1998). Production of herniarin by diploid and tetraploid *Chamomilla recutita*. *Pharmazie* 53: 278–279.

Rey JM, Walter G (1998). *Hypericum perforatum* (St John's wort) in depression: Pest or blessing? *Med J Aust* 169: 583–586.

Rininger JA, Franck Z, Wheelock GD *et al.* (2000a). The value of bioassays in assessing the quality of botanical products. *Pharmacopoeial Forum* 26: 857–864.

Rininger JA, Kickner S, Chigurupathi P *et al.* (2000b). Immunopharmacological activity of Echinacea preparations following simulated digestion on murine macrophages and human peripheral mononuclear cells. *J Leukocyte Biol* 68: 503–510.

Roby CA, Anderson GD, Kantor E *et al.* (2000). St John's wort: Effect on CYP3A4 activity. *Clin Pharmacol Ther* 67: 451–457.

Roitman JN (1981). Comfrey and liver damage. *Lancet* 1: 944.

Roots I, Johne A, Schmider J *et al.* (2000). Interaction of a herbal extract from St. John's Wort with amitriptyline and its metabolites. *Clin Pharmacol Ther* 76: 59.

Roth L, Daunderer M, Kormann K (1984). *Giftpflanzen, Pflanzengifte: Vorkommen, Wirkung, Therapie*. München: Ecomed Verlagsgesellschaft.

Ruschitzka F, Meier PJ, Turina M *et al.* (2000). Acute heart transplant rejection due to Saint John's wort. *Lancet* 355: 548–549.

Sannerstedt R, Berglund F, Flodh H *et al.* (1980). Medication during pregnancy and breast-feeding, a new Swedish system for classifying drugs. *Int J Clin Pharmacol Ther Toxicol* 18: 45–49.

Schimmer O, Häfele F, Krüger A (1988). The mutagenic potencies of plant extracts containing quercetin in *Salmonella typhimurium* TA98 and TA100. *Mutat Res* 206: 201–208.

Schmeiser HH, Bieler CA, Wiessler M *et al.* (1996). Detection of DNA adducts formed by aristolochic acid in renal tissue from patients with Chinese herb nephropathy. *Cancer Res* 56: 2025–2028.

Schöpke T, Bartlakowski J (1997). Effects of saponins on the water solubility of quercetin. *Pharmazie* 52: 232–234.

Schwarz UI, Bueschel B, Kirch W (2003). Unwanted pregnancy on self-medication with St John's wort despite hormonal contraception. *Br J Clin Pharmacol* 55: 112–113.

Sharff JA, Bayer MJ (1982). Acute and chronic digitalis toxicity: presentation and treatment. *Ann Emerg Med* 11: 327–331.

Singh J, Dubey RK, Atal CK (1986). Piperine-mediated inhibition of glucuronidation activity in isolated epithelial cells of the guinea-pig small intestine: evidence that piperine lowers the endogenous UDP-glucuronic acid content. *J Pharmacol Exp Ther* 236: 488–493.

Smith M, Lin KM, Zheng YP (2001). An open trial of nifedipine–herb interactions: nifedipine with St. John's wort, ginseng or *Ginkgo biloba*. *Clin Pharmacol Ther* 69: P86.

Smith P, Bullock JM, Booker BM *et al.* (2004a). The influence of St. John's wort on the pharmacokinetics and protein binding of imatinib mesylate. *Pharmacotherapy* 24: 1508–1514.

Smith PF, Bullock JM, Booker BM *et al.* (2004b). Induction of imatinib metabolism by *hypericum perforatum*. *Blood* 104: 1229–1230.

Spinella M, Eaton LA (2001). Hypomania induced by herbal and pharmaceutical psychotropic medicines following mild traumatic brain injury. *Brain Inj* 16: 359–367.

Stahl E, Keller K (1981). Zur Klassifizierung handelsüblicher Kalmusdrogen. *Planta Med* 43: 128–140.

Steiner GG (2000). The correlation between cancer incidence and kava consumption. *Hawaii Med J* 59: 420–422.

Stickel F, Baumüller HM, Seitz K *et al.* (2003). Hepatitis induced by kava (*Piper methysticum* rhizoma). *J Hepatol* 39: 62–67.

Sugimoto K, Ohmori M, Tsuruoka S *et al.* (2001). Different effects of St John's wort on the pharmacokinetics of simvastatin and pravastatin. *Clin Pharmacol Ther* 70: 518–524.

Tannergren C, Engman H, Knutson L *et al.* (2004). St John's wort decreases the bioavailability of R- and S-verapamil through induction of the first-pass metabolism. *Clin Pharmacol Ther* 75: 298–309.

Thesen R (1988). Phytotherapeutika-nicht immer harmlos. *Pharm Ztg* 133: 38–43.

Thiele KG, Muehrcke RC, Berning H (1967). Nierenerkrankungen durch Medikamenten. *Dtsch Med Wochenschr* 92: 1632–1635.

Turton-Weeks SM, Barone GW, Gurley BJ *et al.* (2001). St John's wort: a hidden risk for transplant patients. *Prog Transplant* 11: 116–120.

Vale S (1998). Subarachnoid haemorrhage associated with *Ginkgo biloba*. *Lancet* 352: 36.

Van den Bout-Van den Beukel CJP, Koopmans PP, Van der Ven AJAM *et al.* (2006). Possible drug–metabolism interactions of medicinal herbs with antiretroviral agents. *Drug Metabol Rev* 38: 477–514.

Vanhaelen M, Vanhaelen-Fastre R, But P *et al.* (1994). Identification of aristolochic acid in Chinese herbs. *Lancet* 343(8890): 174.

Vanherweghem JL, Depierreux M, Tielemans C *et al.* (1993). Rapidly progressive interstitial renal fibrosis in young women: association with slimming regimen including Chinese herbs. *Lancet* 341(8842): 387–391.

Van Roon EN, Flikweer S, Le Comte M *et al.* (2005). Clinical relevance of drug–drug interactions: A structured assessment procedure. *Drug Saf* 28: 1131–1139.

Vogel H, Razmilic I, Munoz M *et al.* (1999). Studies of genetic variation of essential oil and alkaloid content in Boldo (*Peumus boldus*). *Planta Med* 65: 90–91.

Vogler B, Klaiber I, Roos G, *et al.* (1998). Combination of LC-MS and LC-NMR as a tool for the structure determination of natural products. *J Nat Prod* 61: 175–178.

Wagner H, Bladt S, Daily A, *et al.* (1989). *Ginkgo biloba*, DC- und HPLC-Analyse von Ginkgo-Extrakten und Ginkgo-Extrakte enthaltenden Phytopräparaten. *Dtsch Apoth Ztg* 129: 2421–2429.

Wagner H, Jurcic K (1980). In vitro- und in vivo-metabolismus von ^{14}C-didrovaltrate. *Planta Med* 38: 366–376.

Waksman JC, Heard K, Jolliff H *et al.* (2000). Serotonin syndrome associated with the use of St. John's wort (*Hypericum perforatum*) and paroxetine. *J Toxicol Clin Toxicol* 38: 521.

Wang LS, Zhou G, Zhu B *et al.* (2004). St John's wort induces both cytochrome P450 3A4-catalyzed sulfoxidation and 2C19-dependent hydroxylation of omeprazole. *Clin Pharmacol Ther* 75: 191–197.

Wang Z, Gorski JC, Hamman MA *et al.* (2001). The effects of St John's wort (*Hypericum perforatum*) on human cytochrome P450 activity. *Clin Pharmacol Ther* 70: 317–326.

Wang Z, Hamman MA, Huang SM *et al.* (2002). Effect of St John's wort on the pharmacokinetics of fexofenadine. *Clin Pharmacol Ther* 71: 414–420.

Wenk M, Todesco L, Krähenbühl S (2004). Effect of St John's wort on the activities of CYP1A2, CYP3A4, CYP2D6, N-acetyltransferase 2, and xanthine oxidase in healthy males and females. *Br J Clin Pharmacol* 57: 495–499.

Whitton PA, Lau A, Salisbury A *et al.* (2003). Kava lactones and the kava-kava controversy. *Phytochemistry* 64: 673–679.

Wijbenga JA, Zijm FJ, Halkes SBA *et al.* (2004a). Geneesmiddelinteracties met kruiden en kruidenmiddelen (1): Inventarisatie levert ruim 2000 meldingen zonder veel evidence. *Pharm Weekbl* 139: 528–532.

Wijbenga JA, Zijm FJ, van Roon EN *et al.* (2004b). Geneesmiddelinteracties met kruiden en kruidenmiddelen (2): Ginkgo biloba, vermoedens bij antithrombotica. *Pharm Weekbl* 139: 593–596.

Wijbenga JA, Zijm FJ, van Roon EN *et al.* (2004c). Geneesmiddelinteracties met kruiden en kruidenmiddelen (3): Sint-janskruid, relevant bij ciclosporine en anticonceptiva. *Pharm Weekbl* 139: 695–700.

Wijbenga JA, Zijm FJ, van Roon EN *et al.* (2004d). Geneesmiddelinteracties met kruiden en kruidenmiddelen (4): Ginseng, vermoedens bij digoxine. *Pharm Weekbl* 139: 850–853.

Wijbenga JA, Zijm FJ, van Roon EN *et al.* (2004e). Geneesmiddelinteracties met kruiden en kruidenmiddelen (5): Knoflook, vermoedens bij saquinavir. *Pharm Weekbl* 139: 955–957.

Wijbenga JA, Zijm FJ, van Roon EN *et al.* (2004f). Geneesmiddelinteracties met kruiden en kruidenmiddelen (6): Valeriaan en zoethout: kalm en zoet blijven. *Pharm Weekbl* 139: 1034–1036.

Williams AC, Barry BW (1991). Terpenes and the lipid-protein-partitioning theory of skin penetration enhancement. *Pharm Res* 8: 17–24.

Will-Shahab L, Brattström A, Roots I *et al.* (2001). Studie zur Interaktion von Johanniskrautextrakt (Ze 117) mit Kontrazeptiva an Probandinnen. www.phytotherapy.org/kongress2001.pdf (accessed 20 Mar 2003).

Xie HG (2005). Additional discussions regarding the altered metabolism and transport of omeprazole after long-term use of St John's wort. *Clin Pharmacol Ther* 78: 440–441.

Yue QY, Bergquist C, Gerdén B (2000). Safety of St John's wort (*Hypericum perforatum*). *Lancet* 355: 576–577.

Index

Note: page numbers in *italics* refer to figures and tables